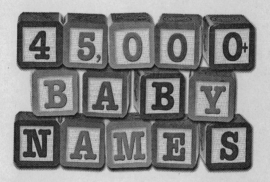

45,000+ BABY NAMES

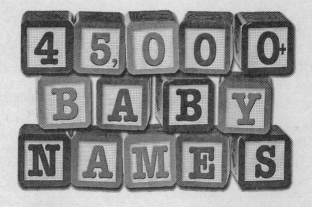

Bruce Lansky

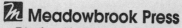 **Meadowbrook Press**
Distributed by Simon & Schuster
New York

Library of Congress Cataloging-in-Publication Data

Lansky, Bruce.
   45,000+ baby names / Bruce Lansky.
        p. cm.
   ISBN 0-88166-478-2 (Meadowbrook) ISBN 0-684-03089-6 (Simon
   & Schuster)
   1. Names, Personal—Dictionaries. I. Title: forty-five thousand plus baby
   names. II. Title.
CS2377L354 2004
929.4'4'03—dc22

                                                                    2004009357

Editorial Director: Christine Zuchora-Walske
Editors: Liya Lev Oertel, Megan McGinnis, Angela Wiechmann
Proofreader: Joseph Gredler
Production Manager: Paul Woods
Graphic Design Manager: Tamara Peterson
Cover Design: Tamara Peterson, Erik Broberg
Cover Photography: Comstock Images, Corbis, Getty Images

© 2004 by Bruce Lansky

All rights reserved. No part of this book may be reproduced or trans-
mitted in any form or by any means, electronic or mechanical, includ-
ing photocopying, recording, or using any information storage and
retrieval system, without written permission from the publisher, except
in the case of brief quotations embodied in critical articles and reviews.

Published by Meadowbrook Press, 5451 Smetana Drive,
Minnetonka, MN 55343

www.meadowbrookpress.com

BOOK TRADE DISTRIBUTION by Simon & Schuster,
a division of Simon and Schuster, Inc., 1230 Avenue
of the Americas, New York, NY 10020

09 08 07 06 05 04   10 9 8 7 6 5 4 3 2 1

Printed in the United States of America

Contents

Introduction

When you think about names for your baby, you'll find yourself daydreaming about what he or she may look like and be like. And you'll find yourself thinking about your hopes and dreams for the newest member of your family.

As you consider and discuss names, you'll find that they conjure up pictures in your mind. Scarlett may bring to mind Scarlett O'Hara of Margaret Mitchell's *Gone with the Wind*. Ronald may call to mind Ronald Reagan or Ronald McDonald.

You'll find yourself putting first, middle, and last names together and saying them out loud. Someone watching you may think you're talking to yourself. You probably are!

You'll also find yourself fascinated by all the names you read in the birth announcements section of the newspaper; names of students in your local day care center, school, church, or favorite team; names you see or hear in the news; and names you see in books, movies, on television, or on the Internet.

Don't be surprised to discover that you've developed a "fashion sense" about which names are currently "in" and which names are currently "out." As a result, you may find yourself considering:

- names from other countries and ethnic groups;

- names that have been recently created (perhaps a name you've made up yourself);

- names that feature new spellings of familiar names;

- names for a girl that once were more often used for boys;

- names that are traditional surnames.

The reasons you'll probably consider some names that your parents never did are simple. Pick up the sports section of your local newspaper and you'll read about Shaquille, Kobe, and LeBron on the basketball court or Andre, Gustavo, and Lleyton on the tennis court. Turn on the television and you'll see Shania, Beyoncé, and Alanis perform. Go to the movies and you can watch Uma, Charlize, and Angelina. Interesting, unusual names from all around the world surround you.

This book was designed to open up the whole world of names to you. I scoured the world for popular and unusual names that just might work for your child. Here are a few of the unusual names I find intriguing:

Native American: Cheyenne and Dakotah
Spanish: Nevada and Sierra
French: Brie and Chardonnay
African: Saki and Simba
Welsh: Bryn and Rhett
Russian: Sasha and Tamara
Gypsy: Chik and Tawny
Italian: Giulia and Matteo
Japanese: Kimiko and Ringo

I could go on for pages.

I created this book to give you the choice of a lifetime—more interesting and unusual names from all around the world than any other book.

My best advice is to:

a) Rate the names you're considering on the rating sheet that follows. It will help you make the very subjective process of selecting a name a little more objective.

b) "Go public" with the naming process. "Test" names you're considering on your friends and relatives. Find out how the names you're considering are perceived and received. What positive or negative associations come to mind?* How do your friends and relatives feel about the names?

Chances are, if a name survives this process, it may well be a name both you and your child can live with happily ever after.

Happy hunting,

Bruce Lansky

---

*If this factor intrigues you, consult *The Baby Name Survey Book* to find how 1,700 popular names are perceived by a sample of 100,000 parents.

Ten Guidelines for Naming Your Baby

A Comparative Scoring System

If you have a name you like, you already know how pleasant it is going through life with a name that "fits" or "feels right." If you don't, you know how unpleasant it is to go through life with a name that, for whatever reason, doesn't work for you.

It may help to test each name you're considering against the list of factors that could affect the way a name will work for your child. This will help make the subjective process of selecting a name more objective for you.

In the chart on the following page, give each name two points for a positive rating on any criterion, one point for a medium rating, and no points for a negative rating.

I realize that this scoring system has a built-in bias toward names that are relatively common and familiar—and therefore easy to spell and pronounce. However, you're free to give extra weight to any factor you like. If, for example, you love exotic names that are unfamiliar (and potentially hard to spell and pronounce), you might want to double the weight of the "uniqueness" and/or "sound/rhythm" factors—in other words, give four points for a positive rating and two points for a medium rating.

Factors	Positive	Medium	Negative
1. Spelling	❑ easy	❑ medium	❑ hard
2. Pronunciation	❑ easy	❑ medium	❑ hard
3. Gender ID	❑ clear		❑ confusing
4. Stereotypes	❑ positive	❑ ok	❑ negative
5. Sound/Rhythm	❑ pleasing	❑ ok	❑ unpleasant
6. Nicknames	❑ appealing	❑ ok	❑ unappealing
7. Meaning	❑ positive	❑ ok	❑ negative
8. Popularity	❑ *not* too popular		❑ too popular
9. Uniqueness	❑ *not* too strange		❑ too strange
10. Initials	❑ pleasing	❑ ok	❑ unpleasant

Top Five Girls' Names

Name 1: _____Score_____

Name 2: _____Score_____

Name 3: _____Score_____

Name 4: _____Score_____

Name 5: _____Score_____

Top Five Boys' Names

Name 1: _____Score_____

Name 2: _____Score_____

Name 3: _____Score_____

Name 4: _____Score_____

Name 5: _____Score_____

Where in the World?

45,000+ Baby Names includes names from over 150 different languages. Some of these languages are quite familiar, while others may be more obscure or exotic. In order to help identify where each language comes from, the following language chart has been provided.

In this chart, the languages used in *45,000+ Baby Names* have been divided up into general geographical categories. Upon encountering a name entry with an unfamiliar language citation, please refer to the chart below to discover what part of the world the name in question originated from.

Languages used in
45,000+ Baby Names:

African
Abaluhya
African
Afrikaans
Akan
Ateso
Bambara
Benin
Egyptian
Ethiopian
Ewe
Fante
Ghanaian
Hausa
Ibo
Kakwa
Kikuyu
Lomwe
Luganda
Luo
Musoga
Mwera

Nguni
Nigerian
North African
Nyakyusa
Ochi
Rhodesian
Rukiga
Runyankore
Runyoro
Rutooro
Shona
Somali
Swahili
Tanzanian
Tiv
Tswana
Twi
Ugandan
Umbundu
Uset
Xhosa
Yao

Yoruba
Zimbabwean
Zulu

Native American
Algonquin
Apache
Arapaho
Ashanti
Blackfoot
Carrier
Cherokee
Cheyenne
Choctaw
Comanche
Coos
Dakota
Dene
Eskimo
Fox
Hopi

Iroquois
Kiowa
Lakota
Mahona
Moquelumnan
Native American
Navajo
Ojibwa
Omaha
Osage
Pawnee
Pomo
Ponca
Quiché
Sauk
Shoshone
Taos
Tupi-Guarani
Watamare
Winnebago
Zuni

East Asian and Pacific
Australian
Burmese
Cambodian
Chinese
Filipino
Fijian
Hawaiian
Japanese
Korean
Malayan
Maori
Polynesian
Tai
Tibetan
Vietnamese

West Australian
    Aboriginal

East European and North Asian
Armenian
Basque
Bulgarian
Czech
Estonian
Hungarian
Latvian
Lithuanian
Mongolian
Polish
Romanian
Russian
Slavic
Turkish
Ukrainian

West European
Cornish
Danish
Dutch
English
Finnish
French
German
Gypsy
Icelandic
Irish
Italian
Norwegian
Portugese
Scandinavian
Scottish
Spanish
Swedish
Swiss

Welsh
Yiddish

Middle and Near Eastern
Afghan
Arabic
Hebrew
Hindi
Pakistani
Persian
Punjabi
Tamil
Todas
Urdu

South and North American
American
Peruvian

Historical
Aramaic
Assyrian
Babylonian
Greek
Latin
Phoenician
Sanskrit
Syrian
Teutonic

Girls

A

Aaleyah (Hebrew) a form of Aliya.
Aalayah, Aalayaha, Aalea, Aaleah, Aaleaha, Aaleeyah, Aaleyiah, Aaleyyah

Aaliah (Hebrew) a form of Aliya.
Aaliaya, Aaliayah

Aalisha (Greek) a form of Alisha.
Aaleasha, Aaliesha

Aaliyah (Hebrew) a form of Aliya.
Aahliyah, Aailiyah, Aailyah, Aalaiya, Aaleah, Aalia, Aalieyha, Aaliya, Aaliyaha, Aaliyha, Aalliah, Aalliyah, Aalyah, Aalyiah

Abagail (Hebrew) a form of Abigale.
Abagael, Abagaile, Abagale, Abagayle, Abageal, Abagil, Abaigael, Abaigeal

Abbagail (Hebrew) a form of Abigale.
Abbagale, Abbagayle, Abbegail, Abbegale, Abbegayle

Abbey, Abbie, Abby (Hebrew) familiar forms of Abigail.
Aabbee, Abbe, Abbea, Abbeigh, Abbi, Abbye, Abeey, Abey, Abi, Abia, Abie, Aby

Abbygail (Hebrew) a form of Abigale.
Abbeygale, Abbygale, Abbygayl, Abbygayle

Abegail (Hebrew) a form of Abigail.
Abegale, Abegaile, Abegayle

Abelina (American) a combination of Abbey + Lina.
Abilana, Abilene

Abia (Arabic) great.
Abbia, Abbiah, Abiah, Abya

Abianne (American) a combination of Abbey + Ann.
Abena, Abeni, Abian, Abinaya

Abida (Arabic) worshiper.
Abedah, Abidah

Abigail (Hebrew) father's joy. Bible: one of the wives of King David. See also Gail.
Abagail, Abbagail, Abbey, Abbiegail, Abbiegayle, Abbigael, Abbigail, Abbigal, Abbigale, Abbigayl, Abbigayle, Abbygail, Abegail, Abgail, Abgale, Abgayle, Abigael, Abigaile, Abigaill, Abigal, Abigale, Abigayil, Abigayl, Abigayle, Abigel, Abigial, Abugail, Abygail, Avigail

Abinaya (American) a form of Abiann.
Abenaa, Abenaya, Abinaa, Abiniaya, Abinayan

Abira (Hebrew) my strength.
*Abbira, Abeer, Abeerah, Abeir,
Abera, Aberah, Abhira, Abiir,
Abir*

Abra (Hebrew) mother of
many nations.
Abree, Abri, Abria

Abria (Hebrew) a form of
Abra.
*Abréa, Abrea, Abreia, Abriah,
Abriéa, Abrya*

Abrial (French) open; secure,
protected.
*Abrail, Abreal, Abreale, Abriale,
Abrielle*

Abriana (Italian) a form of
Abra.
*Abbrienna, Abbryana, Abreana,
Abreanna, Abreanne, Abreeana,
Abreona, Abreonia, Abriann,
Abrianna, Abriannah, Abrieana,
Abrien, Abrienna, Abrienne,
Abrietta, Abrion, Abrionée,
Abrionne, Abriunna, Abryann,
Abryanna, Abryona*

Abrielle (French) a form of
Abrial.
Aabriella, Abriel, Abriell, Abryell

Abril (French) a form of
Abrial.
Abrilla, Abrille

Abygail (Hebrew) a form of
Abigail.
Abygael, Abygale, Abygayle

Acacia (Greek) thorny.
Mythology: the acacia tree
symbolizes immortality and
resurrection. See also Casey.
*Acasha, Acatia, Accassia, Acey,
Acie, Akacia, Cacia, Casia,
Kasia*

Ada (German) a short form of
Adelaide. (English) prosper-
ous; happy.
*Adabelle, Adah, Adan, Adaya,
Adda, Auda*

Adah (Hebrew) ornament.
Ada, Addah

Adair (Greek) a form of
Adara.
Adaire

Adalene (Spanish) a form of
Adalia.
*Adalane, Adalena, Adalin,
Adalina, Adaline, Adalinn,
Adalyn, Adalynn, Adalynne,
Addalyn, Addalynn*

Adalia (German, Spanish)
noble.
*Adal, Adala, Adalea, Adaleah,
Adalee, Adalene, Adali, Adalie,
Adaly, Addal, Addala, Addaly*

Adama (Phoenician, Hebrew)
a form of Adam (see Boys'
Names).

Adamma (Ibo) child of
beauty.

Adana (Spanish) a form of
Adama.

Adanna (Nigerian) her father's daughter.
Adanya

Adara (Greek) beauty. (Arabic) virgin.
Adair, Adaira, Adaora, Adar, Adarah, Adare, Adaria, Adarra, Adasha, Adauré, Adra

Adaya (American) a form of Ada.
Adaija, Adaijah, Adaja, Adajah, Adayja, Adayjah, Adejah

Addie (Greek, German) a familiar form of Adelaide, Adrienne.
Aday, Adde, Addee, Addey, Addi, Addia, Addy, Ade, Adee, Adei, Adey, Adeye, Adi, Adie, Ady, Atti, Attie, Atty

Addison, Addyson (English) child of Adam.
Addis, Addisen, Addisson, Adison

Adela (English) a short form of Adelaide.
Adelae, Adelia, Adelista, Adella

Adelaide (German) noble and serene. See also Ada, Adela, Adeline, Adelle, Ailis, Delia, Della, Ela, Elke, Heidi.
Adelade, Adelaid, Adelaida, Adelei, Adelheid, Adeliade, Adelka, Aley, Laidey, Laidy

Adele (English) a form of Adelle.
Adel, Adelie, Adile

Adelina (English) a form of Adeline.
Adalina, Adeleana, Adelena, Adellyna, Adeliana, Adellena, Adileena, Adlena

Adeline (English) a form of Adelaide.
Adaline, Adelaine, Adelin, Adelina, Adelind, Adelita, Adeliya, Adelle, Adelyn, Adelynn, Adelynne, Adilene, Adlin, Adline, Adlyn, Adlynn, Aline

Adelle (German, English) a short form of Adelaide, Adeline.
Adele, Adell

Adena (Hebrew) noble; adorned.
Adeana, Adeen, Adeena, Aden, Adene, Adenia, Adenna, Adina

Adia (Swahili) gift.
Addia, Adéa, Adea, Adiah

Adila (Arabic) equal.
Adeala, Adeela, Adela, Adelah, Adeola, Adilah, Adileh, Adilia, Adyla

Adilene (English) a form of Adeline.
Adilen, Adileni, Adilenne, Adlen, Adlene

Adina (Hebrew) a form of Adena. See also Dina.
Adeana, Adiana, Adiena, Adinah, Adine, Adinna, Adyna

Adira (Hebrew) strong.
Ader, Adera, Aderah, Aderra,
Adhira, Adirah, Adirana

Adison, Adyson (English)
forms of Addison, Addyson.
Adis, Adisa, Adisen, Adisynne,
Adysen

Aditi (Hindi) unbound.
Religion: the mother of the
Hindu sun gods.
Adithi, Aditti

Adleigh (Hebrew) my ornament.
Adla, Adleni

Adonia (Spanish) beautiful.
Adonica, Adonis, Adonna,
Adonnica, Adonya

Adora (Latin) beloved. See
also Dora.
Adore, Adoree, Adoria

Adra (Arabic) virgin.
Adara

Adreana, Adreanna (Latin)
forms of Adrienne.
Adrean, Adreanne, Adreauna,
Adreeanna, Adreen, Adreena,
Adreeyana, Adrena, Adrene,
Adrenea, Adréona, Adreonia,
Adreonna

Adria (English) a short form
of Adriana, Adriene.
Adrea, Adriani, Adrya

Adriana, Adrianna (Italian)
forms of Adrienne.
Addrianna, Addriyanna,
Adreiana, Adreinna, Adria,
Adriannea, Adriannia, Adrionna

Adriane, Adrianne (English)
forms of Adrienne.
Addrian, Adranne, Adria,
Adrian, Adreinne, Adriann,
Adriayon, Adrion

Adrielle (Hebrew) member of
God's flock.
Adriel, Adrielli, Adryelle

Adrien, Adriene (English)
forms of Adrienne.

Adrienna (Italian) a form of
Adrienne. See also Edrianna.
Adreana, Adrieanna,
Adrieaunna, Adriena, Adrienia,
Adriennah, Adrieunna

Adrienne (Greek) rich. (Latin)
dark. See also Hadriane.
Addie, Adrien, Adriana,
Adriane, Adrianna, Adrianne,
Adrie, Adrieanne, Adrien,
Adrienna, Adriyanna

Adrina (English) a short form
of Adriana.
Adrinah, Adrinne

Adriyanna (American) a form
of Adrienne.
Adrieyana, Adriyana, Adryan,
Adryana, Adryane, Adryanna,
Adryanne

Adya (Hindi) Sunday.
Adia

Aerial, Aeriel (Hebrew) forms of Ariel.
Aeriale, Aeriela, Aerielle, Aeril, Aerile, Aeryal

Afi (African) born on Friday.
Affi, Afia, Efi, Efia

Afra (Hebrew) young doe. (Arabic) earth color. See also Aphra.
Affery, Affrey, Affrie, Afraa

Africa (Irish) pleasant. Geography: one of the seven continents.
Affrica, Afric, Africah, Africaya, Africia, Africiana, Afrika, Aifric

Afrika (Irish) a form of Africa.
Afrikah

Afrodite, Aphrodite (Greek) Mythology: the goddess of love and beauty.
Afrodita

Afton (English) from Afton, England.
Aftan, Aftine, Aftinn, Aftyn

Agate (English) a semiprecious stone.
Aggie

Agatha (Greek) good, kind. Literature: Agatha Christie was a British writer of more than seventy detective novels. See also Gasha.
Agace, Agaisha, Agasha, Agata, Agatah, Agathe, Agathi, Agatka, Agetha, Aggie, Agota, Agotha, Agueda, Atka

Agathe (Greek) a form of Agatha.

Aggie (Greek) a short form of Agatha, Agnes.
Ag, Aggy, Agi

Agnes (Greek) pure. See also Aneesa, Anessa, Anice, Anisha, Ina, Inez, Necha, Nessa, Nessie, Neza, Nyusha, Una, Ynez.
Aganetha, Aggie, Agna, Agne, Agneis, Agnelia, Agnella, Agnés, Agnesa, Agnesca, Agnese, Agnesina, Agness, Agnessa, Agnesse, Agneta, Agneti, Agnetta, Agnies, Agnieszka, Agniya, Agnola, Agnus, Aignéis, Aneska, Anka

Ahava (Hebrew) beloved.
Ahivia

Ahliya (Hebrew) a form of Aliya.
Ahlai, Ahlaia, Ahlaya, Ahleah, Ahleeyah, Ahley, Ahleya, Ahlia, Ahliah, Ahliyah

Aida (Latin) helpful. (English) a form of Ada.
Aidah, Aidan, Aide, Aidee

Aidan, Aiden (Latin) forms of Aida.

Aiesha (Swahili, Arabic) a form of Aisha.
Aeisha, Aeshia, Aieshia, Aieysha, Aiiesha

Aiko (Japanese) beloved.

Ailani (Hawaiian) chief.
Aelani, Ailana

Aileen (Scottish) light bearer.
(Irish) a form of Helen. See
also Eileen.
*Ailean, Aileena, Ailen, Ailene,
Aili, Ailina, Ailinn, Aillen*

Aili (Scottish) a form of Alice.
(Finnish) a form of Helen.
Aila, Ailee, Ailey, Ailie, Aily

Ailis (Irish) a form of
Adelaide.
Ailesh, Ailish, Ailyse, Eilis

Ailsa (Scottish) island dweller.
Geography: Ailsa Craig is an
island in Scotland.
Ailsha

Ailya (Hebrew) a form of
Aliya.
Ailiyah

Aimee (Latin) a form of Amy.
(French) loved.
*Aime, Aimée, Aimey, Aimi,
Aimia, Aimie, Aimy*

Ainsley (Scottish) my own
meadow.
*Ainslee, Ainsleigh, Ainslie, Ainsly,
Ansley, Aynslee, Aynsley, Aynslie*

Airiana (English) a form of
Ariana, Arianna.
*Airana, Airanna, Aireana,
Aireanah, Aireanna, Aireona,
Aireonna, Aireyonna, Airianna,
Airianne, Airiona, Airriana,
Airrion, Airryon, Airyana,
Airyanna*

Airiél (Hebrew) a form of
Ariel.
*Aieral, Aierel, Aiiryel, Aire,
Aireal, Aireale, Aireel, Airel,
Airele, Airelle, Airi, Airial,
Airiale, Airrel*

Aisha (Swahili) life. (Arabic)
woman. See also Asha, Asia,
Iesha, Isha, Keisha, Yiesha.
*Aaisha, Aaishah, Aesha,
Aeshah, Aheesha, Aiasha,
Aiesha, Aieshah, Aisa, Aischa,
Aish, Aishah, Aisheh, Aishia,
Aishiah, Aiysha, Aiyesha,
Ayesha, Aysa, Ayse, Aytza*

Aislinn, Aislynn (Irish) forms
of Ashlyn.
*Aishellyn, Aishlinn, Aislee,
Aisley, Aislin, Aisling, Aislyn,
Aislynne*

Aiyana (Native American) for-
ever flowering.
*Aiyhana, Aiyona, Aiyonia,
Ayana*

Aiyanna (Hindi) a form of
Ayanna.
*Aianna, Aiyannah, Aiyonna,
Aiyunna*

Aja (Hindi) goat.
*Ahjah, Aija, Aijah, Ajá, Ajada,
Ajah, Ajara, Ajaran, Ajare,
Ajaree, Ajha, Ajia*

Ajanae (American) a combination of the letter A + Janae.
Ajahnae, Ajahne, Ajana, Ajanaé, Ajane, Ajané, Ajanee, Ajanique, Ajena, Ajenae, Ajené

Ajia (Hindi) a form of Aja.
Aijia, Ajhia, Aji, Ajjia

Akayla (American) a combination of the letter A + Kayla.
Akaela, Akaelia, Akaila, Akailah, Akala, Akaylah, Akaylia

Akeisha (American) a combination of the letter A + Keisha.
Akaesha, Akaisha, Akasha, Akasia, Akeecia, Akeesha, Akeishia, Akeshia, Akisha

Akela (Hawaiian) noble.
Ahkayla, Ahkeelah, Akelah, Akelia, Akeliah, Akeya, Akeyla, Akeylah

Akeria (American) a form of Akira.
Akera, Akerah, Akeri, Akerra, Akerra

Aki (Japanese) born in autumn.
Akeeye

Akia (American) a combination of the letter A + Kia.
Akaja, Akeia, Akeya, Akiá, Akiah, Akiane, Akiaya, Akiea,
Akiya, Akiyah, Akya, Akyan, Akyia, Akyiah

Akiko (Japanese) bright light.

Akilah (Arabic) intelligent.
Aikiela, Aikilah, Akeela, Akeelah, Akeila, Akeilah, Akeiyla, Akiela, Akielah, Akila, Akilaih, Akilia, Akilka, Akillah, Akkila, Akyla, Akylah

Akili (Tanzanian) wisdom.

Akina (Japanese) spring flower.

Akira (American) a combination of the letter A + Kira.
Akeria, Akiera, Akierra, Akirah, Akire, Akiria, Akirrah, Akyra

Alaina, Alayna (Irish) forms of Alana.
Aalaina, Alainah, Alaine, Alainna, Alainnah, Alane, Alaynah, Alayne, Alaynna, Aleine, Alleyna, Alleynah, Alleyne

Alair (French) a form of Hilary.
Alaira, Ali, Allaire

Alamea (Hawaiian) ripe; precious.

Alameda (Spanish) poplar tree.

Alana (Irish) attractive; peaceful. (Hawaiian) offering. See also Lana.
Alaana, Alaina, Alanae, Alanah, Alane, Alanea, Alani, Alania, Alanis, Alanna, Alawna, Alayna, Allana, Allanah, Allyn, Alonna

Alandra, Alandria (Spanish) forms of Alexandra, Alexandria.
Alandrea, Alantra, Aleandra, Aleandrea

Alani (Hawaiian) orange tree. (Irish) a form of Alana.
Alaini, Alainie, Alania, Alanie, Alaney, Alannie

Alanna (Irish) a form of Alana.
Alannah

Alanza (Spanish) noble and eager.

Alaysha, Alaysia (American) forms of Alicia.
Alaysh, Alayshia

Alba (Latin) from Alba Longa, an ancient city near Rome, Italy.
Albana, Albani, Albanie, Albany, Albeni, Albina, Albine, Albinia, Albinka, Elba

Alberta (German, French) noble and bright. See also Auberte, Bertha, Elberta.
Albertina, Albertine, Albertyna, Albertyne, Alverta

Albreanna (American) a combination of Alberta + Breanna (see Breana).
Albré, Albrea, Albreona, Albreonna, Albreyon

Alcina (Greek) strong-minded.
Alceena, Alcine, Alcinia, Alseena, Alsinia, Alsyna, Alzina

Alda (German) old; elder.
Aldina, Aldine

Alden (English) old; wise protector.
Aldan, Aldon, Aldyn

Aldina, Aldine (Hebrew) forms of Alda.
Aldeana, Aldene, Aldona, Aldyna, Aldyne

Alea, Aleah (Arabic) high, exalted. (Persian) God's being.
Aileah, Aleea, Aleeah, Aleia, Aleiah, Allea, Alleah, Alleea, Alleeah

Aleasha, Aleesha (Greek) forms of Alisha.
Aleashae, Aleashea, Aleashia, Aleassa, Aleeshia

Alecia (Greek) a form of Alicia.
Aalecia, Ahlasia, Aleacia, Aleacya, Aleasia, Alecea, Aleceea, Aleceia, Aleciya, Aleciyah, Alecy, Alecya, Aleeceia, Aleecia, Aleesia, Aleesiya, Aleicia, Alesha, Alesia, Allecia, Alleecia

Aleela (Swahili) she cries.
Aleelah, Alila, Alile

Aleena (Dutch) a form of Aleene.
Ahleena, Aleana, Aleeanna

Aleene (Dutch) alone.
Aleen, Aleena, Alene, Alleen

Aleeya (Hebrew) a form of Aliya.
Alee, Aleea, Aleeyah, Aleiya, Aleiyah

Aleeza (Hebrew) a form of Aliza. See also Leeza.
Aleiza

Alegria (Spanish) cheerful.
Aleggra, Alegra, Allegra, Allegria

Aleisha, Alesha (Greek) forms of Alecia, Alisha.
Aleasha, Aleashea, Aleasia, Aleesha, Aleeshah, Aleeshia, Aleeshya, Aleisa, Alesa, Alesah, Aleisha, Aleshia, Aleshya, Alesia, Alessia

Alejandra (Spanish) a form of Alexandra.
Aleiandra, Alejanda, Alejandr, Alejandrea, Alejandria, Alejandrina, Alejandro

Aleka (Hawaiian) a form of Alice.
Aleeka, Alekah

Aleksandra (Greek) a form of Alexandra.
Alecsandra, Aleksasha, Aleksandrija, Aleksandriya

Alena (Russian) a form of Helen.
Alenah, Alene, Alenea, Aleni, Alenia, Alenka, Alenna, Alennah, Alenya, Alyna

Alesia, Alessia (Greek) forms of Alice, Alicia, Alisha.
Alessea, Alesya, Allesia

Alessa (Greek) a form of Alice.
Alessi, Allessa

Alessandra (Italian) a form of Alexandra.
Alesandra, Alesandrea, Alissandra, Alissondra, Allesand, Allessandra

Aleta (Greek) a form of Alida. See also Leta.
Aletta, Alletta

Alethea (Greek) truth.
Alathea, Alathia, Aletea, Aletha, Aletheia, Alethia, Aletia, Alithea, Alithia

Alette (Latin) wing.

Alex (Greek) a short form of Alexander, Alexandra.
Aleix, Aleks, Alexe, Alexx, Allex, Allexx

Alexa (Greek) a short form of Alexandra.
Aleixa, Alekia, Aleksa, Aleksha, Aleksi, Alexah, Alexsa, Alexssa, Alexxa, Allexa, Alyxa

Alexandra (Greek) defender of humankind. History: the last czarina of Russia. See also Lexia, Lexie, Olesia, Ritsa, Sandra, Sandrine, Sasha, Shura, Sondra, Xandra, Zandra.
Alandra, Alaxandra, Aleczandra, Alejandra, Aleksandra, Alessandra, Alex, Alexa, Alexande, Alexandera,

Alexandre, Alexas, Alexi,
Alexina, Alexine, Alexis,
Alexsandra, Alexius, Alexsis,
Alexus, Alexxandra, Alexys,
Alexzandra, Alix, Alixandra,
Aljexi, Alla, Alyx, Alyxandra,
Lexandra

Alexandrea (Greek) a form of
Alexandria.
Alexandreana, Alexandreia,
Alexandriea, Alexandrieah,
Alexanndrea

Alexandria (Greek) a form of
Alexandra. See also Drinka,
Xandra, Zandra.
Alaxandria, Alecsandria,
Aleczandria, Alexanderia,
Alexanderine, Alexandrea,
Alexandrena, Alexandrie,
Alexandrina, Alexandrine,
Alexanndria, Alexandrya,
Alexendria, Alexendrine, Alexia,
Alixandrea, Alyxandria

Alexandrine (Greek) a form
of Alexandra.
Alexandrina

Alexanne (American) a com-
bination of Alex + Anne.
Alexan, Alexanna, Alexane,
Alexann, Alexanna, Alexian,
Alexiana

Alexas, Alexes (Greek) short
forms of Alexandra.
Alexess

Alexi, Alexie (Greek) short
forms of Alexandra.
Aleksey, Aleksi, Alexey, Alexy

Alexia (Greek) a short form of
Alexandria. See also Lexia.
Aleksia, Aleska, Alexcia, Alexea,
Alexsia, Alexsiya, Allexia,
Alyxia

Alexis (Greek) a short form of
Alexandra.
Aalexis, Ahlexis, Alaxis, Alecsis,
Alecxis, Aleexis, Aleksis, Alexcis,
Alexias, Alexiou, Alexiss,
Alexiz, Alexxis, Alixis, Allexis,
Elexis, Lexis

Alexius, Alexus (Greek) short
forms of Alexandra.
Aalexus, Aalexxus, Aelexus,
Ahlexus, Alecsus, Alexsus,
Alexuss, Alexxus, Alixus,
Allexius, Allexus, Elexus, Lexus

Alexsandra (Greek) a form of
Alexandra.
Alexsandria, Alexsandro,
Alixsandra

Alexsis, Alexxis (Greek) short
forms of Alexandra.
Alexxiz

Alexys (Greek) a short form of
Alexandra.
Alexsys, Alexyes, Alexyis,
Alexyss, Allexys

Alexzandra, Alexzandra
(Greek) forms of Alexandra.
Alexzand, Alexzandrea,
Alexzandriah, Alexzandrya,
Alixzandria

Aleya, Aleyah (Hebrew) forms of Aliya.
Alayah, Aleayah, Aleeya, Aléyah, Aleyia, Aleyiah

Alfie (English) a familiar form of Alfreda.
Alfi, Alfy

Alfreda (English) elf counselor; wise counselor. See also Effie, Elfrida, Freda, Frederica.
Alfie, Alfredda, Alfredia, Alfreeda, Alfreida, Alfrieda

Ali, Aly (Greek) familiar forms of Alice, Alicia, Alisha, Alison.
Allea, Alli, Allie, Ally

Alia, Aliah (Hebrew) forms of Aliya. See also Aaliyah, Alea.
Aelia, Allia, Alya

Alice (Greek) truthful. (German) noble. See also Aili, Aleka, Alie, Alisa, Alison, Alli, Alysa, Alyssa, Alysse, Elke.
Adelice, Alecia, Aleece, Alesia, Alicie, Aliece, Alise, Alix, Alize, Alla, Alleece, Allice, Allis, Allise, Allix

Alicia (English) a form of Alice. See also Elicia, Licia.
Aelicia, Alaysha, Alecea, Alecia, Aleecia, Ali, Alicea, Alicha, Alichia, Aliciah, Alician, Alicja, Alicya, Aliecia, Alisha, Allicea, Allicia, Alycia, Ilysa

Alida (Latin) small and winged. (Spanish) noble. See also Aleta, Lida, Oleda.
Aleda, Aleida, Alidia, Alita, Alleda, Allida, Allidah, Alyda, Alydia, Elida, Elidia

Alie, Allie (Greek) familiar forms of Alice.

Aliesha (Greek) a form of Alisha.
Alieshai, Alieshia, Alliesha

Alika (Hawaiian) truthful. (Swahili) most beautiful.
Aleka, Alica, Alikah, Alike, Alikee, Aliki

Alima (Arabic) sea maiden; musical.

Alina, Alyna (Slavic) bright. (Scottish) fair. (English) short forms of Adeline. See also Alena.
Aliana, Alianna, Alinah, Aline, Alinna, Allyna, Alynna, Alyona

Aline (Scottish) a form of Alina.
Alianne, Allene, Alline, Allyn, Allyne, Alyne, Alynne

Alisa, Alissa (Greek) a form of Alice. See also Elisa, Ilisa.
Aalissah, Aaliysah, Aleessa, Alisah, Alisea, Alisia, Alisza, Alisza, Aliysa, Allissa, Alyssa

Alise, Allise (Greek) forms of Alice.
Alics, Aliese, Alis, Aliss, Alisse, Alisse, Alles, Allesse, Allis, Allisse

Alisha (Greek) truthful.
(German) noble. (English) a
form of Alicia. See also
Elisha, Ilisha, Lisha.
Aalisha, Aleasha, Aleesha,
Aleisha, Alesha, Ali, Aliesha,
Aliscia, Alishah, Alishay,
Alishaye, Alishia, Alishya,
Alitsha, Allisha, Allysha, Alysha

Alishia, Alisia, Alissia
(English) forms of Alisha.
Alishea, Alisheia, Alishiana,
Alyssaya, Alisea, Alissya,
Alisyia, Allissia

Alison, Allison (English)
forms of Alice. See also
Lissie.
Ali, Alicen, Alicyn, Alisan,
Alisann, Alisanne, Alisen,
Alisenne, Alisin, Alision,
Alisonn, Alisson, Alisun, Alles,
Allesse, Alleyson, Allie, Allisson,
Allisyn, Allix, Allsun

Alita (Spanish) a form of
Alida.
Allita

Alivia (Latin) a form of Olivia.
Alivah

Alix (Greek) a short form of
Alexandra, Alice.
Alixe, Alixia, Allix, Alyx

Alixandra, Alixandria (Greek)
forms of Alexandria.
Alixandriya, Allixandra,
Allixandria, Allixandrya

Aliya (Hebrew) ascender.
Aaleyah, Aaliyah, Aeliyah,
Ahliya, Ailya, Alea, Aleya, Alia,
Alieya, Alieyah, Aliyah, Aliyiah,
Aliyyah, Allia, Alliyah, Aly,
Alyah

Aliye (Arabic) noble.
Aliyeh

Aliza (Hebrew) joyful. See also
Aleeza, Eliza.
Alieza, Aliezah, Alitza, Aliz,
Alizah, Alize, Alizee

Alizabeth (Hebrew) a form of
Elizabeth.
Alyzabeth

Allana, Allanah (Irish) forms
of Alana.
Allanie, Allanna, Allauna

Allegra (Latin) cheerful.
Legra

Allena (Irish) a form of Alana.
Alleen, Alleyna, Alleynah

Alli, Ally (Greek) familiar
forms of Alice.
Ali, Alley

Allia, Alliah (Hebrew) forms
of Aliya.

Allissa (Greek) a form of
Alyssa.
Allisa

Alliyah (Hebrew) a form of
Aliya.
Alliya, Alliyha, Alliyia,
Alliyyah, Allya, Allyah

Allysa, Allyssa (Greek) a form of Alyssa.
Allissa, Allyisa, Allysa, Allysah, Allyssah

Allysha (English) a form of Alisha.
Alishia, Allysia

Allyson, Alyson (English) forms of Alison.
Allysen, Allyson, Allysonn, Allysson, Allysun, Alyson

Alma (Arabic) learned. (Latin) soul.
Almah

Almeda (Arabic) ambitious.
Allmeda, Allmedah, Allmeta, Allmita, Almea, Almedah, Almeta, Almida, Almita

Almira (Arabic) aristocratic, princess; exalted. (Spanish) from Almeíra, Spain. See also Elmira, Mira.
Allmeera, Allmeria, Allmira, Almeera, Almeeria, Almeira, Almeria, Almire

Aloha (Hawaiian) loving, kindhearted, charitable.
Alohi

Aloisa (German) famous warrior.
Aloisia, Aloysia

Aloma (Latin) a short form of Paloma.

Alondra (Spanish) a form of Alexandra.
Allandra, Alonda

Alonna (Irish) a form of Alana.
Alona, Alonnah, Alonya, Alonyah

Alonza (English) noble and eager.

Alora (American) a combination of the letter A + Lora.
Alorah, Alorha, Alorie, Aloura, Alouria

Alpha (Greek) first-born. Linguistics: the first letter of the Greek alphabet.
Alphia

Alta (Latin) high; tall.
Allta, Altah, Altana, Altanna, Altea, Alto

Althea (Greek) wholesome; healer. History: Althea Gibson was the first African American to win a major tennis title. See also Thea.
Altha, Altheda, Altheya, Althia, Elthea, Eltheya, Elthia

Alva (Latin, Spanish) white; light skinned. See also Elva.
Alvana, Alvanna, Alvannah

Alvina (English) friend to all; noble friend; friend to elves. See also Elva, Vina.
Alveanea, Alveen, Alveena, Alveenia, Alvenea, Alvie, Alvinae, Alvincia, Alvine,

Alvinea, Alvinesha, Alvinia,
Alvinna, Alvita, Alvona,
Alvyna, Alwin, Alwina, Alwyn

Alyah, Alyiah (Hebrew) forms
of Aliya.
Aly, Alya, Aleah, Alyia

Alycia, Alyssia (English) forms
of Alicia.
Allyce, Alycea, Alyciah, Alyse,
Lycia

Alysa, Alyse, Alysse (Greek)
forms of Alice.
Allys, Allyse, Allyss, Alys, Alyss

Alysha, Alysia (Greek) forms
of Alisha.
Allysea, Allyscia, Alysea,
Alyshia, Alyssha, Alyssia

Alyssa (Greek) rational.
Botany: alyssum is a flower-
ing herb. See also Alice,
Elissa.
Ahlyssa, Alissa, Allissa, Allyssa,
Alyesa, Alyessa, Alyissa, Alysah,
Ilyssa, Lyssa, Lyssah

Alysse (Greek) a form of
Alice.
Allyce, Allys, Allyse, Allyss, Alys,
Alyss

Alyx, Alyxis (Greek) short
forms of Alexandra.

Alyxandra, Alyxandria
(Greek) forms of Alexandria.
Alyxandrea, Alyxzandrya

Am (Vietnamese) lunar; female.

Ama (African) born on Saturday.

Amabel (Latin) lovable. See
also Bel, Mabel.

Amada (Spanish) beloved.
Amadea, Amadi, Amadia,
Amadita

Amairani (Greek) a form of
Amara.
Amairaine, Amairane,
Amairanie, Amairany

Amal (Hebrew) worker.
(Arabic) hopeful.
Amala

Amalia (German) a form of
Amelia.
Ahmalia, Amalea, Amaleah,
Amaleta, Amalija, Amalina,
Amalisa, Amalita, Amaliya,
Amalya, Amalyn

Amalie (German) a form of
Amelia.
Amalee, Amali, Amaly

Aman, Amani (Arabic) forms
of Imani.
Aamani, Ahmani, Amane,
Amanee, Amaney, Amanie,
Ammanu

Amanada (Latin) a form of
Amanda.

Amanda (Latin) lovable. See
also Manda.
Amada, Amanada, Amandah,
Amandalee, Amandalyn,
Amandi, Amandie, Amandine,
Amandy

Amandeep (Punjabi) peaceful light.

Amara (Greek) eternally beautiful. See also Mara.
Amar, Amaira, Amairani, Amarah, Amari, Amaria, Amariah

Amaranta (Spanish) a flower that never fades.

Amari (Greek) a form of Amara.
Amaree, Amarie, Amarii, Amarri

Amaris (Hebrew) promised by God.
Amarissa, Amarys, Maris

Amaryllis (Greek) fresh; flower.
Amarillis, Amarylis

Amaui (Hawaiian) thrush.

Amaya (Japanese) night rain.

Ambar (French) a form of Amber.

Amber (French) amber.
Aamber, Ahmber, Ambar, Amberia, Amberise, Amberly, Ambria, Ambur, Ambyr, Ambyre, Ammber, Ember

Amberly (American) a familiar form of Amber.
Amberle, Amberlea, Amberlee, Amberleigh, Amberley, Amberli, Amberlie, Amberlly, Amberlye

Amberlyn, Amberlynn (American) combinations of Amber + Lynn.
Amberlin, Amberlina, Amberlyne, Amberlynne

Ambria (American) a form of Amber.
Ambrea, Ambra, Ambriah

Amelia (German) hard working. (Latin) a form of Emily. History: Amelia Earhart, an American aviator, was the first woman to fly solo across the Atlantic Ocean. See also Ima, Melia, Millie, Nuela, Yamelia.
Aemilia, Aimilia, Amalia, Amalie, Amaliya, Ameila, Ameilia, Amelie, Amelina, Ameline, Amelisa, Amelita, Amella, Amilia, Amilina, Amilisa, Amilita, Amilyn, Amylia

Amelie (German) a familiar form of Amelia.
Amaley, Amalie, Amelee, Ameleigh, Ameley, Amélie, Amely, Amilie

America (Teutonic) industrious.
Americana, Amerika

Ami, Amie (French) forms of Amy.
Aami, Amiee, Amii, Amiiee, Ammee, Ammie, Ammiee

Amilia, Amilie (Latin, German) forms of Amelia.
Amilee, Amili, Amillia, Amily, Amilya

Amina (Arabic) trustworthy, faithful. History: the mother of the prophet Muhammad.
Aamena, Aamina, Aaminah, Ameena, Ameenah, Aminah, Aminda, Amindah, Aminta, Amintah

Amira (Hebrew) speech; utterance. (Arabic) princess. See also Mira.
Ameera, Ameerah, Amirah

Amissa (Hebrew) truth.
Amissah

Amita (Hebrew) truth.
Amitha

Amity (Latin) friendship.
Amitie

Amlika (Hindi) mother.
Amlikah

Amma (Hindi) god, godlike. Religion: another name for the Hindu goddess Shakti.

Amorie (German) industrious leader.

Amparo (Spanish) protected.

Amrit (Sanskrit) nectar.
Amrita

Amy (Latin) beloved. See also Aimee, Emma, Esmé.
Amata, Ame, Amey, Ami, Amia, Amie, Amio, Ammy, Amye, Amylyn

An (Chinese) peaceful.

Ana (Hawaiian, Spanish) a form of Hannah.
Anai, Anaia

Anaba (Native American) she returns from battle.

Anabel, Anabelle (English) forms of Annabel.
Anabela, Anabele, Anabell, Anabella

Anahita (Persian) a river and water goddess.
Anahai, Anahi, Anahit, Anahy

Anais (Hebrew) gracious.
Anaise, Anaïse

Anala (Hindi) fine.

Analisa, Analise (English) combinations of Ana + Lisa.
Analice, Analicia, Analis, Analisha, Analisia, Analissa

Anamaria (English) a combination of Ana + Maria.
Anamarie, Anamary

Ananda (Hindi) blissful.

Anastacia (Greek) a form of Anastasia.
Anastace, Anastacie

Anastasia (Greek) resurrection. See also Nastasia, Stacey, Stacia, Stasya.
Anastacia, Anastase, Anastascia, Anastasha, Anastashia, Anastasie, Anastasija, Anastassia, Anastassya, Anastasya, Anastatia, Anastaysia, Anastazia, Anastice, Annastasia,

Anastasia *(cont.)*
Annastasija, Annastaysia,
Annastazia, Annstás

Anatola (Greek) from the
east.

Anci (Hungarian) a form of
Hannah.
Annus, Annushka

Andee, Andi, Andie
(American) short forms of
Andrea, Fernanda.
Ande, Andea, Andy

Andrea (Greek) strong; coura-
geous. See also Ondrea.
Aindrea, Andee, Andera,
Anderea, Andra, Andrah,
Andraia, Andraya, Andreah,
Andreaka, Andreana, Andreane,
Andree, Andrée, Andreea,
Andreia, Andreja, Andreka,
Andrel, Andrell, Andrelle,
Andreo, Andressa, Andrette,
Andreya, Andria, Andriana,
Andrieka, Andrietta, Andris,
Aundrea

Andreana, Andreanna
'Greek) forms of Andrea.
Ahndrianna, Andreina,
Andrena, Andreyana,
Andreyonna, Andrina,
Andriona, Andrionna

Andreane, Andreanne
(Greek) forms of Andrea.
Andrean, Andreeanne, Andree
Anne, Andrene, Andrian,
Andrienne

Andria (Greek) a form of
Andrea.
Andri, Andriea

Andriana, Andrianna (Greek)
forms of Andrea.

Aneesa, Aneesha (Greek)
forms of Agnes.
Ahnesha, Ahnesia, Ahnesshia,
Anee, Aneesah, Aneese,
Aneeshah, Aneesia, Aneisa,
Aneisha, Anessa, Anessia

Aneko (Japanese) older sister.

Anela (Hawaiian) angel.
Anel, Anelle

Anessa (Greek) a form of Agnes.
Anesha, Aneshia, Anesia,
Anessia, Annessa

Anetra (American) a form of
Annette.
Anitra

Anezka (Czech) a form of
Hannah.

Angel (Greek) a short form of
Angela.
Angele, Angéle, Angell, Angelle,
Angil, Anjel

Angela (Greek) angel; messen-
ger.
Angala, Anganita, Angel,
Angelanell, Angelanette,
Angelee, Angeleigh, Angeles,
Angeli, Angelia, Angelica,
Angelina, Angelique, Angelita,
Angella, Angellita, Angie,
Anglea, Anjela, Anjelica

Angelia (Greek) a form of
Angela.
Angelea, Angeleah, Angelie

Angelica, Angelika (Greek)
forms of Angela.
*Angalic, Angelic, Angelici,
Angelicia, Angelike, Angeliki,
Angellica, Angilica*

Angelina, Angeline (Russian)
forms of Angela.
*Angalena, Angalina, Angeleen,
Angelena, Angelene, Angeliana,
Angeleana, Angellina, Angelyn,
Angelyna, Angelyne, Angelynn,
Angelynne, Anhelina, Anjelina*

Angelique (French) a form of
Angela.
*Angeliqua, Angélique, Angilique,
Anjelique*

Angeni (Native American)
spirit.

Angie (Greek) a familiar form
of Angela.
Ange, Angee, Angey, Angi, Angy

Ani (Hawaiian) beautiful.
Aany, Aanye

Ania (Polish) a form of
Hannah.
Ahnia, Anaya, Aniah

Anica, Anika (Czech) familiar
forms of Anna.
*Aanika, Anaka, Aneeky, Aneka,
Anekah, Anicka, Anik, Anikah,
Anike, Anikka, Anikke, Aniko,
Anneka, Annik, Annika,
Anouska, Anuska*

Anice (English) a form of
Agnes.
*Anesse, Anis, Anise, Annes,
Annice, Annis, Annus*

Anila (Hindi) Religion: an
attendant of the Hindu god
Vishnu.
Anilla

Anisa, Anisah (Arabic) friendly.
Annissah

Anissa, Anisha (English)
forms of Agnes, Ann.
*Aanisha, Aeniesha, Anis, Anisa,
Anissah, Anise, Annisa,
Annisha, Annissa, Anyssa*

Anita (Spanish) a form of
Ann, Anna. See also Nita.
*Aneeta, Aneetah, Aneethah,
Anetha, Anitha, Anithah,
Anitia, Anitra, Anitte*

Anjelica (Greek) a form of
Angela.
Anjelika

Anka (Polish) a familiar form
of Hannah.
Anke

Ann, Anne (English) gracious.
*Anissa, Anita, Annchen,
Annette, Annie, Annik, Annika,
Annze, Anouche*

Anna (German, Italian, Czech,
Swedish) gracious. Culture:
Anna Pavlova was a famous
Russian ballerina. See also
Anica, Anissa, Nina.
Ahnna, Ana, Anah, Anica,

Anna *(cont.)*
Anita, Annah, Annina, Annora, Anona, Anya, Anyu, Aska

Annabel (English) a combination of Anna + Bel.
Amabel, Anabel, Annabal, Annabelle

Annabelle (English) a form of Annabel.
Anabelle, Annabell, Annabella

Annalie (Finnish) a form of Hannah.
Analee, Annalea, Annaleah, Annalee, Annaleigh, Annaleigha, Annali, Anneli, Annelie

Annalisa, Annalise (English) combinations of Anna + Lisa.
Analisa, Analise, Annaliesa, Annaliese, Annalissa, Annalisse

Annamarie, Annemarie, Annmarie, Anne-Marie (English) combinations of Anne + Marie.
Annamaria, Anna-Maria, Anna-Marie, Annmaria

Anneka (Swedish) a form of Hannah.
Annaka, Anneke, Annika, Anniki, Annikki

Annelisa (English) a combination of Ann + Lisa.
Analiese, Anelisa, Anelise, Anneliese, Annelise

Annette (French) a form of Ann. See also Anetra, Nettie.
Anet, Aneta, Anetra, Anett, Anetta, Anette, Anneth, Annett, Annetta

Annie (English) a familiar form of Ann.
Anni, Anny

Annik, Annika (Russian) forms of Ann.
Aneka, Anekah, Annick, Annicka, Annike, Annikka, Anninka, Anouk

Annjanette (American) a combination of Ann + Janette (see Janett).
Angen, Angenett, Angenette, Anjane, Anjanetta, Anjani

Anona (English) pineapple.

Anouhea (Hawaiian) cool, soft fragrance.

Ansley (Scottish) forms of Ainsley.
Anslea, Anslee, Ansleigh, Anslie

Anthea (Greek) flower.
Antha, Anthe, Anthia, Thia

Antionette (French) a form of Antonia.
Antionet, Antionett, Anntionett

Antoinette (French) a form of Antonia. See also Netti, Toinette, Toni.
Anta, Antanette, Antoinella, Antoinet, Antonella, Antonetta,

Antonette, Antonice, Antonieta,
Antonietta, Antonique

Antonia (Greek) flourishing.
(Latin) praiseworthy. See also
Toni, Tonya, Tosha.
Ansonia, Ansonya, Antania,
Antinia, Antionette, Antoinette,
Antona, Antoñía, Antonice,
Antonie, Antonina, Antonine,
Antoniya, Antonnea, Antonnia,
Antonya

Antonice (Latin) a form of
Antonia.
Antanise, Antanisha, Antonesha,
Antoneshia, Antonise, Antonisha

Anya (Russian) a form of
Anna.
Aaniyah, Aniya, Aniyah, Anja

Anyssa (English) a form of
Anissa.
Anysa, Anysha

'Aolani (Hawaiian) heavenly
cloud.

Aphra (Hebrew) young doe.
See also Afra.

April (Latin) opening. See also
Avril.
Aprele, Aprelle, Apriell, Aprielle,
Aprila, Aprile, Aprilette, Aprili,
Aprill, Apryl

Apryl (Latin) a form of April.
Apryle

Aquene (Native American)
peaceful.

Ara (Arabic) opinionated.
Ahraya, Aira, Arae, Arah, Araya,
Arayah

Arabella (Latin) beautiful altar.
See also Belle, Orabella.
Arabela, Arabele, Arabelle

Araceli, Aracely (Latin) heav-
enly altar.
Aracele, Aracelia, Aracelli,
Araseli, Arasely, Arcelia, Arceli

Ardelle (Latin) warm; enthusiastic.
Ardelia, Ardelis, Ardella

Arden (English) valley of the
eagle. Literature: in
Shakespeare, a romantic place
of refuge.
Ardeen, Ardeena, Ardena,
Ardene, Ardenia, Ardi, Ardin,
Ardina, Ardine

Ardi (Hebrew) a short form of
Arden, Ardice, Ardith.
Ardie, Arti, Artie

Ardice (Hebrew) a form of
Ardith.
Ardis, Artis, Ardiss, Ardyce, Ardys

Ardith (Hebrew) flowering
field.
Ardath, Ardi, Ardice, Ardyth

Areli, Arely (American) forms
of Oralee.
Areil, Areile, Arelee, Areli, Arelis,
Arelli, Arellia, Arelly

Arella (Hebrew) angel; messenger.
Arela, Arelle, Orella, Orelle

Aretha (Greek) virtuous. See also Oretha.
Areatha, Areetha, Areta, Aretina, Aretta, Arette, Arita, Aritha, Retha, Ritha

Ari, Aria, Arie (Hebrew) short forms of Ariel.
Ariah, Ariea, Aryia

Ariadne (Greek) holy. Mythology: the daughter of King Minos of Crete.

Ariana, Arianna (Greek) holy.
Aeriana, Aerianna, Aerionna, Ahreanna, Ahriana, Ahrianna, Airiana, Arieana, Ariona, Arionna, Aryonna

Ariane (French), Arianne (English) forms of Ariana, Arianna.
Aerian, Aeriann, Aerion, Aerionne, Airiann, Ari, Arianie, Ariann, Ariannie, Arieann, Arien, Ariene, Arienne, Arieon, Arionne, Aryane, Aryann, Aryanne

Arica (Scandinavian) forms of Erica.
Aerica, Aericka, Aeryka, Aricca, Aricka, Arika, Arike, Arikka

Ariel (Hebrew) lion of God.
Aerial, Aeriale, Aeriel, Aeriela, Aeryal, Ahriel, Aire, Aireal, Airial, Ari, Aria, Arial, Ariale,

Arieal, Ariela, Arielle, Arrieal, Arriel, Aryel, Auriel

Arielle (French) a form of Ariel.
Aeriell, Ariella, Arriele, Arriell, Arrielle, Aryelle, Aurielle

Arin (Hebrew) enlightened. (Arabic) messenger. See also Erin.
Aaren, Aerin, Aieron, Aieren, Arinn, Aryn

Arista (Greek) best.
Aris, Arissa, Aristana, Aristen

Arla (German) a form of Carla.

Arleigh (English) a form of Harley.
Arlea, Arlee, Arley, Arlie, Arly

Arlene (Irish) pledge. See also Lena, Lina.
Airlen, Arlana, Arleen, Arleene, Arlen, Arlena, Arlenis, Arlette, Arleyne, Arliene, Arlina, Arlinda, Arline, Arlis

Arlette (English) a form of Arlene.
Arleta, Arletta, Arletty

Arlynn (American) a combination of Arlene + Lynn.
Arlyn, Arlyne, Arlynne

Armani (Persian) desire, goal.
Armahni, Arman, Armanee, Armanii

Armine (Latin) noble. (German) soldier. (French) a

form of Herman (see Boys' Names).
Armina

Arnelle (German) eagle.
Arnell, Arnella

Artha (Hindi) wealthy, prosperous.
Arthi, Arti, Artie

Artis (Irish) noble; lofty hill. (Scottish) bear. (English) rock. (Icelandic) follower of Thor.
Arthea, Arthelia, Arthene, Arthette, Arthurette, Arthurina, Arthurine, Artina, Artice

Aryana, Aryanna (Italian) forms of Ariana.
Aryan, Aryanah, Aryannah

Aryn (Hebrew) a form of Arin.
Aerryn, Aeryn, Airyn, Aryne, Arynn, Arynne

Asa (Japanese) born in the morning.

Asha (Arabic, Swahili) a form of Aisha, Ashia.

Ashanti (Swahili) from a tribe in West Africa.
Achante, Achanti, Asante, Ashanta, Ashantae, Ashante, Ashanté, Ashantee, Ashantie, Ashaunta, Ashauntae, Ashauntee, Ashaunti, Ashonti, Ashuntae, Ashunti

Ashely (English) form of Ashley.
Ashelee, Ashelei, Asheley, Ashelie, Ashelley, Ashelly

Ashia (Arabic) life.
Asha, Ashya, Ashyah, Ashyia, Ayshia

Ashlee, Ashli, Ashlie, Ashly (English) forms of Ashley.
Ashle, Ashlea, Ashleah, Ashleeh, Ashliee

Ashleigh (English) a form of Ashley.
Ahsleigh, Asheleigh, Ashlei, Ashliegh

Ashley (English) ash tree meadow. See also Lee.
Ahslee, Aishlee, Ashala, Ashalee, Ashalei, Ashaley, Ashely, Ashla, Ashlay, Ashleay, Ashlee, Ashleigh, Ashleye, Ashli, Ashlie, Ashly, Ashlye

Ashlin (English) a form of Ashlyn.
Ashlean, Ashliann, Ashlianne, Ashline

Ashlyn, Ashlynn (English) ash tree pool. (Irish) vision, dream.
Ashlan, Ashleann, Ashleen, Ashleene, Ashlen, Ashlene, Ashlin, Ashling, Ashlyne, Ashlynne

Ashten, Ashtin (English) forms of Ashton.
Ashtine

Ashton (English) ash-tree *settlement*.
Ashten, Ashtyn

Ashtyn (English) a form of Ashton.
Ashtynne

Asia (Greek) resurrection. (English) eastern sunrise. (Swahili) a form of Aisha.
Ahsia, Aisia, Aisian, Asiah, Asian, Asianae, Asya, Aysia, Aysiah, Aysian, Ayzia

Aspen (English) aspen tree.
Aspin, Aspyn

Aster (English) a form of Astra.
Astera, Asteria, Astyr

Astra (Greek) star.
Asta, Astara, Aster, Astraea, Astrea

Astrid (Scandinavian) divine strength.
Astri, Astrida, Astrik, Astrud, Atti, Estrid

Atalanta (Greek) mighty huntress. Mythology: an athletic young woman who refused to marry any man who could not outrun her in a footrace. See also Lani.
Atalaya, Atlanta, Atlante, Atlee

Atara (Hebrew) crown.
Atarah, Ataree

Athena (Greek) wise. Mythology: the goddess of wisdom.
Athenea, Athene, Athina, Atina

Atira (Hebrew) prayer.

Auberte (French) a form of Alberta.
Auberta, Aubertha, Auberthe, Aubine

Aubree, Aubrie (French) forms of Aubrey.
Auberi, Aubre, Aubrei, Aubreigh, Aubri, Aubrielle

Aubrey (German) noble; bear-like. (French) blond ruler; elf ruler.
Aubary, Aubery, Aubray, Aubrea, Aubreah, Aubree, Aubrette, Aubria, Aubrie, Aubry, Aubury, Avery

Aubriana, Aubrianna (English) combinations of Aubrey + Anna.
Aubreyana, Aubreyanna, Aubreyanne, Aubreyena, Aubrianne

Audey (English) a familiar form of Audrey.
Aude, Audi, Audie

Audra (French) a form of Audrey.
Audria, Audriea

Audreanne (English) a combination of Audrey + Anne.
Audrea, Audreen, Audrianne, Audrienne

Audree, Audrie (English)
forms of Audrey.
Audre, Audri

Audrey (English) noble
strength.
Adrey, Audey, Audra, Audray,
Audree, Audrie, Audrin,
Audriya, Audry, Audrye

Audriana, Audrianna
(English) combinations of
Audrey + Anna.
Audreanna, Audrienna, Audrina

Audris (German) fortunate,
wealthy.
Audrys

Augusta (Latin) a short form
of Augustine. See also Gusta.
Agusta, August, Auguste,
Augustia, Augustus, Austina

Augustine (Latin) majestic.
Religion: Saint Augustine
was the first archbishop of
Canterbury. See also Tina.
Agustina, Augusta, Augustina,
Augustyna, Augustyne, Austin

'Aulani (Hawaiian) royal messenger.
Lani, Lanie

Aundrea (Greek) a form of
Andrea.
Aundreah

Aura (Greek) soft breeze.
(Latin) golden. See also Ora.

Aurelia (Latin) golden. See
also Oralia.
Auralea, Auralia, Aurea, Aureal,
Aurel, Aurele, Aurelea,
Aureliana, Aurelie, Auria, Aurie,
Aurilia, Aurita

Aurelie (Latin) a form of
Aurelia.
Auralee, Auralei, Aurelee,
Aurelei, Aurelle

Aurora (Latin) dawn.
Mythology: Aurora was the
goddess of dawn.
Aurore, Ora, Ori, Orie, Rora

Austin (Latin) a short form of
Augustine.
Austen, Austin, Austyn,
Austynn

Autumn (Latin) autumn.
Autum

Ava (Greek) a form of Eva.
Avada, Avae, Ave, Aveen

Avalon (Latin) island.
Avallon

Avery (English) a form of
Aubrey.
Aivree, Averi, Averie, Avry

Avis (Latin) bird.
Avais, Avi, Avia, Aviana,
Avianca, Aviance, Avianna

Aviva (Hebrew) springtime.
See also Viva.
Aviv, Avivah, Avivi, Avivice,
Avni, Avnit, Avri, Avrit, Avy

Avril (French) a form of April.
Averil, Averyl, Avra, Avri,
Avrilia, Avrill, Avrille, Avrillia,
Avy

Axelle (Latin) axe. (German)
small oak tree; source of life.
Aixa

Aya (Hebrew) bird; fly swiftly.
Aia, Aiah, Aiya, Aiyah

Ayanna (Hindi) innocent.
Ahyana, Aiyanna, Ayan, Ayana,
Ayania, Ayannica, Ayna

Ayesha (Persian) a form of
Aisha.
Ayasha, Ayeshah, Ayessa,
Ayisha, Ayishah, Aysha,
Ayshah, Ayshe, Ayshea, Aysia

Ayita (Cherokee) first in the
dance.

Ayla (Hebrew) oak tree.
Aylana, Aylee, Ayleen, Aylene,
Aylie, Aylin

Aza (Arabic) comfort.
Aiza, Aizha, Aizia, Azia

Aziza (Swahili) precious.
Azize

B

Baba (African) born on
Thursday.
Aba

Babe (Latin) a familiar form
of Barbara. (American) a
form of Baby.
Babby

Babette (French, German) a
familiar form of Barbara.
Babita, Barbette

Babs (American) a familiar
form of Barbara.
Bab

Baby (American) baby.
Babby, Babe, Bebe

Bailee, Bailie (English) forms
of Bailey.
Baelee, Baeli, Bailea, Bailei,
Baillee, Baillie, Bailli

Baileigh, Baleigh (English)
forms of Bailey.
Baeleigh

Bailey (English) bailiff.
Baeley, Bailee, Baileigh, Bailley,
Bailly, Baily, Bali, Balley,
Baylee, Bayley

Baka (Hindi) crane.

Bakula (Hindi) flower.

Bambi (Italian) child.
Bambee, Bambie, Bamby

Bandi (Punjabi) prisoner.
Banda, Bandy

Baptista (Latin) baptizer.
Baptiste, Batista, Battista,
Bautista

Bara, Barra (Hebrew) chosen.
Bára, Bari

Barb (Latin) a short form of Barbara.
Barba, Barbe

Barbara (Latin) stranger, foreigner. See also Bebe, Varvara, Wava.
Babara, Babb, Babbie, Babe, Babette, Babina, Babs, Barb, Barbara-Ann, Barbarit, Barbarita, Barbary, Barbeeleen, Barbera, Barbie, Barbora, Barborah, Barborka, Barbra, Barbraann, Barbro, Barùska, Basha, Bebe, Bobbi, Bobbie

Barbie (American) a familiar form of Barbara.
Barbee, Barbey, Barbi, Barby, Baubie

Barbra (American) a form of Barbara.
Barbro

Barrett (German) strong as a bear.

Barrie (Irish) spear; markswoman.
Bari, Barri, Berri, Berrie, Berry

Basia (Hebrew) daughter of God.
Basya, Bathia, Batia, Batya, Bitya, Bithia

Bathsheba (Hebrew) daughter of the oath; seventh daughter. Bible: a wife of King David. See also Sheba.
Bathshua, Batsheva, Bersaba, Bethsabee, Bethsheba

Batini (Swahili) inner thoughts.

Baylee, Bayleigh, Baylie (English) forms of Bailey.
Bayla, Bayle, Baylea, Bayleah, Baylei, Bayli, Bayliee, Bayliegh

Bayley (English) a form of Bailey.
Bayly

Bayo (Yoruba) joy is found.

Bea, Bee (American) short forms of Beatrice.

Beata (Latin) a short form of Beatrice.
Beatta

Beatrice (Latin) blessed; happy; bringer of joy. See also Trish, Trixie.
Bea, Beata, Beatrica, Béatrice, Beatricia, Beatriks, Beatrisa, Beatrise, Beatrissa, Beatriz, Beattie, Beatty, Bebe, Bee, Trice

Beatriz (Latin) a form of Beatrice.
Beatris, Beatriss, Beatrix, Beitris

Bebe (Spanish) a form of Barbara, Beatrice.
BB, Beebee, Bibi

Becca (Hebrew) a short form of Rebecca.
Beca, Becka, Bekah, Bekka

Becky (American) a familiar form of Rebecca.
Beckey, Becki, Beckie

Bedelia (Irish) a form of
Bridget.
Bedeelia, Biddy, Bidelia

Bel (Hindi) sacred wood of
apple trees. A short form of
Amabel, Belinda, Isabel.

Bela (Czech) white.
(Hungarian) bright.
Belah, Biela

Belen (Greek) arrow. (Spanish)
Bethlehem.
Belina

Belicia (Spanish) dedicated to
God.
Beli, Belia, Belica

Belinda (Spanish) beautiful.
Literature: a name coined by
English poet Alexander Pope
in *The Rape of the Lock*. See
also Blinda, Linda.
Bel, Belindra, Belle, Belynda

Bella (Latin) beautiful.
Bellah

Belle (French) beautiful. A
short form of Arabella,
Belinda, Isabel. See also
Billie.
Belita, Bell, Belli, Bellina

Belva (Latin) beautiful view.
Belvia

Bena (Native American)
pheasant. See also Bina.
Benea

Benecia (Latin) a short form
of Benedicta.
*Beneisha, Benicia, Benish,
Benisha, Benishia, Bennicia*

Benedicta (Latin) blessed.
*Bendite, Benecia, Benedetta,
Benedicte, Benedikta, Bengta,
Benita, Benna, Benni, Bennicia,
Benoîte, Binney*

Benedicte (Latin) a form of
Benedicta.

Benita (Spanish) a form of
Benedicta.
*Beneta, Benetta, Benitta,
Bennita, Neeta*

Bennett (Latin) little blessed
one.
Bennet, Bennetta

Benni (Latin) a familiar form
of Benedicta.
Bennie, Binni, Binnie, Binny

Bente (Latin) blessed.

Berenice (Greek) a form of
Bernice.
*Berenise, Berenisse, Bereniz,
Berenize*

Berget (Irish) a form of
Bridget.
Bergette, Bergit

Berit (German) glorious.
Beret, Berette, Berta

Berkley (Scottish, English)
birch-tree meadow.
Berkeley, Berkly

Berlynn (English) a combination of Bertha + Lynn.
Berla, Berlin, Berlinda, Berline, Berling, Berlyn, Berlyne, Berlynne

Bernadette (French) a form of Bernadine. See also Nadette.
Bera, Beradette, Berna, Bernadet, Bernadete, Bernadett, Bernadetta, Bernarda, Bernardette, Bernedet, Bernedette, Bernessa, Berneta

Bernadine (English, German) brave as a bear.
Bernadene, Bernadette, Bernadin, Bernadina, Bernardina, Bernardine, Berni

Berneta (French) a short form of Bernadette.
Bernatta, Bernetta, Bernette, Bernita

Berni (English) a familiar form of Bernadine, Bernice.
Bernie, Berny

Bernice (Greek) bringer of victory. See also Bunny, Vernice.
Berenice, Berenike, Bernessa, Berni, Bernicia, Bernise, Nixie

Bertha (German) bright; illustrious; brilliant ruler. A short form of Alberta. See also Birdie, Peke.
Barta, Bartha, Berta, Berthe, Bertille, Bertita, Bertrona, Bertus, Birtha

Berti (German, English) a familiar form of Gilberte, Bertina.
Berte, Bertie, Berty

Bertille (French) a form of Bertha.

Bertina (English) bright, shining.
Bertine

Beryl (Greek) sea green jewel.
Beryle

Bess, Bessie (Hebrew) familiar forms of Elizabeth.
Bessi, Bessy

Beth (Hebrew, Aramaic) house of God. A short form of Bethany, Elizabeth.
Betha, Bethe, Bethia

Bethani, Bethanie (Aramaic) forms of Bethany.
Bethanee, Bethania, Bethannie, Bethni, Bethnie

Bethann (English) a combination of Beth + Ann.
Beth-Ann, Bethan, Bethane, Bethanne, Beth-Anne

Bethany (Aramaic) house of figs. Bible: the site of Lazarus's resurrection.
Beth, Bethaney, Bethani, Bethanney, Bethanny, Bethena, Betheny, Bethia, Bethina, Bethney, Bethny, Betthany

Betsy (American) a familiar
form of Elizabeth.
Betsey, Betsi, Betsie

Bette (French) a form of Betty.
Beta, Beti, Betka, Bett, Betta

Bettina (American) a combination of Beth + Tina.
Betina, Betine, Betti, Bettine

Betty (Hebrew) consecrated to
God. (English) a familiar
form of Elizabeth.
*Bette, Bettey, Betti, Bettie,
Bettye, Bettyjean, Betty-Jean,
Bettyjo, Betty-Jo, Bettylou,
Betty-Lou, Bety, Boski, Bözsi*

Betula (Hebrew) girl, maiden.

Beulah (Hebrew) married.
Bible: Beulah is a name for
Israel.
Beula, Beulla, Beullah

Bev (English) a short form of
Beverly.

Bevanne (Welsh) child of Evan.
Bevan, Bevann, Bevany

Beverly (English) beaver field.
See also Buffy.
*Bev, Bevalee, Beverle, Beverlee,
Beverley, Beverlie, Beverlly,
Bevlyn, Bevlynn, Bevlynne,
Bevvy, Verly*

Beverlyann (American) a
combination of Beverly +
Ann.
*Beverliann, Beverlianne,
Beverlyanne*

Bian (Vietnamese) hidden;
secretive.

Bianca (Italian) white. See also
Blanca, Vianca.
*Biancca, Biancha, Biancia,
Bianco, Bianey, Bianica, Bianka,
Biannca, Binney, Bionca,
Blanca, Blanche, Byanca*

Bianka (Italian) a form of
Bianca.
Beyanka, Biannka

Bibi (Latin) a short form of
Bibiana. (Arabic) lady.
(Spanish) a form of Bebe.

Bibiana (Latin) lively.
Bibi

Biddy (Irish) a familiar form
of Bedelia.
Biddie

Billi, Billy (English) forms of
Billie.
Billye

Billie (English) strong willed.
(German, French) a familiar
form of Belle, Wilhelmina.
*Bilee, Bileigh, Bili, Bilie, Billee,
Billi, Billy, Billye*

Billie-Jean (American) a combination of Billie + Jean.
Billiejean, Billyjean, Billy-Jean

Billie-Jo (American) a combination of Billie + Jo.
Billiejo, Billyjo, Billy-Jo

Bina (Hebrew) wise; understanding. (Swahili) dancer.

(Latin) a short form of
Sabina. See also Bena.
Binah, Binney, Binta, Bintah

Binney (English) a familiar
form of Benedicta, Bianca,
Bina.
Binnee, Binni, Binnie, Binny

Bionca (Italian) a form of
Bianca.
*Beonca, Beyonca, Beyonka,
Bioncha, Bionica, Bionka,
Bionnca*

Birdie (English) bird.
(German) a familiar form of
Bertha.
*Bird, Birdee, Birdella, Birdena,
Birdey, Birdi, Birdy, Byrd,
Byrdey, Byrdie, Byrdy*

Birgitte (Swedish) a form of
Bridget.
Birgit, Birgita, Birgitta

Blaine (Irish) thin.
Blane, Blayne

Blair (Scottish) plains dweller.
Blaire

Blaire (Scottish) a form of
Blair.
Blare, Blayre

Blaise (French) one who
stammers.
*Blaize, Blasha, Blasia, Blaza,
Blaze, Blazena*

Blake (English) dark.
Blaque, Blayke

Blakely (English) dark
meadow.
*Blakelea, Blakelee, Blakeleigh,
Blakeley, Blakeli, Blakelyn,
Blakelynn, Blakesley, Blakley,
Blakli*

Blanca (Italian) a form of
Bianca.
Bellanca, Blancka, Blanka

Blanche (French) a form of
Bianca.
Blanch, Blancha, Blinney

Blinda (American) a short
form of Belinda.
Blynda

Bliss (English) blissful, joyful.
Blisse, Blyss, Blysse

Blodwyn (Welsh) flower. See
also Wynne.
Blodwen, Blodwynne, Blodyn

Blondelle (French) blond, fair
haired.
Blondell, Blondie

Blondie (American) a familiar
form of Blondell.
Blondee, Blondey, Blondy

Blossom (English) flower.

Blum (Yiddish) flower.
Bluma

Blythe (English) happy, cheerful.
Blithe, Blyss, Blyth

Bo (Chinese) precious.

Boacha (Hebrew) blessed.

Bobbette (American) a familiar form of Roberta.
Bobbet, Bobbetta

Bobbi, Bobbie (American) familiar forms of Barbara, Roberta.
Baubie, Bobbe, Bobbey, Bobbisue, Bobby, Bobbye, Bobi, Bobie, Bobina, Bobbie-Jean, Bobbie-Lynn, Bobbie-Sue

Bobbi-Ann, Bobbie-Ann (American) combinations of Bobbi + Ann.
Bobbiann, Bobbi-Anne, Bobbianne, Bobbie-Anne, Bobby-Ann, Bobbyann, Bobby-Anne, Bobbyanne

Bobbi-Jo (American) a combination of Bobbi + Jo.
Bobbiejo, Bobbie-Jo, Bobbijo, Bobby-Jo, Bobijo

Bobbi-Lee (American) a combination of Bobbi + Lee.
Bobbie-Lee, Bobbilee, Bobbylee, Bobby-Leigh, Bobile

Bonita (Spanish) pretty.
Bonesha, Bonetta, Bonnetta, Bonnie, Bonny

Bonnie, Bonny (English, Scottish) beautiful, pretty. (Spanish) familiar forms of Bonita.
Boni, Bonie, Bonne, Bonnee, Bonnell, Bonney, Bonni, Bonnin

Bonnie-Bell (American) a combination of Bonnie + Belle.
Bonnebell, Bonnebelle, Bonnibell, Bonnibelle, Bonniebell, Bonniebelle, Bonnybell, Bonnybelle

Bradley (English) broad meadow.
Bradlee, Bradleigh, Bradlie

Brady (Irish) spirited.
Bradee, Bradey, Bradi, Bradie, Braedi, Braidee, Braidi, Braidie, Braidey, Braidy, Braydee

Braeden (English) broad hill.
Bradyn, Bradynn, Braedan, Braedean, Braedyn, Braidan, Braiden, Braidyn, Brayden, Braydn, Braydon

Braelyn (American) a combination of Braeden + Lynn.
Braelee, Braeleigh, Braelin, Braelle, Braelon, Braelynn, Braelynne, Brailee, Brailenn, Brailey, Braili, Brailyn, Braylee, Brayley, Braylin, Braylon, Braylyn, Braylynn

Branda (Hebrew) blessing.

Brandee (Dutch) a form of Brandy.
Brande, Brandea, Brendee

Branden (English) beacon valley.
Brandan, Brandon, Brendan, Brandyn, Brennan

Brandi, Brandie (Dutch) forms of Brandy.
Brandei, Brandice, Brandiee,

Brandii, Brandily, Brandin,
Brandis, Brandise, Brani,
Branndie, Brendi

Brandy (Dutch) an after-dinner drink made from distilled wine.
Brand, Brandace, Brandaise,
Brandala, Brandee, Brandeli,
Brandell, Brandi, Brandye,
Brandylee, Brandy-Lee, Brandy-
Leigh, Brann, Brantley,
Branyell, Brendy

Brandy-Lynn (American) a combination of Brandy + Lynn.
Brandalyn, Brandalynn,
Brandelyn, Brandelynn,
Brandelynne, Brandilyn,
Brandilynn, Brandilynne,
Brandlin, Brandlyn, Brandlynn,
Brandlynne, Brandolyn,
Brandolynn, Brandolynne,
Brandylyn, Brandy-Lyn,
Brandylynne, Brandy-Lynne

Braxton (English) Brock's town.
Braxten, Braxtyn

Brea, Bria (Irish) short forms of Breana, Briana.
Breah, Breea, Briah, Brya

Breana, Breanna (Irish) forms of Briana.
Brea, Breanah, Breanda, Bre-
Anna, Breannah, Breannea,
Breannia, Breasha, Breawna,
Breeanna, Breila

Breann, Breanne (Irish) short forms of Briana.
Breane, Bre-Ann, Bre-Anne,
Breaunne, Bree, Breean,
Breeann, Breeanne, Breelyn,
Breeon, Breiann, Breighann,
Breyenne, Brieann, Brieon

Breasha (Russian) a familiar form of Breana.

Breauna, Breunna, Briauna (Irish) forms of Briana.
Breaunna, Breeauna, Breuna,
Breuna, Briaunna

Breck (Irish) freckled.
Brecken

Bree (English) broth. (Irish) a short form of Breann. See also Brie.
Breay, Brei, Breigh

Breeana, Breeanna (Irish) forms of Briana.
Breeanah, Breeannah

Breena (Irish) fairy palace. A form of Brina.
Breenea, Breene, Breina, Brina

Breiana, Breianna (Irish) forms of Briana.
Breiane, Breiann, Breianne

Brenda (Irish) little raven. (English) sword.
Brendell, Brendelle, Brendette,
Brendie, Brendyl, Brenna

Brenda-Lee (American) a combination of Brenda + Lee.
Brendalee, Brendaleigh, Brendali, Brendaly, Brendalys, Brenlee, Brenley

Brenna (Irish) a form of Brenda.
Bren, Brenie, Brenin, Brenn, Brennah, Brennaugh, Brenne

Brennan (English) a form of Brendan (see Boys' Names).
Brennea, Brennen, Brennon, Brennyn

Breona, Breonna (Irish) forms of Briana.
Breeona, Breiona, Breionna, Breonah, Breonia, Breonie, Breonne

Brett (Irish) a short form of Brittany. See also Brita.
Bret, Brette, Brettin, Bretton

Breyana, Breyann, Breyanna (Irish) forms of Briana.
Breyan, Breyane, Breyannah, Breyanne

Breyona, Breyonna (Irish) forms of Briana.
Breyonia

Briana, Brianna (Irish) strong; virtuous, honorable.
Bhrianna, Brana, Brea, Breana, Breann, Breauna, Breeana, Breiana, Breona, Breyana, Breyona, Bria, Briahna, Brianah, Briand, Brianda, Briannah, Brianne, Brianni, Briannon, Brienna, Brina, Briona, Briyana, Bryanna, Bryona

Brianne (Irish) a form of Briana.
Briane, Briann, Brienne, Bryanne

Briar (French) heather.
Brear, Brier, Bryar

Bridey (Irish) a familiar form of Bridget.
Bridi, Bridie, Brydie

Bridget (Irish) strong. See also Bedelia, Bryga, Gitta.
Berget, Birgitte, Bride, Bridey, Bridger, Bridgete, Bridgett, Bridgette, Bridgid, Bridgot, Brietta, Brigada, Briget, Brigid, Brigida, Brigitte, Brita

Bridgett, Bridgette (Irish) forms of Bridget.
Bridgitte, Brigette, Bridggett, Briggitte, Bridgitt, Brigitta

Brie (French) a type of cheese. Geography: a region in France known for its cheese. See also Bree.
Briea, Brielle, Briena, Brieon, Brietta, Briette

Brieana, Brieanna (American) combinations of Brie + Anna.
Brieannah

Brieann, Brieanne (American) combinations of

Brie + Ann. See also Briana.
Brie-Ann, Brie-Anne

Brielle (French) a form of
Brie.
Briel, Briele, Briell, Briella

Brienna, Brienne (Irish)
forms of Briana.
*Briene, Brieon, Brieona,
Brieonna*

Brienne (French) a form of
Briana.
Brienn

Brigette (French) a form of
Bridget.
*Briget, Brigett, Brigetta,
Brigettee, Brigget*

Brigitte (French) a form of
Bridget.
Briggitte, Brigit, Brigita

Brina (Latin) a short form of
Sabrina. (Irish) a familiar
form of Briana.
*Brin, Brinan, Brinda, Brindi,
Brindy, Briney, Brinia, Brinlee,
Brinly, Brinn, Brinna, Brinnan,
Briona, Bryn, Bryna*

Briona (Irish) a form of
Briana.
*Brione, Brionna, Brionne,
Briony, Briunna, Bryony*

Brisa (Spanish) beloved.
Mythology: Briseis was the
Greek name of Achilles's
beloved.
*Breezy, Breza, Brisha, Brishia,
Brissa, Bryssa*

Brita (Irish) a form of Bridget.
(English) a short form of
Britany.
*Bretta, Brieta, Brietta, Brit,
Britta*

Britaney, Brittaney (English)
forms of Britany, Brittany.
*Britanee, Britanny, Britenee,
Briteny, Britianey, British,
Britkney, Britley, Britlyn,
Britney, Briton*

Britani, Brittani, Brittanie
(English) forms of Britany.
*Brit, Britania, Britanica,
Britanie, Britanii, Britanni,
Britannia, Britatani, Britia,
Britini, Brittane, Brittanee,
Brittanni, Brittannia, Brittannie,
Brittenie, Brittiani, Brittianni*

Britany, Brittany (English)
from Britain. See also Brett.
*Brita, Britana, Britaney, Britani,
Britanna, Britlyn, Britney, Britt,
Brittainny, Brittainy, Brittamy,
Brittana, Brittaney, Brittani,
Brittania, Brittanica, Brittanny,
Brittany-Ann, Brittanyne,
Brittell, Britteny, Brittiany,
Brittini, Brittlin, Brittlynn,
Brittnee, Brittony, Bryttany*

Britin, Brittin (English) from
Britain.
*Britann, Brittan, Brittin,
Brittina, Brittine, Brittini,
Brittiny*

Britney, Brittney, Brittny
(English) forms of Britany.
Bittney, Bridnee, Bridney,
Britnay, Britne, Britnee, Britnei,
Britni, Britny, Britnye, Brittnay,
Brittnaye, Brytnea, Brytni

Britni, Brittni, Brittnie
(English) forms of Britney,
Britney.
Britnie

Briton, Brittin (English) forms
of Britin, Brittin.
Britton

Britt, Britta (Latin) short
forms of Britany, Brittany.
(Swedish) strong.
Brett, Briet, Brit, Brita, Britte

Britteny (English) a form of
Britany, Brittany.
Britten, Brittenay, Brittenee,
Britteney, Brittenie

Brittini, Brittiny (English)
forms of Britany, Brittany.
Brittinee, Brittiney, Brittinie,
Brittiny

Brittnee (English) a form of
Britany, Brittany.
Brittne, Brittnea, Brittnei,
Brittneigh

Briyana, Briyanna (Irish)
forms of Briana.

Brodie (Irish) ditch; canal
builder.
Brodee, Brodi, Brody

Bronnie (Welsh) a familiar
form of Bronwyn.
Bron, Bronia, Bronney, Bronny,
Bronya

Bronwyn (Welsh) white
breasted.
Bronnie, Bronwen, Bronwin,
Bronwynn, Bronwynne

Brook, Brooke (English)
brook, stream.
Bhrooke, Brookelle, Brookie,
Brooks, Brooky

Brooklyn, Brooklynn
(American) combinations of
Brook + Lynn.
Brookellen, Brookelyn,
Brookelyne, Brookelynn,
Brooklen, Brooklin, Brooklyne,
Brooklynne

Bruna (German) a short form
of Brunhilda.
Brona

Brunhilda (German) armored
warrior.
Brinhilda, Brinhilde, Bruna,
Brunhilde, Brünnhilde,
Brynhild, Brynhilda, Brynhilde,
Hilda

Bryana, Bryanna, Bryanne
(Irish) short forms of Bryana.
Bryann, Bryanni

Bryce (Welsh) alert; ambitious.

Bryga (Polish) a form of
Bridget.
Brygid, Brygida, Brygitka

Brylie (American) a combination of the letter B + Riley.
Brylee, Brylei, Bryley, Bryli

Bryn, Brynn (Latin) from the boundary line. (Welsh) mound.
Brinn, Brynee, Brynne

Bryna (Latin, Irish) a form of Brina.
Brynan, Brynna, Brynnan

Bryona, Bryonna (Irish) forms of Briana.
Bryonia, Bryony

Bryttani, Bryttany (English) forms of Britany.
Brytani, Brytanie, Brytanny, Brytany, Brytnee, Brytnie, Bryton, Bryttanee, Bryttanie, Bryttine, Bryttney, Bryttnie, Brytton

Buffy (American) buffalo; from the plains.
Buffee, Buffey, Buffie, Buffye

Bunny (Greek) a familiar form of Bernice. (English) little rabbit. See also Bonnie.
Bunni, Bunnie

Burgundy (French) Geography: a region of France known for its Burgundy wine.
Burgandi, Burgandie, Burgandy, Burgunde

C

Cachet (French) prestigious; desirous.
Cachae, Cache, Cachea, Cachee, Cachée

Cadence (Latin) rhythm.
Cadena, Cadenza, Kadena

Cady (English) a form of Kady.
Cade, Cadee, Cadey, Cadi, Cadie, Cadine, Cadye

Caeley, Cailey, Cayley (American) forms of Kaylee, Kelly.
Caela, Caelee, Caeleigh, Caeley, Caeli, Caelie, Caelly, Caely, Cailee, Caileigh, Caili, Cailie, Cailley, Caillie, Caily, Caylee

Caelin, Caelyn (American) forms of Kaelyn.
Caelan, Caelinn, Caelynn, Cailan, Caylan

Cai (Vietnamese) feminine.
Cae, Cay, Caye

Cailida (Spanish) adoring.
Kailida

Cailin, Cailyn (American) forms of Caitlin.
Caileen, Cailene, Cailine, Cailynn, Cailynne, Calen, Cayleen, Caylen, Caylene, Caylin, Cayline, Caylyn, Caylyne, Caylynne

Caitlan (Irish) a form of
Caitlin.
Caitland, Caitlandt

Caitlin (Irish) pure. See also
Kaitlin, Katalina, Katelin,
Katelyn, Kaytlyn.
*Caetlin, Cailin, Caitlan,
Caitleen, Caitlen, Caitlene,
Caitlenn, Caitline, Caitlinn,
Caitlon, Caitlyn, Catlee,
Catleen, Catleene, Catlin*

Caitlyn, Caitlynn (Irish) forms
of Caitlin. See also Kaitlyn.
*Caitlyne, Caitlynne, Catelyn,
Catlyn, Catlynn, Catlynne*

Cala (Arabic) castle, fortress.
See also Callie, Kala.
Calah, Calan, Calla, Callah

Calandra (Greek) lark.
*Calan, Calandrea, Calandria,
Caleida, Calendra, Calendre,
Kalandra, Kalandria*

Caleigh, Caley (American)
forms of Caeley.
Caileigh, Caleah

Cali, Calli (Greek) forms of
Calie. See also Kali.
Calee

Calida (Spanish) warm; ardent.
*Calina, Calinda, Callida,
Callinda, Kalida*

Callie (Greek, Arabic) a familiar form of Cala, Callista. See
also Kalli.
*Cal, Cali, Calie, Callee, Calley,
Calli, Cally, Caly*

Callista (Greek) most beautiful. See also Kallista.
Calesta, Calista, Callie, Calysta

Calvina (Latin) bald.
Calvine, Calvinetta, Calvinette

Calypso (Greek) concealer.
Botany: a pink orchid native
to northern regions.
Mythology: the sea nymph
who held Odysseus captive
for seven years.
Caly, Lypsie, Lypsy

Cam (Vietnamese) sweet citrus.
Kam

Camara (American) a form of
Cameron.
*Camera, Cameri, Cameria,
Camira, Camry*

Camberly (American) a form
of Kimberly.
*Camber, Camberlee,
Camberleigh*

Cambria (Latin) from Wales.
See also Kambria.
*Camberry, Cambreia, Cambie,
Cambrea, Cambree, Cambrie,
Cambrina, Cambry, Cambrya,
Cami*

Camden (Scottish) winding
valley.
Camdyn

Camellia (Italian) Botany: a
camellia is an evergreen tree
or shrub with fragrant rose-
like flowers.
Camala, Camalia, Camallia,

*Camela, Camelia, Camelita,
Camella, Camellita, Cami,
Kamelia, Kamellia*

*Cameisha, Camesa, Camesha,
Cameshaa, Cameshia,
Camiesha, Camyeshia*

Cameo (Latin) gem or shell
on which a portrait is
carved.
Cami, Kameo

Cameron (Scottish) crooked
nose. See also Kameron,
Kamryn.
*Camara, Cameran, Cameren,
Camira, Camiran, Camiron,
Camryn*

Cami (French) a short form of
Camille. See also Kami.
*Camey, Camie, Cammi,
Cammie, Cammy, Cammye,
Camy*

Camila, Camilla (Italian)
forms of Camille. See also
Kamila, Mila.
*Camia, Camilia, Camillia,
Camilya, Cammilla, Chamelea,
Chamelia, Chamika, Chamila,
Chamilia*

Camille (French) young cere-
monial attendant. See also
Millie.
*Cam, Cami, Camiel, Camielle,
Camil, Camila, Camile,
Camill, Cammille, Cammillie,
Cammilyn, Cammyl, Cammyll,
Camylle, Chamelle, Chamille,
Kamille*

Camisha (American) a combination of Cami + Aisha.
Cameasha, Cameesha,

Camri, Camrie (American)
short forms of Camryn. See
also Kamri.
*Camrea, Camree, Camrey,
Camry*

Camryn (American) a form of
Cameron. See also Kamryn.
*Camri, Camrin, Camron,
Camrynn*

Camylle (French) a form of
Camille.
Camyle, Camyll

Candace (Greek) glittering
white; glowing. History: the
title of the queens of ancient
Ethiopia. See also Dacey,
Kandace.
*Cace, Canace, Canda, Candas,
Candece, Candelle, Candi,
Candiace, Candice, Candyce*

Candi, Candy (American)
familiar forms of Candace,
Candice, Candida. See also
Kandi.
Candee, Candie

Candice, Candis (Greek)
forms of Candace.
*Candes, Candi, Candias,
Candies, Candise, Candiss,
Candus*

Candida (Latin) bright white.
*Candeea, Candi, Candia,
Candide, Candita*

Candra (Latin) glowing. See
also Kandra.
Candrea, Candria

Candyce (Greek) a form of
Candace.
Candys, Candyse, Cyndyss

Cantara (Arabic) small crossing.
Cantarah

Cantrelle (French) song.
Cantrella

Capri (Italian) a short form of
Caprice. Geography: an
island off the west coast of
Italy. See also Kapri.
Capria, Caprie, Capry

Caprice (Italian) fanciful.
*Cappi, Caprece, Caprecia,
Capresha, Capricia, Capriese,
Caprina, Capris, Caprise,
Caprisha, Capritta*

Cara (Latin) dear. (Irish)
friend. See also Karah.
*Caira, Caragh, Carah, Caralee,
Caranda, Carey, Carra*

Caralee (Irish) a form of Cara.
*Caralea, Caraleigh, Caralia,
Caralie, Carely*

Caralyn (English) a form of
Caroline.
*Caralin, Caraline, Caralynn,
Caralynna, Caralynne*

Caressa (French) a form of
Carissa.
Caresa, Carese, Caresse,

*Carissa, Charessa, Charesse,
Karessa*

Carey (Welsh) a familiar form
of Cara, Caroline, Karen,
Katherine. See also Carrie,
Kari.
Caree, Cari, Carrey, Cary

Cari, Carie (Welsh) forms of
Carey, Kari.

Carina (Italian) dear little one.
(Swedish) a form of Karen.
(Greek) a familiar form of
Cora.
*Carena, Carinah, Carine,
Carinna*

Carine (Italian) a form of
Carina.
Carin, Carinn, Carinne

Carisa, Carrisa (Greek) forms
of Carissa.
*Carise, Carisha, Carisia,
Charisa*

Carissa (Greek) beloved. See
also Karissa.
*Caressa, Carisa, Carrissa,
Charissa*

Carita (Latin) charitable.
Caritta, Karita, Karitta

Carla (German) farmer.
(English) strong. (Latin) a
form of Carol, Caroline.
*Carila, Carilla, Carleta, Carlia,
Carliqua, Carliyle, Carlonda,
Carlyjo, Carlyle, Carlysle*

Carlee, Carleigh, Carley
(English) forms of Carly. See
also Karlee.
Carle, Carlea, Carleah, Carleh

Carleen, Carlene (English)
forms of Caroline. See also
Karlene.
*Carlaen, Carlaena, Carleena,
Carlen, Carlena, Carlenna,
Carline, Carlyn, Carlyne*

Carli, Carlie (English) forms
of Carly. See also Karli.

Carlin (Irish) little champion.
(Latin) a short form of
Caroline.
*Carlan, Carlana, Carlandra,
Carlina, Carlinda, Carline,
Carling, Carllan, Carlyn,
Carllen, Carrlin*

Carlisa (American) a form of
Carlissa.
*Carilis, Carilise, Carilyse,
Carleesia, Carlesia, Carletha,
Carlethe, Carlicia, Carlis,
Carlise, Carlisha, Carlisia,
Carlyse*

Carlissa (American) a combi-
nation of Carla + Lissa.
*Carleeza, Carlisa, Carliss,
Carlissah, Carlisse, Carlissia,
Carlista*

Carlotta (Italian) a form of
Charlotte.
Carletta, Carlita, Carlota

Carly (English) a familiar form
of Caroline, Charlotte. See

also Karli.
Carlee, Carli, Carlie, Carlye

Carlyn, Carlynn (Irish) forms
of Carlin.
Carlyna, Carlynne

Carmela, Carmella (Hebrew)
garden; vineyard. Bible:
Mount Carmel in Israel is
often thought of as paradise.
See also Karmel.
*Carma, Carmalla, Carmarit,
Carmel, Carmeli, Carmelia,
Carmelina, Carmelit, Carmelle,
Carmellia, Carmellina,
Carmesa, Carmesha, Carmi,
Carmie, Carmiel, Carmil,
Carmila, Carmile, Carmilla,
Carmille, Carmisha, Leeta, Lita*

Carmelit (Hebrew) a form of
Carmela.
*Carmaletta, Carmalit,
Carmalita, Carmelita,
Carmelitha, Carmelitia,
Carmellit, Carmellita,
Carmellitha, Carmellitia*

Carmen (Latin) song.
Religion: Nuestra Señora del
Carmen—Our Lady of
Mount Carmel—is one of
the titles of the Virgin Mary.
See also Karmen.
*Carma, Carmaine, Carman,
Carmelina, Carmencita,
Carmene, Carmi, Carmia,
Carmin, Carmina, Carmine,
Carmita, Carmon, Carmynn,
Charmaine*

Carol (German) farmer.
(French) song of joy.
(English) strong. See also
Charlene, Kalle, Karoll.
*Carel, Cariel, Caro, Carola,
Carole, Carolenia, Carolinda,
Caroline, Caroll, Carrie, Carrol,
Carroll, Caryl*

**Carolane, Carolann,
Carolanne** (American) com-
binations of Carol + Ann.
Forms of Caroline.
*Carolan, Carol Ann, Carole-
Anne*

Carole (English) a form of
Carol.
Carolee, Karole, Karrole

Carolina (Italian) a form of
Caroline. See also Karolina.
*Carilena, Carlena, Carlina,
Caroleena, Caroleina, Carolena,
Carrolena*

Caroline (French) little and
strong. See also Carla,
Carleen, Carlin, Karolina.
*Caralin, Caraline, Carileen,
Carilene, Carilin, Cariline,
Carling, Carly, Caro, Carolann,
Caroleen, Carolin, Carolina,
Carolyn, Carrie, Carroleen,
Carrolene, Carrolin, Carroline,
Cary, Charlene*

Carolyn (English) a form of
Caroline. See also Karolyn.
*Carilyn, Carilynn, Carilynne,
Carlyn, Carlynn, Carlynne,
Carolyne, Carolynn, Carolynne,*
*Carrolyn, Carrolynn,
Carrolynne*

Caron (Welsh) loving, kindhearted, charitable.
Caronne, Carron, Carrone

Carra (Irish) a form of Cara.
Carrah

Carrie (English) a familiar
form of Carol, Caroline. See
also Carey, Kari, Karri.
*Carree, Carrey, Carri, Carria,
Carry, Cary*

Carson (English) child of
Carr.
Carsen, Carsyn

Carter (English) cart driver.

Caryl (Latin) a form of Carol.
Caryle, Caryll, Carylle

Caryn (Danish) a form of
Karen.
*Caren, Carren, Carrin, Carryn,
Caryna, Caryne, Carynn*

Carys (Welsh) love.
Caris, Caryse, Ceris, Cerys

Casandra (Greek) a form of
Cassandra.
*Casandera, Casandre,
Casandrea, Casandrey,
Casandri, Casandria,
Casanndra, Casaundra,
Casaundre, Casaundri,
Casaundria, Casondra,
Casondre, Casondri, Casondria*

Casey (Irish) brave. (Greek) a
familiar form of Acacia. See

also Kasey.
Cacy, Cascy, Casie, Casse,
Cassee, Cassey, Cassye, Casy,
Cayce, Cayse, Caysee, Caysy

Casidy (Irish) a form of
Cassidy.
Casidee, Casidi

Casie (Irish) a form of Casey.
Caci, Caesi, Caisie, Casci,
Cascie, Casi, Cayci, Caysi,
Caysie, Cazzi

Cass (Greek) a short form of
Cassandra.

Cassady (Irish) a form of
Cassidy.
Casadee, Casadi, Casadie,
Cassaday, Cassadee, Cassadey,
Cassadi, Cassadie, Cassadina

Cassandra (Greek) helper of
men. Mythology: a prophet-
ess of ancient Greece whose
prophesies were not believed.
See also Kassandra, Sandra,
Sandy, Zandra.
Casandra, Cass, Cassandre,
Cassandri, Cassandry,
Cassaundra, Cassie, Cassondra

Cassaundra (Greek) a form of
Cassandra.
Cassaundre, Cassaundri,
Cassundra, Cassundre,
Cassundri, Cassundria

Cassia (Greek) a cinnamon-
like spice. See also Kasia.
Casia, Cass, Casya

Cassidy (Irish) clever. See also
Kassidy.
Casidy, Cassady, Casseday,
Cassiddy, Cassidee, Cassidi,
Cassidie, Cassity

Cassie, Cassey, Cassi (Greek)
familiar forms of Cassandra,
Catherine. See also Kassie.
Cassee, Cassii, Cassy, Casy

Cassiopeia (Greek) clever.
Mythology: the wife of the
Ethiopian king Cepheus; the
mother of Andromeda.
Cassio

Cassondra (Greek) a form of
Cassandra.
Cassondre, Cassondri,
Cassondria

Catalina (Spanish) a form of
Catherine. See also Katalina.
Cataleen, Catalena, Catalene,
Catalin, Catalyn, Catalyna,
Cateline

Catarina (German) a form of
Catherine.
Catarena, Catarin, Catarine,
Caterin, Caterina, Caterine

Catelyn (Irish) a form of
Caitlin.
Catelin, Cateline, Catelyne,
Catelynn

Catharine (Greek) a form of
Catherine.
Catharen, Catharin, Catharina,
Catharyn

Catherine (Greek) pure.
(English) a form of
Katherine.
*Cat, Catalina, Catarina, Cate,
Cathann, Cathanne, Catharine,
Cathenne, Catheren, Catherene,
Catheria, Catherin, Catherina,
Catheryn, Catheryne, Cathi,
Cathleen, Cathrine, Cathryn,
Cathy, Catlaina, Catreeka,
Catrelle, Catrice, Catricia,
Catrika, Catrina*

Cathi, Cathy (Greek) familiar
forms of Catherine,
Cathleen. See also Kathy.
*Catha, Cathe, Cathee, Cathey,
Cathie*

Cathleen (Irish) a form of
Catherine. See also Caitlin,
Kathleen.
*Caithlyn, Cathaleen, Cathelin,
Cathelina, Cathelyn, Cathi,
Cathleana, Cathleene, Cathlene,
Cathleyn, Cathlin, Cathline,
Cathlyn, Cathlyne, Cathlynn,
Cathy*

Cathrine (Greek) a form of
Catherine.

Cathryn (Greek) forms of
Catherine.
Cathryne, Cathrynn, Catryn

Catrina (Slavic) a form of
Catherine, Katrina.
*Caitriana, Caitriona, Catina,
Catreen, Catreena, Catrene,
Catrenia, Catrin, Catrine,
Catrinia, Catriona, Catroina*

Cayla (Hebrew) a form of
Kayla.
Caylea, Caylia

Caylee, Caylie (American)
forms of Caeley, Cailey,
Cayley.
Cayle, Cayleigh, Cayli, Cayly

Ceara (Irish) a form of Ciara.
*Ceaira, Ceairah, Ceairra,
Cearaa, Cearie, Cearah, Cearra,
Cera*

Cecelia (Latin) a form of
Cecilia. See also Sheila.
*Caceli, Cacelia, Cece, Ceceilia,
Ceceli, Cecelia, Cecelie, Cecely,
Cecelyn, Cecette, Cescelia,
Cescelie*

Cecilia (Latin) blind. See also
Cicely, Cissy, Secilia, Selia,
Sissy.
*Cacilia, Caecilia, Cecelia, Cecil,
Cecila, Cecile, Cecilea, Cecilija,
Cecilla, Cecille, Cecillia, Cecily,
Cecilya, Ceclia, Cecylia, Cee,
Ceil, Ceila, Ceilagh, Ceileh,
Ceileigh, Ceilena, Celia,
Cesilia, Cicelia*

Cecily (Latin) a form of
Cecilia.
*Cacilie, Cecilee, Ceciley, Cecilie,
Cescily, Cicely, Cilley*

Ceil (Latin) a short form of
Cecilia.
Ceel, Ciel

Ceira, Ceirra (Irish) forms of Ciara.
Ceire

Celena (Greek) a form of Selena.
Celeena, Celene, Celenia, Celine, Cena

Celene (Greek) a form of Celena.
Celeen

Celeste (Latin) celestial, heavenly.
Cele, Celeeste, Celense, Celes, Celesia, Celesley, Celest, Celesta, Celestia, Celestial, Celestin, Celestina, Celestine, Celestinia, Celestyn, Celestyna, Cellest, Celleste, Selestina

Celia (Latin) a short form of Cecilia.
Ceilia, Celie

Celina (Greek) a form of Celena. See also Selina.
Caleena, Calena, Calina, Celena, Celinda, Celinka, Celinna, Celka, Cellina

Celine (Greek) a form of Celena.
Caline, Celeen, Celene, Céline, Cellinn

Cera (French) a short form of Cerise.
Cerea, Ceri, Ceria, Cerra

Cerella (Latin) springtime.
Cerelisa, Ceres

Cerise (French) cherry; cherry red.
Cera, Cerese, Cerice, Cericia, Cerissa, Cerria, Cerrice, Cerrina, Cerrita, Cerryce, Ceryce, Cherise

Cesilia (Latin) a form of Cecilia.
Cesia, Cesya

Chablis (French) a dry, white wine. Geography: a region in France where wine grapes are grown.
Chabeli, Chabelly, Chabely, Chablee, Chabley, Chabli

Chadee (French) from Chad, a country in north-central Africa. See also Sade.
Chaday, Chadday, Chade, Chadea, Chadi

Chai (Hebrew) life.
Chae, Chaela, Chaeli, Chaella, Chaena, Chaia

Chaka (Sanskrit) a form of Chakra. See also Shaka.
Chakai, Chakia, Chakka, Chakkah

Chakra (Sanskrit) circle of energy.
Chaka, Chakara, Chakaria, Chakena, Chakina, Chakira, Chakrah, Chakria, Chakriya, Chakyra

Chalice (French) goblet.
Chalace, Chalcie, Chalece, Chalicea, Chalie, Chaliese, Chalis, Chalisa, Chalise,

Chalice *(cont.)*
*Chalisk, Chalissa, Chalisse,
Challa, Challaine, Challis,
Challisse, Challysse, Chalsey,
Chalyce, Chalyn, Chalyse,
Chalyssa, Chalysse*

Chalina (Spanish) a form of
Rose.
Chaline, Chalini

Chalonna (American) a com-
bination of the prefix Cha +
Lona.
*Chalon, Chalona, Chalonda,
Chalonn, Chalonne, Chalonte,
Shalon*

Chambray (French) a light-
weight fabric.
*Chambrae, Chambre, Chambree,
Chambrée, Chambrey, Chambria,
Chambrie*

Chan (Cambodian) sweet-
smelling tree.

Chana (Hebrew) a form of
Hannah.
*Chanae, Chanai, Chanay,
Chanea, Chanie*

Chancey (English) chancellor;
church official.
*Chance, Chancee, Chancie,
Chancy*

Chanda (Sanskrit) short tem-
pered. Religion: the demon
defeated by the Hindu goddess
Chamunda. See also Shanda.
*Chandee, Chandey, Chandi,
Chandie, Chandin*

Chandelle (French) candle.
*Chandal, Chandel, Shandal,
Shandel*

Chandler (Hindi) moon. (Old
English) candlemaker.
*Chandlar, Chandlier, Chandlor,
Chandlyr*

Chandra (Sanskrit) moon.
Religion: the Hindu god of
the moon. See also Shandra.
*Chandrae, Chandray, Chandre,
Chandrea, Chandrelle,
Chandria*

Chanel (English) channel. See
also Shanel.
*Chanal, Chaneel, Chaneil,
Chanele, Chanell, Channal,
Channel, Chenelle*

Chanell, Chanelle (English)
forms of Chanel.
Channell, Shanell

Chanise (American) a form of
Shanice.
Chanisse, Chenice, Chenise

Channa (Hindi) chickpea.
Channah

Chantal (French) song.
*Chandal, Chantaal, Chantael,
Chantala, Chantale, Chantall,
Chantalle, Chantara, Chantarai,
Chantasia, Chante, Chanteau,
Chantel, Chantle, Chantoya,
Chantrill, Chauntel*

Chante (French) a short form
of Chantal.
*Chanta, Chantae, Chantai,
Chantay, Chantaye, Chanté,
Chantéa, Chantee, Chanti,
Chantia, Chaunte, Chauntea,
Chauntéa, Chauntee*

Chantel, Chantell, Chantelle
(French) forms of Chantal.
See also Shantel.
*Chanteese, Chantela, Chantele,
Chantella, Chanter, Chantey,
Chantez, Chantrel, Chantrell,
Chantrelle, Chatell*

Chantilly (French) fine lace.
See also Shantille.
*Chantiel, Chantielle, Chantil,
Chantila, Chantilée, Chantill,
Chantille*

Chantrea (Cambodian)
moon; moonbeam.
*Chantra, Chantrey, Chantri,
Chantria*

Chantrice (French) singer. See
also Shantrice.
Chantreese, Chantress

Chardae, Charde (Punjabi)
charitable. (French) short
forms of Chardonnay. See
also Shardae.
*Charda, Chardai, Charday,
Chardea, Chardee, Chardée,
Chardese, Chardey, Chardie*

Chardonnay (French) a dry
white wine.
*Char, Chardae, Chardnay,
Chardney, Chardon, Chardonae,*

*Chardonai, Chardonay,
Chardonaye, Chardonee,
Chardonna, Chardonnae,
Chardonnai, Chardonnee,
Chardonnée, Chardonney,
Shardonay, Shardonnay*

Charis (Greek) grace;
kindness.
*Charece, Chareece, Chareeze,
Charese, Chari, Charice,
Charie, Charish, Charisse*

Charissa, Charisse (Greek)
forms of Charity.
*Charesa, Charese, Charessa,
Charesse, Charis, Charisa,
Charise, Charisha, Charissee,
Charista, Charyssa*

Charity (Latin) charity,
kindness.
*Chariety, Charis, Charissa,
Charisse, Charista, Charita,
Chariti, Charitie, Sharity*

Charla (French, English) a
short form of Charlene,
Charlotte.
Char, Charlea

Charlaine (English) a form of
Charlene.
*Charlaina, Charlane,
Charlanna, Charlayna,
Charlayne*

Charlee, Charley (German,
English) forms of Charlie.
Charle, Charleigh

Charlene (English) a form of Caroline. See also Carol, Karla, Sharlene.
Charla, Charlaine, Charlean, Charleen, Charleene, Charleesa, Charlena, Charlenae, Charlesena, Charline, Charlyn, Charlyne, Charlynn, Charlynne, Charlzina, Charoline

Charlie (German, English) strong.
Charlee, Charley, Charli, Charyl, Chatty, Sharli, Sharlie

Charlotte (French) a form of Caroline. Literature: Charlotte Brontë was a British novelist and poet best known for her novel *Jane Eyre*. See also Karlotte, Lotte, Sharlotte, Tottie.
Carlotta, Carly, Chara, Charil, Charl, Charla, Charlet, Charlett, Charletta, Charlette, Charlisa, Charlita, Charlott, Charlotta, Charlottie, Charlotty, Charolet, Charolette, Charolot, Charolotte

Charmaine (French) a form of Carmen. See also Sharmaine.
Charamy, Charma, Charmae, Charmagne, Charmaigne, Charmain, Chamaine, Charmalique, Charman, Charmane, Charmar, Charmara, Charmayane, Charmayne, Charmeen, Charmeine, Charmene, Charmese, Charmian, Charmin, Charmine, Charmion, Charmisa, Charmon, Charmyn, Charmyne, Charmynne

Charnette (American) a combination of Charo + Annette.
Charnetta, Charnita

Charnika (American) a combination of Charo + Nika.
Charneka, Charniqua, Charnique

Charo (Spanish) a familiar form of Rosa.
Charyanna (American) a combination of Charo + Anna.
Charian, Charyian, Cheryn

Chasidy, Chassidy (Latin) forms of Chastity.
Chasa Dee, Chasadie, Chasady, Chasidee, Chasidey, Chasidie, Chassedi, Chassidi, Chasydi

Chasity (Latin) a form of Chastity.
Chasiti, Chasitie, Chasitty, Chassey, Chassie, Chassiti, Chassity, Chassy

Chastity (Latin) pure.
Chasidy, Chasity, Chasta, Chastady, Chastidy, Chastin, Chastitie, Chastney, Chasty

Chauntel (French) a form of Chantal.
Chaunta, Chauntae, Chauntay,

Chaunte, Chauntell,
Chauntelle, Chawntel,
Chawntell, Chawntelle,
Chontelle

Chava (Hebrew) life. (Yiddish)
bird. Religion: the original
name of Eve.
Chabah, Chavae, Chavah,
Chavalah, Chavarra, Chavarria,
Chave, Chavé, Chavette,
Chaviva, Chavvis, Hava, Kaÿa

Chavella (Spanish) a form of
Isabel.
Chavel, Chaveli, Chavell,
Chavelle, Chevelle, Chavely,
Chevie

Chavi (Gypsy) girl.
Chavali

Chavon (Hebrew) a form of
Jane.
Chavona, Chavonda, Chavonn,
Chavonne, Shavon

Chavonne (Hebrew) a form
of Chavon. (American) a
combination of the prefix
Cha + Yvonne.
Chavondria, Chavonna,
Chevon, Chevonn, Chevonna

Chaya (Hebrew) life; living.
Chaike, Chaye, Chayka,
Chayla, Chaylah, Chaylea,
Chaylee, Chaylene, Chayra

Chelci, Chelcie (English)
forms of Chelsea.
Chelce, Chelcee, Chelcey, Chelcy

Chelsea (English) seaport. See
also Kelsi, Shelsea.
Chelci, Chelese, Chelesia,
Chelsa, Chelsae, Chelsah,
Chelse, Chelseah, Chelsee,
Chelsey, Chelsia, Chelsie,
Chesea, Cheslee, Chessea

Chelsee (English) a form of
Chelsea.
Chelsei, Chelseigh

Chelsey, Chelsy (English)
forms of Chelsea. See also
Kelsey.
Chelcy, Chelsay, Chelssy,
Chelssey, Chelsye, Chesley

Chelsie (English) a form of
Chelsea.
Chelli, Chellie, Chellise,
Chellsie, Chelsi, Chelssie,
Cheslie, Chessie

Chenelle (English) a form of
Chanel.
Chenel, Chenell

Chenoa (Native American)
white dove.
Chenee, Chenika, Chenita,
Chenna, Chenoah

Cher (French) beloved, dear-
est. (English) a short form of
Cherilyn.
Chere, Cheri, Cherie, Sher

Cherelle, Cherrelle (French)
forms of Cheryl. See also
Sherelle.
Charell, Charelle, Cherell,
Cherrel, Cherrell

Cherese (Greek) a form of Cherish.
Chereese, Cheresa, Cheresse, Cherice

Cheri, Cherie (French) familiar forms of Cher.
Cheree, Chérie, Cheriee, Cherri, Cherrie

Cherilyn (English) a combination of Cheryl + Lynn.
Cher, Cheralyn, Chereen, Chereena, Cherilynn, Cherlyn, Cherlynn, Cherralyn, Cherrilyn, Cherrylyn, Cherylene, Cherylin, Cheryline, Cheryl-Lyn, Cheryl-Lynn, Cheryl-Lynne, Cherylyn, Cherylynn, Cherylynne, Sherilyn

Cherise (French) a form of Cherish. See also Sharice, Sherice.
Charisa, Charise, Cherece, Chereese, Cheresa, Cherice, Cheriss, Cherissa, Cherisse, Cherrise

Cherish (English) dearly held, precious.
Charish, Charisha, Cheerish, Cherise, Cherishe, Cherrish, Sherish

Cherokee (Native American) a tribal name.
Cherika, Cherkita, Cherrokee, Sherokee

Cherry (Latin) a familiar form of Charity. (French) cherry; cherry red.
Chere, Cheree, Cherey, Cherida, Cherita, Cherrey, Cherrita, Cherry-Ann, Cherry-Anne, Cherrye, Chery, Cherye

Cheryl (French) beloved. See also Sheryl.
Charel, Charil, Charyl, Cherelle, Cherrelle, Cheryl-Ann, Cheryl-Anne, Cheryle, Cherylee, Cheryll, Cherylle, Cheryl-Lee

Chesarey (American) a form of Desiree.
Chesarae, Chessa

Chesna (Slavic) peaceful.
Chesnee, Chesney, Chesnie, Chesny

Chessa (American) a short form of Chesarey.
Chessi, Chessie, Chessy

Cheyanne (Cheyenne) a form of Cheyenne.
Cheyan, Cheyana, Cheyane, Cheyann, Cheyanna, Cheyeana, Cheyeannna, Cheyeannne

Cheyenne (Cheyenne) a tribal name. See also Shaianne, Sheyenne, Shianne, Shyann.
Cheyanne, Cheyeene, Cheyena, Cheyene, Cheyenna, Cheyna, Chi, Chi-Anna, Chie, Chyanne

Cheyla (American) a form of Sheila.
Cheylan, Cheyleigh, Cheylo

Cheyna (American) a short form of Cheyenne.
Chey, Cheye, Cheyne, Cheynee, Cheyney, Cheynna

Chiara (Italian) a form of Clara.
Cheara, Chiarra

Chika (Japanese) near and dear.
Chikaka, Chikako, Chikara, Chikona

Chiku (Swahili) chatterer.

China (Chinese) fine porcelain. Geography: a country in eastern Asia. See also Ciana, Shina.
Chinaetta, Chinah, Chinasa, Chinda, Chinea, Chinesia, Chinita, Chinna, Chinwa, Chyna, Chynna

Chinira (Swahili) God receives.
Chinara, Chinarah, Chinirah

Chinue (Ibo) God's own blessing.

Chiquita (Spanish) little one. See also Shiquita.
Chaqueta, Chaquita, Chica, Chickie, Chicky, Chikata, Chikita, Chiqueta, Chiquila, Chiquite, Chiquitha, Chiquithe, Chiquitia, Chiquitta

Chiyo (Japanese) eternal.
Chiya

Chloe (Greek) blooming, verdant. Mythology: another name for Demeter, the goddess of agriculture.
Chloé, Chlöe, Chloee, Chloie, Cloe, Kloe

Chloris (Greek) pale. Mythology: the only daughter of Niobe to escape the vengeful arrows of Apollo and Artemis. See also Loris.
Cloris, Clorissa

Cho (Korean) beautiful.
Choe

Cholena (Native American) bird.

Chriki (Swahili) blessing.

Chris (Greek) a short form of Christina. See also Kris.
Chrys, Cris

Chrissa (Greek) a short form of Christina. See also Khrissa.
Chrysa, Chryssa, Crissa, Cryssa

Chrissy (English) a familiar form of Christina.
Chrisie, Chrissee, Chrissie, Crissie, Khrissy

Christa (German) a short form of Christina. History: Christa McAuliffe, an American school teacher, was the first civilian on a U. S. space flight. See also Krista.
Chrysta, Crista, Crysta

Christabel (Latin, French)
beautiful Christian.
*Christabell, Christabella,
Christabelle, Christable,
Cristabel, Kristabel*

Christain (Greek) a form of
Christina.
*Christana, Christann,
Christanna*

Christal (Latin) a form of
Crystal. (Scottish) a form of
Christina.
*Christalene, Christalin,
Christaline, Christall, Christalle,
Christalyn, Christelle, Christle,
Chrystal*

Christelle (French) a form of
Christal.
*Christel, Christele, Christell,
Chrystel, Chrystelle*

Christen, Christin (Greek)
forms of Christina. See also
Kristen.
*Christan, Christyn, Chrystan,
Chrysten, Chrystyn, Crestienne*

Christena, Christen (Greek)
forms of Christina.

Christi, Christie (Greek)
short forms of Christina,
Christine. See also Kristi.
*Christy, Chrysti, Chrystie,
Chrysty, Kristi*

**Christian, Christiana,
Christianna** (Greek) forms
of Christina. See also

Kristian, Krystian.
*Christiane, Christiann, Christi-
Ann, Christianne, Christi-
Anne, Christianni, Christiaun,
Christiean, Christien,
Christiena, Christienne,
Christinan, Christy-Ann,
Christy-Anne, Crystian,
Chrystyann, Chrystyanne,
Crystiann, Crystianne*

Christin (Greek) a short form
of Christina.
Christen, Chrystin

Christina (Greek) Christian;
anointed. See also Khristina,
Kristina, Stina, Tina.
*Chris, Chrissa, Chrissy, Christa,
Christain, Christal, Christeena,
Christella, Christen, Christena,
Christi, Christian, Christie,
Christin, Christinaa, Christine,
Christinea, Christinia,
Christinna, Christinnah,
Christna, Christy, Christyn,
Christyna, Christynna,
Chrystina, Chrystyna,
Cristeena, Cristena, Cristina,
Crystina, Chrystena, Cristena*

Christine (French, English) a
form of Christina. See also
Kirsten, Kristen, Kristine.
*Chrisa, Christeen, Christen,
Christene, Christi, Christie,
Christy, Chrystine, Cristeen,
Cristene, Cristine, Crystine*

Christophe (Greek) Christ-
bearer.

Christy (English) a short form of Christina, Christine.
Cristy

Christyn (Greek) a form of Christina.
Christyne

Chrys (English) a form of Chris.
Krys

Chrystal (Latin) a form of Christal.
Chrystale, Chrystalla, Chrystallina, Chrystallynn,

Chu Hua (Chinese) chrysanthemum.

Chumani (Lakota) dewdrops.
Chumany

Chun (Burmese) nature's renewal.

Chyanne, Chyenne (Cheyenne) forms of Cheyenne.
Chyan, Chyana, Chyane, Chyann, Chyanna, Chyeana, Chyenn, Chyenna, Chyennee

Chyna, Chynna (Chinese) forms of China.

Ciana (Chinese) a form of China. (Italian) a form of Jane.
Cian, Ciandra, Ciann, Cianna

Ciara, Ciarra (Irish) black. See also Sierra.
Ceara, Chiairah, Ciaara, Ciaera, Ciaira, Ciarah, Ciaria, Ciarrah, Cieara, Ciearra, Ciearria, Ciera, Cierra, Cioria, Cyarra

Cicely (English) a form of Cecilia. See also Sissy.
Cicelia, Cicelie, Ciciley, Cicilia, Cicilie, Cicily, Cile, Cilka, Cilla, Cilli, Cillie, Cilly

Cidney (French) a form of Sydney.
Cidnee, Cidni, Cidnie

Ciera, Cierra (Irish) forms of Ciara.
Ceira, Cierah, Ciere, Cieria, Cierrah, Cierre, Cierria, Cierro

Cinderella (French, English) little cinder girl. Literature: a fairy tale heroine.
Cindella

Cindy (Greek) moon. (Latin) a familiar form of Cynthia. See also Sindy.
Cindee, Cindi, Cindie, Cyndi

Cinthia, Cinthya (Greek) forms of Cynthia.
Cinthiya, Cintia

Cira (Spanish) a form of Cyrilla.

Cissy (American) a familiar form of Cecelia, Cicely.
Cissey, Cissi, Cissie

Claire (French) a form of Clara.
Clair, Klaire, Klarye

Clairissa (Greek) a form of
Clarissa.
Clairisa, Clairisse, Claraissa

Clara (Latin) clear; bright.
Music: Clara Shumann was a
famous nineteenth-century
German composer. See also
Chiara, Klara.
*Claira, Claire, Clarabelle, Clare,
Claresta, Clarice, Clarie,
Clarina, Clarinda, Clarine,
Clarissa, Clarita*

Clarabelle (Latin) bright and
beautiful.
Clarabella, Claribel, Claribell

Clare (English) a form of
Clara.

Clarie (Latin) a familiar form
of Clara.
Clarey, Clari, Clary

Clarice (Italian) a form of
Clara.
*Claris, Clarise, Clarisse,
Claryce, Cleriese, Klarice,
Klarise*

Clarisa (Greek) a form of
Clarissa.
Claresa, Clarise, Clarisia

Clarissa (Greek) brilliant.
(Italian) a form of Clara. See
also Klarissa.
*Clairissa, Clarecia, Claressa,
Claresta, Clarisa, Clarissia,
Claritza, Clarizza, Clarrisa,
Clarrissa, Clerissa*

Clarita (Spanish) a form of
Clara.
*Clairette, Clareta, Claretta,
Clarette, Claritza*

Claudette (French) a form of
Claudia.
Clauddetta

Claudia (Latin) lame. See also
Gladys, Klaudia.
*Claudeen, Claudel, Claudelle,
Claudette, Claudex, Claudiana,
Claudiane, Claudie, Claudie-
Anne, Claudina, Claudine*

Claudie (Latin) a form of
Claudia.
Claudee

Clea (Greek) a form of Cleo,
Clio.

Clementine (Latin) merciful.
*Clemence, Clemencia,
Clemencie, Clemency,
Clementia, Clementina,
Clemenza, Clemette*

Cleo (Greek) a short form of
Cleopatra.
Chleo, Clea

Cleone (Greek) famous.
Cleonie, Cleonna, Cliona

Cleopatra (Greek) her father's
fame. History: a great
Egyptian queen.
Cleo

Cleta (Greek) illustrious.

Clio (Greek) proclaimer; glorifier. Mythology: the Muse of history.
Clea

Cloe (Greek) a form of Chloe.
Clo, Cloei, Cloey, Cloie

Clotilda (German) heroine.

Coco (Spanish) coconut. See also Koko.

Codi, Cody (English) cushion. See also Kodi.
Coady, Codee, Codey, Codia, Codie

Colby (English) coal town. Geography: a region in England known for cheese-making. See also Kolby.
Cobi, Cobie, Colbi, Colbie

Colette (Greek, French) a familiar form of Nicole.
Coe, Coetta, Coletta, Collet, Collete, Collett, Colletta, Collette, Kolette, Kollette

Colleen (Irish) girl. See also Kolina.
Coe, Coel, Cole, Coleen, Colene, Coley, Coline, Colleene, Collen, Collene, Collie, Collina, Colline, Colly

Collina (Irish) a form of Colleen.
Colena, Colina, Colinda

Concetta (Italian) pure.
Concettina, Conchetta

Conchita (Spanish) conception.
Chita, Conceptia, Concha, Conciana

Concordia (Latin) harmonious. Mythology: the goddess governing the peace after war.
Con, Cordae, Cordaye

Connie (Latin) a familiar form of Constance.
Con, Connee, Conni, Conny, Konnie, Konny

Connor (Scottish) wise. (Irish) praised; exhalted.
Connar, Conner, Connery, Conor

Constance (Latin) constant; firm. History: Constance Motley was the first African-American woman to be appointed as a U. S. federal judge. See also Konstance, Kosta.
Connie, Constancia, Constancy, Constanta, Constantia, Constantina, Constantine, Constanza, Constynse

Constanza (Spanish) a form of Constance.
Constanz, Constanze

Consuelo (Spanish) consolation. Religion: Nuestra Señora del Consuelo—Our Lady of Consolation—is a name for the Virgin Mary.
Consolata, Consuela, Consuella, Consula, Conzuelo, Konsuela, Konsuelo

Cora (Greek) maiden.
Mythology: Kore is another
name for Persephone, the
goddess of the underworld.
See also Kora.
*Corah, Coralee, Coretta,
Corissa, Corey, Corra*

Corabelle (American) a combination of Cora + Belle.
Corabel, Corabella

Coral (Latin) coral. See also
Koral.
Coraal, Corral

Coralee (American) a combi-
nation of Cora + Lee.
*Coralea, Cora-Lee, Coralena,
Coralene, Coraley, Coralie,
Coraline, Coraly, Coralyn,
Corella, Corilee, Koralie*

Coralie (American) a form of
Coralee.
*Corali, Coralia, Coralina,
Coralynn, Coralynne*

Corazon (Spanish) heart.

Corbin (Latin) raven.
*Corbe, Corbi, Corby, Corbyn,
Corbynn*

Cordasha (American) a combination of Cora + Dasha.

Cordelia (Latin) warm-
hearted. (Welsh) sea jewel.
See also Delia, Della.
*Cordae, Cordelie, Cordett,
Cordette, Cordi, Cordilia,
Cordilla, Cordula, Kordelia,
Kordula*

Cordi (Welsh) a short form of
Cordelia.
Cordey, Cordia, Cordie, Cordy

Coretta (Greek) a familiar
form of Cora.
*Coreta, Corette, Correta,
Corretta, Corrette, Koretta,
Korretta*

Corey, Cory (Irish) from the
hollow. (Greek) familiar
forms of Cora. See also Kori.
*Coree, Cori, Correy, Correye,
Corry*

Cori, Corie, Corrie (Irish)
forms of Corey.

Coriann, Corianne
(American) combinations of
Cori + Ann, Cori + Anne.
*Corian, Coriane, Cori-Ann,
Corri, Corrie-Ann, Corrianne,
Corrie-Anne*

Corina, Corinna (Greek)
familiar forms of Corinne.
See also Korina.
*Coreena, Coriana, Corianna,
Corinda, Correna, Corrinna,
Coryna*

Corinne (Greek) maiden.
*Coreen, Coren, Corin, Corina,
Corine, Corinee, Corinn,
Corinna, Corrina, Coryn,
Corynn, Corynne*

Corissa (Greek) a familiar
form of Cora.
*Coresa, Coressa, Corisa,
Coryssa, Korissa*

Corliss (English) cheerful;
goodhearted.
*Corlisa, Corlise, Corlissa, Corly,
Korliss*

Cornelia (Latin) horn colored.
See also Kornelia, Nelia, Nellie.
*Carna, Carniella, Corneilla,
Cornela, Cornelie, Cornella,
Cornelle, Cornie, Cornilear,
Cornisha, Corny*

Corrina, Corrine (Greek)
forms of Corinne.
*Correen, Corren, Corrin,
Corrinn, Corrinna, Corrinne,
Corrinne, Corryn*

Cortney (English) a form of
Courtney.
*Cortne, Cortnea, Cortnee,
Cortneia, Cortni, Cortnie,
Cortny, Cortnye, Corttney*

Cosette (French) a familiar
form of Nicole.
*Cosetta, Cossetta, Cossette,
Cozette*

Courtenay (English) a form of
Courtney.
*Courtaney, Courtany,
Courteney, Courteny*

Courtnee, Courtnie (English)
forms of Courtney.
*Courtne, Courtnée, Courtnei,
Courtneigh, Courtni, Courtnii*

Courtney (English) from the
court. See also Kortney,
Kourtney.
Cortney, Courtena, Courtenay,
*Courtene, Courtnae, Courtnay,
Courtnee, Courtny, Courtonie*

Crisbell (American) a combination of Crista + Belle.
Crisbel, Cristabel

Crista, Crysta (Italian) forms
of Christa.
Cristah

Cristal (Latin) a form of Crystal.
*Cristalie, Cristalina, Cristalle,
Cristel, Cristela, Cristelia,
Cristella, Cristelle, Cristhie, Cristle*

Cristen, Cristin (Irish) forms
of Christen, Christin. See
also Kristin.
*Cristan, Cristyn, Crystan,
Crysten, Crystin, Crystyn*

Cristina, Cristine (Greek)
forms of Christina. See also
Kristina.
Cristiona, Cristy

Cristy (English) a familiar
form of Cristina. A form of
Christy. See also Kristy.
*Cristey, Cristi, Cristie, Crysti,
Crystie, Crysty*

Crystal (Latin) clear, brilliant
glass. See also Kristal, Krystal.
*Christal, Chrystal, Chrystal-
Lynn, Chrystel, Cristal,
Crystala, Crystale, Crystalee,
Crystalin, Crystall, Crystalle,
Crystaly, Crystel, Crystela,
Crystelia, Crystelle, Crysthelle,
Crystl, Crystle, Crystol,
Crystole, Crystyl*

Crystalin (Latin) crystal pool.
*Crystal-Ann, Cristalanna,
Crystal-Anne, Cristalina,
Cristallina, Cristalyn,
Crystallynn, Crystallynne,
Cristilyn, Crystalina, Crystal-
Lee, Crystal-Lynn, Crystalyn,
Crystalynn*

Crystina (Greek) a form of
Christina.
*Crystin, Crystine, Crystyn,
Crystyna, Crystyne*

Curran (Irish) heroine.
Cura, Curin, Curina, Curinna

Cybele (Greek) a form of
Sybil.
Cybel, Cybil, Cybill, Cybille

Cydney (French) a form of
Sydney.
*Cydne, Cydnee, Cydnei,
Cydni, Cydnie*

Cyerra (Irish) a form of Ciara.
Cyera, Cyerria

Cyndi (Greek) a form of Cindy.
*Cynda, Cyndal, Cyndale,
Cyndall, Cyndee, Cyndel,
Cyndia, Cyndie, Cyndle, Cyndy*

Cynthia (Greek) moon.
Mythology: another name
for Artemis, the moon god-
dess. See also Hyacinth,
Kynthia.
*Cindy, Cinthia, Cyneria,
Cynethia, Cynithia, Cynthea,
Cynthiana, Cynthiann,
Cynthie, Cynthria, Cynthy,
Cynthya, Cyntia, Cyntreia,
Cythia, Synthia*

Cyrilla (Greek) noble.
*Cerelia, Cerella, Cira, Cirilla,
Cyrella, Cyrille*

D

Dacey (Irish) southerner.
(Greek) a familiar form of
Candace.
*Dacee, Dacei, Daci, Dacia,
Dacie, Dacy, Daicee, Daici,
Daicie, Daicy, Daycee, Daycie,
Daycy*

Dacia (Irish) a form of Dacey.
Daciah

Dae (English) day. See also
Dai.

Daeja (French) a form of
Déja.
Daejah, Daejia

Daelynn (American) a combi-
nation of Dae + Lynn.
*Daeleen, Daelena, Daelin,
Daelyn, Daelynne*

Daeshandra (American) a
combination of Dae +
Shandra.
*Daeshandria, Daeshaundra,
Daeshaundria, Daeshawndra,
Daeshawndria, Daeshondra,
Daeshondria*

Daeshawna (American) a
combination of Dae +
Shawna.
Daeshan, Daeshaun,
Daeshauna, Daeshavon,
Daeshawn, Daeshawntia,
Daeshon, Daeshona

Daeshonda (American) a
combination of Dae +
Shonda.
Daeshanda, Daeshawnda

Dafny (American) a form of
Daphne.
Dafany, Daffany, Daffie, Daffy,
Dafna, Dafne, Dafney, Dafnie

Dagmar (German) glorious.
Dagmara

Dagny (Scandinavian) day.
Dagna, Dagnanna, Dagne,
Dagney, Dagnie

Dahlia (Scandinavian) valley.
Botany: a perennial flower.
See also Daliah.
Dahliah, Dahlya, Dahlye

Dai (Japanese) great. See also
Dae.
Day, Daye

Daija, Daijah (French) forms
of Déja.
Daijaah, Daijea, Daijha,
Daijhah, Dayja

Daisha (American) a form of
Dasha.
Daesha, Daishae, Daishia,
Daishya, Daisia

Daisy (English) day's eye.
Botany: a white and yellow
flower.
Daisee, Daisey, Daisi, Daisia,
Daisie, Dasey, Dasi, Dasie,
Dasy, Daysi, Deisy

Daja, Dajah (French) forms of
Déja.
Dajae, Dajai, Daje, Dajha,
Dajia

Dakayla (American) a combi-
nation of the prefix Da +
Kayla.
Dakala, Dakila

Dakira (American) a combina-
tion of the prefix Da + Kira.
Dakara, Dakaria, Dakarra,
Dakirah, Dakyra

Dakota (Native American) a
tribal name.
Dakkota, Dakoda, Dakotah,
Dakotha, Dakotta, Dekoda,
Dekota, Dekotah, Dekotha

Dale (English) valley.
Dael, Dahl, Daile, Daleleana,
Dalena, Dalina, Dayle

Dalia, Daliah (Hebrew)
branch. See also Dahlia.
Daelia, Dailia, Daleah, Daleia,
Dalialah, Daliyah

Dalila (Swahili) gentle.
Dalela, Dalida, Dalilah, Dalilia

Dalisha (American) a form of
Dallas.
Dalisa, Dalishea, Dalishia,
Dalishya, Dalisia, Dalissia

Dallas (Irish) wise.
*Dalis, Dalise, Dalisha, Dalisse,
Dallace, Dallis, Dallise, Dallus,
Dallys, Dalyce, Dalys*

Damaris (Greek) gentle girl.
See also Maris.
*Dama, Damar, Damara,
Damarius, Damary, Damarylis,
Damarys, Dameress, Dameris,
Damiris, Dammaris, Dammeris,
Damris, Demaras, Demaris*

Damiana (Greek) tamer,
soother.
*Daimenia, Daimiona, Damia,
Damiann, Damianna,
Damianne, Damien, Damienne,
Damiona, Damon, Demion*

Damica (French) friendly.
*Damee, Dameeka, Dameka,
Damekah, Damicah, Damicia,
Damicka, Damie, Damieka,
Damika, Damikah, Damyka,
Demeeka, Demeka, Demekah,
Demica, Demicah*

Damita (Spanish) small noble-
woman.
*Damee, Damesha, Dameshia,
Damesia, Dametia, Dametra,
Dametrah*

Damonica (American) a com-
bination of the prefix Da +
Monica.
*Damonec, Damoneke,
Damonik, Damonika,
Damonique, Diamoniqua,
Diamonique*

Dana (English) from
Denmark; bright as day.
*Daina, Dainna, Danah,
Danaia, Danan, Danarra,
Dane, Danean, Danna, Dayna*

Danae (Greek) Mythology:
the mother of Perseus.
*Danaë, Danay, Danayla,
Danays, Danai, Danea, Danee,
Dannae, Denae, Denee*

Danalyn (American) a combination of Dana + Lynn.
Danalee, Donaleen

Daneil (Hebrew) a form of
Danielle.
*Daneal, Daneala, Daneale,
Daneel, Daneela, Daneila*

Danella (American) a form of
Danielle.
*Danayla, Danela, Danelia,
Danelle, Danna, Donella,
Donnella*

Danelle (Hebrew) a form of
Danielle.
*Danael, Danalle, Danel,
Danele, Danell, Danella,
Donelle, Donnelle*

Danesha, Danisha (American)
forms of Danessa.
*Daneisha, Daneshia, Daniesha,
Danishia*

Danessa (American) a combi-
nation of Danielle + Vanessa.
See also Doneshia.
*Danasia, Danesa, Danesha,
Danessia, Daniesa, Danisa, Danissa*

Danessia (American) a form of Danessa.
Danesia, Danieshia, Danisia, Danissia

Danette (American) a form of Danielle.
Danetra, Danett, Danetta, Donnita

Dani (Hebrew) a familiar form of Danielle.
Danee, Danie, Danne, Dannee, Danni, Dannie, Danny, Dannye, Dany

Dania, Danya (Hebrew) short forms of Danielle.
Daniah, Danja, Dannia, Danyae

Danica, Danika (Slavic) morning star. (Hebrew) forms of Danielle.
Daneca, Daneeka, Daneekah, Danicah, Danicka, Danieka, Danikah, Danikla, Danneeka, Dannica, Dannika, Dannikah, Danyka, Denica, Donica, Donika, Donnaica, Donnica, Donnika

Danice (American) a combination of Danielle + Janice.
Donice

Daniela (Italian) a form of Danielle.
Daniellah, Dannilla, Danijela

Danielan (Spanish) a form of Danielle.

Daniella (English) a form of Dana.
Danka, Danniella, Danyella

Danielle (Hebrew, French) God is my judge.
Daneen, Daneil, Daneille, Danelle, Dani, Danial, Danialle, Danica, Daniel, Daniela, Danielan, Daniele, Danielka, Daniell, Daniella, Danilka, Danille, Danit, Dannielle, Danyel, Donniella

Danille (American) a form of Danielle.
Danila, Danile, Danilla, Dannille

Danit (Hebrew) a form of Danielle.
Danett, Danis, Danisha, Daniss, Danita, Danitra, Danitrea, Danitria, Danitza, Daniz

Danna (Hebrew) a short form of Danella.
Dannah

Dannielle (Hebrew, French) a form of Danielle.
Danniel, Danniele, Danniell

Danyel, Danyell, Danyelle (American) forms of Danielle.
Daniyel, Danyae, Danyail, Danyaile, Danyal, Danyale, Danyea, Danyele, Danyiel, Danyielle, Danyle, Donnyale, Donnyell, Donyale, Donyell

Daphne (Greek) laurel tree.
Dafny, Daphane, Daphany,
Dapheney, Daphna, Daphnee,
Daphnique, Daphnit, Daphny

Daphnee (Greek) a form of
Daphne.
Daphaney, Daphanie, Daphney,
Daphni, Daphnie

Dara (Hebrew) compassionate.
Dahra, Daira, Dairah, Darah,
Daraka, Daralea, Daralee,
Daraleigh, Daralie, Daravie,
Darda, Darice, Darisa, Darissa,
Darja, Darra, Darrah

Darby (Irish) free.
(Scandinavian) deer estate.
Darb, Darbe, Darbee, Darbi,
Darbie, Darbra, Darbye

Darcelle (French) a form of
Darci.
Darcel, Darcell, Darcella,
Darselle

Darci, Darcy (Irish) dark.
(French) fortress.
Darcee, Darcelle, Darcey, Darcie,
Darsey, Darsi, Darsie

Daria (Greek) wealthy.
Dari, Dariya, Darria, Darya,
Daryia

Darian, Darrian (Greek)
forms of Daron.
Dariana, Dariane, Dariann,
Darianna, Darianne, Dariyan,
Dariyanne, Darriana, Darriane,
Darriann, Darrianna,
Darrianne, Derrian, Driana

Darielle (French) a form of
Daryl.
Dariel, Dariela, Dariell, Darriel,
Darrielle

Darien, Darrien (Greek)
forms of Daron.
Dariene, Darienne, Darriene

Darilynn (American) a form
of Darlene.
Daralin, Daralyn, Daralynn,
Daralynne, Darilin, Darilyn,
Darilynne, Darlin, Darlyn,
Darlynn, Darlynne, Darylin,
Darylyn, Darylynn, Darylynne

Darion, Darrion (Irish) forms
of Daron.
Dariona, Darione, Darionna,
Darionne, Darriona, Darrionna

Darla (English) a short form
of Darlene.
Darlecia, Darli, Darlice, Darlie,
Darlis, Darly, Darlys

Darlene (French) little darling.
See also Daryl.
Darilynn, Darla, Darlean, Darlee,
Darleen, Darleene, Darlena,
Darlenia, Darlenne, Darletha,
Darlin, Darline, Darling, Darlyn,
Darlynn, Darlynne

Darnee (Irish) a familiar form
of Darnelle.

Darnelle (English) hidden place.
Darnee, Darnel, Darnell,
Darnella, Darnesha, Darnetta,
Darnette, Darnice, Darniece,
Darnita, Darnyell

Darnesha, Darnisha
(American) forms of Darnelle.
Darneisha, Darneishia,
Darneshea, Darneshia,
Darnesia, Darniesha, Darnishia,
Darnisia, Darrenisha

Daron (Irish) great.
Darian, Darien, Darion,
Daronica, Daronice, Darron,
Daryn

Darselle (French) a form of
Darcelle.
Darsel, Darsell, Darsella

Daru (Hindi) pine tree.

Daryl (English) beloved.
(French) a short form of
Darlene.
Darelle, Darielle, Daril,
Darilynn, Darrel, Darrell,
Darrelle, Darreshia, Darryl,
Darryll, Daryll, Darylle

Daryn (Greek) gifts. (Irish) great.
Daron, Daryan, Daryne,
Darynn, Darynne

Dasha, Dasia (Russian) forms
of Dorothy.
Daisha, Dashae, Dashenka,
Dashia, Dashiah, Dasiah,
Daysha

Dashawna (American) a com-
bination of the prefix Da +
Shawna.
Dashawn, Dashawnna, Dashay,
Dashell, Dayshana,
Dayshawnna, Dayshona,
Deshawna

Dashiki (Swahili) loose-fitting
shirt worn in Africa.
Dashi, Dashika, Dashka,
Desheka, Deshiki

Dashonda (American) a com-
bination of the prefix Da +
Shonda.
Dashawnda, Dishante

Davalinda (American) a com-
bination of Davida + Linda.
Davalynda, Davelinda,
Davilinda, Davylinda

Davalynda (American) a form
of Davalinda.
Davelynda, Davilynda,
Davylynda

Davalynn (American) a com-
bination of Davida + Lynn.
Davalin, Davalyn, Davalynne,
Davelin, Davelyn, Davelynn,
Davelynne, Davilin, Davilyn,
Davilynn, Davilynne, Dayleen,
Devlyn

Davida (Hebrew) beloved.
Bible: David was the second
king of Israel. See also Vida.
Daveta, Davetta, Davette,
Davika, Davita

Davina (Scottish) a form of
Davida. See also Vina.
Dava, Davannah, Davean, Davee,
Daveen, Daveena, Davene,
Daveon, Davey, Davi, Daviana,
Davie, Davin, Davinder, Davine,
Davineen, Davinia, Davinna,
Davonna, Davria, Devean,
Deveen, Devene, Devina

Davisha (American) a combination of the prefix Da + Aisha.
Daveisha, Davesia, Davis, Davisa

Davonna (Scottish, English) a form of Davina, Devonna.
Davion, Daviona, Davionna, Davon, Davona, Davonda, Davone, Davonia, Davonne, Davonnia

Dawn (English) sunrise, dawn.
Dawana, Dawandrea, Dawanna, Dawin, Dawna, Dawne, Dawnee, Dawnetta, Dawnisha, Dawnlynn, Dawnn, Dawnrae

Dawna (English) a form of Dawn.
Dawnna, Dawnya

Dawnyelle (American) a combination of Dawn + Danielle.
Dawnele, Dawnell, Dawnelle, Dawnyel, Dawnyella

Dawnisha (American) a form of Dawn.
Dawnesha, Dawni, Dawniell, Dawnielle, Dawnisia, Dawniss, Dawnita, Dawnnisha, Dawnysha, Dawnysia

Dayana (Latin) a form of Diana.
Dayanara, Dayani, Dayanna, Dayanne, Dayanni, Deyanaira, Dyani, Dyanna, Dyia

Dayle (English) a form of Dale.
Dayla, Daylan, Daylea, Daylee

Dayna (Scandinavian) a form of Dana.
Daynah, Dayne, Daynna, Deyna

Daysha (American) a form of Dasha.
Daysa, Dayshalie, Daysia, Deisha

Daysi, Deysi (English) forms of Daisy.
Daysee, Daysia, Daysie, Daysy, Deysia, Deysy

Dayton, Daytona (English) day town; bright, sunny town.
Daytonia

Deana (Latin) divine. (English) valley.
Deanah, Deane, Deanielle, Deanisha, Deanna, Deeana, Deeann, Deeanna, Deena

Deandra (American) a combination of Dee + Andrea.
Dandrea, Deandre, Deandré, Deandrea, Deandree, Deandreia, Deandria, Deanndra, Deaundra, Deaundria, Deeandra, Deyaneira, Deondra, Diandra, Diandre, Diandrea, Diondria, Dyandra

Deangela (Italian) a combination of the prefix De + Angela.
Deangala, Deangalique, Deangle

Deanna (Latin) a form of Deana, Diana.
Deaana, Deahana, Deandra, Deandre, Déanna, Deannia, Deeanna, Deena

Deanne (Latin) a form of Diane.
Deahanne, Deane, Deann, Déanne, Deeann, Dee-Ann, Deeanne

Debbie (Hebrew) a short form of Deborah.
Debbee, Debbey, Debbi, Debby, Debee, Debi, Debie

Deborah (Hebrew) bee. Bible: a great Hebrew prophetess.
Deb, Debbie, Debbora, Debborah, Deberah, Debor, Debora, Deboran, Deborha, Deborrah, Debra, Debrena, Debrina, Debroah, Devora, Dobra

Debra (American) a form of Deborah.
Debbra, Debbrah, Debrah, Debrea, Debria

Dedra (American) a form of Deirdre.
Deeddra, Deedra, Deedrea, Deedrie

Dedriana (American) a combination of Dedra + Adriana.
Dedranae

Dee (Welsh) black, dark.
De, Dea, Deah, Dede, Dedie, Deea, Deedee, Dee Dee, Didi

Deena (American) a form of Deana, Dena, Dinah.

Deidra, Deidre (Irish) forms of Deirdre.
Deidrah, Deidrea, Deidrie, Diedra, Diedre, Dierdra

Deirdre (Irish) sorrowful; wanderer.
Dedra, Deerdra, Deerdre, Deidra, Deidre, Deirdree, Didi, Diedra, Dierdre, Diérdre, Dierdrie

Deisy (English) a form of Daisy.
Deisi, Deissy

Deitra (Greek) a short form of Demetria.
Deetra, Detria

Déja (French) before.
Daeja, Daija, Deejay, Dejae, Déjah, Dejai, Dejanae, Dejanelle, Dejon

Dejanae (French) a form of Déja.
Dajahnae, Dajona, Dejana, Dejanah, Dejanae, Dejanai, Dejanay, Dejane, Dejanea, Dejanee, Dejanna, Dejannaye, Dejena, Dejonae

Dejon (French) a form of Déja.
Daijon, Dajan, Dejone, Dejonee, Dejonelle, Dejonna

Deka (Somali) pleasing.
Dekah

Delacy (American) a combination of the prefix De + Lacy.
Delaceya

Delainey (Irish) a form of Delaney.
Delaine, Delainee, Delaini, Delainie, Delainy

Delana (German) noble protector.
Dalanna, Dalayna, Daleena, Dalena, Dalenna, Dalina, Dalinda, Dalinna, Delaina, Delania, Delanya, Delayna, Deleena, Delena, Delenya, Delina, Dellaina

Delaney (Irish) descendant of the challenger. (English) a form of Adeline.
Dalaney, Dalania, Dalene, Daleney, Daline, Del, Delainey, Delane, Delanee, Delanie, Delany, Delayne, Delayney, Delaynie, Deleani, Déline, Della, Dellaney

Delanie (Irish) a form of Delaney.
Delani

Delfina (Greek) a form of Delphine. (Spanish) dolphin.
Delfeena, Delfine

Delia (Greek) visible; from Delos, Greece. (German, Welsh) a short form of Adelaide, Cordelia. Mythology: a festival of Apollo held in ancient Greece.
Dehlia, Delea, Deli, Deliah, Deliana, Delianne, Delinda, Dellia, Dellya, Delya

Delicia (English) delightful.
Delecia, Delesha, Delice, Delisa, Delise, Delisha, Delishia, Delisiah, Delya, Delys, Delyse, Delysia, Doleesha

Delilah (Hebrew) brooder. Bible: the companion of Samson. See also Lila.
Dalialah, Dalila, Daliliah, Delila, Delilia

Della (English) a short form of Adelaide, Cordelia, Delaney.
Del, Dela, Dell, Delle, Delli, Dellie, Dells

Delores (Spanish) a form of Dolores.
Delora, Delore, Deloria, Delories, Deloris, Delorise, Delorita, Delsie

Delphine (Greek) from Delphi, Greece. See also Delfina.
Delpha, Delphe, Delphi, Delphia, Delphina, Delphinia, Delvina

Delsie (English) a familiar form of Delores.
Delsa, Delsey, Delza

Delta (Greek) door. Linguistics: the fourth letter in the Greek alphabet.

Geography: a triangular land mass at the mouth of a river.
Delte, Deltora, Deltoria, Deltra

Demetria (Greek) cover of the earth. Mythology: Demeter was the Greek goddess of the harvest.
Deitra, Demeta, Demeteria, Demetra, Demetriana, Demetrianna, Demetrias, Demetrice, Demetriona, Demetris, Demetrish, Demetrius, Demi, Demita, Demitra, Demitria, Dymitra

Demi (French) half. (Greek) a short form of Demetria.
Demia, Demiah, Demii, Demmi, Demmie, Demy

Dena (English, Native American) valley. (Hebrew) a form of Dinah. See also Deana.
Deane, Deena, Deeyn, Denae, Denah, Dene, Denea, Deney, Denna, Deonna

Denae (Hebrew) a form of Dena.
Denaé, Denay, Denee, Deneé

Deni (French) a short form of Denise.
Deney, Denie, Denni, Dennie, Denny, Dinnie, Dinny

Denica, Denika (Slavic) forms of Danica.
Denikah, Denikia

Denise (French) Mythology: follower of Dionysus, the god of wine.
Danice, Danise, Denese, Deni, Denice, Denicy, Deniece, Denisha, Denisse, Denize, Dennise, Dennys, Denyce, Denys, Denyse

Denisha (American) a form of Denise.
Deneesha, Deneichia, Deneisha, Deneishea, Denesha, Deneshia, Deniesha, Denishia

Denisse (French) a form of Denise.
Denesse, Denissa

Deonna (English) a form of Dena.
Deon, Deona, Deonah, Deondra, Deonne

Derika (German) ruler of the people.
Dereka, Derekia, Derica, Dericka, Derrica, Derricka, Derrika

Derry (Irish) redhead.
Deri, Derie

Deryn (Welsh) bird.
Derien, Derienne, Derion, Derin, Deron, Derren, Derrin, Derrine, Derrion, Derriona, Deryne

Desarae (French) a form of Desiree.
Desara, Desarai, Desaraie, Desaray, Desare, Desaré, Desarea, Desaree, Desarie, Dezarae

Deserae, Desirae (French) forms of Desiree.
Desera, Deserai, Deseray, Desere, Deseree, Deseret, Deseri, Deserie, Deserrae, Deserray, Deserré, Dessirae, Dezeray, Dezere, Dezerea, Dezrae, Dezyrae

Deshawna (American) a combination of the prefix De + Shawna.
Dashawna, Deshan, Deshane, Deshaun, Deshawn, Desheania, Deshona, Deshonna

Deshawnda (American) a combination of the prefix De + Shawnda.
Deshanda, Deshandra, Deshaundra, Deshawndra, Deshonda

Desi (French) a short form of Desiree.
Désir, Desira, Dezi, Dezia, Dezzia, Dezzie

Desiree (French) desired, longed for. See also Dessa.
Chesarey, Desarae, Deserae, Desi, Desirae, Desirah, Desirai, Desiray, Desire, Desirea, Desireah, Desirée, Désirée, Desirey, Desiri, Desray, Desree,

Dessie, Dessire, Dezarae, Dezirae, Deziree

Dessa (Greek) wanderer. (French) a form of Desiree.
Desta (Ethiopian) happy. (French) a short form of Destiny.
Desti, Destie, Desty

Destany (French) a form of Destiny.
Destanee, Destaney, Destani, Destanie, Destannee, Destannie

Destinee, Destini, Destinie (French) forms of Destiny.
Desteni, Destiana, Destine, Destinée, Destnie

Destiney (French) a form of Destiny.

Destiny (French) fate.
Desnine, Desta, Destany, Destenee, Destenie, Desteny, Destin, Destinee, Destiney, Destini, Destinie, Destonie, Destynee, Dezstany

Destynee, Destyni (French) forms of Destiny.
Desty, Destyn, Destyne, Destyne, Destynie

Deva (Hindi) divine.
Deeva

Devan (Irish) a form of Devin.
Devana, Devane, Devanee, Devaney, Devani, Devanie, Devann, Devanna, Devannae, Devanne, Devany

Devi (Hindi) goddess.
Religion: the Hindu goddess
of power and destruction.

Devin (Irish) poet.
*Devan, Deven, Devena,
Devenje, Deveny, Devine,
Devinn, Devinne, Devyn*

Devon (English) a short form
of Devonna. (Irish) a form of
Devin.
*Deaven, Devion, Devione,
Devionne, Devone, Devoni,
Devonne*

Devonna (English) from
Devonshire.
*Davonna, Devon, Devona,
Devonda, Devondra, Devonia*

Devora (Hebrew) a form of
Deborah.
Deva, Devorah, Devra, Devrah

Devyn (Irish) a form of
Devin.
*Deveyn, Devyne, Devynn,
Devynne*

Dextra (Latin) adroit, skillful.
Dekstra, Dextria

Dezarae, Dezirae, Deziree
(French) forms of Desiree.
*Dezaraee, Dezarai, Dezaray,
Dezare, Dezaree, Dezarey,
Dezerie, Deziray, Dezirea,
Dezirée, Dezorae, Dezra*

Di (Latin) a short form of
Diana, Diane.
Dy

Dia (Latin) a short form of
Diana, Diane.

Diamond (Latin) precious
gem.
*Diamantina, Diamon,
Diamonda, Diamonde,
Diamonia, Diamonique,
Diamonte, Diamontina,
Dyamond*

Diana (Latin) divine.
Mythology: the goddess of
the hunt, the moon, and fer-
tility. See also Deanna,
Deanne, Dyan.
*Daiana, Daianna, Dayana,
Dayanna, Di, Dia, Dianah,
Dianalyn, Dianarose, Dianatris,
Dianca, Diandra, Diane,
Dianelis, Diania, Dianielle,
Dianita, Dianna, Dianys, Didi*

Diane, Dianne (Latin) short
forms of Diana.
*Deane, Deanne, Deeane,
Deeanne, Di, Dia, Diahann,
Dian, Diani, Dianie, Diann*

Dianna (Latin) a form of
Diana.
Diahanna, Diannah

Diantha (Greek) divine
flower.
Diandre, Dianthe

Diedra (Irish) a form of
Deirdre.
Didra, Diedre

Dillan (Irish) loyal, faithful.
Dillon, Dillyn

Dilys (Welsh) perfect; true.

Dina (Hebrew) a form of Dinah.
Dinna, Dyna

Dinah (Hebrew) vindicated. Bible: a daughter of Jacob and Leah.
Dina, Dinnah, Dynah

Dinka (Swahili) people.

Dionna (Greek) an alternative form of Dionne.
Deona, Deondra, Deonia, Deonna, Deonyia, Diona, Diondra, Diondrea

Dionne (Greek) divine queen. Mythology: Dione was the mother of Aphrodite, the goddess of love.
Deonne, Dion, Dione, Dionee, Dionis, Dionna, Dionte

Dior (French) golden.
Diora, Diore, Diorra, Diorre

Dita (Spanish) a form of Edith.
Ditka, Ditta

Divinia (Latin) divine.
Devina, Devinae, Devinia, Devinie, Devinna, Diveena, Divina, Divine, Diviniea, Divya

Dixie (French) tenth. (English) wall; dike. Geography: a nickname for the American South.
Dix, Dixee, Dixi, Dixy

Diza (Hebrew) joyful.
Ditza, Ditzah, Dizah

Dodie (Hebrew) beloved. (Greek) a familiar form of Dorothy.
Doda, Dode, Dodee, Dodi, Dody

Dolly (American) a short form of Dolores, Dorothy.
Dol, Doll, Dollee, Dolley, Dolli, Dollie, Dollina

Dolores (Spanish) sorrowful. Religion: Nuestra Señora de los Dolores—Our Lady of Sorrows—is a name for the Virgin Mary. See also Lola.
Delores, Deloria, Dolly, Dolorcitas, Dolorita, Doloritas

Dominica, Dominika (Latin) belonging to the Lord. See also Mika.
Domenica, Domenika, Domineca, Domineka, Dominga, Domini, Dominick, Dominicka, Dominique, Dominixe, Domino, Dominyika, Domka, Domnicka, Domonica, Domonice, Domonika

Dominique, Domonique (French) forms of Dominica, Dominika.
Domanique, Domeneque, Domenique, Domineque, Dominiqua, Domino, Dominoque, Dominque, Dominuque, Domique, Domminique, Domoniqua

Domino (English) a short
form of Dominica,
Dominique.

Dona (English) world leader;
proud ruler. (Italian) a form
of Donna.
*Donae, Donah, Donalda,
Donaldina, Donelda, Donellia,
Doni*

Doña (Italian) a form of
Donna.
*Donail, Donalea, Donalisa,
Donay, Doni, Donia, Donie,
Donise, Donitrae*

Donata (Latin) gift.
*Donatha, Donato, Donatta,
Donetta, Donette, Donita,
Donnette, Donnita, Donte*

Dondi (American) a familiar
form of Donna.
Dondra, Dondrea, Dondria

Doneshia, Donisha
(American) forms of
Danessa.
*Donasha, Donashay, Doneisha,
Doneishia, Donesha, Donisa,
Donisha, Donishia, Donneshia,
Donnisha*

Donna (Italian) lady.
*Doña, Dondi, Donnae,
Donnalee, Donnalen, Donnay,
Donne, Donnell, Donni,
Donnie, Donnise, Donny,
Dontia, Donya*

Donniella (American) a form
of Danielle.
*Donella, Doniele, Doniell,
Doniella, Donielle, Donnella,
Donnielle, Donnyella, Donyelle*

Dora (Greek) gift. A short
form of Adora, Eudora,
Pandora, Theodora.
*Dorah, Doralia, Doralie,
Doralisa, Doraly, Doralynn,
Doran, Dorchen, Dore, Dorece,
Doree, Doreece, Doreen, Dorelia,
Dorella, Dorelle, Doresha,
Doressa, Doretta, Dori, Dorielle,
Dorika, Doriley, Dorilis,
Dorinda, Dorion, Dorita, Doro,
Dory*

Doralynn (English) a combi-
nation of Dora + Lynn.
*Doralin, Doralyn, Doralynne,
Dorlin*

Doreen (Irish) moody, sullen.
(French) golden. (Greek) a
form of Dora.
*Doreena, Dorena, Dorene,
Dorina, Dorine*

Doretta (American) a form of
Dora, Dorothy.
Doretha, Dorette, Dorettie

Dori, Dory (American) famil-
iar forms of Dora, Doria,
Doris, Dorothy.
*Dore, Dorey, Dorie, Dorree,
Dorri, Dorrie, Dorry*

Doria (Greek) a form of
Dorian.
Dori

Dorian (Greek) from Doris, Greece.
Dorean, Doriana, Doriane, Doriann, Dorianna, Dorianne, Dorin, Dorina, Dorriane

Dorinda (Spanish) a form of Dora.

Doris (Greek) sea. Mythology: wife of Nereus and mother of the Nereids or sea nymphs.
Dori, Dorice, Dorisa, Dorise, Dorris, Dorrise, Dorrys, Dory, Dorys

Dorothea (Greek) a form of Dorothy. See also Thea.
Dorethea, Dorotea, Doroteya, Dorotha, Dorothia, Dorotthea, Dorthea, Dorthia

Dorothy (Greek) gift of God. See also Dasha, Dodie, Lolotea, Theodora.
Dasya, Do, Doa, Doe, Dolly, Doortje, Dorathy, Dordei, Dordi, Doretta, Dori, Dorika, Doritha, Dorka, Dorle, Dorlisa, Doro, Dorolice, Dorosia, Dorota, Dorothea, Dorothee, Dorothi, Dorothie, Dorottya, Dorte, Dortha, Dorthy, Dory, Dosi, Dossie, Dosya, Dottie

Dorrit (Greek) dwelling. (Hebrew) generation.
Dorit, Dorita, Doritt

Dottie, Dotty (Greek) familiar forms of Dorothy.
Dot, Dottee

Drew (Greek) courageous; strong. (Latin) a short form of Drusilla.
Dru, Drue

Drinka (Spanish) a form of Alexandria.
Dreena, Drena, Drina

Drusi (Latin) a short form of Drusilla.
Drucey, Druci, Drucie, Drucy, Drusey, Drusie, Drusy

Drusilla (Latin) descendant of Drusus, the strong one. See also Drew.
Drewsila, Drucella, Drucill, Drucilla, Druscilla, Druscille, Drusi

Dulce (Latin) sweet.
Delcina, Delcine, Douce, Doucie, Dulcea, Dulcey, Dulci, Dulcia, Dulciana, Dulcibel, Dulcibella, Dulcie, Dulcine, Dulcinea, Dulcy, Dulse, Dulsea

Dulcinea (Spanish) sweet. Literature: Don Quixote's love interest.

Duscha (Russian) soul; sweetheart; term of endearment.
Duschah, Dusha, Dushenka

Dusti, Dusty (English) familiar forms of Dustine.
Dustee, Dustie

Dustine (German) valiant fighter. (English) brown rock quarry.
Dusteena, Dusti, Dustin, Dustina, Dustyn

Dyamond, Dymond (Latin)
forms of Diamond.
Dyamin, Dyamon, Dyamone,
Dymin, Dymon, Dymonde,
Dymone, Dymonn

Dyana (Latin) a form of
Diana. (Native American)
deer.
Dyan, Dyane, Dyani, Dyann,
Dyanna, Dyanne

Dylan (Welsh) sea.
Dylaan, Dylaina, Dylana,
Dylane, Dylanee, Dylanie,
Dylann, Dylanna, Dylen,
Dylin, Dyllan, Dylynn

Dyllis (Welsh) sincere.
Dilys, Dylis, Dylys

Dynasty (Latin) powerful
ruler.
Dynastee, Dynasti, Dynastie

Dyshawna (American) a com-
bination of the prefix Dy +
Shawna.
Dyshanta, Dyshawn,
Dyshonda, Dyshonna

E

Earlene (Irish) pledge.
(English) noblewoman.
Earla, Earlean, Earlecia,
Earleen, Earlena, Earlina,
Earlinda, Earline, Erla, Erlana,
Erlene, Erlenne, Erlina, Erlinda,
Erline, Erlisha

Eartha (English) earthy.
Ertha

Easter (English) Easter time.
History: a name for a child
born on Easter.
Eastan, Eastlyn, Easton

Ebone, Ebonee (Greek) forms
of Ebony.
Abonee, Ebanee, Eboné,
Ebonea, Ebonne, Ebonnee

Eboni, Ebonie (Greek) forms
of Ebony.
Ebanie, Ebeni, Ebonni, Ebonnie

Ebony (Greek) a hard, dark
wood.
Abony, Eban, Ebanie, Ebany,
Ebbony, Ebone, Eboney, Eboni,
Ebonie, Ebonique, Ebonisha,
Ebonye, Ebonyi

Echo (Greek) repeated sound.
Mythology: the nymph who
pined for the love of
Narcissus until only her
voice remained.
Echoe, Ecko, Ekko, Ekkoe

Eda (Irish, English) a short
form of Edana, Edith.

Edana (Irish) ardent; flame.
Eda, Edan, Edanna

Edda (German) a form of
Hedda.
Etta

Eddy (American) a familiar
form of Edwina.
Eady, Eddi, Eddie, Edy

Edeline (English) noble; kind.
*Adeline, Edelyne, Ediline,
Edilyne*

Eden (Babylonian) a plain.
(Hebrew) delightful. Bible:
the earthly paradise.
*Eaden, Ede, Edena, Edene,
Edenia, Edin, Edyn*

Edie (English) a familiar form
of Edith.
*Eadie, Edi, Edy, Edye, Eyde,
Eydie*

Edith (English) rich gift. See
also Dita.
*Eadith, Eda, Ede, Edetta,
Edette, Edie, Edit, Edita, Edite,
Editha, Edithe, Editta, Ediva,
Edyta, Edyth, Edytha, Edythe*

Edna (Hebrew) rejuvenation.
Religion: the wife of Enoch,
according to the Book of
Enoch.
*Adna, Adnisha, Ednah,
Edneisha, Edneshia, Ednisha,
Ednita, Edona*

Edrianna (Greek) a form of
Adrienne.
Edria, Edriana, Edrina

Edwina (English) prosperous
friend. See also Winnie.
*Eddy, Edina, Edweena,
Edwena, Edwine, Edwyna,
Edwynn*

Effia (Ghanaian) born on
Friday.

Effie (Greek) spoken well of.
(English) a short form of
Alfreda, Euphemia.
Effi, Effia, Effy, Ephie

Eileen (Irish) a form of Helen.
See also Aileen, Ilene.
*Eilean, Eileena, Eileene, Eilena,
Eilene, Eiley, Eilie, Eilieh,
Eilina, Eiline, Eilleen, Eillen,
Eilyn, Eleen, Elene*

Ekaterina (Russian) a form of
Katherine.
Ekaterine, Ekaterini

Ela (Polish) a form of
Adelaide.

Elaina (French) a form of
Helen.
Elainea, Elainia, Elainna

Elaine (French) a form of
Helen. See also Lainey, Laine.
*Eilane, Elain, Elaina, Elaini,
Elan, Elana, Elane, Elania,
Elanie, Elanit, Elauna, Elayna,
Ellaine*

Elana (Greek) a short form of
Eleanor. See also Ilana, Lana.
*Elan, Elanee, Elaney, Elani,
Elania, Elanie, Elanna, Elanni*

Elayna (French) a form of
Elaina.
Elayn, Elaynah, Elayne, Elayni

Elberta (English) a form of
Alberta.
*Elbertha, Elberthina, Elberthine,
Elbertina, Elbertine*

Eldora (Spanish) golden, gilded.
Eldoree, Eldorey, Eldori,
Eldoria, Eldorie, Eldory

Eleanor (Greek) light. History:
Anna Eleanor Roosevelt was a
U. S. delegate to the United
Nations, a writer, and the
thirty-second First Lady of the
United States. See also Elana,
Ella, Ellen, Leanore, Lena,
Lenore, Leonore, Leora, Nellie,
Nora, Noreen.
Elana, Elanor, Elanore, Eleanora,
Eleanore, Elena, Eleni, Elenor,
Elenorah, Elenore, Eleonor,
Eleonore, Elianore, Elinor, Elinore,
Elladine, Ellenor, Ellie, Elliner,
Ellinor, Ellinore, Elna, Elnore,
Elynor, Elynore

Eleanora (Greek) a form of
Eleanor. See also Lena.
Elenora, Eleonora, Elianora,
Ellenora, Ellenorah, Elnora,
Elynora

Electra (Greek) shining; brilliant. Mythology: the daughter of Agamemnon, leader of
the Greeks in the Trojan War.
Elektra

Elena (Greek) a form of Eleanor.
(Italian) a form of Helen.
Eleana, Eleen, Eleena, Elen, Elene,
Elenitsa, Elenka, Elenna, Elenoa,
Elenola, Elina, Ellena, Lena

Eleni (Greek) a familiar form
of Eleanor.
Elenie, Eleny

Eleora (Hebrew) the Lord is
my light.
Eliora, Elira, Elora

Elexis (Greek) a form of Alexis.
Elexas, Elexes, Elexess, Elexeya,
Elexia, Elexiah

Elexus (Greek) a form of
Alexius, Alexus.
Elexius, Elexsus, Elexxus, Elexys

Elfrida (German) peaceful. See
also Freda.
Elfrea, Elfreda, Elfredda,
Elfreeda, Elfreyda, Elfrieda,
Elfryda

Elga (Norwegian) pious.
(German) a form of Helga.
Elgiva

Elia (Hebrew) a short form of
Eliana.
Eliah

Eliana (Hebrew) my God has
answered me. See also Iliana.
Elia, Eliane, Elianna, Ellianna,
Liana, Liane

Eliane (Hebrew) a form of Eliana.
Elianne, Elliane, Ellianne

Elicia (Hebrew) a form of
Elisha. See also Alicia.
Elecia, Elica, Elicea, Elicet,
Elichia, Eliscia, Elisia, Elissia,
Ellecia, Ellicia

Elida, Elide (Latin) forms of
Alida.
Elidee, Elidia, Elidy

Elisa (Spanish, Italian, English) a short form of Elizabeth. See also Alisa, Ilisa.
Elecea, Eleesa, Elesa, Elesia, Elisia, Elisya, Ellisa, Ellisia, Ellissa, Ellissia, Ellissya, Ellisya, Elysa, Elysia, Elyssia, Elyssya, Elysya, Lisa

Elisabeth (Hebrew) a form of Elizabeth.
Elisabet, Elisabeta, Elisabethe, Elisabetta, Elisabette, Elisabith, Elisebet, Elisheba, Elisheva

Elise (French, English) a short form of Elizabeth, Elysia. See also Ilise, Liese, Lisette, Lissie.
Eilis, Eilise, Elese, Élise, Elisee, Elisie, Elisse, Elizé, Ellice, Ellise, Ellyce, Ellyse, Ellyze, Elsey, Elsie, Elsy, Elyce, Elyci, Elyse, Elyze, Lisel, Lisl, Lison

Elisha (Hebrew) consecrated to God. (Greek) a form of Alisha. See also Ilisha, Lisha.
Eleacia, Eleasha, Eleesha, Eleisha, Elesha, Eleshia, Eleticia, Elicia, Elishah, Elisheva, Elishia, Elishua, Eliska, Ellesha, Ellexia, Ellisha, Elsha, Elysha, Elyshia

Elissa, Elyssa (Greek, English) forms of Elizabeth. Short forms of Melissa. See also Alissa, Alyssa, Lissa.
Elissah, Ellissa, Ellyssa, Ilissa, Ilyssa

Elita (Latin, French) chosen. See also Lida, Lita.
Elitia, Elitia, Elitie, Ellita, Ellitia, Ellitie, Ilida, Ilita, Litia

Eliza (Hebrew) a short form of Elizabeth. See also Aliza.
Eliz, Elizaida, Elizalina, Elize, Elizea

Elizabet (Hebrew) a form of Elizabeth.
Elizabete, Elizabette

Elizabeth (Hebrew) consecrated to God. Bible: the mother of John the Baptist. See also Bess, Beth, Betsy, Betty, Elsa, Ilse, Libby, Liese, Liesel, Lisa, Lisbeth, Lisette, Lissa, Lissie, Liz, Liza, Lizabeta, Lizabeth, Lizbeth, Lizina, Lizzy, Veta, Yelisabeta, Zizi.
Alizabeth, Eliabeth, Elisa, Elisabeth, Elise, Elissa, Eliza, Elizabee, Elizabet, Elizaveta, Elizebeth, Elka, Elsabeth, Elsbeth, Elschen, Elspeth, Elysabeth, Elzbieta, Elzsébet, Helsa, Ilizzabet, Lusa

Elizaveta (Polish, English) a form of Elizabeth.
Elisavet, Elisaveta, Elisavetta, Elisveta, Elizavet, Elizavetta, Elizveta, Elsveta, Elzveta

Elka (Polish) a form of Elizabeth.
Ilka

Elke (German) a form of Adelaide, Alice.
Elki, Ilki

Ella (English) elfin; beautiful fairy-woman. (Greek) a short form of Eleanor.
Ellah, Ellamae, Ellia, Ellie

Elle (Greek) a short form of Eleanor. (French) she.
El, Ele, Ell

Ellen (English) a form of Eleanor, Helen.
Elen, Elenee, Eleny, Elin, Elina, Elinda, Ellan, Ellena, Ellene, Ellie, Ellin, Ellon, Ellyn, Ellynn, Ellynne, Elyn

Ellice (English) a form of Elise.
Ellecia, Ellyce, Elyce

Ellie, Elly (English) short forms of Eleanor, Ella, Ellen.
Ele, Elie, Ellee, Elleigh, Elli

Elma (Turkish) sweet fruit.

Elmira (Arabic, Spanish) a form of Almira.
Elmeera, Elmera, Elmeria, Elmyra

Elnora (American) a combination of Ella + Nora.

Elodie (American) a form of Melody. (English) a form of Alodie.
Elodee, Elodia, Elody

Eloise (French) a form of Louise.
Elois, Eloisa, Eloisia

Elora (American) a short form of Elnora.
Ellora, Elloree, Elorie

Elsa (German) noble. (Hebrew) a short form of Elizabeth. See also Ilse.
Ellsa, Ellse, Else, Elsia, Elsie, Elsje

Elsbeth (German) a form of Elizabeth.
Elsbet, Elzbet, Elzbieta

Elsie (German) a familiar form of Elsa, Helsa.
Ellsie, Ellsie, Ellsy, Elsi, Elsy

Elspeth (Scottish) a form of Elizabeth.
Elspet, Elspie

Elva (English) elfin. See also Alva, Alvina.
Elvia, Elvie

Elvina (English) a form of Alvina.
Elvenea, Elvinea, Elvinia, Elvinna

Elvira (Latin) white; blond. (German) closed up. (Spanish) elfin. Geography: the town in Spain that hosted a Catholic synod in 300 A.D.
Elva, Elvera, Elvire, Elwira, Vira

Elyse (Latin) a form of Elysia.
Ellysa, Ellyse, Elyce, Elys,
Elysee, Elysse

Elysia (Greek) sweet; blissful.
Mythology: Elysium was the
dwelling place of happy
souls.
Elise, Elishia, Ellicia, Elycia,
Elyssa, Ilysha, Ilysia

Elyssa (Latin) a form of Elysia.
Ellyssa

Emalee (Latin) a form of
Emily.
Emaili, Emalea, Emaleigh,
Emali, Emalia, Emalie

Emani (Arabic) a form of
Iman.
Eman, Emane, Emaneé,
Emanie, Emann

Emanuelle (Hebrew) a form
of Emmanuelle.
Emanual, Emanuel, Emanuela,
Emanuella

Ember (French) a form of
Amber.
Emberlee, Emberly

Emelia, Emelie (Latin) forms
of Emily.
Emellie

Emely (Latin) a form of Emily.
Emelly

Emerald (French) bright
green gemstone.
Emelda, Esmeralda

Emery (German) industrious
leader.
Emeri, Emerie

Emilee, Emilie (English) forms
of Emily.
Emile, Emilea, Emileigh, Émi-
lie, Emiliee, Emillee, Emillie,
Emmélie, Emmilee, Emylee

Emilia (Italian) a form of
Amelia, Emily.
Emalia, Emelia, Emila

Emily (Latin) flatterer.
(German) industrious. See
also Amelia, Emma, Millie.
Eimile, Em, Emaily, Emalee,
Emeli, Emelia, Emelie, Emelita,
Emely, Emilee, Emiley, Emili,
Emilia, Emilie, Émilie, Emilis,
Emilka, Emillie, Emilly,
Emmaline, Emmaly, Emmélie,
Emmey, Emmi, Emmie,
Emmilly, Emmily, Emmy,
Emmye, Emyle

Emilyann (American) a com-
bination of Emily + Ann.
Emileane, Emileann,
Emileanna, Emileanne,
Emiliana, Emiliann, Emilianna,
Emilianne, Emillyane,
Emillyann, Emillyanna,
Emillyanne, Emliana, Emliann,
Emlianna, Emlianne

Emma (German) a short form
of Emily. See also Amy.
Em, Ema, Emmah, Emmy

Emmalee (American) a combination of Emma + Lee. A

form of Emily.
Emalea, Emalee, Emilee,
Emmalea, Emmalei,
Emmaleigh, Emmaley, Emmali,
Emmalia, Emmalie, Emmaliese,
Emmalyse, Emylee

Emmaline (French) a form of
Emily.
Emalina, Emaline, Emelina,
Emeline, Emilienne, Emilina,
Emiline, Emmalina, Emmalene,
Emmeline, Emmiline

Emmalynn (American) a
combination of Emma +
Lynn.
Emelyn, Emelyne, Emelynne,
Emilyn, Emilynn, Emilynne,
Emlyn, Emlynn, Emlynne,
Emmalyn, Emmalynne

Emmanuelle (Hebrew) God is
with us.
Emanuelle, Emmanuela,
Emmanuella

Emmy (German) a familiar
form of Emma.
Emi, Emie, Emiy, Emmi,
Emmie, Emmye, Emy

Emmylou (American) a com-
bination of Emmy + Lou.
Emlou, Emmalou, Emmelou,
Emmilou, Emylou

Ena (Irish) a form of Helen.
Enna

Enid (Welsh) life; spirit.

Enrica (Spanish) a form of
Henrietta. See also Rica.
Enrieta, Enrietta, Enrika,
Enriqua, Enriqueta, Enriquetta,
Enriquette

Eppie (English) a familiar
form of Euphemia.
Effie, Effy, Eppy

Erica (Scandinavian) ruler of
all. (English) brave ruler. See
also Arica, Rica, Ricki.
Ericca, Ericha, Ericka, Errica

Ericka, Erika (Scandanavian)
forms of Erica.
Erickah, Erikaa, Erikah,
Erikka, Erricka, Errika, Eyka,
Erykka, Eyrika

Erin (Irish) peace. History:
another name for Ireland.
See also Arin.
Earin, Earrin, Eran, Eren,
Erena, Erene, Ereni, Eri, Erian,
Erina, Erine, Erinetta, Erinn,
Errin, Eryn

Erinn (Irish) a form of Erin.
Erinna, Erinne

Erma (Latin) a short form of
Ermine, Hermina. See also
Irma.
Ermelinda

Ermine (Latin) a form of
Hermina.
Erma, Ermin, Ermina,
Erminda, Erminia, Erminie

Erna (English) a short form of
Ernestine.

Ernestine (English) earnest, sincere.
Erna, Ernaline, Ernesia, Ernesta, Ernestina, Ernesztina

Eryn (Irish) a form of Erin.
Eiryn, Eryne, Erynn, Erynne

Eshe (Swahili) life.
Eisha, Esha

Esmé (French) a familiar form of Esmeralda. A form of Amy.
Esma, Esme, Esmëe

Esmeralda (Greek, Spanish) a form of Emerald.
Emelda, Esmé, Esmerelda, Esmerilda, Esmiralda, Ezmerelda, Ezmirilda

Esperanza (Spanish) hope. See also Speranza.
Esparanza, Espe, Esperance, Esperans, Esperansa, Esperanta, Esperanz, Esperenza

Essence (Latin) life; existence.
Essa, Essenc, Essencee, Essences, Essenes, Essense, Essynce

Essie (English) a short form of Estelle, Esther.
Essa, Essey, Essie, Essy

Estee (English) a short form of Estelle, Esther.
Esta, Estée, Esti

Estefani, Estefania, Estefany (Spanish) forms of Stephanie.
Estafania, Estefana, Estefane, Estefanie

Estelle (French) a form of Esther. See also Stella, Trella.
Essie, Estee, Estel, Estela, Estele, Esteley, Estelina, Estelita, Estell, Estella, Estellina, Estellita, Esthella

Estephanie (Spanish) a form of Stephanie.
Estephania, Estephani, Estephany

Esther (Persian) star. Bible: the Jewish captive whom Ahasuerus made his queen. See also Hester.
Essie, Estee, Ester, Esthur, Eszter, Eszti

Estrella (French) star.
Estrela, Estrelinha, Estrell, Estrelle, Estrellita

Ethana (Hebrew) strong; firm.

Ethel (English) noble.
Ethelda, Ethelin, Etheline, Ethelle, Ethelyn, Ethelynn, Ethelynne, Ethyl

Étoile (French) star.

Etta (German) little. (English) a short form of Henrietta.
Etka, Etke, Etti, Ettie, Etty, Itke, Itta

Eudora (Greek) honored gift. See also Dora.

Eugenia (Greek) born to nobility. See also Gina.
Eugenie, Eugenina, Eugina, Evgenia

Eugenie (Greek) a form of
Eugenia.
Eugenee, Eugénie

Eulalia (Greek) well spoken.
See also Ula.
*Eula, Eulalee, Eulalie, Eulalya,
Eulia*

Eun (Korean) silver.

Eunice (Greek) happy; victori-
ous. Bible: the mother of
Saint Timothy. See also
Unice.
Euna, Eunique, Eunise, Euniss

Euphemia (Greek) spoken
well of, in good repute.
History: a fourth-century
Christian martyr.
*Effam, Effie, Eppie, Eufemia,
Euphan, Euphemie, Euphie*

Eurydice (Greek) wide, broad.
Mythology: the wife of
Orpheus.
Euridice, Euridyce, Eurydyce

Eustacia (Greek) productive.
(Latin) stable; calm. See also
Stacey.
Eustasia

Eva (Greek) a short form of
Evangelina. (Hebrew) a form
of Eve. See also Ava, Chava.
*Éva, Evah, Evalea, Evalee,
Evike*

Evaline (French) a form of
Evelyn.
Evalin, Evalina, Evalyn,
*Evalynn, Eveleen, Evelene,
Evelina, Eveline*

Evangelina (Greek) bearer of
good news.
*Eva, Evangelene, Evangelia,
Evangelica, Evangeline,
Evangelique, Evangelyn,
Evangelynn*

Evania (Irish) young warrior.
*Evan, Evana, Evanka, Evann,
Evanna, Evanne, Evany,
Eveania, Evvanne, Evvunea,
Evyan*

Eve (Hebrew) life. Bible: the
first woman created by God.
(French) a short form of
Evonne. See also Chava,
Hava, Naeva, Vica, Yeva.
*Eva, Evie, Evita, Evuska,
Evyn, Ewa, Yeva*

Evelin (English) a form of
Evelyn.
Evelina, Eveline

Evelyn (English) hazelnut.
*Avalyn, Aveline, Evaleen,
Evalene, Evaline, Evalyn,
Evalynn, Evalynne, Eveleen,
Evelin, Evelyna, Evelyne,
Evelynn, Evelynne, Evline,
Ewalina*

Everett (German) courageous
as a boar.

Evette (French) a form of
Yvette. A familiar form of
Evonne. See also Ivette.
Evett

Evie (Hungarian) a form of
Eve.
*Evey, Evi, Evicka, Evike, Evka,
Evuska, Evvie, Evvy, Evy, Ewa*

Evita (Spanish) a form of Eve.

Evline (English) a form of
Evelyn.
*Evleen, Evlene, Evlin, Evlina,
Evlyn, Evlynn, Evlynne*

Evonne (French) a form of
Yvonne. See also Ivonne.
*Evanne, Eve, Evenie, Evenne,
Eveny, Evette, Evin, Evon,
Evona, Evone, Evoni, Evonna,
Evonnie, Evony, Evyn, Evynn,
Eyona, Eyvone*

Ezri (Hebrew) helper; strong.
Ezra, Ezria

F

Fabia (Latin) bean grower.
*Fabiana, Fabienne, Fabiola,
Fabra, Fabria*

Fabiana (Latin) a form of Fabia.
Fabyana

Fabienne (Latin) a form of
Fabia.
*Fabian, Fabiann, Fabianne,
Fabiene, Fabreanne*

Fabiola, Faviola (Latin) forms
of Fabia.
*Fabiole, Fabyola, Faviana,
Faviolha*

Faith (English) faithful; fidelity.
See also Faye, Fidelity.
Fayth, Faythe

Faizah (Arabic) victorious.

Falda (Icelandic) folded wings.
Faida, Fayda

Faline (Latin) catlike.
*Faleen, Falena, Falene, Falin,
Falina, Fallyn, Fallyne, Faylina,
Fayline, Faylyn, Faylynn,
Faylynne, Felenia, Felina*

Fallon (Irish) grandchild of the
ruler.
*Falan, Falen, Fallan, Fallen,
Fallonne, Falon, Falyn, Falynn,
Falynne, Phalon*

Fancy (French) betrothed.
(English) whimsical; decora-
tive.
*Fanchette, Fanchon, Fanci,
Fancia, Fancie*

Fannie, Fanny (American)
familiar forms of Frances.
*Fan, Fanette, Fani, Fania,
Fannee, Fanney, Fanni, Fannia,
Fany, Fanya*

Fantasia (Greek) imagination.
*Fantasy, Fantasya, Fantaysia,
Fantazia, Fiantasi*

Farah, Farrah (English) beautiful; pleasant.
Fara, Farra, Fayre

Faren, Farren (English) wanderer.
Faran, Fare, Farin, Faron,

Farrahn, Farran, Farrand, Farrin,
Farron, Farryn, Farye, Faryn,
Feran, Ferin, Feron, Ferran,
Ferren, Ferrin, Ferron, Ferryn

Fatima (Arabic) daughter of
the Prophet. History: the
daughter of Muhammad.
Fatema, Fathma, Fatimah,
Fatime, Fatma, Fatmah, Fatme,
Fattim

Fawn (French) young deer.
Faun, Fawna, Fawne

Fawna (French) a form of Fawn.
Fauna, Fawnia, Fawnna

Faye (French) fairy; elf.
(English) a form of Faith.
Fae, Fay, Fayann, Fayanna,
Fayette, Fayina, Fey

Fayola (Nigerian) lucky.
Fayla, Feyla

Felecia (Latin) a form of Felicia.
Flecia

Felica (Spanish) a short form
of Felicia.
Falisa, Felisa, Felisca, Felissa,
Feliza

Felice (Latin) a short form of
Felicia.
Felece, Felicie, Felise, Felize,
Felyce, Felysse

Felicia (Latin) fortunate;
happy. See also Lecia,
Phylicia.
Falecia, Faleshia, Falicia, Fela,
Felecia, Felica, Felice, Felicidad,

Feliciona, Felicity, Felicya,
Felisea, Felisha, Felisia,
Felisiana, Felissya, Felita,
Felixia, Felizia, Felka, Fellcia,
Felycia, Felysia, Felyssia,
Fleasia, Fleichia, Fleishia,
Flichia

Felicity (English) a form of
Felicia.
Falicity, Felicita, Felicitas,
Félicité, Feliciti, Felisita, Felisity

Felisha (Latin) a form of
Felicia.
Faleisha, Falesha, Falisha,
Falleshia, Feleasha, Feleisha,
Felesha, Felishia, Fellishia,
Felysha, Flisha

Femi (French) woman.
(Nigerian) love me.
Femie, Femmi, Femmie, Femy

Feodora (Greek) gift of God.
Fedora, Fedoria

Fern (English) fern. (German)
a short form of Fernanda.
Ferne, Ferni, Fernlee, Fernleigh,
Fernley, Fernly

Fernanda (German) daring,
adventurous. See also Andee,
Nan.
Ferdie, Ferdinanda, Ferdinande,
Fern, Fernande, Fernandette,
Fernandina, Nanda

Fiala (Czech) violet

Fidelia (Latin) a form of
Fidelity.
Fidela, Fidele, Fidelina

Fidelity (Latin) faithful, true.
See also Faith.
Fidelia, Fidelita

Fifi (French) a familiar form of
Josephine.
Feef, Feefee, Fifine

Filippa (Italian) a form of
Philippa.
Felipa, Filipa, Filippina, Filpina

Filomena (Italian) a form of
Philomena.
Fila, Filah, Filemon

Fiona (Irish) fair, white.
Fionna

Fionnula (Irish) white shoul-
dered. See also Nola, Nuala.
*Fenella, Fenula, Finella, Finola,
Finula*

Flair (English) style; verve.
Flaire, Flare

Flannery (Irish) redhead.
Literature: Flannery
O'Connor was a renowned
American writer.
Flan, Flann, Flanna

Flavia (Latin) blond, golden
haired.
*Flavere, Flaviar, Flavie, Flavien,
Flavienne, Flaviere, Flavio,
Flavyere, Fulvia*

Flavie (Latin) a form of Flavia.
Flavi

Fleur (French) flower.
Fleure, Fleuree, Fleurette

Flo (American) a short form
of Florence.

Flora (Latin) flower. A short
form of Florence. See also
Lore.
*Fiora, Fiore, Fiorenza, Flor,
Florann, Florella, Florelle,
Floren, Floria, Floriana,
Florianna, Florica, Florimel*

Florence (Latin) blooming;
flowery; prosperous. History:
Florence Nightingale, a
British nurse, is considered
the founder of modern nurs-
ing. See also Florida.
*Fiorenza, Flo, Flora, Florance,
Florencia, Florency, Florendra,
Florentia, Florentina,
Florentyna, Florenza, Floretta,
Florette, Florie, Florina, Florine,
Floris, Flossie*

Floria (Basque) a form of
Flora.
Flori, Florria

Florida (Spanish) a form of
Florence.
Floridia, Florinda, Florita

Florie (English) a familiar
form of Florence.
*Flore, Flori, Florri, Florrie,
Florry, Flory*

Floris (English) a form of
Florence.
Florisa, Florise

Flossie (English) a familiar form of Florence.
Floss, Flossi, Flossy

Fola (Yoruba) honorable.

Fonda (Latin) foundation. (Spanish) inn.
Fondea, Fonta

Fontanna (French) fountain.
Fontaine, Fontana, Fontane, Fontanne, Fontayne

Fortuna (Latin) fortune; fortunate.
Fortoona, Fortune

Fran (Latin) a short form of Frances.
Frain, Frann

Frances (Latin) free; from France. See also Paquita.
Fanny, Fran, Franca, France, Francee, Francena, Francesca, Francess, Francesta, Franceta, Francetta, Francette, Francine, Francis, Francisca, Françoise, Frankie, Frannie, Franny

Francesca (Italian) a form of Frances.
Franceska, Francessca, Francesta, Franchesca, Franzetta

Franchesca (Italian) a form of Francesca.
Cheka, Chekka, Chesca, Cheska, Francheca, Francheka, Franchelle, Franchesa, Francheska, Franchessca, Franchesska

Franci (Hungarian) a familiar form of Francine.
Francey, Francie, Francy

Francine (French) a form of Frances.
Franceen, Franceine, Franceline, Francene, Francenia, Franci, Francin, Francina, Francyne

Francis (Latin) a form of Frances.
Francise, Franncia, Francys

Francisca (Italian) a form of Frances.
Franciska, Franciszka, Frantiska, Franziska

Françoise (French) a form of Frances.
Frankie (American) a familiar form of Frances.
Francka, Francki, Franka, Frankey, Franki, Frankia, Franky, Frankye

Frannie, Franny (English) familiar forms of Frances.
Frani, Frania, Franney, Franni, Frany

Freda, Freida, Frida (German) short forms of Alfreda, Elfrida, Frederica, Sigfreda.
Frayda, Fredda, Fredella, Fredia, Fredra, Freeda, Freeha, Freia, Frida, Frideborg, Frieda

Freddi, Freddie (English)
familiar forms of Frederica,
Winifred.
*Fredda, Freddy, Fredi, Fredia,
Fredy, Frici*

Frederica (German) peaceful
ruler. See also Alfreda, Rica,
Ricki.
*Farica, Federica, Freda,
Fredalena, Fredaline, Freddi,
Freddie, Frederickina, Frederika,
Frederike, Frederina, Frederine,
Frederique, Fredith, Fredora,
Fredreca, Fredrica, Fredricah,
Fredricia, Freida, Fritzi,
Fryderica*

Frederika (German) a form of
Frederica.
*Fredericka, Fredreka, Fredricka,
Fredrika, Fryderyka*

Frederike (German) a form of
Frederica.
Fredericke, Friederike

Frederique (French) a form of
Frederica.
Frédérique, Rike

Freja (Scandinavian) a form of
Freya.

Freya (Scandinavian) noble-
woman. Mythology: the
Norse goddess of love.
Fraya, Freya

Fritzi (German) a familiar
form of Frederica.
*Friezi, Fritze, Fritzie, Fritzinn,
Fritzline, Fritzy*

G

Gabriel, Gabriele (French)
forms of Gabrielle.
*Gabbriel, Gabbryel, Gabreal,
Gabreale, Gabreil, Gabrial,
Gabryel*

Gabriela, Gabriella (Italian)
forms of Gabrielle.
*Gabriala, Gabrialla, Gabrielia,
Gabriellia, Gabrila, Gabrilla,
Gabryella*

Gabrielle (French) devoted to
God.
*Gabbrielle, Gabielle, Gabrealle,
Gabriana, Gabriel, Gabriela,
Gabriele, Gabriell, Gabriella,
Gabrille, Gabrina, Gabriylle,
Gabryell, Gabryelle, Gaby,
Gavriella*

Gaby (French) a familiar form
of Gabrielle.
*Gabbey, Gabbi, Gabbie, Gabby,
Gabey, Gabi, Gabie, Gavi, Gavy*

Gada (Hebrew) lucky.
Gadah

Gaea (Greek) planet Earth.
Mythology: the Greek god-
dess of Earth.
Gaia, Gaiea, Gaya

Gaetana (Italian) from Gaeta.
Geography: a city in south-
ern Italy.
Gaetan, Gaétane, Gaetanne

Gagandeep (Sikh) sky's light.
*Gagandip, Gagnadeep,
Gagndeep*

Gail (Hebrew) a short form of
Abigail.(English) merry, lively.
*Gael, Gaela, Gaelle, Gaila,
Gaile, Gale, Gayla, Gayle*

Gala (Norwegian) singer.
Galla

Galen (Greek) healer; calm.
(Irish) little and lively.
*Gaelen, Gaellen, Galyn,
Gaylaine, Gayleen, Gaylen,
Gaylene, Gaylyn*

Galena (Greek) healer; calm.

Gali (Hebrew) hill; fountain;
spring.
Galice, Galie

Galina (Russian) a form of
Helen.
*Gailya, Galayna, Galenka,
Galia, Galiana, Galiena,
Galinka, Galochka, Galya,
Galyna*

Ganesa (Hindi) fortunate.
Religion: Ganesha was the
Hindu god of wisdom.

Ganya (Hebrew) garden of the
Lord. (Zulu) clever.
*Gana, Gani, Gania, Ganice,
Ganit*

Gardenia (English) Botany: a
sweet-smelling flower.
*Deeni, Denia, Gardena,
Gardinia*

Garland (French) wreath of
flowers.

Garnet (English) dark red gem.
Garnetta, Garnette

Garyn (English) spear carrier.
Garan, Garen, Garra, Garryn

Gasha (Russian) a familiar
form of Agatha.
Gashka

Gavriella (Hebrew) a form of
Gabrielle.
*Gavila, Gavilla, Gavrid,
Gavrieela, Gavriela, Gavrielle,
Gavrila, Gavrilla*

Gay (French) merry.
Gae, Gai, Gaye

Gayle (English) a form of Gail.
Gayla

Gayna (English) a familiar
form of Guinevere.
Gaynah, Gayner, Gaynor

Geela (Hebrew) joyful.
Gela, Gila

Geena (American) a form of
Gena.
Geania, Geeana, Geeanna

Gelya (Russian) angelic.

Gema, Gemma (Latin, Italian)
jewel, precious stone. See also
Jemma.
*Gem, Gemmey, Gemmie,
Gemmy*

Gemini (Greek) twin.
Gemelle, Gemima, Gemina,
Geminine, Gemmina

Gen (Japanese) spring. A short
form of names beginning
with "Gen."

Gena (French) a form of Gina.
A short form of Geneva,
Genevieve, Iphigenia.
Geanna, Geena, Geenah, Gen,
Genae, Genah, Genai, Genea,
Geneja, Geni, Genia, Genie

Geneen (Scottish) a form of
Jeanine.
Geanine, Geannine, Gen,
Genene, Genine, Gineen,
Ginene

Genell (American) a form of
Jenelle.

Genesis (Latin) origin; birth.
Genes, Genese, Genesha,
Genesia, Genesiss, Genessa,
Genesse, Genessie, Genessis,
Genicis, Genises, Genysis,
Yenesis

Geneva (French) juniper tree.
A short form of Genevieve.
Geography: a city in
Switzerland.
Geena, Gen, Gena, Geneieve,
Geneiva, Geneive, Geneve,
Ginneva, Janeva, Jeaneva, Jeneva

Genevieve (German, French)
a form of Guinevere. See also
Gwendolyn.
Gen, Gena, Genaveeve,

Genaveve, Genavie, Genavieve,
Genavive, Geneva, Geneveve,
Genevie, Geneviéve, Genevievre,
Genevive, Genovieve, Genvieve,
Ginette, Gineveve, Ginevieve,
Ginevive, Guinevieve,
Guinivive, Gwenevieve,
Gwenivive, Jennavieve

Genevra (French, Welsh) a
form of Guinevere.
Gen, Genever, Genevera,
Ginevra

Genice (American) a form of
Janice.
Gen, Genece, Geneice, Genesa,
Genesee, Genessia, Genis,
Genise

Genita (American) a form of
Janita.
Gen, Genet, Geneta

Genna (English) a form of
Jenna.
Gen, Gennae, Gennay, Genni,
Gennie, Genny

Gennifer (American) a form
of Jennifer.
Gen, Genifer, Ginnifer

Genovieve (French) a form of
Genevieve.
Genoveva, Genoveve, Genovive

Georgeanna (English) a com-
bination of Georgia + Anna.
Georgana, Georganna,
Georgeana, Georgiana,
Georgianna, Georgyanna,
Giorgianna

Georgeanne (English) a combination of Georgia + Anne.
Georgann, Georganne, Georgean, Georgeann, Georgie, Georgyann, Georgyanne

Georgene (English) a familiar form of Georgia.
Georgeena, Georgeina, Georgena, Georgenia, Georgiena, Georgienne, Georgina, Georgine

Georgette (French) a form of Georgia.
Georgeta, Georgett, Georgetta, Georjetta

Georgia (Greek) farmer. Art: Georgia O'Keeffe was an American painter known especially for her paintings of flowers. Geography: a southern American state; a country in Eastern Europe. See also Jirina, Jorja.
Georgene, Georgette, Georgie, Giorgia

Georgianna (English) a form of Georgeanna.
Georgiana, Georgiann, Georgianne, Georgie, Georgieann, Georgionna

Georgie (English) a familiar form of Georgeanne, Georgia, Georgianna.
Georgi, Georgy, Giorgi

Georgina (English) a form of Georgia.
Georgena, Georgene, Georgine, Giorgina, Jorgina

Geraldine (German) mighty with a spear. See also Dena, Jeraldine.
Geralda, Geraldina, Geraldyna, Geraldyne, Gerhardine, Geri, Gerianna, Gerianne, Gerrilee, Giralda

Geralyn (American) a combination of Geraldine + Lynn.
Geralisha, Geralynn, Gerilyn, Gerrilyn

Gerardo (English) brave spearwoman.
Gerardine

Gerda (Norwegian) protector. (German) a familiar form of Gertrude.
Gerta

Geri (American) a familiar form of Geraldine. See also Jeri.
Gerri, Gerrie, Gerry

Germaine (French) from Germany. See also Jermaine.
Germain, Germana, Germanee, Germani, Germanie, Germaya, Germine

Gertie (German) a familiar form of Gertrude.
Gert, Gertey, Gerti, Gerty

Gertrude (German) beloved warrior. See also Trudy.
Gerda, Gerta, Gertie, Gertina, Gertraud, Gertrud, Gertruda

Gervaise (French) skilled with a spear.

Gessica (Italian) a form of Jessica.
Gesica, Gesika, Gess, Gesse, Gessy

Geva (Hebrew) hill.
Gevah

Ghada (Arabic) young; tender.
Gada

Ghita (Italian) pearly.
Gita

Gianna (Italian) a short form of Giovanna. See also Jianna, Johana.
Geona, Geonna, Giana, Gianella, Gianetta, Gianina, Gianinna, Gianne, Giannee, Giannella, Giannetta, Gianni, Giannie, Giannina, Gianny, Gianoula

Gigi (French) a familiar form of Gilberte.
Geegee, G. G., Giggi

Gilana (Hebrew) joyful.
Gila, Gilah

Gilberte (German) brilliant; pledge; trustworthy. See also Berti.
Gigi, Gilberta, Gilbertina, Gilbertine, Gill

Gilda (English) covered with gold.
Gilde, Gildi, Gildie, Gildy

Gill (Latin, German) a short form of Gilberte, Gillian.
Gili, Gilli, Gillie, Gilly

Gillian (Latin) a form of Jillian.
Gila, Gilana, Gilenia, Gili, Gilian, Gill, Gilliana, Gilliane, Gilliann, Gillianna, Gillianne, Gillie, Gilly, Gillyan, Gillyane, Gillyann, Gillyanne, Gyllian, Lian

Gin (Japanese) silver. A short form of names beginning with "Gin."

Gina (Italian) a short form of Angelina, Eugenia, Regina, Virginia. See also Jina.
Gena, Gin, Ginah, Ginai, Ginna

Ginette (English) a form of Genevieve.
Gin, Ginata, Ginett, Ginetta, Ginnetta, Ginnette

Ginger (Latin) flower; spice. A familiar form of Virginia.
Gin, Ginja, Ginjer, Ginny

Ginia (Latin) a familiar form of Virginia.
Gin

Ginnifer (English) white; smooth; soft. (Welsh) a form of Jennifer.
Gin, Ginifer

Ginny (English) a familiar form of Ginger, Virginia. See also Jin, Jinny.
Gin, Gini, Ginney, Ginni, Ginnie, Giny, Gionni, Gionny

Giordana (Italian) a form of Jordana.

Giorgianna (English) a form of Georgeanna.
Giorgina

Giovanna (Italian) a form of Jane.
Geovana, Geovanna, Geovonna, Giavanna, Giavonna, Giovana, Giovanne, Giovanni, Giovannica, Giovonna, Givonnie, Jeveny

Gisa (Hebrew) carved stone.
Gazit, Gissa

Gisela (German) a form of Giselle.
Gisella, Gissela, Gissella

Giselle (German) pledge; hostage. See also Jizelle.
Ghisele, Gisel, Gisela, Gisele, Geséle, Giseli, Gisell, Gissell, Gisselle, Gizela, Gysell

Gissel, Gisselle (German) forms of Giselle.
Gissell

Gita (Yiddish) good. (Polish) a short form of Margaret.
Gitka, Gitta, Gituska

Gitana (Spanish) gypsy; wanderer.

Gitta (Irish) a short form of Bridget.
Getta

Giulia (Italian) a form of Julia.
Giulana, Giuliana, Giulianna, Giulliana, Guila, Guiliana, Guilietta

Gizela (Czech) a form of Giselle.
Gizel, Gizele, Gizella, Gizelle, Gizi, Giziki, Gizus

Gladis (Irish) a form of Gladys.
Gladi, Gladiz

Gladys (Latin) small sword. (Irish) princess. (Welsh) a form of Claudia.
Glad, Gladis, Gladness, Gladwys, Glady, Gwladys

Glenda (Welsh) a form of Glenna.
Glanda, Glennda, Glynda

Glenna (Irish) valley, glen. See also Glynnis.
Glenda, Glenetta, Glenina, Glenine, Glenn, Glenne, Glennesha, Glennia, Glennie, Glenora, Gleny, Glyn

Glennesha (American) a form of Glenna.
Glenesha, Glenisha, Glennisha, Glennishia

Gloria (Latin) glory. History: Gloria Steinem, a leading American feminist, founded *Ms.* magazine.
Gloresha, Gloriah, Gloribel,

Gloria *(cont.)*
Gloriela, Gloriella, Glorielle,
Gloris, Glorisha, Glorvina, Glory

Glorianne (American) a com-
bination of Gloria + Anne.
Gloriana, Gloriane, Gloriann,
Glorianna

Glory (Latin) a form of Gloria.

Glynnis (Welsh) a form of
Glenna.
Glenice, Glenis, Glenise,
Glenyse, Glennis, Glennys,
Glenwys, Glenys, Glenyss,
Glinnis, Glinys, Glynesha,
Glynice, Glynis, Glynisha,
Glyniss, Glynitra, Glynys,
Glynyss

Golda (English) gold. History:
Golda Meir was a Russian-
born politician who served
as prime minister of Israel.
Goldarina, Golden, Goldie,
Goldina

Goldie (English) a familiar
form of Golda.
Goldi, Goldy

Goma (Swahili) joyful dance.

Grace (Latin) graceful.
Engracia, Graca, Gracia, Gracie,
Graciela, Graciella, Gracinha,
Graice, Grata, Gratia, Gray,
Grayce, Grecia

Graceanne (English) a combination of Grace + Anne.
Graceann, Graceanna, Gracen,

Graciana, Gracianna, Gracin,
Gratiana

Gracia (Spanish) a form of
Grace.
Gracea, Grecia

Gracie (English) a familiar
form of Grace.
Gracee, Gracey, Graci, Gracy,
Graecie, Graysie

Grant (English) great; giving.

Grayson (English) bailiff's
child.
Graison, Graisyn, Grasien,
Grasyn, Graysen

Grazia (Latin) a form of
Grace.
Graziella, Grazielle, Graziosa,
Grazyna

Grecia (Latin) a form of
Grace.

Greer (Scottish) vigilant.
Grear, Grier

Greta (German) a short form
of Gretchen, Margaret.
Greatal, Greatel, Greeta,
Gretal, Grete, Gretel, Gretha,
Grethal, Grethe, Grethel,
Gretta, Grette, Grieta, Gryta,
Grytta

Gretchen (German) a form of
Margaret.
Greta, Gretchin, Gretchyn

Gricelda (German) a form of
Griselda.
Gricelle

Grisel (German) a short form
of Griselda.
Grisell, Griselle, Grissel,
Grissele, Grissell, Grizel

Griselda (German) gray
woman warrior. See also
Selda, Zelda.
Gricelda, Grisel, Griseldis,
Griseldys, Griselys, Grishilda,
Grishilde, Grisselda, Grissely,
Grizelda

Guadalupe (Arabic) river of
black stones. See also Lupe.
Guadalup, Guadelupe,
Guadlupe, Guadulupe,
Gudalupe

Gudrun (Scandinavian) battler.
See also Runa.
Gudren, Gudrin, Gudrinn,
Gudruna

Guillerma (Spanish) a short
form of Guillermina.
Guilla, Guillermina

Guinevere (French, Welsh)
white wave; white phantom.
Literature: the wife of King
Arthur. See also Gayna,
Genevieve, Genevra, Jennifer,
Winifred, Wynne.
Generva, Genn, Ginette,
Guenevere, Guenna, Guinivere,
Guinna, Gwen, Gwenevere,
Gwenivere, Gwynnevere

Gunda (Norwegian) female
warrior.
Gundala, Gunta

Gurit (Hebrew) innocent baby.

Gurleen (Sikh) follower of the
guru.

Gurpreet (Punjabi) religion.
Gurprit

Gusta (Latin) a short form of
Augusta.
Gus, Gussi, Gussie, Gussy,
Gusti, Gustie, Gusty

Gwen (Welsh) a short form of
Guinevere, Gwendolyn.
Gwenesha, Gweness, Gweneta,
Gwenetta, Gwenette, Gweni,
Gwenisha, Gwenita, Gwenn,
Gwenna, Gwennie, Gwenny

Gwenda (Welsh) a familiar
form of Gwendolyn.
Gwinda, Gwynda, Gwynedd

Gwendolyn (Welsh) white
wave; white browed; new
moon. Literature:
Gwendoloena was the wife
of Merlin, the magician. See
also Genevieve, Gwyneth,
Wendy.
Guendolen, Gwen, Gwendalin,
Gwenda, Gwendalee,
Gwendaline, Gwendalyn,
Gwendalynn, Gwendela,
Gwendelyn, Gwendelynn,
Gwendilyn, Gwendolen,
Gwendolene, Gwendolin,
Gwendoline, Gwendolyne,
Gwendolynn, Gwendolynne,
Gwendylan, Gwyndolyn,
Gwynndolen

Gwyn (Welsh) a short form of Gwyneth.
Gwinn, Gwinne, Gwynn, Gwynne

Gwyneth (Welsh) a form of Gwendolyn. See also Winnie, Wynne.
Gweneth, Gwenith, Gwenneth, Gwennyth, Gwenyth, Gwyn, Gwynneth

Gypsy (English) wanderer.
Gipsy, Gypsie, Jipsi

H

Habiba (Arabic) beloved.
Habibah, Habibeh

Hachi (Japanese) eight; good luck.
Hachiko, Hachiyo

Hadara (Hebrew) adorned with beauty.
Hadarah

Hadassah (Hebrew) myrtle tree.
Hadas, Hadasah, Hadassa, Haddasa, Haddasah

Hadiya (Swahili) gift.
Hadaya, Hadia, Hadiyah, Hadiyyah

Hadley (English) field of heather.
Hadlea, Hadlee, Hadleigh, Hadli, Hadlie, Hadly

Hadriane (Greek, Latin) a form of Adrienne.
Hadriana, Hadrianna, Hadrianne, Hadriene, Hadrienne

Haeley (English) a form of Hailey.
Haelee, Haeleigh, Haeli, Haelie, Haelleigh, Haelli, Haellie, Haely

Hagar (Hebrew) forsaken; stranger. Bible: Sarah's handmaiden, the mother of Ishmael.
Haggar

Haidee (Greek) modest.
Hady, Haide, Haidi, Haidy, Haydee, Haydy

Haiden (English) heather-covered hill.
Haden, Hadyn, Haeden, Haidn, Haidyn

Hailee (English) a form of Hayley.
Haile, Hailei, Haileigh, Haillee

Hailey (English) a form of Hayley.
Haeley, Haiely, Hailea, Hailley, Hailly, Haily

Haili, Hailie (English) forms of Hayley.
Haille, Hailli, Haillie

Haldana (Norwegian) half-Danish.

Halee (English) a form of Haley.
Hale, Halea, Haleah, Haleh, Halei

Haleigh (English) a form of Haley.

Haley (Scandinavian) heroine. See also Hailey, Hayley.
Halee, Haleigh, Hali, Halley, Hallie, Haly, Halye

Hali, Halie (English) forms of Haley.
Haliegh

Halia (Hawaiian) in loving memory.

Halimah (Arabic) gentle; patient.
Halima, Halime

Halina (Hawaiian) likeness. (Russian) a form of Helen.
Haleen, Haleena, Halena, Halinka

Halla (African) unexpected gift.
Hala, Hallah, Halle

Halley (English) a form of Haley.
Hally, Hallye

Hallie (Scandinavian) a form of Haley.
Hallee, Hallei, Halleigh, Halli

Halona (Native American) fortunate.
Halonah, Haloona, Haona

Halsey (English) Hall's island.
Halsea, Halsie

Hama (Japanese) shore.

Hana, Hanah (Japanese) flower. (Arabic) happiness. (Slavic) forms of Hannah.
Hanae, Hanan, Haneen, Hanicka, Hanin, Hanita, Hanka

Hanako (Japanese) flower child.

Hania (Hebrew) resting place.
Haniya, Hanja, Hannia, Hanniah, Hanya

Hanna (Hebrew) a form of Hannah.

Hannah (Hebrew) gracious. Bible: the mother of Samuel. See also Anci, Anezka, Ania, Anka, Ann, Anna, Annalie, Anneka, Chana, Nina, Nusi.
Hana, Hanna, Hanneke, Hannele, Hanni, Hannon, Honna

Hanni (Hebrew) a familiar form of Hannah.
Hani, Hanne, Hannie, Hanny

Happy (English) happy.
Happi

Hara (Hindi) tawny. Religion: another name for the Hindu god Shiva, the destroyer.

Harlee, Harleigh, Harlie (English) forms of Harley.
Harlei, Harli

Harley (English) meadow of
the hare. See also Arleigh.
Harlee, Harleey, Harly

Harleyann (English) a combi-
nation of Harley + Ann.
*Harlann, Harlanna, Harlanne,
Harleen, Harlene, Harleyanna,
Harleyanne, Harliann,
Harlianna, Harlianne, Harlina,
Harline*

Harmony (Latin) harmonious.
*Harmene, Harmeni, Harmon,
Harmonee, Harmonei,
Harmoni, Harmonia, Harmonie*

Harpreet (Punjabi) devoted to
God.
Harprit

Harriet (French) ruler of the
household. (English) a form
of Henrietta. Literature:
Harriet Beecher Stowe was
an American writer noted
for her novel *Uncle Tom's
Cabin*.
*Harri, Harrie, Harriett,
Harrietta, Harriette, Harriot,
Harriott, Hattie*

Haru (Japanese) spring.

Hasana (Swahili) she arrived
first. Culture: a name used
for the first-born female
twin. See also Huseina.
*Hasanna, Hasna, Hassana,
Hassna, Hassona*

Hasina (Swahili) good.
Haseena, Hasena, Hassina

Hateya (Moquelumnan) foot-
prints.

Hattie (English) familiar forms
of Harriet, Henrietta.
*Hatti, Hatty, Hetti, Hettie,
Hetty*

Hausu (Moquelumnan) like a
bear yawning upon awaken-
ing.

Hava (Hebrew) a form of
Chava. See also Eve.
Havah, Havvah

Haven (English) a form of
Heaven.
*Havan, Havana, Havanna,
Havannah, Havyn*

Haviva (Hebrew) beloved.
Havalee, Havelah, Havi, Hayah

Hayden (English) a form of
Haiden.
*Hayde, Haydin, Haydn,
Haydon*

Hayfa (Arabic) shapely.

Haylee, Hayleigh, Haylie
(English) forms of Hayley.
*Hayle, Haylea, Haylei, Hayli,
Haylle, Hayllie*

Hayley (English) hay meadow.
See also Hailey, Haley.
Hailee, Haili, Haylee, Hayly

Hazel (English) hazelnut tree;
commanding authority.
*Hazal, Hazaline, Haze,
Hazeline, Hazell, Hazelle,
Hazen, Hazyl*

Heather (English) flowering heather.
Heath, Heatherlee, Heatherly

Heaven (English) place of beauty and happiness. Bible: where God and angels are said to dwell.
Haven, Heavan, Heavenly, Heavin, Heavon, Heavyn, Hevean, Heven, Hevin

Hedda (German) battler. See also Edda, Hedy.
Heda, Hedaya, Hedia, Hedvick, Hedvig, Hedvika, Hedwig, Hedwiga, Heida, Hetta

Hedy (Greek) delightful; sweet. (German) a familiar form of Hedda.
Heddey, Heddi, Heddie, Heddy, Hede, Hedi

Heidi, Heidy (German) short forms of Adelaide.
Heida, Heide, Heidee, Heidie, Heydy, Hidee, Hidi, Hidie, Hidy, Hiede, Hiedi, Hydi

Helen (Greek) light. See also Aileen, Aili, Alena, Eileen, Elaina, Elaine, Eleanor, Ellen, Galina, Ila, Ilene, Ilona, Jelena, Leanore, Leena, Lelya, Lenci, Lene, Liolya, Nellie, Nitsa, Olena, Onella, Yalena, Yelena.
Elana, Ena, Halina, Hela, Hele, Helena, Helene, Helle, Hellen, Helli, Hellin, Hellon, Hellyn, Helon

Helena (Greek) a form of Helen. See also Ilena.
Halena, Halina, Helaina, Helana, Helania, Helayna, Heleana, Heleena, Helenia, Helenka, Helenna, Helina, Hellanna, Hellena, Hellenna, Helona, Helonna

Helene (French) a form of Helen.
Helaine, Helanie, Helayne, Heleen, Heleine, Héléne, Helenor, Heline, Hellenor

Helga (German) pious. (Scandinavian) a form of Olga. See also Elga.

Helki (Native American) touched.
Helkey, Helkie, Helky

Helma (German) a short form of Wilhelmina.
Halma, Helme, Helmi, Helmine, Hilma

Heloise (French) a form of Louise.
Héloïse, Hlois

Helsa (Danish) a form of Elizabeth.
Helse, Helsey, Helsi, Helsie, Helsy

Heltu (Moquelumnan) like a bear reaching out.

Henna (English) a familiar form of Henrietta.
Hena, Henaa, Henah, Heni, Henia, Henny, Henya

Henrietta (English) ruler of the household. See also Enrica, Etta, Yetta.
Harriet, Hattie, Hatty, Hendrika, Heneretta, Henka, Henna, Hennrietta, Hennriette, Henretta, Henrica, Henrie, Henrieta, Henriete, Henriette, Henrika, Henrique, Henriquetta, Henryetta, Hetta, Hettie

Hera (Greek) queen; jealous. Mythology: the queen of heaven and the wife of Zeus.

Hermia (Greek) messenger.

Hermina (Latin) noble. (German) soldier. See also Erma, Ermine, Irma.
Herma, Hermenia, Hermia, Herminna

Hermione (Greek) earthy.
Hermalina, Hermia, Hermina, Hermine, Herminia

Hermosa (Spanish) beautiful.

Hertha (English) child of the earth.
Heartha, Hirtha

Hester (Dutch) a form of Esther.
Hessi, Hessie, Hessye, Hesther, Hettie

Hestia (Persian) star. Mythology: the Greek goddess of the hearth and home.
Hestea, Hesti, Hestie, Hesty

Heta (Native American) racer.

Hetta (German) a form of Hedda. (English) a familiar form of Henrietta.

Hettie (German) a familiar form of Henrietta, Hester.
Hetti, Hetty

Hilary, Hillary (Greek) cheerful, merry. See also Alair.
Hilaree, Hilari, Hilaria, Hilarie, Hilery, Hiliary, Hillaree, Hillari, Hillarie, Hilleary, Hilleree, Hilleri, Hillerie, Hillery, Hillianne, Hilliary, Hillory

Hilda (German) a short form of Brunhilda, Hildegarde.
Helle, Hilde, Hildey, Hildie, Hildur, Hildy, Hulda, Hylda

Hildegarde (German) fortress.
Hilda, Hildagard, Hildagarde, Hildegard, Hildred

Hinda (Hebrew) hind; doe.
Hindey, Hindie, Hindy, Hynda

Hisa (Japanese) long lasting.
Hisae, Hisako, Hisay

Hiti (Eskimo) hyena.
Hitty

Hoa (Vietnamese) flower; peace.
Ho, Hoai

Hola (Hopi) seed-filled club.

Holley (English) a form of Holly.
Holleah, Hollee

Holli, Hollie (English) forms of Holly.
Holeigh, Holleigh

Hollis (English) near the holly bushes.
Hollise, Hollyce, Holyce

Holly (English) holly tree.
Holley, Holli, Hollie, Hollye

Hollyann (English) a combination of Holly + Ann.
Holliann, Hollianna, Hollianne, Hollyanne, Hollyn

Hollyn (English) a short form of Hollyann.
Holin, Holeena, Hollina, Hollynn

Honey (English) sweet. (Latin) a familiar form of Honora.
Honalee, Hunney, Hunny

Hong (Vietnamese) pink.

Honora (Latin) honorable. See also Nora, Onora.
Honey, Honner, Honnor, Honnour, Honor, Honorah, Honorata, Honore, Honoree, Honoria, Honorina, Honorine, Honour, Honoure

Hope (English) hope.
Hopey, Hopi, Hopie

Hortense (Latin) gardener. See also Ortensia.
Hortencia, Hortensia

Hoshi (Japanese) star.
Hoshie, Hoshiko, Hoshiyo

Hua (Chinese) flower.

Huata (Moquelumnan) basket carrier.

Hunter (English) hunter.
Hunta, Huntar, Huntter

Huong (Vietnamese) flower.

Huseina (Swahili) a form of Hasana.

Hyacinth (Greek) Botany: a plant with colorful, fragrant flowers. See also Cynthia, Jacinda.
Giacinta, Hyacintha, Hyacinthe, Hyacinthia, Hyacinthie, Hycinth, Hycynth

Hydi, Hydeia (German) forms of Heidi.
Hyde, Hydea, Hydee, Hydia, Hydie, Hydiea

Hye (Korean) graceful.

I

Ian (Hebrew) God is gracious.
Iaian, Iain, Iana, Iann, Ianna, Iannel, Iyana

Ianthe (Greek) violet flower.
Iantha, Ianthia, Ianthina

Icess (Egyptian) a form of Isis.
Ices, Icesis, Icesse, Icey, Icia, Icis, Icy

Ida (German) hard working.
(English) prosperous.
Idah, Idaia, Idalia, Idalis, Idaly,
Idamae, Idania, Idarina, Idarine,
Idaya, Ide, Idelle, Idette, Idys

Idalina (English) a combination of Ida + Lina.
Idaleena, Idaleene, Idalena,
Idalene, Idaline

Idalis (English) a form of Ida.
Idalesse, Idalise, Idaliz, Idallas,
Idallis, Idelis, Idelys, Idialis

Ideashia (American) a combination of Ida + Iesha.
Idasha, Idaysha, Ideesha, Idesha

Idelle (Welsh) a form of Ida.
Idell, Idella, Idil

Iesha (American) a form of Aisha.
Ieachia, Ieaisha, Ieasha, Ieashe,
Ieesha, Ieeshia, Ieisha, Ieishia,
Iescha, Ieshah, Ieshea, Iesheia,
Ieshia, Iiesha, Iisha

Ignacia (Latin) fiery, ardent.
Ignacie, Ignasha, Ignashia,
Ignatia, Ignatzia

Ikia (Hebrew) God is my salvation. (Hawaiian) a form of Isaiah (see Boys' Names).
Ikaisha, Ikea, Ikeea, Ikeia,
Ikeisha, Ikeishi, Ikeishia, Ikesha,
Ikeshia, Ikeya, Ikeyia, Ikiea,
Ikiia

Ila (Hungarian) a form of Helen.

Ilana (Hebrew) tree.
Ilaina, Ilane, Ilani, Ilania,
Ilainie, Illana, Illane, Illani,
Ilania, Illanie, Ilanit

Ileana (Hebrew) a form of Iliana.
Ilea, Ileah, Ileane, Ileanna,
Ileanne, Illeana

Ilena (Greek) a form of Helena.
Ileana, Ileena, Ileina, Ilina, Ilyna

Ilene (Irish) a form of Helen.
See also Aileen, Eileen.
Ileen, Ileene, Iline, Ilyne

Iliana (Greek) from Troy.
Ileana, Ili, Ilia, Iliani, Illiana,
Illiani, Illianna, Illyana, Illyanna

Ilima (Hawaiian) flower of Oahu.

Ilisa (Scottish, English) a form of Alisa, Elisa.
Ilicia, Ilissa, Iliza, Illisa, Illissa,
Illysa, Illyssa, Ilycia, Ilysa, Ilysia,
Ilyssa, Ilyza

Ilise (German) a form of Elise.
Ilese, Illytse, Ilyce, Ilyse

Ilisha (Hebrew) a form of Alisha, Elisha. See also Lisha.
Ileshia, Ilishia, Ilysha, Ilyshia

Ilka (Hungarian) a familiar form of Ilona.
Ilke, Milka, Milke

Ilona (Hungarian) a form of Helen.
Ilka, Illona, Illonia, Illonya,
Ilonka, Ilyona

Ilse (German) a form of
Elizabeth. See also Elsa.
Ilsa, Ilsey, Ilsie, Ilsy

Ima (Japanese) presently.
(German) a familiar form of
Amelia.

Imala (Native American)
strong-minded.

Iman (Arabic) believer.
Aman, Imana, Imane, Imani

Imani (Arabic) a form of
Iman.
*Amani, Emani, Imahni, Imanie,
Imanii, Imonee, Imoni*

Imelda (German) warrior.
Imalda, Irmhilde, Melda

Imena (African) dream.
Imee, Imene

Imogene (Latin) image, like-
ness.
*Emogen, Emogene, Imogen,
Imogenia, Imojean, Imojeen,
Innogen, Innogene*

Ina (Irish) a form of Agnes.
Ena, Inanna, Inanne

India (Hindi) from India.
*Indea, Indeah, Indee, Indeia,
Indeya, Indi, Indiah, Indian,
Indiana, Indianna, Indie,
Indieya, Indiya, Indy, Indya*

Indigo (Latin) dark blue color.
Indiga, Indygo

Indira (Hindi) splendid.
History: Indira Nehru Gandhi
was an Indian politician and
prime minister.
Indiara, Indra, Indre, Indria

Ines, Inez (Spanish) forms of
Agnes. See also Ynez.
*Inés, Inesa, Inesita, Inésita,
Inessa*

Inga (Scandinavian) a short
form of Ingrid.
*Ingaberg, Ingaborg, Inge,
Ingeberg, Ingeborg, Ingela*

Ingrid (Scandinavian) hero's
daughter; beautiful daughter.
Inga, Inger

Inoa (Hawaiian) name.

Ioana (Romanian) a form of
Joan.
Ioani, Ioanna

Iola (Greek) dawn; violet col-
ored. (Welsh) worthy of the
Lord.
Iole, Iolee, Iolia

Iolana (Hawaiian) soaring like
a hawk.

Iolanthe (English) a form of
Yolanda. See also Jolanda.
Iolanda, Iolande

Iona (Greek) violet flower.
*Ione, Ioney, Ioni, Ionia, Iyona,
Iyonna*

Iphigenia (Greek) sacrifice.
Mythology: the daughter of
the Greek leader
Agamemnon. See also Gena.

Irene (Greek) peaceful.
Mythology: the goddess of
peace. See also Orina, Rena,
Rene, Yarina.
Irén, Irien, Irina, Jereni

Irina (Russian) a form of
Irene.
*Eirena, Erena, Ira, Irana,
Iranda, Iranna, Irena, Irenea,
Irenka, Iriana, Irin, Irinia,
Irinka, Irona, Ironka, Irusya,
Iryna, Irynka, Rina*

Iris (Greek) rainbow.
Mythology: the goddess of
the rainbow and messenger
of the gods.
*Irisa, Irisha, Irissa, Irita, Irys,
Iryssa*

Irma (Latin) a form of Erma.
Irmina, Irminia

Isabeau (French) a form of
Isabel.

Isabel (Spanish) consecrated
to God. See also Bel, Belle,
Chavella, Ysabel.
*Isabal, Isabeau, Isabeli, Isabelita,
Isabella, Isabelle, Ishbel, Isobel,
Issie, Izabel, Izabele, Izabella*

Isabella (Italian) a form of
Isabel.
Isabela, Isabelia, Isabello

Isabelle (French) a form of
Isabel.
Isabele, Isabell

Isadora (Latin) gift of Isis.
Isidora

Isela (Scottish) a form of Isla.
Isel

Isha (American) a form of
Aisha.
*Ishae, Ishana, Ishanaa, Ishanda,
Ishanee, Ishaney, Ishani,
Ishanna, Ishaun, Ishawna,
Ishaya, Ishenda, Ishia, Iysha*

Ishi (Japanese) rock.
Ishiko, Ishiyo, Shiko, Shiyo

Isis (Egyptian) supreme goddess. Mythology: the goddess
of nature and fertility.
Icess, Issis, Isys

Isla (Scottish) Geography: the
River Isla is in Scotland.
Isela

Isobel (Spanish) a form of
Isabel.
Isobell, Isobella, Isobelle

Isoka (Benin) gift from god.
Soka

Isolde (Welsh) fair lady.
Literature: a princess in the
Arthurian legends; a heroine
in the medieval romance
Tristan and Isolde. See also
Yseult.
Isolda, Isolt, Izolde

Issie (Spanish) a familiar form
of Isabel.
Isa, Issi, Issy, Iza

Ita (Irish) thirsty.

Italia (Italian) from Italy.
Itali, Italie, Italy, Italya

Itamar (Hebrew) palm island.
*Isamar, Isamari, Isamaria,
Ithamar, Ittamar*

Itzel (Spanish) protected.
*Itcel, Itchel, Itesel, Itsel, Itssel,
Itza, Itzallana, Itzayana, Itzell,
Ixchel*

Iva (Slavic) a short form of Ivana.
Ivah

Ivana (Slavic) God is gracious.
See also Yvanna.
*Iva, Ivanah, Ivania, Ivanka,
Ivanna, Ivannia, Ivany*

Iverem (Tiv) good fortune;
blessing.

Iverna (Latin) from Ireland.
Ivernah

Ivette (French) a form of
Yvette. See also Evette.
*Ivet, Ivete, Iveth, Ivetha, Ivett,
Ivetta*

Ivonne (French) a form of
Yvonne. See also Evonne.
*Ivon, Ivona, Ivone, Ivonna,
Iwona, Iwonka, Iwonna, Iwonne*

Ivory (Latin) made of ivory.
Ivoory, Ivori, Ivorie, Ivorine, Ivree

Ivria (Hebrew) from the land
of Abraham.
Ivriah, Ivrit

Ivy (English) ivy tree.
Ivey, Ivie

Iyabo (Yoruba) mother has
returned.

Iyana, Iyanna (Hebrew) forms
of Ian.
Iyanah, Iyannah, Iyannia

Izabella (Spanish) a form of
Isabel.
*Izabela, Izabell, Izabellah,
Izabelle, Izobella*

Izusa (Native American) white
stone.

J

Jabrea, Jabria (American)
combinations of the prefix Ja
+ Brea.
*Jabreal, Jabree, Jabreea, Jabreena,
Jabrelle, Jabreona, Jabri, Jabriah,
Jabriana, Jabrie, Jabriel, Jabrielle,
Jabrienna, Jabrina*

Jacalyn (American) a form of
Jacqueline.
*Jacalynn, Jacolyn, Jacolyne,
Jacolynn*

Jacelyn (American) a form of
Jocelyn.
*Jaceline, Jacelyne, Jacelynn,
Jacilyn, Jacilyne, Jacilynn,
Jacylyn, Jacylyne, Jacylynn*

Jacey, Jacy (Greek) familiar forms of Jacinda. (American) combinations of the initials J. + C.
Jace, Jac-E, Jacee, Jaci, Jacie, Jacylin, Jaice, Jaicee

Jaci, Jacie (Greek) forms of Jacey.
Jacci, Jacia, Jacie, Jaciel, Jaici, Jaicie

Jacinda, Jacinta (Greek) beautiful, attractive. (Spanish) forms of Hyacinth.
Jacenda, Jacenta, Jacey, Jacinthe, Jacintia, Jacynthe, Jakinda, Jaxine

Jacinthe (Spanish) a form of Jacinda.
Jacinte, Jacinth, Jacintha

Jackalyn (American) a form of Jacqueline.
Jackalene, Jackalin, Jackaline, Jackalynn, Jackalynne, Jackelin, Jackeline, Jackelyn, Jackelynn, Jackelynne, Jackilin, Jackilyn, Jackilynn, Jackilynne, Jackolin, Jackoline, Jackolyn, Jackolynn, Jackolynne

Jackeline, Jackelyn (American) forms of Jacqueline.
Jackelin, Jackelline, Jackellyn, Jockeline

Jacki, Jackie (American) familiar forms of Jacqueline.
Jackee, Jackey, Jackia, Jackielee, Jacky, Jackye

Jacklyn (American) a form of Jacqueline.
Jacklin, Jackline, Jacklyne, Jacklynn, Jacklynne

Jackquel (French) a short form of Jacqueline.
Jackqueline, Jackquetta, Jackquiline, Jackquilyn, Jackquilynn, Jackquilynne

Jaclyn (American) a short form of Jacqueline.
Jacleen, Jaclin, Jacline, Jaclyne, Jaclynn

Jacobi (Hebrew) supplanter, substitute. Bible: Jacob was the son of Isaac, brother of Esau.
Coby, Jacoba, Jacobee, Jacobette, Jacobia, Jacobina, Jacoby, Jacolbi, Jacolbia, Jacolby

Jacqualine (French) a form of Jacqueline.
Jacqualin, Jacqualine, Jacqualyn, Jacqualyne, Jacqualynn

Jacquelin (French) a form of Jacqueline.
Jacquelina

Jacqueline (French) supplanter, substitute; little Jacqui.
Jacalyn, Jackalyn, Jackeline, Jacki, Jacklyn, Jackquel, Jaclyn, Jacqueena, Jacqueine, Jacquel, Jacqueleen, Jacquelene, Jacquelin, Jacquelyn, Jacquelynn, Jacquena, Jacquene, Jacquenetta, Jacquenette, Jacqui, Jacquiline, Jacquine, Jakelin, Jaquelin, Jaqueline, Jaquelyn, Jocqueline

Jacquelyn, Jacquelynn
(French) forms of Jacqueline.
Jackquelyn, Jackquelynn,
Jacquelyne, Jacquelynne

Jacqui (French) a short form
of Jacqueline.
Jacquay, Jacqué, Jacquee,
Jacqueta, Jacquete, Jacquetta,
Jacquette, Jacquie, Jacquise,
Jacquita, Jaquay, Jaqui, Jaquie,
Jaquiese, Jaquina, Jaquita

Jacqulin, Jacqulyn (American)
forms of Jacqueline.
Jackquilin, Jacqul, Jacqulin,
Jacqulyne, Jacqulynn, Jacqulynne,
Jacquoline

Jacquiline (French) a form of
Jacqueline.
Jacquil, Jacquilin, Jacquilyn,
Jacquilyne, Jacquilynn

Jacynthe (Spanish) a form of
Jacinda.
Jacynda, Jacynta, Jacynth,
Jacyntha

Jada (Spanish) a form of Jade.
Jadah, Jadda, Jadae, Jadzia,
Jadziah, Jaeda, Jaedra, Jayda

Jade (Spanish) jade.
Jada, Jadea, Jadeann, Jadee,
Jaden, Jadera, Jadi, Jadie,
Jadienne, Jady, Jadyn, Jaedra,
Jaida, Jaide, Jaiden, Jayde, Jayden

Jadelyn (American) a combi-
nation of Jade + Lynn.
Jadalyn, Jadelaine, Jadeline,
Jadelyne, Jadelynn, Jadielyn

Jaden (Spanish) a form of
Jade.
Jadeen, Jadena, Jadene, Jadeyn,
Jadin, Jadine, Jaeden, Jaedine

Jadyn (Spanish) a form of Jade.
Jadynn, Jaedyn, Jaedynn

Jae (Latin) jaybird. (French) a
familiar form of Jacqueline.
Jaea, Jaey, Jaya

Jael (Hebrew) mountain goat;
climber. See also Yael.
Jaela, Jaelee, Jaeli, Jaelie, Jaelle,
Jahla, Jahlea

Jaelyn, Jaelynn (American)
combinations of Jae + Lynn.
Jaeleen, Jaelin, Jaelinn, Jaelyn,
Jailyn, Jalyn, Jalynn, Jayleen,
Jaylyn, Jaylynn, Jaylynne

Jaffa (Hebrew) a form of Yaffa.
Jaffice, Jaffit, Jafit, Jafra

Jaha (Swahili) dignified.
Jahaida, Jahaira, Jaharra,
Jahayra, Jahida, Jahira, Jahitza

Jai (Tai) heart. (Latin) a form
of Jaye.

Jaida, Jaide (Spanish) forms of
Jade.
Jaidah, Jaidan

Jaiden, Jaidyn (Spanish) forms
of Jade.
Jaidey, Jaidi, Jaidin, Jaidon

Jailyn (American) a form of
Jaelyn.
Jaileen, Jailen, Jailene, Jailin,
Jailine

Jaime (French) I love.
Jaima, Jaimee, Jaimey, Jaimie, Jaimini, Jaimme, Jaimy, Jamee

Jaimee (French) a form of Jaime.

Jaimie (French) a form of Jaime.
Jaimi, Jaimmie

Jaira (Spanish) Jehovah teaches.
Jairah, Jairy

Jakeisha (American) a combination of Jakki + Aisha.
Jakeisia, Jakesha, Jakisha

Jakelin (American) a form of Jacqueline.
Jakeline, Jakelyn, Jakelynn, Jakelynne

Jakki (American) a form of Jacki.
Jakala, Jakea, Jakeela, Jakeida, Jakeita, Jakela, Jakelia, Jakell, Jakena, Jaketta, Jakevia, Jaki, Jakia, Jakiah, Jakira, Jakita, Jakiya, Jakiyah, Jakke, Jakkia

Jaleesa (American) a form of Jalisa.
Jaleasa, Jalece, Jalecea, Jaleesah, Jaleese, Jaleesia, Jaleisa, Jaleisha, Jaleisya

Jalena (American) a combination of Jane + Lena.
Jalaina, Jalana, Jalani, Jalanie, Jalayna, Jalean, Jaleen, Jaleena, Jaleene, Jalen, Jalene, Jalina, Jaline, Jallena, Jalyna, Jelayna, Jelena, Jelina, Jelyna

Jalesa, Jalessa (American) forms of Jalisa.
Jalese, Jalesha, Jaleshia, Jalesia

Jalia, Jalea (American) combinations of Jae + Leah.
Jaleah, Jalee, Jaleea, Jaleeya, Jaleia, Jalitza

Jalila (Arabic) great.
Jalile

Jalisa, Jalissa (American) combinations of Jae + Lisa.
Jaleesa, Jalesa, Jalise, Jalisha, Jalisia, Jalysa

Jalyn, Jalynn (American) combinations of Jae + Lynn. See also Jaylyn.
Jaelin, Jaeline, Jaelyn, Jaelyne, Jaelynn, Jaelynne, Jalin, Jaline, Jalyne, Jalynne

Jalysa (American) a form of Jalisa.
Jalyse, Jalyssa, Jalyssia

Jamaica (Spanish) Geography: an island in the Caribbean.
Jameca, Jamecia, Jameica, Jameika, Jameka, Jamica, Jamika, Jamoka, Jemaica, Jemika, Jemyka

Jamani (American) a form of Jami.
Jamana

Jamaria (American) combinations of Jae + Maria.
Jamar, Jamara, Jamarea, Jamaree, Jamari, Jamarie, Jameira, Jamerial, Jamira

Jamecia (Spanish) a form of Jamaica.

Jamee (French) a form of Jaime.

Jameika, Jameka (Spanish) forms of Jamaica.
Jamaika, Jamaka, Jamecka, Jamekia, Jamekka

Jamesha (American) a form of Jami.
Jameisha, Jamese, Jameshia, Jameshyia, Jamesia, Jamesica, Jamesika, Jamesina, Jamessa, Jameta, Jametta, Jamiesha, Jamisha, Jammesha, Jammisha

Jamey (English) a form of Jami, Jamie.

Jami, Jamie (Hebrew, English) supplanter, substitute.
Jama, Jamani, Jamay, Jamesha, Jamey, Jamia, Jamii, Jamis, Jamise, Jammie, Jamy, Jamye, Jayme, Jaymee, Jaymie

Jamia (English) a form of Jami, Jamie.
Jamea, Jamiah, Jamiea, Jamiya, Jamiyah, Jamya, Jamyah

Jamica (Spanish) a form of Jamaica.
Jamika

Jamila (Arabic) beautiful. See also Yamila.
Jahmela, Jahmelia, Jahmil, Jahmilla, Jameela, Jameelah, Jameeliah, Jameila, Jamela, Jamelia, Jameliah, Jamell, Jamella, Jamelle, Jamely, Jamelya, Jamiela, Jamielee, Jamilah, Jamilee, Jamilia, Jamiliah, Jamilla, Jamillah, Jamille, Jamillia, Jamilya, Jamyla, Jemeela, Jemelia, Jemila, Jemilla

Jamilynn (English) a combination of Jami + Lynn.
Jamielin, Jamieline, Jamielyn, Jamielyne, Jamielynn, Jamielynne, Jamilin, Jamiline, Jamilyn, Jamilyne, Jamilynne

Jammie (American) a form of Jami.
Jammi, Jammice, Jammise

Jamonica (American) a combination of Jami + Monica.
Jamoni

Jamylin (American) a form of Jamilynn.
Jamylin, Jamyline, Jamylyn, Jamylyne, Jamylynn, Jamylynne, Jaymylin, Jaymyline, Jaymylyn, Jaymylyne, Jaymylynn, Jaymylynne

Jan (English) a short form of Jane, Janet, Janice.
Jania, Jandy

Jana (Hebrew) gracious, merciful. (Slavic) a form of Jane. See also Yana.
Janalee, Janalisa, Janna, Janne

Janae, Janay (American) forms of Jane.
Janaé, Janaea, Janaeh, Janah, Janai, Janaya, Janaye, Janea, Janee, Janée, Jannae, Jannay, Jenae, Jenay, Jenaya, Jennae, Jennay, Jennaya, Jennaye

Janai (American) a form of Janae.
Janaiah, Janaira, Janaiya

Janalynn (American) a combination of Jana + Lynn.
Janalin, Janaline, Janalyn, Janalyne, Janalynne

Janan (Arabic) heart; soul.
Jananee, Janani, Jananie, Janann, Jananni

Jane (Hebrew) God is gracious. See also Chavon, Jean, Joan, Juanita, Seana, Shana, Shawna, Sheena, Shona, Shunta, Sinead, Zaneta, Zanna, Zhana.
Jaine, Jan, Jana, Janae, Janay, Janelle, Janessa, Janet, Jania, Janice, Janie, Janika, Janine, Janis, Janka, Jannie, Jasia, Jayna, Jayne, Jenica

Janel, Janell (French) forms of Janelle.
Janiel, Jannel, Jannell, Janyll, Jaynel, Jaynell

Janelle (French) a form of Jane.
Janel, Janela, Janele, Janelis, Janell, Janella, Janelli, Janellie, Janelly, Janely, Janelys, Janielle, Janille, Jannelle, Jannellies, Jaynelle

Janesha (American) a form of Janessa.
Janeisha, Janeshia, Janiesha, Janisha, Janishia, Jannesha,

Jannisha, Janysha, Jenesha, Jenisha, Jennisha

Janessa (American) a form of Jane.
Janeesa, Janesa, Janesea, Janesha, Janesia, Janeska, Janessi, Janessia, Janiesa, Janissa, Jannesa, Jannessa, Jannisa, Jannissa, Janyssa, Jenesa, Jenessa, Jenissa, Jennisa, Jennissa

Janet (English) a form of Jane. See also Jessie, Yanet.
Jan, Janeta, Janete, Janeth, Janett, Janette, Jannet, Janot, Jante, Janyte

Janeth (English) a form of Janet.
Janetha, Janith, Janneth

Janette, Jannette (French) forms of Janet.
Janett, Janetta, Jannett, Jannetta

Janice (Hebrew) God is gracious. (English) a familiar form of Jane. See also Genice.
Jan, Janece, Janecia, Janeice, Janiece, Janizzette, Jannice, Janniece, Janyce, Jenice, Jhanice, Jynice

Janie (English) a familiar form of Jane.
Janey, Jani, Janiyh, Jannie, Janny, Jany

Janika (Slavic) a form of Jane.
Janaca, Janeca, Janecka, Janeika, Janeka, Janica, Janick, Janicka,

Janieka, Janikka, Janikke, Janique, Janka, Jankia, Jannica, Jannick, Jannika, Janyca, Jenica, Jenicka, Jenika, Jeniqua, Jenique, Jennica, Jennika, Jonika

Janine (French) a form of Jane.
Janean, Janeann, Janeanne, Janeen, Janenan, Janene, Janina, Jannen, Jannina, Jannine, Jannyne, Janyne, Jeannine, Jeneen, Jenine

Janis (English) a form of Jane.
Janees, Janese, Janesey, Janess, Janesse, Janise, Jannis, Jannise, Janys, Jenesse, Jenis, Jennise, Jennisse

Janita (American) a form of Juanita. See also Genita.
Janitra, Janitza, Janneta, Jaynita, Jenita, Jennita

Janna (Arabic) harvest of fruit. (Hebrew) a short form of Johana.
Janaya, Janaye, Jannae, Jannah, Jannai

Jannie (English) a familiar form of Jan, Jane.
Janney, Janny

Jaquana (American) a combination of Jacqueline + Anna.
Jaqua, Jaquai, Jaquanda, Jaquania, Jaquanna

Jaquelen (American) a form of Jacqueline.
Jaquala, Jaquera, Jaqulene, Jaquonna

Jaquelin, Jaqueline (French) forms of Jacqueline.
Jaqualin, Jaqualine, Jaquelina, Jaquline, Jaquella

Jaquelyn (French) a form of Jacqueline.
Jaquelyne, Jaquelynn, Jaquelynne

Jardena (Hebrew) a form of Jordan. (French, Spanish) garden.
Jardan, Jardana, Jardane, Jarden, Jardenia, Jardin, Jardine, Jardyn, Jardyne

Jarian (American) a combination of Jane + Marian.

Jarita (Arabic) earthen water jug.
Jara, Jaretta, Jari, Jaria, Jarica, Jarida, Jarietta, Jarika, Jarina, Jaritta, Jaritza, Jarixa, Jarnita, Jarrika, Jarrine

Jas (American) a short form of Jasmine.
Jase, Jass, Jaz, Jazz, Jazze, Jazzi

Jasia (Polish) a form of Jane.
Jaisha, Jasa, Jasea, Jasha, Jashae, Jashala, Jashona, Jashonte, Jasie, Jassie, Jaysa

Jasleen, Jaslyn (Latin) forms of Jocelyn.
Jaslene, Jaslien, Jaslin, Jasline, Jaslynn, Jaslynne

Jasmain (Persian) a short form of Jasmine.
Jasmaine, Jasmane, Jassmain, Jassmaine

Jasmarie (American) a combination of Jasmine + Marie.
Jasmari

Jasmin (Persian) a form of Jasmine.
Jasimin, Jasman, Jasmeen, Jasmen, Jasmon, Jassmin, Jassminn

Jasmine (Persian) jasmine flower. See also Jessamine, Yasmin.
Jas, Jasma, Jasmain, Jasme, Jasmeet, Jasmene, Jasmin, Jasmina, Jasminne, Jasmira, Jasmit, Jasmyn, Jassma, Jassmin, Jassmine, Jassmit, Jassmon, Jassmyn, Jazmin, Jazmyn, Jazzmin

Jasmyn, Jasmyne (Persian) forms of Jasmine.
Jasmynn, Jasmynne, Jassmyn

Jaspreet (Punjabi) virtuous.
Jaspar, Jasparit, Jasparita, Jasper, Jasprit, Jasprita, Jasprite

Jatara (American) a combination of Jane + Tara.
Jataria, Jatarra, Jatori, Jatoria

Javana (Malayan) from Java.
Javanna, Javanne, Javona, Javonna, Jawana, Jawanna, Jawn

Javiera (Spanish) owner of a new house. See also Xaviera.
Javeera, Viera

Javona, Javonna (Malayan) forms of Javana.
Javon, Javonda, Javone, Javoni, Javonne, Javonni, Javonya

Jaya (Hindi) victory.
Jaea, Jaia

Jaycee (American) a combination of the initials J. + C.
Jacee, Jacey, Jaci, Jacie, Jacy, Jayce, Jaycey, Jayci, Jaycie, Jaycy

Jayda (Spanish) a form of Jada.
Jaydah, Jeyda

Jayde (Spanish) a form of Jade.
Jayd

Jaydee (American) a combination of the initials J. + D.
Jadee, Jadey, Jadi, Jadie, Jady, Jaydey, Jaydi, Jaydie, Jaydy

Jayden (Spanish) a form of Jade.
Jaydeen, Jaydene, Jaydin, Jaydn, Jaydon

Jaye (Latin) jaybird.
Jae, Jay

Jayla (American) a short form of Jaylene.
Jaylaa, Jaylah, Jayli, Jaylia, Jayliah, Jaylie

Jaylene (American) forms of Jaylyn.
Jayelene, Jayla, Jaylan, Jayleana, Jaylee, Jayleen, Jayleene, Jaylen, Jaylenne

Jaylin (American) a form of Jaylyn.
Jayline, Jaylinn

Jaylyn, Jaylynn (American) combinations of Jaye +

Lynn. See also Jalyn.
Jaylene, Jaylin, Jaylyne, Jaylynne

Jayme, Jaymie (English) forms
of Jami.
Jaymi, Jaymia, Jaymine, Jaymini

Jaymee, Jaymi (English) forms
of Jami.

Jayna (Hebrew) a form of Jane.
Jaynae, Jaynah, Jaynna

Jayne (Hindi) victorious.
(English) a form of Jane.
Jayn, Jaynie, Jaynne

Jaynie (English) a familiar
form of Jayne.
Jaynee, Jayni

Jazlyn (American) a combina-
tion of Jazmin + Lynn.
*Jasleen, Jazaline, Jazalyn,
Jazleen, Jazlene, Jazlin, Jazline,
Jazlon, Jazlynn, Jazlynne,
Jazzalyn, Jazzleen, Jazzlene,
Jazzlin, Jazzline, Jazzlyn,
Jazzlynn, Jazzlynne*

Jazmin, Jazmine (Persian)
forms of Jasmine.
*Jazmaine, Jazman, Jazmen,
Jazminn, Jazmon, Jazzmit*

Jazmyn, Jazmyne (Persian)
forms of Jasmine.
*Jazmynn, Jazmynne, Jazzmyn,
Jazzmyne*

Jazzmin, Jazzmine (Persian)
forms of Jasmine.
*Jazzman, Jazzmeen, Jazzmen,
Jazzmene, Jazzmenn, Jazzmon*

Jean, Jeanne (Scottish) God is
gracious. See also Kini.
*Jeana, Jeanann, Jeancie, Jeane,
Jeaneia, Jeanette, Jeaneva,
Jeanice, Jeanie, Jeanine,
Jeanmaria, Jeanmarie, Jeanna,
Jeanné, Jeannie, Jeannita,
Jeannot, Jeantelle*

Jeana, Jeanna (Scottish) forms
of Jean.
Jeanae, Jeannae, Jeannia

Jeanette, Jeannett (French)
forms of Jean.
*Jeanet, Jeanete, Jeanett, Jeanetta,
Jeanita, Jeannete, Jeannetta,
Jeannette, Jeannita, Jenet, Jenett,
Jenette, Jennet, Jennett, Jennetta,
Jennette, Jennita, Jinetta, Jinette*

Jeanie, Jeannie (Scottish)
familiar forms of Jean.
*Jeannee, Jeanney, Jeani, Jeanny,
Jeany*

Jeanine, Jenine (Scottish)
forms of Jean. See also
Geneen.
*Jeaneane, Jeaneen, Jeanene,
Jeanina, Jeannina, Jeannine,
Jennine*

Jelena (Russian) a form of
Helen. See also Yelena.
*Jalaine, Jalane, Jalani, Jalanna,
Jalayna, Jalayne, Jaleen, Jaleena,
Jaleene, Jalena, Jalene, Jelaina,
Jelaine, Jelana, Jelane, Jelani,
Jelanni, Jelayna, Jelayne, Jelean,
Jeleana, Jeleen, Jeleena, Jelene*

Jelisa (American) a combination of Jean + Lisa.
Jalissa, Jelesha, Jelessa, Jelise, Jelissa, Jellese, Jellice, Jelysa, Jelyssa, Jillisa, Jillissa, Julissa

Jem (Hebrew) a short form of Jemima.
Gem, Jemi, Jemia, Jemiah, Jemie, Jemm, Jemmi, Jemmy

Jemima (Hebrew) dove.
Jamim, Jamima, Jem, Jemimah, Jemma

Jemma (Hebrew) a short form of Jemima. (English) a form of Gemma.
Jemmia, Jemmiah, Jemmie, Jemmy

Jena, Jenae (Arabic) forms of Jenna.
Jenah, Jenai, Jenal, Jenay, Jenaya, Jenea

Jendaya (Zimbabwean) thankful.
Daya, Jenda, Jendayah

Jenelle (American) a combination of Jenny + Nell.
Genell, Jeanell, Jeanelle, Jenall, Jenalle, Jenel, Jenela, Jenele, Jenell, Jenella, Jenille, Jennel, Jennell, Jennella, Jennelle, Jennielle, Jennille, Jinelle, Jinnell

Jenessa (American) a form of Jenisa.
Jenesa, Jenese, Jenesia, Jenessia, Jennesa, Jennese, Jennessa, Jinessa

Jenica (Romanian) a form of Jane.
Jeneca, Jenika, Jenikka, Jennica, Jennika

Jenifer, Jeniffer (Welsh) forms of Jennifer.
Jenefer

Jenilee (American) a combination of Jennifer + Lee.
Jenalea, Jenalee, Jenaleigh, Jenaly, Jenelea, Jenelee, Jeneleigh, Jenely, Jenelly, Jenileigh, Jenily, Jennalee, Jennely, Jennielee, Jennilea, Jennilee, Jennilie

Jenisa (American) a combination of Jennifer + Nisa.
Jenessa, Jenisha, Jenissa, Jenisse, Jennisa, Jennise, Jennisha, Jennissa, Jennisse, Jennysa, Jennyssa, Jenysa, Jenyse, Jenyssa, Jenysse

Jenka (Czech) a form of Jane.

Jenna (Arabic) small bird. (Welsh) a short form of Jennifer. See also Gen.
Jena, Jennae, Jennah, Jennai, Jennat, Jennay, Jennaya, Jennaye, Jhenna

Jenni, Jennie (Welsh) familiar forms of Jennifer.
Jeni, Jenne, Jenné, Jennee, Jenney, Jennia, Jennier, Jennita, Jennora, Jensine

Jennifer (Welsh) white wave; white phantom. A form of Guinevere. See also Gennifer,

Ginnifer, Yenifer.
Jen, Jenifer, Jeniffer, Jenipher, Jenna, Jennafer, Jenni, Jenniferanne, Jenniferlee, Jenniffe, Jenniffer, Jenniffier, Jennifier, Jennilee, Jenniphe, Jennipher, Jenny, Jennyfer

Jennilee (American) a combination of Jenny + Lee.
Jennalea, Jennalee, Jennielee, Jennilea, Jennilie, Jinnalee

Jennilyn, Jennilynn
(American) combinations of Jenni + Lynn.
Jennalin, Jennaline, Jennalyn, Jenalynann, Jenelyn, Jenilyn, Jennalyne, Jennalynn, Jennalynne, Jennilin, Jenniline, Jennilyne, Jennilynne

Jenny (Welsh) a familiar form of Jennifer.
Jenney, Jenni, Jennie, Jeny, Jinny

Jennyfer (Welsh) a form of Jennifer.
Jenyfer

Jeraldine (English) a form of Geraldine.
Jeraldeen, Jeraldene, Jeraldina, Jeraldyne, Jeralee, Jeri

Jereni (Russian) a form of Irene.
Jerena, Jerenae, Jerina

Jeri, Jerri, Jerrie (American) short forms of Jeraldine. See also Geri.
Jera, Jerae, JeRae, Jeree, Jeriel,

Jerilee, Jerinda, Jerra, Jerrah, Jerrece, Jerree, Jerriann, Jerrilee, Jerrine, Jerry, Jerrylee, Jerryne, Jerzy

Jerica (American) a combination of Jeri + Erica.
Jereca, Jerecka, Jerice, Jericka, Jerika, Jerrica, Jerrice, Jeryka

Jerilyn (American) a combination of Jeri + Lynn.
Jeralin, Jeraline, Jeralyn, Jeralyne, Jeralynn, Jeralynne, Jerelin, Jereline, Jerelyn, Jerelyne, Jerelynn, Jerelynne, Jerilin, Jeriline, Jerilyne, Jerilynn, Jerilynne, Jerrilin, Jerriline, Jerrilyn, Jerrilyne, Jerrilynn, Jerrilynne, Jerrylea

Jermaine (French) a form of Germaine.
Jermain, Jerman, Jermanay, Jermanaye, Jermane, Jermanee, Jermani, Jermanique, Jermany, Jermayne, Jermecia, Jermia, Jermice, Jermicia, Jermika, Jermila

Jerrica (American) a form of Jerica.
Jerreka, Jerricah, Jerricca, Jerricha, Jerricka, Jerrieka, Jerrika

Jerusha (Hebrew) inheritance.
Jerushah, Yerusha

Jesenia, Jessenia (Arabic) flower.
Jescenia, Jessennia, Jessenya

Jesica, Jesika (Hebrew) forms of Jessica.
Jesicca, Jesikah, Jesikkah

Jessa (American) a short form of Jessalyn, Jessamine, Jessica.
Jesa, Jesha, Jessah

Jessalyn (American) a combination of Jessica + Lynn.
Jesalin, Jesaline, Jesalyn, Jesalyne, Jesalynn, Jesalynne, Jesilin, Jesiline, Jesilyn, Jesilyne, Jesilynn, Jesilynne, Jessa, Jessalin, Jessaline, Jessalyne, Jessalynn, Jessalynne, Jesselin, Jesseline, Jesselyn, Jesselyne, Jesselynn, Jesselynne, Jesslyn

Jessamine (French) a form of Jasmine.
Jessa, Jessamin, Jessamon, Jessamy, Jessamyn, Jessemin, Jessemine, Jessimin, Jessimine, Jessmin, Jessmine, Jessmon, Jessmy, Jessmyn

Jesse, Jessi (Hebrew) forms of Jessie.
Jese, Jesi, Jesie

Jesseca (Hebrew) a form of Jessica.

Jessica (Hebrew) wealthy. Literature: a name perhaps invented by Shakespeare for a character in his play *The Merchant of Venice*. See also Gessica, Yessica.
Jesica, Jesika, Jessa, Jessaca, Jessca, Jesscia, Jesseca, Jessia, Jessicah, Jessicca, Jessicia, Jessicka, Jessie,

Jessika, Jessiqua, Jessy, Jessyca, Jessyka, Jezeca, Jezica, Jezika, Jezyca

Jessie, Jessy (Hebrew) short forms of Jessica. (Scottish) forms of Janet.
Jescie, Jesey, Jess, Jesse, Jessé, Jessee, Jessey, Jessi, Jessia, Jessiya, Jessye

Jessika (Hebrew) a form of Jessica.
Jessieka

Jesslyn (American) a short form of Jessalyn.
Jessilyn, Jessilynn, Jesslin, Jesslynn, Jesslynne

Jessyca, Jessyka (Hebrew) forms of Jessica.

Jésusa (Hebrew, Spanish) God is my salvation.

Jetta (English) jet black mineral. (American) a familiar form of Jevette.
Jeta, Jetia, Jetje, Jette, Jettie

Jevette (American) a combination of Jean + Yvette.
Jetta, Jeva, Jeveta, Jevetta

Jewel (French) precious gem.
Jewelann, Jewelia, Jeweliana, Jeweliann, Jewelie, Jewell, Jewelle, Jewellee, Jewellene, Jewellie, Juel, Jule

Jezebel (Hebrew) unexalted; impure. Bible: the wife of King Ahab.
Jesibel, Jessabel, Jessebel, Jez,

*Jezabel, Jezabella, Jezabelle,
Jezebell, Jezebella, Jezebelle*

Jianna (Italian) a form of
Giana.
*Jiana, Jianina, Jianine, Jianni,
Jiannini*

Jibon (Hindi) life.

Jill (English) a short form of
Jillian.
Jil, Jilli, Jillie, Jilly

Jillaine (Latin) a form of
Jillian.
*Jilaine, Jilane, Jilayne, Jillana,
Jillane, Jillann, Jillanne, Jillayne*

Jilleen (Irish) a form of Jillian.
*Jileen, Jilene, Jiline, Jillene,
Jillenne, Jilline, Jillyn*

Jillian (Latin) youthful. See
also Gillian.
*Jilian, Jiliana, Jiliann, Jilianna,
Jilianne, Jilienna, Jilienne, Jill,
Jillaine, Jilliana, Jilliane, Jilliann,
Jillianne, Jileen, Jillien, Jillienne,
Jillion, Jilliyn*

Jimi (Hebrew) supplanter, sub-
stitute.
*Jimae, Jimaria, Jimee, Jimella,
Jimena, Jimia, Jimiah, Jimie,
Jimiyah, Jimmeka, Jimmet,
Jimmi, Jimmia, Jimmie*

Jimisha (American) a combi-
nation of Jimi + Aisha.
*Jimica, Jimicia, Jimmicia,
Jimysha*

Jin (Japanese) tender.
(American) a short form of
Ginny, Jinny.

Jina (Swahili) baby with a
name. (Italian) a form of
Gina.
*Jena, Jinae, Jinan, Jinda, Jinna,
Jinnae*

Jinny (Scottish) a familiar form
of Jenny. (American) a familiar form of Virginia. See also
Ginny.
Jin, Jinnee, Jinney, Jinni, Jinnie

Jirina (Czech) a form of
Georgia.
Jirah, Jireh

Jizelle (American) a form of
Giselle.
*Jessel, Jezel, Jezell, Jezella,
Jezelle, Jisel, Jisela, Jisell, Jisella,
Jiselle, Jissel, Jissell, Jissella,
Jisselle, Jizel, Jizella, Joselle*

Jo (American) a short form of
Joanna, Jolene, Josephine.
Joangie, Joetta, Joette, Joey

Joan (Hebrew) God is
gracious. History: Joan of Arc
was a fifteenth-century hero-
ine and resistance fighter. See
also Ioana, Jean, Juanita,
Siobahn.
*Joane, Joaneil, Joanel, Joanelle,
Joanie, Joanmarie, Joann,
Joannanette, Joanne, Joannel,
Joanny, Jonni*

Joana, Joanna (English) a
form of Joan. See also
Yoanna.
*Janka, Jhoana, Jo, Jo-Ana,
Joandra, Joanka, Joananna, Jo-
Anie, Joanka, Jo-Anna,
Joannah, Jo-Annie, Joeana,
Joeanna, Johana, Johanna,
Johannah*

Joanie, Joannie (Hebrew)
familiar forms of Joan.
*Joanee, Joani, Joanni, Joenie,
Johanie, Johnnie, Joni*

Joanne (English) a form of
Joan.
*Joanann, Joananne, Joann, Jo-
Ann, Jo-Anne, Joayn, Joeann,
Joeanne*

Joanny (Hebrew) a familiar
form of Joan.
Joany

Joaquina (Hebrew) God will
establish.
Joaquine

Jobeth (English) a combination of Jo + Beth.
Joby

Joby (Hebrew) afflicted.
(English) a familiar form of
Jobeth.
*Jobey, Jobi, Jobie, Jobina, Jobita,
Jobrina, Jobye, Jobyna*

Jocacia (American) a combination of Joy + Acacia.

Jocelin, Joceline (Latin) forms
of Jocelyn.
Jocelina, Jocelinn

Jocelyn (Latin) joyous. See also
Yocelin, Yoselin.
*Jacelyn, Jasleen, Jocelin, Jocelle,
Jocelyne, Jocelynn, Joci, Jocia,
Jocilyn, Jocilynn, Jocinta, Joclyn,
Joclynn, Josalyn, Joscelin, Joselin,
Joselyn, Joshlyn, Josilin, Jossalin,
Josselyn, Joycelyn*

Jocelyne (Latin) a form of
Jocelyn.
Joceline, Jocelynne, Joclynne

Jodi, Jodie, Jody (American)
familiar forms of Judith.
*Jodee, Jodele, Jodell, Jodelle,
Jodevea, Jodey, Jodia, Jodiee,
Jodilee, Jodi-Lee, Jodilynn, Jodi-
Lynn, Joedi, Joedy*

Jodiann (American) a combi-
nation of Jodi + Ann.
*Jodene, Jodi-Ann, Jodianna,
Jodi-Anna, Jodianne, Jodi-Anne,
Jodine, Jodyann, Jody-Ann,
Jodyanna, Jody-Anna, Jodyanne,
Jody-Anne, Jodyne*

Joelle (Hebrew) God is will-
ing.
*Joela, Joele, Joelee, Joeli, Joelia,
Joelie, Joell, Joella, Joëlle, Joelli,
Joelly, Joely, Joyelle*

Joelynn (American) a combi-
nation of Joelle + Lynn.
*Joeleen, Joelene, Joeline, Joellen,
Joellyn, Joelyn, Joelyne*

Johana, Johanna, Johannah
(German) forms of Joana.
Janna, Joahna, Johanah,
Johanka, Johanne, Johnna,
Johonna, Jonna, Joyhanna,
Joyhannah

Johanie, Johannie (Hebrew)
forms of Joanie.
Johani, Johanni, Johanny, Johany

Johnna, Jonna (American)
forms of Johana, Joanna.
Jahna, Jahnaya, Jhona, Jhonna,
Johna, Johnda, Johnnielynn,
Johnnie-Lynn, Johnnquia,
Joncie, Jonda, Jondrea, Jontel,
Jutta

Johnnie (Hebrew) a form of
Joanie.
Johni, Johnie, Johnni, Johnny

Johnnessa (American) a com-
bination of Johnna + Nessa.
Jahnessa, Johneatha, Johnecia,
Johnesha, Johnetra, Johnisha,
Johnishi, Johnnise, Jonyssa

Joi (Latin) a form of Joy.
Joia, Joie

Jokla (Swahili) beautiful robe.

Jolanda (Greek) a form of
Yolanda. See also Iolanthe.
Jola, Jolan, Jolán, Jolande,
Jolander, Jolanka, Jolánta,
Jolantha, Jolanthe

Joleen, Joline (English) forms
of Jolene.
Joleena, Joleene, Jolleen, Jollene

Jolene (Hebrew) God will
add, God will increase.
(English) a form of
Josephine.
Jo, Jolaine, Jolana, Jolane,
Jolanna, Jolanne, Jolanta,
Jolayne, Jole, Jolean, Joleane,
Joleen, Jolena, Joléne, Jolenna,
Jolin, Jolina, Jolinda, Joline,
Jolinn, Jolinna, Jolleane, Jolleen,
Jolline

Jolie (French) pretty.
Jole, Jolea, Jolee, Joleigh, Joley,
Joli, Jolibeth, Jollee, Jollie, Jolly,
Joly, Jolye

Jolisa (American) a combina-
tion of Jo + Lisa.
Joleesa, Joleisha, Joleishia,
Jolieasa, Jolise, Jolisha, Jolisia,
Jolissa, Jolysa, Jolyssa, Julissa

Jolynn (American) a combination of Jo + Lynn.
Jolyn, Jolyne, Jolynne

Jonatha (Hebrew) gift of God.
Johnasha, Johnasia, Jonesha,
Jonisha

Jonelle (American) a combi-
nation of Joan + Elle.
Jahnel, Jahnell, Jahnelle, Johnel,
Johnell, Johnella, Johnelle, Jonel,
Jonell, Jonella, Jonyelle, Jynell,
Jynelle

Jonesha, Jonisha (American)
forms of Jonatha.
Joneisha, Jonesa, Joneshia,
Jonessa, Jonisa, Jonishia,
Jonneisha, Jonnesha, Jonnessia

Joni (American) a familiar
form of Joan.
*Jona, Jonae, Jonai, Jonann,
Jonati, Joncey, Jonci, Joncie,
Jonice, Jonie, Jonilee, Joni-lee,
Jonis, Jony*

Jonika (American) a form of
Janika.
*Johnica, Johnique, Johnquia,
Johnnica, Johnnika, Joneeka,
Joneika, Jonica, Joniqua, Jonique*

Jonina (Hebrew) dove. See
also Yonina.
Jona, Jonita, Jonnina

Jonita (Hebrew) a form of
Jonina. See also Yonita.
*Johnetta, Johnette, Johnita,
Johnittia, Jonati, Jonetia, Jonetta,
Jonette, Jonit, Jonnita, Jonta,
Jontae, Jontaé, Jontaya*

Jonni, Jonnie (American)
familiar forms of Joan.
Jonny

Jonquil (Latin, English) Botany:
an ornamental plant with fragrant yellow flowers.
*Jonquelle, Jonquie, Jonquill,
Jonquille*

Jontel (American) a form of
Johna.
*Jontaya, Jontell, Jontelle, Jontia,
Jontila, Jontrice*

Jora (Hebrew) autumn rain.
Jorah

Jordan (Hebrew) descending.
See also Jardena.
*Jordain, Jordaine, Jordana,
Jordane, Jordann, Jordanna,
Jordanne, Jordany, Jordea, Jordee,
Jorden, Jordi, Jordian, Jordie,
Jordin, Jordon, Jordyn, Jori, Jorie,
Jourdan*

Jordana, Jordanna (Hebrew)
forms of Jordan. See also
Giordana, Yordana.
*Jordannah, Jordina, Jordonna,
Jourdana, Jourdanna*

Jorden, Jordin, Jordon
(Hebrew) forms of Jordan.
Jordenne, Jordine

Jordyn (Hebrew) a form of
Jordan.
Jordyne, Jordynn, Jordynne

Jori, Jorie (Hebrew) familiar
forms of Jordan.
*Jorai, Jorea, Joree, Jorée, Jorey,
Jorian, Jorin, Jorina, Jorine,
Jorita, Jorre, Jorrey, Jorri, Jorrian,
Jorrie, Jorry, Jory*

Joriann (American) a combi-
nation of Jori + Ann.
*Jori-Ann, Jorianna, Jori-Anna,
Jorianne, Jori-Anne, Jorriann,
Jorrianna, Jorrianne, Jorryann,
Jorryanna, Jorryanne, Joryann,
Joryanna, Joryanne*

Jorja (American) a form of
Georgia.
*Jeorgi, Jeorgia, Jorgana, Jorgi,
Jorgia, Jorgina, Jorjana, Jorji*

Josalyn (Latin) a form of Jocelyn.
Josalene, Josalin, Josalind, Josaline, Josalynn, Joshalyne

Joscelin, Joscelyn (Latin) forms of Jocelyn.
Josceline, Joscelyne, Joscelynn, Joscelynne, Joselin, Joseline, Joselyn, Joselyne, Joselynn, Joselynne, Joshlyn

Josee, Josée (American) familiar forms of Josephine.
Joesee, Josey, Josi, Josina, Josy, Jozee

Josefina (Spanish) a form of Josephine.
Josefa, Josefena, Joseffa, Josefine

Joselin, Joseline (Latin) forms of Jocelyn.
Joselina, Joselinne, Josielina

Joselle (American) a form of Jizelle.
Joesell, Jozelle

Joselyn, Joslyn (Latin) forms of Jocelyn.
Joselene, Joselyne, Joselynn, Joshely, Josiline, Josilyn

Josephine (French) God will add, God will increase. See also Fifi, Pepita, Yosepha.
Fina, Jo, Joey, Josee, Josée, Josefina, Josepha, Josephe, Josephene, Josephin, Josephina, Josephyna, Josephyne, Josette, Josey, Josie, Jozephine, Jozie, Sefa

Josette (French) a familiar form of Josephine.
Joesette, Josetta, Joshetta, Jozette

Josey, Josie (Hebrew) familiar forms of Josephine.
Josi, Josse, Jossee, Jossie, Josy, Josye

Joshann (American) a combination of Joshlyn + Ann.
Joshana, Joshanna, Joshanne

Joshlyn (Latin) a form of Jocelyn. (Hebrew) God is my salvation.
Joshalin, Joshalyn, Joshalynn, Joshalynne, Joshelle, Joshleen, Joshlene, Joshlin, Joshline, Joshlyne, Joshlynn, Joshlynne

Josiane, Josianne (American) combinations of Josie + Anne.
Josian, Josie-Ann, Josieann

Josilin, Joslin (Latin) forms of Jocelyn.
Josielina, Josiline, Josilyn, Josilyne, Josilynn, Josilynne, Joslin, Josline, Joslyn, Joslyne, Joslynn, Joslynne

Jossalin (Latin) a form of Jocelyn.
Jossaline, Jossalyn, Jossalynn, Jossalynne, Josselyn, Josslin, Jossline

Josselyn (Latin) a form of Jocelyn.
Josselen, Josselin, Josseline, Jossellen, Jossellin, Jossellyn, Josselyne, Josselynn, Josselynne, Josslyn, Josslyne, Josslynn, Josslynne

Jourdan (Hebrew) a form of
Jordan.
Jourdain, Jourdann, Jourdanne,
Jourden, Jourdian, Jourdon,
Jourdyn

Jovana (Latin) a form of
Jovanna.
Jeovana, Jouvan, Jovan, Jovanah,
Jovena, Jovian, Jowan, Jowana

Jovanna (Latin) majestic.
(Italian) a form of Giovanna.
Mythology: Jove, also known
as Jupiter, was the supreme
Roman god.
Jeovanna, Jovado, Joval, Jovana,
Jovann, Jovannie, Jovena, Jovina,
Jovon, Jovonda, Jovonia,
Jovonna, Jovonnah, Jovonne,
Jowanna

Jovannie (Italian) a familiar
form of Jovanna.
Jovanee, Jovani, Jovanie, Jovanne,
Jovanni, Jovanny, Jovonnie

Jovita (Latin) jovial.
Joveda, Joveta, Jovetta, Jovida,
Jovitta

Joy (Latin) joyous.
Joe, Joi, Joya, Joye, Joyeeta,
Joyella, Joyia, Joyous, Joyvina

Joyanne (American) a combination of Joy + Anne.
Joyan, Joyann, Joyanna,

Joyce (Latin) joyous. A short
form of Joycelyn.
Joice, Joycey, Joycie, Joyous, Joysel

Joycelyn (American) a form of
Jocelyn.
Joycelin, Joyceline, Joycelyne,
Joycelynn, Joycelynne

Joylyn (American) a combina-
tion of Joy + Lynn.
Joyleen, Joylene, Joylin, Joyline,
Joylyne, Joylynn, Joy-Lynn,
Joylynne

Jozie (Hebrew) a familiar form
of Josephine.
Jozee, Jozée, Jozi, Jozy

Juana (Spanish) a short form
of Juanita.
Juanell, Juaney, Juanika, Juanit,
Juanna, Juannia

Juandalyn (Spanish) a form of
Juanita.
Jualinn, Juandalin, Juandaline,
Juandalyne, Juandalynn,
Juandalynne

Juanita (Spanish) a form of
Jane, Joan. See also Kwanita,
Nita, Waneta, Wanika.
Juana, Juandalyn, Juaneice,
Juanequa, Juanesha, Juanice,
Juanicia, Juaniqua, Juanisha,
Juanishia

Juci (Hungarian) a form of Judy.
Jucika

Judith (Hebrew) praised.
Mythology: the slayer of
Holofernes, according to
ancient Jewish legend. See
also Yehudit, Yudita.
Giuditta, Ioudith, Jodi, Jodie, Jody,

Jude, Judine, Judit, Judita, Judite, Juditha, Judithe, Judy, Judyta, Jutka

Judy (Hebrew) a familiar form of Judith.
Juci, Judi, Judie, Judye

Judyann (American) a combination of Judy + Ann.
Judana, Judiann, Judianna, Judianne, Judyanna, Judyanne

Jula (Polish) a form of Julia.
Julca, Julcia, Juliska, Julka

Julene (Basque) a form of Julia. See also Yulene.
Julena, Julina, Juline, Julinka, Juliska, Julleen, Jullena, Jullene, Julyne

Julia (Latin) youthful. See also Giulia, Jill, Jillian, Sulia, Yulia.
Iulia, Jula, Julea, Juleah, Julene, Juliah, Juliana, Juliann, Julica, Julie, Juliea, Juliet, Julija, Julina, Juline, Julisa, Julissa, Julita, Juliya, Julka, Julyssa

Juliana, Julianna (Czech, Spanish, Hungarian) forms of Julia.
Julieana, Julieanna, Juliena, Julliana, Jullianna, Julyana, Julyanna, Yuliana

Juliann, Julianne (English) forms of Julia.
Julean, Juleann, Julian, Juliane, Julieann, Julie-Ann, Julieanne, Julie-Anne, Julien, Juliene, Julienn, Julienne, Jullian

Julie (English) a form of Julia.
Juel, Jule, Julee, Juli, Julie-Lynn, Julie-Mae, Julle, Jullee, Jullie, Jully, July

Juliet, Juliette (French) forms of Julia.
Julet, Julieta, Juliett, Julietta, Jullet, Julliet, Jullietta

Julisa, Julissa (Latin) forms of Julia.
Julis, Julisha, Julysa, Julyssa

Julita (Spanish) a form of Julia.
Julitta, Julyta

Jumaris (American) a combination of Julie + Maris.

Jun (Chinese) truthful.

June (Latin) born in the sixth month.
Juna, Junea, Junel, Junell, Junella, Junelle, Junette, Juney, Junia, Junie, Juniet, Junieta, Junietta, Juniette, Junina, Junita

Juno (Latin) queen. Mythology: the supreme Roman goddess.

Justice (Latin) just, righteous.
Justis, Justise, Justiss, Justisse, Justus, Justyce, Justys

Justina (Italian) a form of Justine.
Jestena, Jestina, Justinna, Justyna

Justine (Latin) just, righteous.
Giustina, Jestine, Juste, Justi, Justice, Justie, Justina, Justinn, Justy, Justyn, Justyne, Justynn, Justynne

K

Kacey, Kacy (Irish) brave. (American) forms of Casey. Combinations of the initials K. + C.
K. C., Kace, Kacee, Kaci, Kacie, Kaicee, Kaicey, Kasey, Kasie, Kaycee, Kayci, Kaycie

Kachina (Native American) sacred dancer.
Kachine

Kaci, Kacie (American) forms of Kacey, Kacy.
Kasci, Kaycie, Kaysie

Kacia (Greek) a short form of Acacia.
Kaycia, Kaysia

Kadedra (American) a combination of Kady + Dedra.
Kadeadra, Kadedrah, Kadedria, Kadeedra, Kadeidra, Kadeidre, Kadeidria

Kadejah (Arabic) a form of Kadijah.
Kadeija, Kadeijah, Kadejá, Kadejia

Kadelyn (American) a combination of Kady + Lynn.

Kadesha (American) a combination of Kady + Aisha.
Kadeesha, Kadeeshia, Kadeesia, Kadeesiah, Kadeezia, Kadesa, Kadesheia, Kadeshia, Kadesia, Kadessa, Kadezia

Kadie (English) a form of Kady.
Kadi, Kadia, Kadiah

Kadijah (Arabic) trustworthy.
Kadajah, Kadeeja, Kadeejah, Kadija

Kadisha (American) a form of Kadesha.
Kadiesha, Kadieshia, Kadishia, Kadisia, Kadysha, Kadyshia

Kady (English) a form of Katy. A combination of the initials K. + D. See also Cady.
K. D., Kade, Kadee, Kadey, Kadie, Kadya, Kadyn, Kaidi, Kaidy, Kayde, Kaydee, Kaydey, Kaydi, Kaydie, Kaydy

Kaedé (Japanese) maple leaf.

Kaela (Hebrew, Arabic) beloved, sweetheart. A short form of Kalila, Kelila.
Kaelah, Kaelea, Kaeleah, Kaelee, Kaeli, Kayla

Kaelee, Kaeli (American) forms of Kaela.
Kaelei, Kaeleigh, Kaeley, Kaelia, Kaelie, Kaelii, Kaelly, Kaely, Kaelye

Kaelin (American) a form of Kaelyn.
Kaeleen, Kaelene, Kaelina, Kaelinn, Kalan

Kaelyn (American) a combination of Kae + Lynn. See also Caelin, Kaylyn.
Kaelan, Kaelen, Kaelin, Kaelynn, Kaelynne

Kaetlyn (Irish) a form of Kaitlin.
Kaetlin, Kaetlynn

Kagami (Japanese) mirror.

Kahsha (Native American) fur robe.
Kasha, Kashae, Kashia

Kai (Hawaiian) sea. (Hopi, Navaho) willow tree.
Kae, Kaie

Kaia (Greek) earth. Mythology: Gaea was the earth goddess.
Kaiah, Kaija

Kaila (Hebrew) laurel; crown.
Kailah, Kailea, Kaileah, Kailee, Kailey, Kayla

Kailee, Kailey (American) familiar forms of Kaila. Forms of Kaylee.
Kaile, Kaileh, Kaileigh, Kaili, Kailia, Kailie, Kailli, Kaillie, Kaily, Kailya

Kailyn, Kailynn (American) forms of Kaitlin.
Kailan, Kaileen, Kaileena, Kailen, Kailena, Kailene, Kaileyne, Kailin, Kailina, Kailon, Kailynne

Kairos (Greek) last, final, complete. Mythology: the last goddess born to Jupiter.
Kaira, Kairra

Kaishawn (American) a combination of Kai + Shawna.
Kaeshun, Kaisha, Kaishala, Kaishon

Kaitlin (Irish) pure. See also Katelin.
Kaetlyn, Kailyn, Kailynn, Kaitlan, Kaitland, Kaitleen, Kaitlen, Kaitlind, Kaitlinn, Kaitlinne, Kaitlon, Kaytlin

Kaitlyn, Kaitlynn (Irish) forms of Caitlyn.
Kaitelynne, Kaitlynne

Kaiya (Japanese) forgiveness.
Kaiyah, Kaiyia

Kala (Arabic) a short form of Kalila. A form of Cala.
Kalah, Kalla, Kallah

Kalama (Hawaiian) torch.

Kalani (Hawaiian) chieftain; sky.
Kailani, Kalanie, Kaloni

Kalare (Latin, Basque) bright; clear.

Kalea (Hawaiian) bright; clear.
Kahlea, Kahleah, Kailea, Kaileah, Kaleah, Kaleeia, Kaleia, Kalia, Kallea, Kalleah, Kaylea, Kayleah, Khalea, Khaleah

Kalee, Kaleigh, Kaley, Kalie
(American) forms of Caley,
Kaylee.
*Kalei, Kalleigh, Kalley, Kally,
Kaly*

Kalei (Hawaiian) flower
wreath.
*Kahlei, Kailei, Kallei, Kaylei,
Khalei*

Kalena (Hawaiian) pure. See
also Kalina.
*Kaleen, Kaleena, Kalene,
Kalenea, Kalenna*

Kalere (Swahili) short woman.
Kaleer

Kali (Hindi) the black one.
(Hawaiian) hesitating.
Religion: a form of the
Hindu goddess Devi. See
also Cali.
*Kalee, Kaleigh, Kaley, Kalie,
Kallee, Kalley, Kalli, Kallie,
Kally, Kallye, Kaly*

Kalia (Hawaiian) a form of
Kalea.
Kaliah, Kaliea, Kalieya

Kalifa (Somali) chaste; holy.

Kalila (Arabic) beloved, sweet-
heart. See also Kaela.
*Kahlila, Kala, Kaleela, Kalilla,
Kaylil, Kaylila, Kelila, Khalila,
Khalilah, Khalillah, Kylila,
Kylilah, Kylillah*

Kalina (Slavic) flower.
(Hawaiian) a form of Karen.
See also Kalena.
*Kalin, Kalinna, Kalyna,
Kalynah, Kalynna*

Kalinda (Hindi) sun.
*Kaleenda, Kalindi, Kalynda,
Kalyndi*

Kalisa (American) a combination of Kate + Lisa.
Kalise, Kalissa, Kalysa, Kalyssa

Kalisha (American) a combination of Kate + Aisha.
Kaleesha, Kaleisha, Kalishia

Kaliska (Moquelumnan) coyote chasing deer.

Kallan (Slavic) stream, river.
*Kalahn, Kalan, Kalen, Kallen,
Kallon, Kalon*

Kalle (Finnish) a form of
Carol.
Kaille, Kaylle

Kalli, Kallie (Greek) forms of
Callie. Familiar forms of
Kalliope, Kallista, Kalliyan.
*Kalle, Kallee, Kalley, Kallita,
Kally*

Kalliope (Greek) a form of
Calliope.
Kalli, Kallie, Kallyope

Kallista (Greek) a form of
Callista.
*Kalesta, Kalista, Kallesta, Kalli,
Kallie, Kallysta, Kaysta*

Kalliyan (Cambodian) best.
Kalli, Kallie

Kaltha (English) marigold,
yellow flower.

Kaluwa (Swahili) forgotten
one.
Kalua

Kalyca (Greek) rosebud.
Kalica, Kalika, Kaly

Kalyn, Kalynn (American)
forms of Kaylyn.
Kalin, Kallen, Kallin, Kallon,
Kallyn, Kalyne, Kalynne

Kama (Sanskrit) loved one.
Religion: the Hindu god of
love.

Kamala (Hindi) lotus.
Kamalah, Kammala

Kamali (Mahona) spirit guide;
protector.
Kamalie

Kamaria (Swahili) moonlight.
Kamar, Kamara, Kamarae,
Kamaree, Kamari, Kamariah,
Kamarie, Kamariya,
Kamariyah, Kamarya

Kamata (Moquelumnan)
gambler.

Kambria (Latin) a form of
Cambria.
Kambra, Kambrie, Kambriea,
Kambry

Kamea (Hawaiian) one and
only; precious.
Kameah, Kameo, Kamiya

Kameke (Swahili) blind.

Kameko (Japanese) turtle
child. Mythology: the turtle
symbolizes longevity.

Kameron (American) a form
of Cameron.
Kameran, Kamri

Kami (Japanese) divine aura.
(Italian, North African) a
short form of Kamila,
Kamilah. See also Cami.
Kamie, Kammi, Kammie,
Kammy, Kammye, Kamy

Kamila (Slavic) a form of
Camila. See also Millie.
Kameela, Kamela, Kamelia,
Kamella, Kami, Kamilah,
Kamilia, Kamilka, Kamilla,
Kamille, Kamma, Kammilla,
Kamyla

Kamilah (North African)
perfect.
Kameela, Kameelah, Kami,
Kamillah, Kammilah

Kamiya (Hawaiian) a form of
Kamea.
Kamia, Kamiah, Kamiyah

Kamri (American) a short
form of Kameron. See also
Camri.
Kamree, Kamrey, Kamrie,
Kamry, Kamrye

Kamryn (American) a short form of Kameron. See also Camryn.
Kameryn, Kamren, Kamrin, Kamron, Kamrynn

Kanani (Hawaiian) beautiful.
Kana, Kanae, Kanan

Kanda (Native American) magical power.

Kandace, Kandice (Greek) glittering white; glowing. (American) forms of Candace, Candice.
Kandas, Kandess, Kandi, Kandis, Kandise, Kandiss, Kandus, Kandyce, Kandys, Kandyse

Kandi (American) a familiar form of Kandace, Kandice. See also Candi.
Kandhi, Kandia, Kandie, Kandy, Kendi, Kendie, Kendy, Kenndi, Kenndie, Kenndy

Kandra (American) a form of Kendra. See also Candra.
Kandrea, Kandree, Kandria

Kane (Japanese) two right hands.

Kaneisha, Kanisha (American) forms of Keneisha.
Kaneasha, Kanecia, Kaneesha, Kanesah, Kanesha, Kaneshea, Kaneshia, Kanessa, Kaneysha, Kaniece, Kanishia

Kanene (Swahili) a little important thing.

Kani (Hawaiian) sound.

Kanika (Mwera) black cloth.
Kanica, Kanicka

Kannitha (Cambodian) angel.

Kanoa (Hawaiian) free.

Kanya (Hindi) virgin. (Tai) young lady. Religion: a form of the Hindu goddess Devi.
Kanea, Kania, Kaniya, Kanyia

Kapri (American) a form of Capri.
Kapre, Kapree, Kapria, Kaprice, Kapricia, Kaprisha, Kaprisia

Kapua (Hawaiian) blossom.

Kapuki (Swahili) first-born daughter.

Kara (Greek, Danish) pure.
Kaira, Kairah, Karah, Karalea, Karaleah, Karalee, Karalie, Kari, Karra

Karah (Greek, Danish) a form of Kara. (Irish, Italian) a form of Cara.
Karrah

Karalynn (English) a combination of Kara + Lynn.
Karalin, Karaline, Karalyn, Karalyne, Karalynne

Karelle (American) a form of Carol.
Karel, Kareli, Karell, Karely

Karen (Greek) pure. See also
Carey, Carina, Caryn.
*Kaaren, Kalina, Karaina,
Karan, Karena, Karin, Karina,
Karine, Karna, Karon, Karren,
Karron, Karyn, Kerron, Koren*

Karena (Scandinavian) a form
of Karen.
*Kareen, Kareena, Kareina,
Karenah, Karene, Karreen,
Karreena, Karrena, Karrene*

Karessa (French) a form of
Caressa.

Kari (Greek) pure. (Danish) a
form of Caroline, Katherine.
See also Carey, Cari, Carrie.
*Karee, Karey, Karia, Kariah,
Karie, Karrey, Karri, Karrie,
Karry, Kary*

Kariane, Karianne
(American) combinations of
Kari + Ann.
*Karian, Kariana, Kariann,
Karianna*

Karida (Arabic) untouched,
pure.
Kareeda, Karita

Karilynn (American) a combi-
nation of Kari + Lynn.
*Kareelin, Kareeline, Kareelinn,
Kareelyn, Kareelyne, Kareelynn,
Kareelynne, Karilin, Kariline,
Karilinn, Karilyn, Karilyne,
Karilynne, Karylin, Karyline,
Karylinn, Karylyn, Karylyne,
Karylynn, Karylynne*

Karimah (Arabic) generous.
*Kareema, Kareemah, Karima,
Karime*

Karin (Scandinavian) a form
of Karen.
*Kaarin, Kareen, Karina,
Karine, Karinne, Karrin, Kerrin*

Karina (Russian) a form of
Karen.
*Kaarina, Karinna, Karrina,
Karryna, Karyna, Karynna*

Karine (Russian) a form of
Karen.
Karrine, Karryne, Karyne

Karis (Greek) graceful.
*Karess, Karice, Karise, Karisse,
Karris, Karys, Karyss*

Karissa (Greek) a form of
Carissa.
*Karese, Karesse, Karisa,
Karisha, Karishma, Karisma,
Karissimia, Kariza, Karrisa,
Karrissa, Karysa, Karyssa,
Kerisa*

Karla (German) a form of
Carla. (Slavic) a short form
of Karoline.
*Karila, Karilla, Karle, Karlene,
Karlicka, Karlinka, Karlisha,
Karlisia, Karlitha, Karlla,
Karlon, Karlyn*

Karlee, Karleigh (American)
forms of Karley, Karly. See
also Carlee.
Karlea, Karleah, Karlei

Karlene, Karlyn (American)
forms of Karla. See also
Carleen.
*Karleen, Karlen, Karlena,
Karlign, Karlin, Karlina,
Karlinna, Karlyan, Karlynn,
Karlynne*

Karley, Karly (Latin) little and
strong. (American) forms of
Carly.
*Karlee, Karley, Karlie, Karlyan,
Karlye*

Karli, Karlie (American)
forms of Karley, Karly. See
also Carli.

Karlotte (American) a form of
Charlotte.
*Karlita, Karletta, Karlette,
Karlotta*

Karma (Hindi) fate, destiny;
action.

Karmel (Hebrew) a form of
Carmela.
*Karmeita, Karmela, Karmelina,
Karmella, Karmelle, Karmiella,
Karmielle, Karmyla*

Karmen (Latin) song.
*Karman, Karmencita, Karmin,
Karmina, Karmine, Karmita,
Karmon, Karmyn, Karmyne*

Karolane (American) a com-
bination of Karoll + Anne.
*Karolan, Karolann, Karolanne,
Karol-Anne*

Karolina, Karoline (Slavic)
forms of Caroline. See also
Carolina.
*Karaleen, Karalena, Karalene,
Karalin, Karaline, Karileen,
Karilena, Karilene, Karilin,
Karilina, Kariline, Karleen,
Karlen, Karlena, Karlene,
Karling, Karoleena, Karolena,
Karolinka, Karroleen,
Karrolena, Karrolene, Karrolin,
Karroline*

Karoll (Slavic) a form of
Carol.
*Karel, Karilla, Karily, Karol,
Karola, Karole, Karoly, Karrol,
Karyl, Kerril*

Karolyn (American) a form of
Carolyn.
*Karalyn, Karalyna, Karalynn,
Karalynne, Karilyn, Karilyna,
Karilynn, Karilynne, Karlyn,
Karlynn, Karlynne, Karolyna,
Karolynn, Karolynne, Karrolyn,
Karrolyna, Karrolynn,
Karrolynne*

Karri, Karrie (American)
forms of Carrie.
Kari, Karie, Karry, Kary

Karsen, Karsyn (English) child
of Kar. Forms of Carson.
Karson

Karuna (Hindi) merciful.

Karyn (American) a form of
Karen.
*Karyne, Karynn, Karynna,
Kerrynn, Kerrynne*

Kasa (Hopi) fur robe.

Kasandra (Greek) a form of
Kassandra.
Kasander, Kasandria, Kasandra,
Kasaundra, Kasondra,
Kasoundra

Kasey, Kasie (Irish) brave.
(American) forms of Casey,
Kacey.
Kaisee, Kaisie, Kasci, Kascy,
Kasee, Kasi, Kassee, Kassey,
Kasy, Kasya, Kaysci, Kaysea,
Kaysee, Kaysey, Kaysi, Kaysie,
Kaysy

Kashawna (American) a com-
bination of Kate + Shawna.
Kasha, Kashae, Kashana,
Kashanna, Kashauna,
Kashawn, Kasheana,
Kasheanna, Kasheena,
Kashena, Kashonda, Kashonna

Kashmir (Sanskrit)
Geography: a region located
between India and Pakistan.
Cashmere, Kashmear, Kashmere,
Kashmia, Kashmira, Kasmir,
Kasmira, Kazmir, Kazmira

Kasi (Hindi) from the holy
city.

Kasia (Polish) a form of
Katherine. See also Cassia.
Kashia, Kasiah, Kasian,
Kasienka, Kasja, Kaska, Kassa,
Kassia, Kassya, Kasya

Kasinda (Umbundu) our last
baby.

Kassandra (Greek) a form of
Cassandra.
Kassandr, Kassandre, Kassandré,
Kassaundra, Kassi, Kassondra,
Kassondria, Kassundra,
Kazandra, Khrisandra,
Krisandra, Krissandra

Kassi, Kassie (American)
familiar forms of Kassandra,
Kassidy. See also Cassie.
Kassey, Kassia, Kassy

Kassidy (Irish) clever.
(American) a form of
Cassidy.
Kassadee, Kassadi, Kassadie,
Kassadina, Kassady, Kasseday,
Kassedee, Kassi, Kassiddy,
Kassidee, Kassidi, Kassidie,
Kassity, Kassydi

Katalina (Irish) a form of
Caitlin. See also Catalina.
Kataleen, Kataleena, Katalena,
Katalin, Katalyn, Katalynn

Katarina (Czech) a form of
Katherine.
Kata, Katareena, Katarena,
Katarin, Katarine, Katarinna,
Katarinne, Katarrina, Kataryna,
Katarzyna, Katinka, Katrika,
Katrinka

Kate (Greek) pure. (English) a
short form of Katherine.
Kait, Kata, Katee, Kati, Katica,
Katie, Katka, Katy, Katya

Katee, Katey (English) familiar forms of Kate, Katherine.

Katelin (Irish) a form of
Caitlin. See also Kaitlin.
Kaetlin, Katalin, Katelan,
Kateland, Kateleen, Katelen,
Katelene, Katelind, Kateline,
Katelinn, Katelun, Kaytlin

Katelyn, Katelynn (Irish)
forms of Caitlin.
Kaetlyn, Kaetlynn, Kaetlynne,
Katelyne, Katelynne, Kaytlyn,
Kaytlynn, Kaytlynne

Katerina (Slavic) a form of
Katherine.
Katenka, Katerine, Katerini,
Katerinka

Katharine (Greek) a form of
Katherine.
Katharaine, Katharin,
Katharina, Katharyn

Katherine (Greek) pure. See
also Carey, Catherine,
Ekaterina, Kara, Karen, Kari,
Kasia, Katerina, Yekaterina.
Ekaterina, Ekatrinna, Kasienka,
Kasin, Kat, Katarina, Katchen,
Kate, Katee, Kathann,
Kathanne, Katharine,
Kathereen, Katheren, Katherene,
Katherenne, Katherin,
Katherina, Katheryn,
Katheryne, Kathi, Kathleen,
Kathrine, Kathryn, Kathy,
Kathyrine, Katia, Katina,
Katlaina, Katoka, Katreeka,
Katrina, Kay, Kitty

Kathi, Kathy (English) familiar forms of Katherine,

Kathleen. See also Cathi.
Kaethe, Katha, Kathe, Kathee,
Kathey, Kathi, Kathie, Katka,
Katla, Kató

Kathleen (Irish) a form of
Katherine. See also Cathleen.
Katheleen, Kathelene, Kathi,
Kathileen, Kathlean, Kathleena,
Kathleene, Kathlene, Kathlin,
Kathlina, Kathlyn, Kathlyne,
Kathlynn, Kathy, Katleen

Kathrine (Greek) a form of
Katherine.
Kathreen, Kathreena, Kathrene,
Kathrin, Kathrina

Kathryn (English) a form of
Katherine.
Kathren, Kathryne, Kathrynn,
Kathrynne

Kati (Estonian) a familiar form
of Kate.
Katja, Katya, Katye

Katia, Katya (Russian) forms
of Katherine.
Cattiah, Katiya, Kattia,
Kattiah, Katyah

Katie (English) a familiar form
of Kate.
Katee, Kati, Kãtia, Katti,
Kattie, Katy, Kayte, Kaytee,
Kaytie

Katilyn (Irish) a form of
Katlyn.
Katilin, Katilynn

Katlin (Irish) a form of Katlyn.
Katlina, Katline

Katlyn (Greek) pure. (Irish) a
form of Katelin.
*Kaatlain, Katilyn, Katland,
Katlin, Katlynd, Katlyne,
Katlynn, Katlynne*

Katriel (Hebrew) God is my
crown.
*Katrelle, Katri, Katrie, Katry,
Katryel*

Katrina (German) a form of
Katherine. See also Catrina,
Trina.
*Katreen, Katreena, Katrene,
Katri, Katrice, Katricia, Katrien,
Katrin, Katrine, Katrinia,
Katriona, Katryn, Katryna,
Kattrina, Kattryna, Katus,
Katuska*

Katy (English) a familiar form
of Kate. See also Cady.
Kady, Katey, Katty, Kayte

Kaulana (Hawaiian) famous.
Kaula, Kauna, Kahuna

Kaveri (Hindi) Geography: a
sacred river in India.

Kavindra (Hindi) poet.

Kawena (Hawaiian) glow.
Kawana, Kawona

Kay (Greek) rejoicer.
(Teutonic) a fortified place.
(Latin) merry. A short form
of Katherine.
Caye, Kae, Kai, Kaye, Kayla

Kaya (Hopi) wise child.
(Japanese) resting place.
Kaja, Kayah, Kayia

Kaycee (American) a combi-
nation of the initials K. + C.
*Kayce, Kaysee, Kaysey, Kaysi,
Kaysie, Kaysii*

Kaydee (American) a combi-
nation of the initials K. + D.
*Kayda, Kayde, Kayden, Kaydi,
Kaydie*

Kayla (Arabic, Hebrew) laurel;
crown. A form of Kaela,
Kaila. See also Cayla.
*Kaylah, Kaylea, Kaylee,
Kayleen, Kaylene, Kaylia,
Keila, Keyla*

Kaylah (Arabic, Hebrew) a
form of Kayla.
Kayleah, Kaylia, Keylah

Kaylan, Kaylen (Hebrew)
forms of Kayleen.
*Kaylana, Kayland, Kaylani,
Kaylann, Kaylean, Kayleana,
Kayleanna, Kaylenn*

Kaylee (American) a form of
Kayla. See also Caeley, Kalee.
*Kailee, Kayle, Kayleigh, Kayley,
Kayli, Kaylie*

Kayleen, Kaylene (Hebrew)
beloved, sweetheart. Forms of
Kayla.
*Kaylan, Kayleena, Kayleene,
Kaylen, Kaylena*

Kayleigh (American) a form
of Kaylee.
Kaylei

Kayley, Kayli, Kaylie
(American) forms of Kaylee.

Kaylin (American) a form of
Kaylyn.
Kaylon

Kaylyn, Kaylynn (American)
combinations of Kay +
Lynn. See also Kaelyn.
*Kalyn, Kalynn, Kayleen,
Kaylene, Kaylin, Kaylyna,
Kaylyne, Kaylynne*

Kaytlin, Kaytlyn (Irish) forms
of Kaitlin.
*Kaytlan, Kaytlann, Kaytlen,
Kaytlyne, Kaytlynn, Kaytlynne*

Keaira (Irish) a form of Keara.
*Keair, Keairah, Keairra, Keairre,
Keairrea*

Keala (Hawaiian) path.

Keana, Keanna (German)
bold; sharp. (Irish) beautiful.
*Keanah, Keanne, Keanu,
Keenan, Keeyana, Keeyanah,
Keeyanna, Keeyona. Keeyonna,
Keiana, Keianna, Keona,
Keonna*

Keandra, Keondra
(American) forms of Kenda.
*Keandrah, Keandre, Keandrea,
Keandria, Kedeana, Kedia,
Keonda, Keondre, Keondria*

Keara (Irish) dark; black.
Religion: an Irish saint.
*Keaira, Kearah, Kearia, Kearra,
Keera, Keerra, Keiara, Keiarah,
Keiarra, Keira, Kera*

Kearsten, Keirsten (Greek)
forms of Kirstin.
*Kearstin, Kearston, Kearstyn,
Keirstan, Keirstein, Keirstin,
Keirston, Keirstyn, Keirstynne*

Keeley, Keely (Irish) forms of
Kelly.
*Kealee, Kealey, Keali, Kealie,
Keallie, Kealy, Keela, Keelan,
Keele, Keelee, Keeleigh, Keeli,
Keelia, Keelie, Keellie, Keelye,
Keighla, Keilee, Keileigh,
Keiley, Keilly, Kiela, Kiele,
Kieley, Kielly, Kiely*

Keelyn (Irish) a form of
Kellyn.
Kealyn, Keelin, Keilan, Kielyn

Keena (Irish) brave.
Keenya, Kina

Keesha (American) a form of
Keisha.
*Keesa, Keeshae, Keeshana,
Keeshanne, Keeshawna,
Keeshonna, Keeshya, Keiosha*

Kei (Japanese) reverent.

Keiana, Keianna (Irish) forms
of Keana. (American) forms
of Kiana.
Keiann, Keiannah, Keionna

Keiki (Hawaiian) child.
Keikana, Keikann, Keikanna, Keikanne

Keiko (Japanese) happy child.

Keila (Arabic, Hebrew) a form of Kayla.
Keilah, Kela, Kelah

Keilani (Hawaiian) glorious chief.
Kaylani, Keilan, Keilana, Keilany, Kelana, Kelanah, Kelane, Kelani, Kelanie

Keira (Irish) a form of Keara.
Keiara, Keiarra, Keirra, Keirrah, Kera, Keyeira

Keisha (American) a short form of Keneisha.
Keasha, Keashia, Keesha, Keishaun, Keishauna, Keishawn, Kesha, Keysha, Kiesha, Kisha, Kishanda

Keita (Scottish) woods; enclosed place.
Keiti

Kekona (Hawaiian) second-born child.

Kelcey, Kelci, Kelcie (Scottish) forms of Kelsey.
Kelse, Kelcee, Kelcy

Kelila (Hebrew) crown, laurel. See also Kaela, Kayla, Kalila.
Kelilah, Kelula

Kelley (Irish) a form of Kelly.

Kelli, Kellie (Irish) familiar forms of Kelly.
Keleigh, Keli, Kelia, Keliah, Kelie, Kellee, Kelleigh, Kellia, Kellisa

Kelly (Irish) brave warrior. See also Caeley.
Keeley, Keely, Kelley, Kelley, Kelli, Kellie, Kellye

Kellyanne (Irish) a combination of Kelly + Anne.
Kelliann, Kellianne, Kellyann

Kellyn (Irish) a combination of Kelly + Lyn.
Keelyn, Kelleen, Kellen, Kellene, Kellina, Kelline, Kellynn, Kellynne

Kelsea (Scottish) a form of Kelsey.
Kelcea, Kelcia, Kelsa, Kelsae, Kelsay, Kelse

Kelsey (Scandinavian, Scottish) ship island. (English) a form of Chelsea.
Kelcey, Kelda, Kellsee, Kellsei, Kellsey, Kellsie, Kellsy, Kelsea, Kelsei, Kelsey, Kelsi, Kelsie, Kelsy, Kelsye

Kelsi, Kelsie, Kelsy (Scottish) forms of Chelsea.
Kalsie, Kelci, Kelcie, Kellsi

Kenda (English) water baby. (Dakota) magical power.
Keandra, Kendra, Kennda

Kendal (English) a form of
Kendall.
*Kendahl, Kendale, Kendalie,
Kendalin, Kendalyn,
Kendalynn, Kendel, Kendele,
Kendil, Kindal*

Kendall (English) ruler of the
valley.
*Kendal, Kendalla, Kendalle,
Kendell, Kendelle, Kendera,
Kendia, Kendyl, Kinda,
Kindall, Kindi, Kindle, Kynda,
Kyndal, Kyndall, Kyndel*

Kendra (English) a form of
Kenda.
*Kandra, Kendrah, Kendre,
Kendrea, Kendreah, Kendria,
Kenndra, Kentra, Kentrae,
Kindra, Kyndra*

Kendyl (English) a form of
Kendall.
Kendyle, Kendyll

Keneisha (American) a com-
bination of the prefix Ken +
Aisha.
*Kaneisha, Keisha, Keneesha,
Kenesha, Keneshia, Kenisha,
Kenneisha, Kennesha,
Kenneshia, Keosha, Kineisha*

Kenenza (English) a form of
Kennice.
Kenza

Kenia (Hebrew) a form of
Kenya.
Keniya, Kennia

Kenisha (American) a form of
Keneisha.
*Kenisa, Kenise, Kenishia,
Kenissa, Kennisa, Kennisha,
Kennysha*

Kenna (Irish) a short form of
Kennice.

Kennedy (Irish) helmeted
chief. History: John F.
Kennedy was the thirty-fifth
U. S. president.
*Kenedee, Kenedey, Kenedi,
Kenedie, Kenedy, Kenidee,
Kenidi, Kenidie, Kenidy,
Kennadee, Kennadi, Kennadie,
Kennady, Kennedee, Kennedey,
Kennedi, Kennedie, Kennidee,
Kennidi, Kennidy, Kynnedi*

Kennice (English) beautiful.
*Kanice, Keneese, Kenenza,
Kenese, Kennise*

Kenya (Hebrew) animal horn.
Geography: a country in
Africa.
*Keenya, Kenia, Kenja, Kenyah,
Kenyana, Kenyatta, Kenyia*

Kenyatta (American) a form
of Kenya.
*Kenyata, Kenyatah, Kenyatte,
Kenyattia, Kenyatta, Kenyette*

Kenzie (Scottish) light
skinned. (Irish) a short form
of Mackenzie.
*Kenzea, Kenzee, Kenzey,
Kenzi, Kenzia, Kenzy, Kinzie*

Keona, Keonna (Irish) forms of Keana.
Keiona, Keionna, Keoana, Keoni, Keonia, Keonnah, Keonni, Keonnia

Keosha (American) a short form of Keneisha.
Keoshae, Keoshi, Keoshia, Keosia

Kerani (Hindi) sacred bells. See also Rani.
Kera, Kerah, Keran, Kerana

Keren (Hebrew) animal's horn.
Kerrin, Keryn

Kerensa (Cornish) a form of Karenza.
Karensa, Karenza, Kerenza

Keri, Kerri, Kerrie (Irish) forms of Kerry.
Keriann, Kerianne, Kerriann, Kerrianne

Kerry (Irish) dark haired. Geography: a county in Ireland.
Keary, Keiry, Keree, Kerey, Keri, Kerri, Kerrie, Kerryann, Kerryanne, Kery, Kiera, Kierra

Kerstin (Scandinavian) a form of Kirsten.
Kerstan, Kerste, Kerstein, Kersten, Kerstie, Kerstien, Kerston, Kerstyn, Kerstynn

Kesare (Latin) long haired. (Russian) a form of Caesar (see Boys' Names).

Kesha (American) a form of Keisha.
Keshah, Keshal, Keshala, Keshan, Keshana, Keshara, Keshawn, Keshawna, Keshawnna

Keshia (American) a form of Keisha. A short form of Keneisha.
Kecia, Keishia, Keschia, Keshea, Kesia, Kesiah, Kessia, Kessiah

Kesi (Swahili) born during difficult times.

Kessie (Ashanti) chubby baby.
Kess, Kessa, Kesse, Kessey, Kessi

Kevyn (Irish) beautiful.
Keva, Kevan, Keven, Kevia, Keviana, Kevinna, Kevina, Kevion, Kevionna, Kevon, Kevona, Kevone, Kevonia, Kevonna, Kevonne, Kevonya, Kevynn

Keyana, Keyanna (American) forms of Kiana.
Keya, Keyanah, Keyanda, Keyandra, Keyannah

Keyara (Irish) a form of Kiara.
Keyarah, Keyari, Keyarra, Keyera, Keyerah, Keyerra

Keyona, Keyonna (American) forms of Kiana.
Keyonda, Keyondra, Keyonnia, Keyonnie

Keysha (American) a form of
Keisha.
Keyosha, Keyoshia, Keyshana,
Keyshanna, Keyshawn,
Keyshawna, Keyshia, Keyshla,
Keyshona, Keyshonna

Keziah (Hebrew) cinnamon-
like spice. Bible: one of the
daughters of Job.
Kazia, Kaziah, Ketzi, Ketzia,
Ketziah, Kezi, Kezia, Kizzy

Khadijah (Arabic) trustworthy.
History: Muhammed's first
wife.
Khadaja, Khadajah, Khadeeja,
Khadeejah, Khadeja, Khadejah,
Khadejha, Khadija, Khadije,
Khadijia, Khadijiah

Khalida (Arabic) immortal,
everlasting.
Khali, Khalia, Khaliah,
Khalidda, Khalita

Khrissa (American) a form of
Chrissa. (Czech) a form of
Krista.
Khrishia, Khryssa, Krisha,
Krisia, Krissa, Krysha, Kryssa

Khristina (Russian,
Scandinavian) a form of
Kristina, Christina.
Khristeen, Khristen, Khristin,
Khristine, Khyristya,
Khristyana, Khristyna,
Khrystyne

Ki (Korean) arisen.

Kia (African) season's beginning. (American) a short
form of Kiana.
Kiah

Kiana (American) a combina-
tion of the prefix Ki + Ana.
Keanna, Keiana, Keyana,
Keyona, Khiana, Khianah,
Khianna, Ki, Kiahna, Kiane,
Kiani, Kiania, Kianna, Kiauna,
Kiandra, Kiandria, Kiauna,
Kiaundra, Kiyana, Kyana

Kianna (American) a form of
Kiana.
Kiannah, Kianne, Kianni

Kiara (Irish) little and dark.
Keyara, Kiarra, Kieara, Kiearah,
Kiearra, Kyara

Kiaria, Kiarra, Kichi
(Japanese) fortunate.

Kiele (Hawaiian) gardenia;
fragrant blossom.
Kiela, Kieley, Kieli, Kielli,
Kielly

Kiera, Kierra (Irish) forms of
Kerry.
Kierana, Kieranna, Kierea

Kiersten, Kierstin
(Scandanavian) forms of
Kirsten.
Keirstan, Kerstin, Kierstan,
Kierston, Kierstyn, Kierstynn

Kiki (Spanish) a familiar form
of names ending in "queta."

Kiku (Japanese) chrysanthemum.
Kiko

Kiley (Irish) attractive; from
the straits.
*Kilea, Kilee, Kileigh, Kili, Kilie,
Kylee, Kyli, Kylie*

Kim (Vietnamese) needle.
(English) a short form of
Kimberly.
Kima, Kimette, Kym

Kimana (Shoshone) butterfly.
Kiman, Kimani

Kimber (English) a short form
of Kimberly.
Kimbra

Kimberlee, Kimberley
(English) forms of Kimberly.
*Kimbalee, Kimberlea, Kimberlei,
Kimberleigh, Kimbley*

Kimberly (English) chief,
ruler.
*Cymberly, Cymbre, Kim,
Kimba, Kimbely, Kimber,
Kimbereley, Kimberely,
Kimberlee, Kimberli, Kimberlie,
Kimberlyn, Kimbery, Kimbria,
Kimbrie, Kimbry, Kimmie,
Kymberly*

Kimberlyn (English) a form of
Kimberly.
Kimberlin, Kimberlynn

Kimi (Japanese) righteous.
*Kimia, Kimika, Kimiko,
Kimiyo, Kimmi, Kimmie,
Kimmy*

Kimmie (English) a familiar
form of Kimberly.
*Kimee, Kimme, Kimmee,
Kimmi, Kimmy, Kimy*

Kina (Hawaiian) from China.

Kineisha (American) a form
of Keneisha.
*Kineesha, Kinesha, Kineshia,
Kinisha, Kinishia*

Kineta (Greek) energetic.
Kinetta

Kini (Hawaiian) a form of Jean.
Kina

Kinsey (English) offspring;
relative.
*Kinsee, Kinsley, Kinza, Kinze,
Kinzee, Kinzey, Kinzi, Kinzie,
Kinzy*

Kinsley (American) a form of
Kinsey.
Kinslee, Kinslie, Kinslyn

Kioko (Japanese) happy child.
Kiyo, Kiyoko

Kiona (Native American)
brown hills.
Kionah, Kioni, Kionna

Kira (Persian) sun. (Latin) light.
*Kirah, Kiri, Kiria, Kiro, Kirra,
Kirrah, Kirri*

Kiran (Hindi) ray of light.

Kirby (Scandinavian) church
village. (English) cottage by
the water.
Kirbee, Kirbi

Kirima (Eskimo) hill.

Kirsi (Hindi) amaranth blossoms.
Kirsie

Kirsta (Scandinavian) a form of Kirsten.

Kirsten (Greek) Christian; annointed. (Scandinavian) a form of Christine.
Karsten, Kearsten, Keirstan, Kerstin, Kiersten, Kirsteni, Kirsta, Kirstan, Kirstene, Kirstie, Kirstin, Kirston, Kirsty, Kirstyn, Kjersten, Kursten, Kyersten, Kyrsten, Kyrstin

Kirstin (Scandinavian) a form of Kirsten.
Karstin, Kirsteen, Kirstien, Kirstine

Kirstie, Kirsty (Scandinavian) familiar forms of Kirsten.
Kerstie, Kirsta, Kirste, Kirstee, Kirstey, Kirsti, Kjersti, Kyrsty

Kirstyn (Greek) a form of Kirsten.
Kirstynn

Kisa (Russian) kitten.
Kisha, Kiska, Kissa, Kiza

Kishi (Japanese) long and happy life.

Kissa (Ugandan) born after twins.

Kita (Japanese) north.

Kitra (Hebrew) crowned.

Kitty (Greek) a familiar form of Katherine.
Ketter, Ketti, Ketty, Kit, Kittee, Kitteen, Kittey, Kitti, Kittie

Kiwa (Japanese) borderline.

Kiyana (American) a form of Kiana.
Kiya, Kiyah, Kiyan, Kiyani, Kiyanna, Kiyenna

Kizzy (American) a familiar form of Keziah.
Kezi, Kissie, Kizzi, Kizzie

Klara (Hungarian) a form of Clara.
Klára, Klari, Klarika

Klarise (German) a form of Klarissa.
Klarice, Kláris, Klaryce

Klarissa (German) clear, bright. (Italian) a form of Clarissa.
Klarisa, Klarise, Klarrisa, Klarrissa, Klarrissia, Klarisza, Klarysa, Klaryssa, Kleresa

Klaudia (American) a form of Claudia.
Klaudija

Kloe (American) a form of Chloe.
Khloe, Kloee, Kloey, Klohe, Kloie

Kodi (American) a form of Codi.
Kodee, Kodey, Kodie, Kody, Kodye, Koedi

Koffi (Swahili) born on Friday.
Kaffe, Kaffi, Koffe, Koffie

Koko (Japanese) stork. See also Coco.

Kolby (American) a form of Colby.
Kobie, Koby, Kolbee, Kolbey, Kolbi, Kolbie

Kolina (Swedish) a form of Katherine. See also Colleen.
Koleen, Koleena, Kolena, Kolene, Koli, Kolleen, Kollena, Kollene, Kolyn, Kolyna

Kona (Hawaiian) lady. (Hindi) angular.
Koni, Konia

Konstance (Latin) a form of Constance.
Konstantina, Konstantine, Konstanza, Konstanze

Kora (Greek) a form of Cora.
Korah, Kore, Koren, Koressa, Koretta, Korra

Koral (American) a form of Coral.
Korel, Korele, Korella, Korilla, Korral, Korrel, Korrell, Korrelle

Kori (American) a short form of Korina. See also Corey, Cori.
Koree, Korey, Koria, Korie, Korri, Korrie, Korry, Kory

Korina (Greek) a form of Corina.
Koreena, Korena, Koriana, Korianna, Korine, Korinna, Korreena, Korrina, Korrinna, Koryna, Korynna

Korine (Greek) a form of Korina.
Koreen, Korene, Koriane, Korianne, Korin, Korinn, Korinne, Korrin, Korrine, Korrinne, Korryn, Korrynne, Koryn, Koryne, Korynn

Kornelia (Latin) a form of Cornelia.
Karniela, Karniella, Karnis, Kornelija, Kornelis, Kornelya, Korny

Kortney (English) a form of Courtney.
Kortnay, Kortnee, Kortni, Kortnie, Kortny

Kosma (Greek) order; universe.
Cosma

Kosta (Latin) a short form of Constance.
Kostia, Kostusha, Kostya

Koto (Japanese) harp.

Kourtney (American) a form of Courtney.
Kourtnay, Kourtne, Kourtnee, Kourtnei, Kourtneigh, Kourtni, Kourtny, Kourtynie

Kris (American) a short form of Kristine. A form of Chris.
Khris, Krissy

Krissy (American) a familiar
form of Kris.
Krissey, Krissi, Krissie

Krista (Czech) a form of
~Christina. See also Christa.
*Khrissa, Khrista, Khryssa,
Khrysta, Krissa, Kryssa, Krysta*

Kristal (Latin) a form of
Crystal.
*Kristale, Kristall, Kristill, Kristl,
Kristle, Kristy*

Kristan (Greek) a form of
Kristen.
*Kristana, Kristanna, Kristanne,
Kriston, Krystan, Krystane*

Kristen (Greek) Christian;
annointed. (Scandinavian) a
form of Christine.
*Christen, Kristan, Kristene,
Kristien, Kristin, Kristyn,
Krysten*

Kristi, Kristie (Scandinavian)
short forms of Kristine.
Christi

Kristian, Kristiana (Greek)
Christian; anointed. Forms of
Christian.
*Khristian, Kristian, Kristiane,
Kristiann, Kristi-Ann,
Kristianna, Kristianne, Kristi-
Anne, Kristienne, Kristyan,
Kristyana, Kristy-Ann, Kristy-
Anne*

Kristin (Scandinavian) a form
of Kristen. See also Cristen.
Kristiin, Krystin

Kristina (Greek) Christian;
annointed. (Scandinavian) a
form of Christina. See also
Cristina.
*Khristina, Kristena, Kristina,
Kristeena, Kristena, Kristinka,
Krystina*

Kristine (Scandinavian) a
form of Christine.
*Kris, Kristeen, Kristene, Kristi,
Kristie, Kristy, Krystine,
Krystyne*

Kristy (American) a familiar
form of Kristine, Krystal. See
also Cristy.
*Kristi, Kristia, Kristie, Krysia,
Krysti*

Kristyn (Greek) a form of
Kristen.
Kristyne, Kristynn

Krysta (Polish) a form of
Krista.
Krystah, Krystka

Krystal (American) clear, bril-
liant glass.
*Kristabel, Kristal, Krystalann,
Krystalanne, Krystale, Krystall,
Krystalle, Krystel, Krystil,
Krystle, Krystol*

Krystalee (American) a com-
bination of Krystal + Lee.
*Kristalea, Kristaleah, Kristalee,
Krystalea, Krystaleah, Krystlea,
Krystleah, Krystlee, Krystlelea,
Krystleleah, Krystlelee*

Krystalynn (American) a combination of Krystal + Lynn.
Kristaline, Kristalyn, Kristalynn, Kristilyn, Kristilynn, Kristlyn, Krystaleen, Krystalene, Krystalin, Krystalina, Krystallyn, Krystalyn, Krystalynne

Krystel (Latin) a form of Krystal.
Kristel, Kristell, Kristelle, Krystelle

Krysten (Greek) a form of Kristen.
Krystene, Krystyn, Krystyne

Krystian, Krystiana (Greek) forms of Christian.
Krystiana, Krystianna, Krystianne, Krysty-Ann, Krystyan, Kristyana, Krystyanna, Krystyanne, Krysty-Anne, Krystyen

Krystin (Czech) a form of Kristin.

Krystina (Greek) a form of Kristina.
Krysteena, Krystena, Krystyna, Krystynka

Krystle (American) a form of Krystal.
Krystl, Krystyl

Kudio (Swahili) born on Monday.

Kuma (Japanese) bear. (Tongan) mouse.

Kumiko (Japanese) girl with braids.
Kumi

Kumuda (Sanskrit) lotus flower.

Kuniko (Japanese) child from the country.

Kunto (Twi) third-born.

Kuri (Japanese) chestnut.

Kusa (Hindi) God's grass.

Kwanita (Zuni) a form of Juanita.

Kwashi (Swahili) born on Sunday.

Kwau (Swahili) born on Thursday.

Kyana (American) a form of Kiana.
Kyanah, Kyani, Kyann, Kyanna, Kyanne, Kyanni, Kyeana, Kyeanna

Kyara (Irish) a form of Kiara.
Kiyara, Kiyera, Kiyerra, Kyarah, Kyaria, Kyarie, Kyarra, Kyera, Kyerra

Kyla (Irish) attractive. (Yiddish) crown; laurel.
Khyla, Kylah, Kylea, Kyleah, Kylia

Kyle (Irish) attractive.
Kial, Kiele, Kylee, Kyleigh, Kylene, Kylie

Kylee (Irish) a familiar form of
Kyle.
Kylea, Kyleah, Kylie, Kyliee

Kyleigh (Irish) a form of Kyle.
Kyliegh

Kylene (Irish) a form of Kyle.
Kyleen, Kylen, Kylyn, Kylynn

Kylie (West Australian
Aboriginal) curled stick;
boomerang. (Irish) a familiar
form of Kyle.
*Keiley, Keilley, Keilly, Keily,
Kiley, Kye, Kylee, Kyley, Kyli,
Kyllie*

Kymberly (English) a form of
Kimberly.
*Kymber, Kymberlee,
Kymberleigh, Kymberley,
Kymberli, Kymberlie,
Kymberlyn, Kymberlynn,
Kymberlynne*

Kyndal, Kyndall (English)
forms of Kendall.
*Kyndahl, Kyndalle, Kyndel,
Kyndell, Kyndelle, Kyndle,
Kyndol*

Kynthia (Greek) a form of
Cynthia.
Kyndi

Kyoko (Japanese) mirror.

Kyra (Greek) ladylike. A form
of Cyrilla.
*Keera, Keira, Kira, Kyrah,
Kyrene, Kyria, Kyriah, Kyriann,
Kyrie*

L

Lacey, Lacy (Latin) cheerful.
(Greek) familiar forms of
Larissa.
Lacee, Laci, Lacie, Lacye

Lachandra (American) a com-
bination of the prefix La +
Chandra.
Lachanda, Lachandice

Laci, Lacie (Latin) forms of
Lacey.
Lacia, Laciann, Lacianne

Lacrecia (Latin) a form of
Lucretia.
*Lacrasha, Lacreash, Lacreasha,
Lacreashia, Lacreisha, Lacresha,
Lacreshia, Lacresia, Lacretia,
Lacricia, Lacriesha, Lacrisah,
Lacrisha, Lacrishia, Lacrissa*

Lada (Russian) Mythology:
the Slavic goddess of beauty.

Ladasha (American) a combi-
nation of the prefix La +
Dasha.
*Ladaesha, Ladaisa, Ladaisha,
Ladaishea, Ladaishia,
Ladashiah, Ladaseha, Ladashia,
Ladasia, Ladassa, Ladaysha,
Ladesha, Ladisha, Ladosha*

Ladeidra (American) a combi-
natione of the prefix La +
Deidra.
Ladedra, Ladiedra

Ladonna (American) a com-
bination of the prefix La +
Donna.
*Ladan, Ladana, Ladon,
Ladona, Ladonne, Ladonya*

Laela (Arabic, Hebrew) a form
of Leila.
Lael, Laelle

Lahela (Hawaiian) a form of
Rachel.

Laila (Arabic) a form of Leila.
Lailah, Laili, Lailie

Laine, Layne (French) short
forms of Elaine.
*Lain, Laina, Lainah, Lainee,
Lainna, Layna*

Lainey, Layney (French)
familiar forms of Elaine.
*Laini, Lainie, Laynee, Layni,
Laynie*

Lajila (Hindi) shy, coy.

Lajuana (American) a combi-
nation of the prefix La +
Juana.
*Lajuanna, Lawana, Lawanna,
Lawanza, Lawanze, Laweania*

Laka (Hawaiian) attractive;
seductive; tame. Mythology:
the goddess of the hula.

Lakayla (American) a combi-
nation of the prefix La +
Kayla.
*Lakala, Lakaya, Lakeila,
Lakela, Lakella*

Lakeisha (American) a combi-
nation of the prefix La +
Keisha. See also Lekasha.
*Lakaiesha, Lakaisha, Lakasha,
Lakashia, Lakaysha, Lakaysia,
Lakeasha, Lakecia, Lakeesh,
Lakeesha, Lakeeshia, Lakesha,
Lakeshia, Lakeysha, Lakezia,
Lakicia, Lakieshia, Lakisha*

Laken, Lakin, Lakyn
(American) short forms of
Lakendra.
Lakena, Lakyna, Lakynn

Lakendra (American) a com-
bination of the prefix La +
Kendra.
*Lakanda, Lakedra, Laken,
Lakenda*

Lakenya (American) a combina-
tion of the prefix La + Kenya.
*Lakeena, Lakeenna, Lakeenya,
Lakena, Lakenia, Lakinja,
Lakinya, Lakwanya, Lekenia,
Lekenya*

Lakesha, Lakeshia, Lakisha
(American) forms of Lakeisha.
*Lakecia, Lakeesha, Lakesa,
Lakese, Lakeseia, Lakeshya,
Lakesi, Lakesia, Lakeyshia,
Lakiesha*

Laketa (American) a combina-
tion of the prefix La + Keita.
*Lakeeta, Lakeetah, Lakeita,
Lakeitha, Lakeithia, Laketha,
Laketia, Laketta, Lakieta,
Lakietha, Lakita, Lakitia,
Lakitra, Lakitri, Lakitta*

Lakia (Arabic) found treasure.
Lakiea, Lakkia

Lakota (Dakota) a tribal name.
Lakoda, Lakohta, Lakotah

Lakresha (American) a form
of Lucretia.
*Lacresha, Lacreshia, Lacresia,
Lacretia, Lacrisha, Lakreshia,
Lakrisha, Lekresha, Lekresia*

Lakya (Hindi) born on
Thursday.
*Lakeya, Lakeyah, Lakieya,
Lakiya, Lakyia*

Lala (Slavic) tulip.
Lalah, Lalla

Lalasa (Hindi) love.

Laleh (Persian) tulip.
Lalah

Lali (Spanish) a form of
Lulani.
Lalia, Lalli, Lally

Lalita (Greek) talkative.
(Sanskrit) charming; candid.

Lallie (English) babbler.
Lalli, Lally

Lamesha (American) a com-
bination of the prefix La +
Mesha.
*Lamees, Lameesha, Lameise,
Lameisha, Lameshia, Lamisha,
Lamishia, Lemisha*

Lamia (German) bright land.
Lama, Lamiah

Lamis (Arabic) soft to the touch.
Lamese, Lamise

Lamonica (American) a com-
bination of the prefix La +
Monica.
Lamoni, Lamonika

Lamya (Arabic) dark lipped.
Lama

Lan (Vietnamese) flower.

Lana (Latin) woolly. (Irish)
attractive, peaceful. A short
form of Alana, Elana.
(Hawaiian) floating; bouyant.
*Lanae, Lanai, Lanata, Lanay,
Laneah, Laneetra, Lanette,
Lanna, Lannah*

Landa (Basque) another name
for the Virgin Mary.

Landon (English) open, grassy
meadow.
*Landan, Landen, Landin,
Landyn, Landynne*

Landra (German, Spanish)
counselor.
Landrea

Lane (English) narrow road.
Laina, Laney, Layne

Laneisha (American) a com-
bination of the prefix La +
Keneisha.
*Laneasha, Lanecia, Laneesha,
Laneise, Laneishia, Lanesha,
Laneshe, Laneshea, Laneshia,
Lanesia, Lanessa, Lanesse,
Lanisha, Lanishia*

Laney (English) a familiar
form of Lane.
Lanie, Lanni, Lanny, Lany

Lani (Hawaiian) sky; heaven. A
short form of Atalanta,
'Aulani, Leilani.
*Lanee, Lanei, Lania, Lanie,
Lanita, Lanney, Lanni, Lannie*

Laporsha (American) a com-
bination of the prefix La +
Porsha.
*Laporcha, Laporche, Laporscha,
Laporsche, Laporschia, Laporshe,
Laporshia, Laportia*

Laqueena (American) a com-
bination of the prefix La +
Queenie.
*Laqueen, Laquena, Laquenetta,
Laquinna*

Laquinta (American) a com-
bination of the prefix La +
Quintana.
*Laquanta, Laqueinta,
Laquenda, Laquenta, Laquinda*

Laquisha (American) a com-
bination of the prefix La +
Queisha.
*Laquasha, Laquaysha,
Laqueisha, Laquesha, Laquiesha*

Laquita (American) a combi-
nation of the prefix La +
Queta.
*Laqeita, Laqueta, Laquetta,
Laquia, Laquiata, Laquieta,
Laquitta, Lequita*

Lara (Greek) cheerful. (Latin)
shining; famous. Mythology:
a Roman nymph. A short
form of Laraine, Larissa,
Laura.
Larae, Larah, Laretta, Larette

Laraine (Latin) a form of
Lorraine.
*Lara, Laraene, Larain, Larane,
Larayn, Larayne, Laraynna,
Larein, Lareina, Lareine, Laren,
Larenn, Larenya, Lauraine,
Laurraine*

Larina (Greek) seagull.
Larena, Larine

Larisa (Greek) a form of
Larissa.
*Lareesa, Lareese, Laresa, Laris,
Larise, Larisha, Larrisa, Larysa,
Laurisa*

Larissa (Greek) cheerful. See
also Lacey.
*Lara, Laressa, Larisa, Larissah,
Larrissa, Larryssa, Laryssa,
Laurissa, Laurissah*

Lark (English) skylark.

Lashae, Lashay (American)
combinations of the prefix
La + Shay.
*Lasha, Lashai, Lashaia,
Lashaya, Lashaye, Lashea*

Lashana (American) a combi-
nation of the prefix La +
Shana.
*Lashanay, Lashane, Lashanna,
Lashannon, Lashona, Lashonna*

Lashanda (American) a combination of the prefix La + Shanda.
Lashandra, Lashanta, Lashante

Lashawna (American) a combination of the prefix La + Shawna.
Lashaun, Lashauna, Lashaune, Lashaunna, Lashaunta, Lashawn, Lashawnd, Lashawnda, Lashawndra, Lashawne, Lashawnia, Leshawn, Leshawna

Lashonda (American) a combination of the prefix La + Shonda.
Lachonda, Lashaunda, Lashaundra, Lashon, Lashond, Lashonde, Lashondia, Lashondra, Lashonta, Lashunda, Lashundra, Lashunta, Lashunte, Leshande, Leshandra, Leshondra, Leshundra

Latanya (American) a combination of the prefix La + Tanya.
Latana, Latandra, Latania, Latanja, Latanna, Latanua, Latonshia

Latara (American) a combination of the prefix La + Tara.

Latasha (American) a combination of the prefix La + Tasha.
Latacha, Latacia, Latai, Lataisha, Latashia, Latasia, Lataysha, Letasha, Letashia, Letasiah

Latavia (American) a combination of the prefix La + Tavia.

Lateefah (Arabic) pleasant. (Hebrew) pat, caress.
Lateefa, Latifa, Latifah, Latipha

Latesha (American) a form of Leticia.
Lataeasha, Lateasha, Lateashia, Latecia, Lateicia, Lateisha, Latesa, Lateshia, Latessa, Lateysha, Latisa, Latissa, Leteisha, Leteishia

Latia (American) a combination of the prefix La + Tia.
Latea, Lateia, Lateka

Latika (Hindi) elegant.
Lateeka, Lateka

Latisha (Latin) joy. (American) a combination of the prefix La + Tisha.
Laetitia, Laetizia, Latashia, Lateasha, Lateashia, Latecia, Lateesha, Lateicia, Lateisha, Latice, Laticia, Latiesha, Latishia, Latishya, Latissha, Latitia, Latysha

Latona (Latin) Mythology: the powerful goddess who bore Apollo and Diana.
Latonna, Latonnah

Latonya (American) a combination of the prefix La + Tonya. (Latin) a form of Latona.
Latoni, Latonia

Latoria (American) a combination of the prefix La + Tori.
Latoira, Latorio, Latorja, Latorray, Latorreia, Latory, Latorya, Latoyra, Latoyria

Latosha (American) a combination of the prefix La + Tosha.
Latoshia, Latoshya, Latosia

Latoya (American) a combination of the prefix La + Toya.
Latoia, Latoiya, LaToya, Latoyia, Latoye, Latoyia, Latoyita, Latoyo

Latrice (American) a combination of the prefix La + Trice.
Latrece, Latreece, Latreese, Latresa, Latrese, Latressa, Letreece, Letrice

Latricia (American) a combination of the prefix La + Tricia.
Latrecia, Latresh, Latresha, Latreshia, Latrica, Latrisha, Latrishia

Laura (Latin) crowned with laurel.
Lara, Laurah, Lauralee, Laurelen, Laurella, Lauren, Lauricia, Laurie, Laurka, Laury, Lauryn, Lavra, Lolly, Lora, Loretta, Lori, Lorinda, Lorna, Loura

Laurel (Latin) laurel tree.
Laural, Laurell, Laurelle, Lorel, Lorelle

Lauren (English) a form of Laura.
Lauran, Laureen, Laurena, Laurene, Laurien, Laurin, Laurine, Lawren, Loren, Lorena

Laurence (Latin) crowned with laurel.
Laurencia, Laurens, Laurent, Laurentana, Laurentina, Lawrencia

Laurianna (English) a combination of Laurie + Anna.
Laurana, Laurann, Laureana, Laureanne, Laureen, Laureena, Laurian, Lauriana, Lauriane, Laurianna, Laurie Ann, Laurie Anne, Laurina

Laurie (English) a familiar form of Laura.
Lari, Larilia, Laure, Lauré, Lauri, Lawrie

Laury (English) a familiar form of Laura.

Lauryn (English) a familiar form of Laura.
Laurynn

Laveda (Latin) cleansed, purified.
Lavare, Lavetta, Lavette

Lavelle (Latin) cleansing.
Lavella

Lavena (Irish, French) joy. (Latin) a form of Lavina.

Laverne (Latin) springtime. (French) grove of alder trees. See also Verna.
Laverine, Lavern, Laverna, La Verne

Lavina (Latin) purified; woman of Rome. See also Vina.
Lavena, Lavenia, Lavinia, Lavinie, Levenia, Levinia, Livinia, Louvinia, Lovina, Lovinia

Lavonna (American) a combination of the prefix La + Yvonne.
Lavon, Lavonda, Lavonder, Lavondria, Lavone, Lavonia, Lavonica, Lavonn, Lavonne, Lavonnie, Lavonya

Lawan (Tai) pretty.
Lawanne

Lawanda (American) a combination of the prefix La + Wanda.
Lawonda, Lawynda

Layce (American) a form of Lacey.
Laycee, Layci, Laycia, Laycie, Laysa, Laysea, Laysie

Layla (Hebrew, Arabic) a form of Leila.
Laylah, Layli, Laylie

Le (Vietnamese) pearl.

Lea (Hawaiian) Mythology: the goddess of canoe makers. (Hebrew) a form of Leah.

Leah (Hebrew) weary. Bible: the first wife of Jacob. See also Lia.
Lea, Léa, Lee, Leea, Leeah, Leia

Leala (French) faithful, loyal.
Lealia, Lealie, Leial

Lean, Leann, Leanne (English) forms of Leeann, Lian.
Leana, Leane, Leanna

Leandra (Latin) like a lioness.
Leanda, Leandre, Leandrea, Leandria, Leeanda, Leeandra

Leanna, Leeanna (English) forms of Liana.
Leana, Leeana, Leianna

Leanore (Greek) a form of Eleanor. (English) a form of Helen.
Leanora, Lanore

Lecia (Latin) a short form of Felecia.
Leasia, Leecia, Leesha, Leesia, Lesha, Leshia, Lesia

Leda (Greek) lady. Mythology: the queen of Sparta and the mother of Helen of Troy.
Ledah, Lyda, Lydah

Lee (Chinese) plum. (Irish) poetic. (English) meadow. A short form of Ashley, Leah.
Lea, Leigh

Leeann, Leeanne (English) combinations of Lee + Ann. Forms of Lian.
Leane, Leean, Leian, Leiann, Leianne

Leena (Estonian) a form of Helen. (Greek, Latin, Arabic) a form of Lina.

Leeza (Hebrew) a short form of Aleeza. (English) a form of Lisa, Liza.
Leesa

Lei (Hawaiian) a familiar form of Leilani.

Leigh, Leigha (English) forms of Leah.
Leighann, Leighanna, Leighanne

Leiko (Japanese) arrogant.

Leila (Hebrew) dark beauty; night. (Arabic) born at night. See also Laela, Layla, Lila.
Laila, Leela, Leelah, Leilah, Leilia, Lela, Lelah, Leland, Lelia, Leyla

Leilani (Hawaiian) heavenly flower; heavenly child.
Lailanee, Lailani, Lailanie, Lailany, Lailoni, Lani, Lei, Leilany, Leiloni, Leilony, Lelani, Lelania

Lekasha (American) a form of Lakeisha.
Lekeesha, Lekeisha, Lekesha, Lekeshia, Lekesia, Lekicia, Lekisha

Leli (Swiss) a form of Magdalen.
Lelie

Lelia (Greek) fair speech. (Hebrew, Arabic) a form of Leila.
Leliah, Lelika, Lelita, Lellia

Lelya (Russian) a form of Helen.

Lena (Hebrew) dwelling or lodging. (Latin) temptress. (Norwegian) illustrious. (Greek) a short form of Eleanor. Music: Lena Horne, a well-known African American singer and actress.
Lenah, Lene, Lenee, Leni, Lenka, Lenna, Lennah, Lina, Linah

Lenci (Hungarian) a form of Helen.
Lency

Lene (German) a form of Helen.
Leni, Line

Leneisha (American) a combination of the prefix Le + Keneisha.
Lenece, Lenesha, Leniesha, Lenieshia, Leniesia, Leniessia, Lenisa, Lenise, Lenisha, Lennise, Lennisha, Lynesha

Lenia (German) a form of Leona.
Lenayah, Lenda, Lenea, Leneen, Lenna, Lennah, Lennea, Leny

Lenita (Latin) gentle.
Leneta, Lenette, Lennette

Lenore (Greek, Russian) a form of Eleanor.
Lenni, Lenor, Lenora, Lenorah

Leona (German) brave as a lioness. See also Lona.
Lenia, Leoine, Leola, Leolah, Leonae, Leonah, Leondra, Leone, Leonelle, Leonia, Leonice, Leonicia, Leonie, Leonissa, Leonna, Leonne, Liona

Leonie (German) a familiar form of Leona.
Leoni, Léonie, Leony

Leonore (Greek) a form of Eleanor. See also Nora.
Leonor, Leonora, Leonorah, Léonore

Leontine (Latin) like a lioness.
Leona, Leonine, Leontyne, Léontyne

Leora (Hebrew) light. (Greek) a familiar form of Eleanor. See also Liora.
Leorah, Leorit

Leotie (Native American) prairie flower.

Lera (Russian) a short form of Valera.
Lerka

Lesley (Scottish) gray fortress.
Leslea, Leslee, Leslie, Lesly, Lezlee, Lezley

Leslie (Scottish) a form of Lesley.
Leslei, Lesleigh, Lesli, Lesslie, Lezli

Lesly (Scottish) a form of Lesley.
Leslye, Lessly, Lezly

Leta (Latin) glad. (Swahili) bringer. (Greek) a short form of Aleta.
Lita, Lyta

Leticia (Latin) joy. See also Latisha, Tisha.
Laticia, Leisha, Leshia, Let, Leta, Letesa, Letesha, Leteshia, Letha, Lethia, Letice, Letichia, Letisha, Letishia, Letisia, Letissa, Letita, Letitia, Letiticia, Letiza, Letizia, Letty, Letycia, Loutitia

Letty (English) a familiar form of Leticia.
Letta, Letti, Lettie

Levana (Hebrew) moon; white. (Latin) risen. Mythology: the goddess of newborn babies.
Lévana, Levania, Levanna, Levenia, Lewana, Livana

Levani (Fijian) anointed with oil.

Levia (Hebrew) joined, attached.
Leevya, Levi, Levie

Levina (Latin) flash of lightning.
Levene

Levona (Hebrew) spice;
incense.
*Leavonia, Levonat, Levonna,
Levonne, Livona*

Lewana (Hebrew) a form of
Levana.
Lebhanah, Lewanna

Lexandra (Greek) a short
form of Alexandra.
Lisandra

Lexi, Lexie (Greek) familiar
forms of Alexandra.
Leksi, Lexey, Lexy

Lexia (Greek) a familiar form
of Alexandra.
*Leska, Lesya, Lexa, Lexane,
Lexina, Lexine*

Lexis (Greek) a short form of
Alexius, Alexus.
Laexis, Lexius, Lexsis, Lexxis

Lexus (Greek) a short form of
Alexis.
Lexuss, Lexxus, Lexyss

Leya (Spanish) loyal. (Tamil)
the constellation Leo.
Leyah, Leyla

Lia (Greek) bringer of good
news. (Hebrew, Dutch,
Italian) dependent. See also
Leah.
Liah

Lian (Chinese) graceful wil-
low. (Latin) a short form of
Gillian, Lillian.
*Lean, Leeann, Liane, Liann,
Lianne*

Liana, Lianna (Latin) youth.
(French) bound, wrapped up;
tree covered with vines.
(English) meadow. (Hebrew)
short forms of Eliana.
Leanna

Liane, Lianne (Hebrew) short
forms of Eliane. (English)
forms of Lian.
Leeanne

Libby (Hebrew) a familiar
form of Elizabeth.
Ibby, Lib, Libbee, Libbey, Libbie

Liberty (Latin) free.
Liberti, Libertie

Licia (Greek) a short form of
Alicia.
Licha, Lishia, Lisia, Lycia

Lida (Greek) happy. (Slavic)
loved by people. (Latin) a
short form of Alida, Elita.
Leeda, Lidah, Lidochka, Lyda

Lide (Latin, Basque) life.

Lidia (Greek) a form of Lydia.
*Lidea, Lidi, Lidija, Lidiya,
Lidka, Lidya*

Lien (Chinese) lotus.
Lienne

Liesabet (German) a short
form of Elizabeth.
Liesbeth, Lisbete

Liese (German) a familiar
form of Elise, Elizabeth.
Liesa, Lieschen, Lise

Liesel (German) a familiar
form of Elizabeth.
*Leesel, Leesl, Leezel, Leezl,
Liesl, Liezel, Liezl, Lisel*

Lila (Arabic) night. (Hindi)
free will of God. (Persian)
lilac. A short form of Dalila,
Delilah, Lillian.
Lilah, Lilia, Lyla, Lylah

Lilac (Sanskrit) lilac; blue purple.

Lilia (Persian) a form of Lila.
Lili

Lilian (Latin) a form of Lillian.
Liliane, Liliann, Lilianne

Liliana (Latin) a form of Lillian.
*Lileana, Lilliana, Lilianna,
Lilliana, Lillianna*

Lilibeth (English) a combina-
tion of Lilly + Beth.
*Lilibet, Lillibeth, Lillybeth,
Lilybet, Lilybeth*

Lilith (Arabic) of the night;
night demon. Mythology: the
first wife of Adam, according
to ancient Jewish legends.
Lillis, Lily

Lillian (Latin) lily flower.
*Lian, Lil, Lila, Lilas, Lileane,
Lilia, Lilian, Liliana, Lilias,*

*Liliha, Lilja, Lilla, Lilli, Lillia,
Lilliane, Lilliann, Lillianne,
Lillyann, Lis, Liuka*

Lillyann (English) a combina-
tion of Lilly + Ann. (Latin) a
form of Lillian.
*Lillyan, Lillyanne, Lily, Lilyan,
Lilyana, Lilyann, Lilyanna,
Lilyanne*

Lily (Latin, Arabic) a familiar
form of Lilith, Lillian,
Lillyann.
*Lil, Líle, Lili, Lilie, Lilijana,
Lilika, Lilike, Liliosa, Lilium,
Lilka, Lille, Lilli, Lillie, Lilly*

Limber (Tiv) joyful.

Lin (Chinese) beautiful jade.
(English) a form of Lynn.
Linh, Linn

Lina (Greek) light. (Arabic)
tender. (Latin) a form of
Lena.

Linda (Spanish) pretty.
Lind, Lindy, Linita, Lynda

Lindsay (English) a form of
Lindsey.
Lindsi, Linsay, Lyndsay

Lindsey (English) linden tree
island; camp near the stream.
*Lind, Lindsea, Lindsee, Lindsi,
Linsey, Lyndsey, Lynsey*

Lindsi (American) a familiar
form of Lindsay, Lindsey.
*Lindsie, Lindsy, Lindze,
Lindzee, Lindzey, Lindzy*

Lindy (Spanish) a familiar
form of Linda.
*Linde, Lindee, Lindey, Lindi,
Lindie*

Linette (Welsh) idol. (French)
bird.
*Lanette, Linet, Linnet, Linnetta,
Linnette, Lyannette, Lynette*

Ling (Chinese) delicate, dainty.

Linnea (Scandinavian) lime
tree. Botany: the national
flower of Sweden.
*Lin, Linae, Linea, Linnae,
Linnaea, Linneah, Lynea,
Lynnea*

Linsey (English) a form of
Lindsey.
*Linsea, Linsee, Linsi, Linsie,
Linsy, Linzee, Linzey, Linzi,
Linzie, Linzy, Linzzi, Lynsey*

Liolya (Russian) a form of
Helen.

Liora (Hebrew) light. See also
Leora.

Lirit (Hebrew) poetic; lyrical,
musical.

Liron (Hebrew) my song.
Leron, Lerone, Lirone

Lisa (Hebrew) consecrated to
God. (English) a short form
of Elizabeth.
*Leeza, Liesa, Liisa, Lise,
Lisenka, Lisette, Liszka, Litsa,
Lysa*

Lisbeth (English) a short form
of Elizabeth.
Lisbet

Lise (German) a form of Lisa.

Lisette, Lissette (French)
forms of Lisa. (English)
familiar forms of Elise,
Elizabeth.
*Liset, Liseta, Lisete, Liseth,
Lisett, Lisetta, Lisettina, Lisset,
Lissete, Lissett, Lizet, Lizette,
Lysette*

Lisha (Arabic) darkness before
midnight. (Hebrew) a short
form of Alisha, Elisha, Ilisha.
Lishe

Lissa (Greek) honey bee. A
short form of Elissa,
Elizabeth, Melissa, Millicent.
Lyssa

Lissie (American) a familiar
form of Allison, Elise,
Elizabeth.
Lissee, Lissey, Lissi, Lissy, Lissye

Lita (Latin) a familiar form of
names ending in "lita."
Leta, Litah, Litta

Litonya (Moquelumnan) dart-
ing hummingbird.

Liv (Latin) a short form of
Livia, Olivia.

Livana (Hebrew) a form of
Levana.
Livna, Livnat

Livia (Hebrew) crown. A familiar form of Olivia. (Latin) olive.
Levia, Liv, Livie, Livy, Livya, Livye

Liviya (Hebrew) brave lioness; royal crown.
Leviya, Levya, Livya

Livona (Hebrew) a form of Levona.

Liz (English) a short form of Elizabeth.

Liza (American) a short form of Elizabeth.
Leeza, Lizela, Lizka, Lyza

Lizabeta (Russian) a form of Elizabeth.
Lizabetah, Lizaveta, Lizonka

Lizabeth (English) a short form of Elizabeth.
Lisabet, Lisabeth, Lisabette, Lizabette

Lizbeth (English) a short form of Elizabeth.
Lizbet, Lizbett

Lizet, Lizette (French) forms of Lisette.
Lizet, Lizete, Lizeth, Lizett, Lizzet, Lizzeth, Lizzette

Lizina (Latvian) a familiar form of Elizabeth.

Lizzy (American) a familiar form of Elizabeth.
Lizzie, Lizy

Logan (Irish) meadow.
Logann, Loganne, Logen, Loghan, Logun, Logyn, Logynn

Lois (German) famous warrior.

Lola (Spanish) a familiar form of Carlota, Dolores, Louise.
Lolah, Lolita

Lolita (Spanish) sorrowful. A familiar form of Lola.
Lita, Lulita

Lolly (English) sweet; candy. A familiar form of Laura.

Lolotea (Zuni) a form of Dorothy.

Lomasi (Native American) pretty flower.

Lona (Latin) lioness. (English) solitary. (German) a short form of Leona.
Loni, Lonna

London (English) fortress of the moon. Geography: the capital of the United Kingdom.
Landyn, Londen, Londun, Londyn

Loni (American) a form of Lona.
Lonee, Lonie, Lonni, Lonnie

Lora (Latin) crowned with laurel. (American) a form of Laura.
Lorah, Lorane, Lorann, Lorra, Lorrah, Lorrane

Lore (Basque) flower. (Latin) a
short form of Flora.
Lor

Lorelei (German) alluring.
Mythology: the siren of the
Rhine River who lured
sailors to their deaths. See
also Lurleen.
*Loralee, Loralei, Lorali, Loralie,
Loralyn, Loreal, Lorelea, Loreli,
Lorilee, Lorilyn*

Lorelle (American) a form of
Laurel.

Loren (American) a form of
Lauren.
*Loreen, Lorena, Lorin, Lorne,
Lorren, Lorrin, Lorryn, Loryn,
Lorynn, Lorynne*

Lorena (English) a form of
Lauren.
*Lorene, Lorenea, Lorenia,
Lorenna, Lorina, Lorrina,
Lorrine, Lurana*

Lorenza (Latin) a form of
Laura.
Laurencia, Laurentia, Laurentina

Loretta (English) a familiar
form of Laura.
*Larretta, Lauretta, Laurette,
Loretah, Lorette, Lorita,
Lorretta, Lorrette*

Lori (Latin) crowned with lau-
rel. (French) a short form of
Lorraine. (American) a famil-
iar form of Laura.
Loree, Lorey, Loria, Lorianna,
*Lorianne, Lorie, Lorree, Lorri,
Lorrie, Lory*

Lorin (American) a form of
Loren.
Lorine

Lorinda (Spanish) a form of
Laura.

Loris (Latin) thong. (Dutch)
clown. (Greek) a short form
of Chloris.
Laurice, Laurys, Lorice

Lorna (Latin) crowned with
laurel. Literature: probably
coined by Richard Blackmore
in his novel *Lorna Doone*.
Lorna

Lorraine (Latin) sorrowful.
(French) from Lorraine, a
former province of France.
See also Rayna.
*Laraine, Lorain, Loraine,
Lorayne, Lorein, Loreine, Lori,
Lorine, Lorrain, Lorraina,
Lorrayne, Lorreine*

Lotte (German) a short form
of Charlotte.
*Lotie, Lotta, Lottchen, Lottey,
Lottie, Lotty, Loty*

Lotus (Greek) lotus.

Lou (American) a short form
of Louise, Luella.
Lu

Louam (Ethiopian) sleep well.

Louisa (English) a familiar form of Louise. Literature: Louisa May Alcott was an American writer and reformer best known for her novel *Little Women*.
Aloisa, Eloisa, Heloisa, Lou, Louisian, Louisane, Louisina, Louiza, Lovisa, Luisa, Luiza, Lujza, Lujzika

Louise (German) famous warrior. See also Alison, Eloise, Heloise, Lois, Lola, Ludovica, Luella, Lulu.
Loise, Lou, Louisa, Louisette, Louisiane, Louisine, Lowise, Loyce, Loyise, Luise

Lourdes (French) from Lourdes, France. Religion: a place where the Virgin Mary was said to have appeared.

Love (English) love, kindness, charity.
Lovely, Lovewell, Lovey, Lovie, Lovy, Luv, Luvvy

Lovisa (German) a form of Louisa.

Luann (Hebrew, German) graceful woman warrior. (Hawaiian) happy; relaxed. (American) a combination of Louise + Ann.
Louann, Louanne, Lu, Lua, Luan, Luane, Luanna, Luanne, Luanni, Luannie

Luanna (German) a form of Luann.
Lewanna, Louanna, Luana, Luwana

Lubov (Russian) love.
Luba, Lubna, Lubochka, Lyuba, Lyubov

Lucerne (Latin) lamp; circle of light. Geography: the Lake of Lucerne is in Switzerland.
Lucerna, Lucero

Lucero (Latin) a form of Lucerne.

Lucetta (English) a familiar form of Lucy.
Lucette

Lucia (Italian, Spanish) a form of Lucy.
Luciana, Lucianna

Lucie (French) a familiar form of Lucy.

Lucille (English) a familiar form of Lucy.
Lucila, Lucile, Lucilla

Lucinda (Latin) a form of Lucy. See also Cindy.

Lucine (Arabic) moon. (Basque) a form of Lucy.
Lucienne, Lucina, Lucyna, Lukene, Lusine, Luzine

Lucita (Spanish) a form of Lucy.
Lusita

Lucretia (Latin) rich; rewarded.
*Lacrecia, Lucrece, Lucréce, Lucrecia,
Lucreecia, Lucresha, Lucreshia,
Lucrezia, Lucrisha, Lucrishia*

Lucrezia (Italian) a form of
Lucretia. History: Lucrezia
Borgia was the Duchess of
Ferrara and a patron of
learning and the arts.

Lucy (Latin) light; bringer of
light.
*Luca, Luce, Lucetta, Luci, Lucia,
Lucida, Lucie, Lucija, Lucika,
Lucille, Lucinda, Lucine, Lucita,
Luciya, Lucya, Luzca, Luzi*

Ludmilla (Slavic) loved by the
people. See also Mila.
*Ludie, Ludka, Ludmila, Lyuba,
Lyudmila*

Ludovica (German) a form of
Louise.
Ludovika, Ludwiga

Luella (English) elf. (German)
a familiar form of Louise.
*Loella, Lou, Louella, Ludella,
Luelle, Lula, Lulu*

Luisa (Spanish) a form of Louisa.

Lulani (Polynesian) highest
point of heaven.

Lulu (Arabic) pearl. (English)
soothing, comforting. (Native
American) hare. (German) a
familiar form of Louise,
Luella.
Loulou, Lula, Lulie

Luna (Latin) moon.
*Lunetta, Lunette, Lunneta,
Lunnete*

Lupe (Latin) wolf. (Spanish) a
short form of Guadalupe.
Lupi, Lupita, Luppi

Lupita (Latin) a form of Lupe.

Lurleen, Lurlene
(Scandinavian) war horn.
(German) forms of Lorelei.
Lura, Lurette, Lurline

Lusa (Finnish) a form of
Elizabeth.

Lusela (Moquelumnan) like a
bear swinging its foot when
licking it.

Luvena (Latin, English) little;
beloved.
Lovena, Lovina, Luvenia, Luvina

Luyu (Moquelumnan) like a
pecking bird.

Luz (Spanish) light. Religion:
Nuestra Señora de Luz—Our
Lady of the Light—is another
name for the Virgin Mary.
Luzi, Luzija

Lycoris (Greek) twilight.

Lyda (Greek) a short form of
Lidia, Lydia.

Lydia (Greek) from Lydia, an
ancient land in Asia. (Arabic)
strife.
*Lidia, Lidija, Lidiya, Lyda,
Lydie, Lydië*

Lyla (French) island. (English) a form of Lyle (see Boys' Names). (Arabic, Hindi, Persian) a form of Lila.
Lila, Lilah

Lynda (Spanish) pretty. (American) a form of Linda.
Lyndah, Lynde, Lyndi, Lynnda

Lyndell (English) a form of Lynelle.
Lyndall, Lyndel, Lyndella

Lyndi (Spanish) a familiar form of Lynda.
Lyndee, Lindie, Lyndy, Lynndie, Lynndy

Lyndsay (American) a form of Lindsay.
Lyndsaye

Lyndsey (English) linden tree island; camp near the stream. (American) a form of Lindsey.
Lyndsea, Lyndsee, Lyndsi, Lyndsie, Lyndsy, Lyndzee, Lyndzey, Lyndzi, Lyndzie, Lynndsie

Lynelle (English) pretty.
Linel, Linell, Linnell, Lyndell, Lynel, Lynell, Lynella, Lynnell

Lynette (Welsh) idol. (English) a form of Linette.
Lynett, Lynetta, Lynnet, Lynnette

Lynn, Lynne (English) waterfall; pool below a waterfall.
Lin, Lina, Linley, Linn, Lyn, Lynlee, Lynley, Lynna, Lynnae, Lynnea

Lynnell (English) a form of Lynelle.
Linnell, Lynnelle

Lynsey (American) a form of Lyndsey.
Lynnsey, Lynnzey, Lynsie, Lynsy, Lynzee, Lynzey, Lynzi, Lynzie, Lynzy

Lyra (Greek) lyre player.
Lyre, Lyric, Lyrica, Lyrie, Lyris

Lysandra (Greek) liberator.
Lisandra, Lysandre, Lytle

Lysanne (American) a combination of Lysandra + Anne.
Lisanne, Lizanne

M

Mab (Irish) joyous. (Welsh) baby. Literature: queen of the fairies.
Mabry

Mabel (Latin) lovable. A short form of Amabel.
Mabelle, Mable, Mabyn, Maible, Maybel, Maybeline, Maybelle, Maybull

Macawi (Dakota) generous; motherly.

Macayla (American) a form of Michaela.
Macaela, Macaila, Macala, Macalah, Macaylah, Macayle, Macayli, Mackayla

Macey, Macie, Macy (Polish) familiar forms of Macia.
Macee, Maci, Macye

Machaela (Hebrew) a form of Michaela.
Machael, Machaelah, Machaelie, Machaila, Machala, Macheala

Machiko (Japanese) fortunate child.
Machi

Macia (Polish) a form of Miriam.
Macelia, Macey, Machia, Macie, Macy, Masha, Mashia

Mackenna (American) a form of Mackenzie.
Mackena, Makenna, Mckenna

Mackenzie (Irish) child of the wise leader. See also Kenzie.
Macenzie, Mackenna, Mackensi, Mackensie, Mackenze, Mackenzee, Mackenzey, Mackenzi, Mackenzia, Mackenzy, Mackenzye, Mackinsey, Mackynze, Makenzie, McKenzie, Mckinzie, Mekenzie, Mykenzie

Mackinsey (Irish) a form of Mackenzie.
Mackinsie, Mackinze, Mackinzee, Mackinzey, Mackinzi, Mackinzie

Mada (English) a short form of Madaline, Magdalen.
Madda, Mahda

Madaline (English) a form of Madeline.
Mada, Madailéin, Madaleen, Madaleine, Madalene, Madalin, Madaline

Madalyn (Greek) a form of Madeline.
Madalyne, Madalynn, Madalynne

Maddie (English) a familiar form of Madeline.
Maddi, Maddy, Mady, Maidie, Maydey

Maddison (English) a form of Madison.
Maddisan, Maddisen, Maddisson, Maddisyn, Maddyson

Madelaine (French) a form of Madeline.
Madelane, Madelayne

Madeleine (French) a form of Madeline.
Madalaine, Madalayne, Madelaine, Madelein, Madeliene

Madelena (English) a form of Madeline.
Madalaina, Madalena, Madalina, Maddalena, Madelaina, Madeleina, Madelina, Madelyna

Madeline (Greek) high tower.
See also Lena, Lina, Maud.
*Madaline, Madalyn, Maddie,
Madel, Madelaine, Madeleine,
Madelena, Madelene, Madelia,
Madella, Madelle, Madelon,
Madelyn, Madge, Madilyn,
Madlen, Madlin, Madline,
Madlyn, Madolyn, Maida*

Madelyn (Greek) a form of
Madeline.
*Madelyne, Madelynn, Madelynne,
Madilyn, Madlyn, Madolyn*

Madge (Greek) a familiar
form of Madeline, Margaret.
Madgi, Madgie, Mady

Madilyn (Greek) a form of
Madeline.
*Madilen, Madiline, Madilyne,
Madilynn*

Madisen (English) a form of
Madison.
*Madisan, Madisin, Madissen,
Madisun*

Madison (English) good; child
of Maud.
*Maddison, Madisen, Madisson,
Madisyn, Madyson, Mattison*

Madisyn (English) a form of
Madison.
*Madissyn, Madisynn,
Madisynne*

Madolyn (Greek) a form of
Madeline.
*Madoline, Madolyne,
Madolynn, Madolynne*

Madonna (Latin) my lady.
Madona

Madrona (Spanish) mother.
Madre, Madrena

Madyson (English) a form of
Madison.
Madysen, Madysun

Mae (English) a form of May.
History: Mae Jemison was
the first African American
woman in space.
*Maelea, Maeleah, Maelen,
Maelle, Maeona*

Maegan (Irish) a form of
Megan.
Maegen, Maeghan, Maegin

Maeko (Japanese) honest
child.
Mae, Maemi

Maeve (Irish) joyous.
Mythology: a legendary
Celtic queen. See also Mavis.
Maevi, Maevy, Maive, Mayve

Magali, Magaly (Hebrew)
from the high tower.
Magalie, Magally

Magan, Magen (Greek) forms
of Megan.
Maggen, Maggin

Magda (Czech, Polish, Russian)
a form of Magdalen.
Mahda, Makda

Magdalen (Greek) high tower.
Bible: Magdala was the home
of Saint Mary Magdalen. See

also Madeline, Malena,
Marlene.
Mada, Magda, Magdala,
Magdaleen, Magdalena,
Magdalene, Magdaline,
Magdalyn, Magdalynn,
Magdelane, Magdelene,
Magdeline, Magdelyn, Magdlen,
Magdolna, Maggie, Magola,
Maighdlin, Mala, Malaine

Magdalena (Greek) a form of
Magdalen.
Magdalina, Magdelana,
Magdelena, Magdelina

Magena (Native American)
coming moon.

Maggie (Greek) pearl.
(English) a familiar form of
Magdalen, Margaret.
Mag, Magge, Maggee, Maggi,
Maggia, Maggie, Maggiemae,
Maggy, Magi, Magie, Mags

Maggy, Meggy (English)
forms of Maggie.
Maggey, Magy

Magnolia (Latin) flowering
tree. See also Nollie.
Nola

Mahal (Filipino) love.

Mahala (Arabic) fat, marrow;
tender. (Native American)
powerful woman.
Mahalah, Mahalar, Mahalla,
Mahela, Mahila, Mahlah,
Mahlaha, Mehala, Mehalah

Mahalia (American) a form of
Mahala.
Mahaley, Mahaliah, Mahalie,
Mahayla, Mahaylah, Mahaylia,
Mahelea, Maheleah, Mahelia,
Mahilia, Mehalia

Maharene (Ethiopian) forgive
us.

Mahesa (Hindi) great lord.
Religion: a name for the
Hindu god Shiva.
Maheesa, Mahisa

Mahila (Sanskrit) woman.

Mahina (Hawaiian) moon
glow.

Mahira (Hebrew) energetic.
Mahri

Mahogony (Spanish) rich;
strong.
Mahagony, Mahoganey,
Mahogani, Mahoganie,
Mahogany, Mahogney,
Mahogny, Mohogany, Mohogony

Mai (Japanese) brightness.
(Vietnamese) flower.
(Navajo) coyote.

Maia (Greek) mother; nurse.
(English) kinswoman;
maiden. Mythology: the
loveliest of the Pleiades, the
seven daughters of Atlas, and
the mother of Hermes. See
also Maya.
Maiah, Maie, Maiya

Maida (English) maiden.
*(Greek) a short form of
Madeline.
Maidel, Mayda, Maydena

Maija (Finnish) a form of
Mary.
Maiji, Maikki

Maika (Hebrew) a familiar
form of Michaela.
Maikala, Maikka, Maiko

Maira, Maire (Irish) forms of
Mary.
*Maairah, Mair, Mairi, Mairim,
Mairin, Mairona, Mairwen*

Maisie (Scottish) familiar
forms of Margaret.
*Maisa, Maise, Maisey, Maisi,
Maisy, Maizie, Maycee, Maysie,
Mayzie, Mazey, Mazie, Mazy,
Mazzy, Mysie, Myzie*

Maita (Spanish) a form of
Martha.
Maite, Maitia

Maitlyn (American) a combi-
nation of Maita + Lynn.
*Maitlan, Maitland, Maitlynn,
Mattilyn*

Maiya (Greek) a form of
Maia.
Maiyah

Maja (Arabic) a short form of
Majidah.
*Majal, Majalisa, Majalyn,
Majalynn*

Majidah (Arabic) splendid.
Maja, Majida

Makaela, Makaila (American)
forms of Michaela.
*Makaelah, Makaelee, Makaella,
Makaely, Makail, Makailah,
Makailee, Makailla, Makaillah,
Makealah, Makell*

Makala (Hawaiian) myrtle.
(Hebrew) a form of
Michaela.
*Makalae, Makalah, Makalai,
Makalea, Makalee, Makaleh,
Makaleigh, Makaley, Makalia,
Makalie, Makalya, Makela,
Makelah, Makell, Makella*

Makana (Hawaiian) gift, present.

Makani (Hawaiian) wind.

Makara (Hindi) Astrology:
another name for the zodiac
sign Capricorn.

Makayla (American) a form of
Michaela.
*Macayla, Makaylah, Makaylee,
Makayleigh, Makayli,
Makaylia, Makaylla, Makell,
Makyla, Makylah, Mckayla,
Mekayla, Mikayla*

Makell (American) a short
form of Makaela, Makala,
Makayla.
Makele, Makelle, Mckell, Mekel

Makenna (American) a form
of Mackenna.
Makena, Makennah, Mikenna

Makenzie (Irish) a form of
Mackenzie.
Makense, Makensey, Makensie,
Makenze, Makenzee,
Makenzey, Makenzi, Makenzy,
Makenzye, Makinzey,
Makynzey, Mekenzie,
Mykenzie

Mala (Greek) a short form of
Magdalen.
Malana, Malee, Mali

Malana (Hawaiian) bouyant,
light.

Malaya (Filipino) free.
Malayaa, Malayah, Malayna,
Malea, Maleah

Malena (Swedish) a familiar
form of Magdalen.
Malen, Malenna, Malin,
Malina, Maline, Malini,
Malinna

Malha (Hebrew) queen.
Maliah, Malkah, Malkia,
Malkiah, Malkie, Malkiya,
Malkiyah, Miliah

Mali (Tai) jasmine flower.
(Tongan) sweet. (Hungarian)
a short form of Malika.
Malea, Malee, Maley

Malia (Hawaiian, Zuni) a form
of Mary. (Spanish) a form of
Maria.
Malea, Maleah, Maleeya,
Maleeyah, Maleia, Maliah,
Maliasha, Malie, Maliea,
Maliya, Maliyah, Malli, Mally

Malika (Hungarian) industri-
ous. (Arabic) queen.
Malak, Maleeka, Maleka, Mali,
Maliaka, Malik, Malikah,
Malikee, Maliki, Malikia,
Malky

Malina (Hebrew) tower.
(Native American) soothing.
(Russian) raspberry.
Malin, Maline, Malina,
Malinna, Mallie

Malinda (Greek) a form of
Melinda.
Malinde, Malinna, Malynda

Malini (Hindi) gardener.
Maliny

Malissa (Greek) a form of
Melissa.
Malisa, Malisah, Malyssa

Mallalai (Pashto) beautiful.

Malley (American) a familiar
form of Mallory.
Mallee, Malli, Mallie, Mally,
Maly

Mallorie (French) a form of
Mallory.
Malerie, Mallari, Mallerie,
Malloreigh, Mallori

Mallory (German) army
counselor. (French) unlucky.
Maliri, Mallary, Mallauri,
Mallery, Malley, Malloree,
Mallorey, Mallorie, Malorie,
Malory, Malorym, Malree,
Malrie, Mellory

Malorie, Malory (German) forms of Mallory.
Malarie, Maloree, Malori, Melorie, Melory

Malva (English) a form of Melba.
Malvi, Malvy

Malvina (Scottish) a form of Melvina. Literature: a name created by the eighteenth-century romantic poet James Macpherson.
Malvane, Malvi

Mamie (American) a familiar form of Margaret.
Mame, Mamee, Mami, Mammie, Mamy, Mamye

Mamo (Hawaiian) saffron flower; yellow bird.

Mana (Hawaiian) psychic; sensitive.
Manal, Manali, Manna, Mannah

Manar (Arabic) guiding light.
Manayra

Manda (Spanish) woman warrior. (Latin) a short form of Amanda.
Mandy

Mandara (Hindi) calm.

Mandeep (Punjabi) enlightened.

Mandisa (Xhosa) sweet.

Mandy (Latin) lovable. A familiar form of Amanda, Manda, Melinda.
Mandee, Mandi, Mandie

Manette (French) a form of Mary.

Mangena (Hebrew) song, melody.
Mangina

Mani (Chinese) a mantra repeated in Tibetan Buddhist prayer to impart understanding.
Manee

Manka (Polish, Russian) a form of Mary.

Manon (French) a familiar form of Marie.
Mannon

Manpreet (Punjabi) mind full of love.
Manprit

Mansi (Hopi) plucked flower.
Mancey, Manci, Mancie, Mansey, Mansie, Mansy

Manuela (Spanish) a form of Emmanuelle.
Manuala, Manuelita, Manuella, Manuelle

Manya (Russian) a form of Mary.

Mara (Hebrew) melody. (Greek) a short form of Amara. (Slavic) a form of Mary.
Mahra, Marae, Marah, Maralina, Maraline, Marra

Marabel (English) a form of Mirabel.
Marabella, Marabelle

Maranda (Latin) a form of Miranda.

Maraya (Hebrew) a form of Mariah.
Mareya

Marcela (Latin) a form of Marcella.
Marcele, Marcelen, Marcelia, Marcelina, Marceline, Maricela

Marcelen (English) a form of Marcella.
Marcelen, Marcelin, Marcelina, Marceline, Marcellin, Marcellina, Marcelline, Marcelyn, Marcilen

Marcella (Latin) martial, warlike. Mythology: Mars was the god of war.
Mairsil, Marca, Marce, Marceil, Marcela, Marcelen, Marcell, Marcelle, Marcello, Marcena, Marchella, Marchelle, Marci, Marcia, Marcie, Marciella, Marcile, Marcilla, Marcille, Marella, Marsella, Marselle, Marsiella

Marcena (Latin) a form of Marcella, Marcia.
Maracena, Marceen, Marcene, Marcenia, Marceyne, Marcina

Marci, Marcie (English) familiar forms of Marcella, Marcia.
Marca, Marcee, Marcita, Marcy, Marsi, Marsie

Marcia (Latin) martial, warlike. See also Marquita.
Marcena, Marchia, Marci, Marciale, Marcie, Marcsa, Marsha, Martia

Marciann (American) a combination of Marci + Ann.
Marciane, Marcianna, Marcianne, Marcyane, Marcyanna, Marcyanne

Marcilynn (American) a combination of Marci + Lynn.
Marcilen, Marcilin, Marciline, Marcilyn, Marcilyne, Marcilynne, Marcylen, Marcylin, Marcyline, Marcylyn, Marcylyne, Marcylynn, Marcylynne

Marcy (English) a form of Marci.
Marsey, Marsy

Mardi (French) born on Tuesday. (Aramaic) a familiar form of Martha.

Mare (Irish) a form of Mary.
Mair, Maire

Marelda (German) renowned warrior.
Marella, Marilda

Maren (Latin) sea. (Aramaic) a form of Mary. See also Marina.
Marin, Marine, Marinn, Miren

Maresa, Maressa (Latin)
forms of Marisa.
Maresha, Meresa

Maretta (English) a familiar
form of Margaret.
Maret, Marette

Margaret (Greek) pearl.
History: Margaret Hilda
Thatcher served as British
prime minister. See also Gita,
Greta, Gretchen, Marjorie,
Markita, Meg, Megan, Peggy,
Reet, Rita.
*Madge, Maergrethe, Maggie,
Maisie, Mamie, Maretta, Marga,
Margalo, Marganit, Margara,
Maretha, Margarett, Margarette,
Margarida, Margarit, Margarita,
Margaro, Margaux, Marge,
Margeret, Margeretta,
Margerette, Margery, Margetta,
Margiad, Margie, Margisia,
Margit, Margo, Margot, Margret,
Marguerite, Meta*

Margarit (Greek) a form of
Margaret.
*Margalide, Margalit, Margalith,
Margarid, Margaritt, Margerit*

Margarita (Italian, Spanish) a
form of Margaret.
*Margareta, Margaretta,
Margarida, Margaritis,
Margaritta, Margeretta,
Margharita, Margherita,
Margrieta, Margrita,
Marguarita, Marguerita,
Margurita*

Margaux (French) a form of
Margaret.
Margeaux

Marge (English) a short form
of Margaret, Marjorie.
Margie

Margery (English) a form of
Margaret.
Margerie, Margorie

Margie (English) a familiar
form of Marge, Margaret.
Margey, Margi, Margy

Margit (Hungarian) a form of
Margaret.
Marget, Margette, Margita

Margo, Margot (French)
forms of Margaret.
Mago, Margaro

Margret (German) a form of
Margaret.
*Margreta, Margrete, Margreth,
Margrett, Margretta, Margrette,
Margrieta, Margrita*

Marguerite (French) a form
of Margaret.
*Margarete, Margaretha,
Margarethe, Margarite,
Margerite, Marguaretta,
Marguarette, Marguarite,
Marguerette, Margurite*

Mari (Japanese) ball. (Spanish)
a form of Mary.

Maria (Hebrew) bitter; sea of bitterness. (Italian, Spanish) a form of Mary.
Maie, Malia, Marea, Mareah, Mariabella, Mariae, Mariesa, Mariessa, Mariha, Marija, Mariya, Mariyah, Marja, Marya

Mariah (Hebrew) a form of Mary. See also Moriah.
Maraia, Maraya, Mariyah, Marriah, Meriah

Mariam (Hebrew) a form of Miriam.
Mariama, Mariame, Mariem, Meryam

Marian (English) a form of Maryann.
Mariana, Mariane, Mariann, Marianne, Mariene, Marion, Marrian, Marriann

Mariana, Marianna (Spanish) forms of Marian.
Marriana, Marrianna, Maryana, Maryanna

Mariane, Marianne (English) forms of Marian.
Marrianne, Maryanne

Maribel (French) beautiful. (English) a combination of Maria + Bell.
Marabel, Marbelle, Mariabella, Maribella, Maribelle, Maridel, Marybel, Marybella, Marybelle

Marice (Italian) a form of Mary. See also Maris.
Marica, Marise, Marisse

Maricela (Latin) a form of Marcella.
Maricel, Mariceli, Maricelia, Maricella, Maricely

Maridel (English) a form of Maribel.

Marie (French) a form of Mary.
Maree, Marietta, Marrie

Mariel, Marielle (German, Dutch) forms of Mary.
Marial, Marieke, Marielana, Mariele, Marieli, Marielie, Marieline, Mariell, Mariellen, Marielsie, Mariely, Marielys

Mariela, Mariella (German, Dutch) forms of Mary.

Marietta (Italian) a familiar form of Marie.
Maretta, Marette, Mariet, Mariette, Marrietta

Marieve (American) a combination of Mary + Eve.

Marigold (English) Mary's gold. Botany: a plant with yellow or orange flowers.
Marygold

Marika (Dutch, Slavic) a form of Mary.
Marica, Marieke, Marija, Marijke, Marikah, Marike, Marikia, Marikka, Mariska, Mariske, Marrika, Maryk, Maryka, Merica, Merika

Mariko (Japanese) circle.

Marilee (American) a combi-
nation of Mary + Lee.
*Marili, Marilie, Marily,
Marrilee, Marylea, Marylee,
Merrilee, Merrili, Merrily*

Marilla (Hebrew, German) a
form of Mary.
Marella, Marelle

Marilou (American) a form of
Marylou.
Marilu, Mariluz

Marilyn (Hebrew) Mary's line
of descendants. See also
Merilyn.
*Maralin, Maralyn, Maralyne,
Maralynn, Maralynne, Marelyn,
Marilin, Marillyn, Marilyne,
Marilynn, Marilynne, Marlyn,
Marolyn, Marralynn, Marrilin,
Marrilyn, Marrilynn,
Marrilynne, Marylin, Marylinn,
Marylyn, Marylyne, Marylynn,
Marylynne*

Marina (Latin) sea. See also
Maren.
*Mareena, Marena, Marenka,
Marinae, Marinah, Marinda,
Marindi, Marinka, Marinna,
Marrina, Maryna, Merina,
Mirena*

Marini (Swahili) healthy;
pretty.

Marion (French) a form of
Mary.
*Marrian, Marrion, Maryon,
Maryonn*

Maris (Latin) sea. (Greek) a
short form of Amaris,
Damaris. See also Marice.
*Maries, Marise, Marris, Marys,
Maryse, Meris*

Marisa (Latin) sea.
*Maresa, Mariesa, Mariessa,
Marisela, Marissa, Marita,
Mariza, Marrisa, Marrissa,
Marysa, Maryse, Maryssa,
Merisa*

Marisela (Latin) a form of
Marisa.
*Mariseli, Marisella, Marishelle,
Marissela*

Marisha (Russian) a familiar
form of Mary.
*Mareshah, Marishenka,
Marishka, Mariska*

Marisol (Spanish) sunny sea.
Marise, Marizol, Marysol

Marissa (Latin) a form of
Maris, Marisa.
*Maressa, Marisa, Marisha,
Marissah, Marisse, Marizza,
Marrissa, Marrissia, Maryssa,
Merissa, Morissa*

Marit (Aramaic) lady.
Marita, Marite

Marita (Spanish) a form of
Marisa. (Aramaic) a form of
Marit.
Marité, Maritha

Maritza (Arabic) blessed.
Maritsa, Maritssa

Mariyan (Arabic) purity.
*Mariya, Mariyah, Mariyana,
Mariyanna*

Marja (Finnish) a form of
Mary.
Marjae, Marjatta, Marjie

Marjan (Persian) coral. (Polish)
a form of Mary.
Marjaneh, Marjanna

Marjie (Scottish) a familiar
form of Marjorie.
Marje, Marjey, Marji, Marjy

Marjolaine (French) marjo-
ram.

Marjorie (Greek) a familiar
form of Margaret. (Scottish)
a form of Mary.
*Majorie, Marge, Margeree,
Margerey, Margerie, Margery,
Margorie, Margory, Marjarie,
Marjary, Marjerie, Marjery,
Marjie, Marjorey, Marjori,
Marjory*

Markayla (American) a com-
bination or Mary + Kayla.
*Marka, Markaiah, Markaya,
Markayel, Markeela, Markel*

Markeisha (English) a combi-
nation of Mary + Keisha.
*Markasha, Markeisa, Markeisia,
Markeisha, Markeshia,
Markesia, Markiesha, Markisha,
Markishia, Marquesha*

Markita (Czech) a form of
Margaret.
Marka, Markeah, Markeda,

*Markee, Markeeta, Marketa,
Marketta, Marki, Markia,
Markie, Markieta, Markita,
Markitha, Markketta, Merkate*

Marla (English) a short form
of Marlena, Marlene.
Marlah, Marlea, Marleah

Marlana (English) a form of
Marlena.
*Marlaena, Marlaina, Marlainna,
Marlania, Marlanna, Marlayna,
Marleana*

Marlee (English) a form of
Marlene.
Marlea, Marleah, Marleigh

Marlena (German) a form of
Marlene.
*Marla, Marlaina, Marlana,
Marlanna, Marleena, Marlina,
Marlinda, Marlyna, Marna*

Marlene (Greek) high tower.
(Slavic) a form of Magdalen.
*Marla, Marlaine, Marlane,
Marlayne, Marlee, Marleen,
Marleene, Marlen, Marlena,
Marlenne, Marley, Marlin,
Marline, Marlyne*

Marley (English) a familiar
form of Marlene.
Marlee, Marli, Marlie, Marly

Marlis (English) a combina-
tion of Maria + Lisa.
*Marles, Marlisa, Marlise,
Marlys, Marlyse, Marlyssa*

Marlo (English) a form of Mary.
Marlon, Marlow, Marlowe

Marlyn (Hebrew) a short form of Marilyn. (Greek, Slavic) a form of Marlene.
Marlynn, Marlynne

Marmara (Greek) sparkling, shining.
Marmee

Marni (Hebrew) a form of Marnie.
Marnia, Marnique

Marnie (Hebrew) a short form of Marnina.
Marna, Marnay, Marne, Marnee, Marney, Marni, Marnisha, Marnja, Marny, Marnya, Marnye

Marnina (Hebrew) rejoice.

Maroula (Greek) a form of Mary.

Marquise (French) noblewoman.
Markese, Marquees, Marquese, Marquice, Marquies, Marquiese, Marquis, Marquisa, Marquisee, Marquisha, Marquisse, Marquiste

Marquisha (American) a form of Marquise.
Marquiesha, Marquisia

Marquita (Spanish) a form of Marcia.
Marquatte, Marqueda,

Marquedia, Marquee, Marqueita, Marquet, Marqueta, Marquetta, Marquette, Marquia, Marquida, Marquietta, Marquitra, Marquitia, Marquitta

Marrim (Chinese) tribal name in Manpur state.

Marsala (Italian) from Marseilles, France.
Marsali, Marseilles

Marsha (English) a form of Marcia.
Marcha, Marshae, Marshay, Marshel, Marshele, Marshell, Marshia, Marshiela

Marta (English) a short form of Martha, Martina.
Martá, Martä, Marte, Martia, Marttaha, Merta

Martha (Aramaic) lady; sorrowful. Bible: a friend of Jesus. See also Mardi.
Maita, Marta, Martaha, Marth, Marthan, Marthe, Marthy, Marti, Marticka, Martita, Mattie, Matty, Martus, Martuska, Masia

Marti (English) a familiar form of Martha, Martina.
Martie, Marty

Martina (Latin) martial, warlike. See also Tina.
Marta, Martel, Martella, Martelle, Martene, Marthena, Marthina, Marthine, Marti, Martine, Martinia, Martino,

Martisha, Martosia, Martoya,
Martricia, Martrina, Martyna,
Martyne, Martynne

Martiza (Arabic) blessed.

Maru (Japanese) round.

Maruca (Spanish) a form of
Mary.
Maruja, Maruska

Marvella (French) marvelous.
Marva, Marvel, Marvela,
Marvele, Marvelle, Marvely,
Marvetta, Marvette, Marvia,
Marvina

Mary (Hebrew) bitter; sea of
bitterness. Bible: the mother
of Jesus. See also Maija,
Malia, Maren, Mariah,
Marjorie, Maura, Maureen,
Miriam, Mitzi, Moira,
Mollie, Muriel.
Maira, Maire, Manette, Manka,
Manon, Manya, Mara, Mare,
Maree, Maren, Marella, Marelle,
Mari, Maria, Maricara, Marice,
Marie, Mariel, Mariela, Marika,
Marilla, Marilyn, Marion,
Mariquilla, Mariquita, Marisha,
Marja, Marjan, Marlo, Maroula,
Maruca, Marye, Maryla,
Marynia, Masha, Mavra,
Mendi, Mérane, Meridel,
Mhairie, Mirja, Molara, Morag,
Moya

Marya (Arabic) purity; bright
whiteness.
Maryah

Maryam (Hebrew) a form of
Miriam.
Maryama

Maryann, Maryanne (English)
combinations of Mary +
Ann.
Marian, Marryann, Maryan,
Meryem

Marybeth (American) a combination of Mary + Beth.
Maribeth, Maribette

Maryellen (American) a combination of Mary + Ellen.
Mariellen

Maryjane (American) a combination of Mary + Jane.

Maryjo (American) a combination of Mary + Jo.
Marijo, Maryjoe

Marykate (American) a combination of Mary + Kate.
Mary-Kate

Marylou (American) a combination of Mary + Lou.
Marilou, Marylu

Maryssa (Latin) a form of
Marissa.
Maryse, Marysia

Masago (Japanese) sands of
time.

Masani (Luganda) gap
toothed.

Masha (Russian) a form of Mary.
Mashka, Mashenka

Mashika (Swahili) born during the rainy season.
Masika

Matana (Hebrew) gift.
Matat

Mathena (Hebrew) gift of God.

Mathilde (German) a form of Matilda.
Mathilda

Matilda (German) powerful battler. See also Maud, Tilda, Tillie.
Máda, Mahaut, Maitilde, Malkin, Mat, Matelda, Mathilde, Matilde, Mattie, Matty, Matusha, Matylda

Matrika (Hindi) mother. Religion: a name for the Hindu goddess Shakti in the form of the letters of the alphabet.
Matrica

Matsuko (Japanese) pine tree.

Mattea (Hebrew) gift of God.
Matea, Mathea, Mathia, Matia, Matte, Matthea, Matthia, Mattia, Matya

Mattie, Matty (English) familiar forms of Martha, Matilda.
Matte, Mattey, Matti, Mattye

Matusha (Spanish) a form of Matilda.
Matuja, Matuxa

Maud, Maude (English) short forms of Madeline, Matilda. See also Madison.
Maudie, Maudine, Maudlin

Maura (Irish) dark. A form of Mary, Maureen. See also Moira.
Maurah, Maure, Maurette, Mauricette, Maurita

Maureen (French) dark. (Irish) a form of Mary.
Maura, Maurene, Maurine, Mo, Moreen, Morena, Morene, Morine, Morreen, Moureen

Maurelle (French) dark; elfin.
Mauriel, Mauriell, Maurielle

Maurise (French) dark skinned; moor; marshland.
Maurisa, Maurissa, Maurita, Maurizia

Mausi (Native American) plucked flower.

Mauve (French) violet colored.

Mavis (French) thrush, songbird. See also Maeve.
Mavies, Mavin, Mavine, Mavon, Mavra

Maxie (English) a familiar form of Maxine.
Maxi, Maxy

Maxine (Latin) greatest.
Max, Maxa, Maxeen, Maxena,
Maxene, Maxie, Maxima,
Maxime, Maximiliane, Maxina,
Maxna, Maxyne

May (Latin) great. (Arabic)
discerning. (English) flower;
month of May. See also Mae,
Maia.
Maj, Mayberry, Maybeth,
Mayday, Maydee, Maydena,
Maye, Mayela, Mayella,
Mayetta, Mayrene

Maya (Hindi) God's creative
power. (Greek) mother;
grandmother. (Latin) great. A
form of Maia.
Mayam, Mya

Maybeline (Latin) a familiar
form of Mabel.

Maygan, Maygen (Irish) forms
of Megan.
Mayghan, Maygon

Maylyn (American) a combi-
nation of May + Lynn.
Mayelene, Mayleen, Maylen,
Maylene, Maylin, Maylon,
Maylynn, Maylynne

Mayoree (Tai) beautiful.
Mayra, Mayree, Mayariya

Mayra (Tai) a form of
Mayoree.

Maysa (Arabic) walks with a
proud stride.

Maysun (Arabic) beautiful.

Mazel (Hebrew) lucky.
Mazal, Mazala, Mazella

Mckayla (American) a form of
Makayla.
Mckaela, Mckaila, Mckala,
Mckaylah, Mckayle, Mckaylee,
Mckayleh, Mckayleigh, Mckayli,
Mckaylia, Mckaylie

Mckell (American) a form of
Makell.
Mckelle

Mckenna (American) a form
of Mackenna.
Mckena, Mckennah, Mckinna,
Mckinnah

Mckenzie (Scottish) a form of
Mackenzie.
Mckennzie, Mckensee,
Mckensey, McKensi, Mckensi,
Mckensie, Mckensy, Mckenze,
Mckenzee, Mckenzey, Mckenzi,
Mckenzy, Mckenzye, Mekensie,
Mekenzi, Mekenzie

Mckinley (Irish) daughter of
the learned ruler.
Mckinlee, Mckinleigh, Mckinlie,
Mckinnley

Mckinzie (American) a form
of Mackenzie.
Mckinsey, Mckinze, Mckinzea,
Mckinzee, Mckinzi, Mckinzy,
Mckynze, Mckynzie

Mead, Meade (Greek) honey
wine.

Meagan (Irish) a form of
Megan.
*Maegan, Meagain, Meagann,
Meagen, Meagin, Meagnah,
Meagon*

Meaghan (Welsh) a form of
Megan.
*Maeghan, Meaghann, Meaghen,
Meahgan*

Meara (Irish) mirthful.

Meda (Native American)
prophet; priestess.

Medea (Greek) ruling. (Latin)
middle. Mythology: a sorcer-
ess who helped Jason get the
Golden Fleece.
Medeia

Medina (Arabic) History: the
site of Muhammed's tomb.
Medinah

Medora (Greek) mother's gift.
Literature: a character in
Lord Byron's poem *The
Corsair.*

Meena (Hindi) blue
semiprecious stone; bird.
(Greek, German, Dutch) a
form of Mena.

Meg (English) a short form of
Margaret, Megan.

Megan (Greek) pearl; great.
(Irish) a form of Margaret.
*Maegan, Magan, Magen,
Meagan, Meaghan, Magen,
Maygan, Maygen, Meg, Megane,*

*Megann, Megean, Megen,
Meggan, Meggen, Meggie,
Meghan, Megyn, Meygan*

Megane (Irish) a form of
Megan.
Magana, Meganna, Meganne

Megara (Greek) first.
Mythology: Heracles's first
wife.

Meggie (English) a familiar
form of Margaret, Megan.
Meggi, Meggy

Meghan (Welsh) a form of
Megan.
*Meeghan, Meehan, Megha,
Meghana, Meghane, Meghann,
Meghanne, Meghean, Meghen,
Mehgan, Mehgen*

Mehadi (Hindi) flower.

Mehira (Hebrew) speedy;
energetic.
Mahira

Mehitabel (Hebrew) benefited
by trusting God.
*Mehetabel, Mehitabelle, Hetty,
Hitty*

Mehri (Persian) kind; lovable;
sunny.

Mei (Hawaiian) great. (Chinese)
a short form of Meiying.
Meiko

Meira (Hebrew) light.
Meera

Meit (Burmese) affectionate.

Meiying (Chinese) beautiful flower.
Mei

Meka (Hebrew) a familiar form of Michaela.

Mekayla (American) a form of Michaela.
Mekaela, Mekaila, Mekayela, Mekaylia

Mel (Portuguese, Spanish) sweet as honey.

Mela (Hindi) religious service. (Polish) a form of Melanie.

Melana (Russian) a form of Melanie.
Melanna, Melashka, Melenka, Milana

Melanie (Greek) dark skinned.
Malania, Malanie, Meila, Meilani, Meilin, Melaine, Melainie, Melana, Melane, Melanee, Melaney, Melani, Melania, Mélanie, Melanka, Melanney, Melannie, Melany, Melanya, Melasya, Melayne, Melenia, Mella, Mellanie, Melonie, Melya, Milena, Milya

Melantha (Greek) dark flower.

Melba (Greek) soft; slender. (Latin) mallow flower.
Malva, Melva

Mele (Hawaiian) song; poem.

Melesse (Ethiopian) eternal.
Mellesse

Melia (German) a short form of Amelia.
Melcia, Melea, Meleah, Meleia, Meleisha, Meli, Meliah, Melida, Melika, Mema

Melina (Latin) canary yellow. (Greek) a short form of Melinda.
Melaina, Meleana, Meleena, Melena, Meline, Melinia, Melinna, Melynna

Melinda (Greek) honey. See also Linda, Melina, Mindy.
Maillie, Malinda, Melinde, Melinder, Mellinda, Melynda, Melyne, Milinda, Milynda, Mylenda, Mylinda, Mylynda

Meliora (Latin) better.
Melior, Meliori, Mellear, Melyor, Melyora

Melisa (Greek) a form of Melissa.
Melesa, Mélisa, Melise, Melisha, Melishia, Melisia, Meliza, Melizah, Mellisa, Melosa, Milisa, Mylisa, Mylisia

Melisande (French) a form of Melissa, Millicent.
Lisandra, Malisande, Malissande, Malyssandre, Melesande, Melisandra, Melisandre, Mélisandré, Melisenda, Melissande, Melissandre, Mellisande, Melond, Melysande, Melyssandre

Melissa (Greek) honey bee.
See also Elissa, Lissa,
Melisande, Millicent.
*Malissa, Mallissa, Melessa,
Meleta, Melisa, Mélissa,
Melisse, Melissia, Mellie,
Mellissa, Melly, Melyssa,
Milissa, Millie, Milly, Missy,
Molissia, Mollissa, Mylissa,
Mylissia*

Melita (Greek) a form of
Melissa. (Spanish) a short
form of Carmelita.
*Malita, Meleeta, Melitta,
Melitza, Melletta, Molita*

Melly (American) a familiar
form of names beginning
with "Mel." See also Millie.
Meli, Melie, Melli, Mellie

Melody (Greek) melody. See
also Elodie.
*Meladia, Melodee, Melodey,
Melodi, Melodia, Melodie,
Melodyann, Melodye*

Melonie (American) a form of
Melanie.
*Melloney, Mellonie, Mellony,
Melonee, Meloney, Meloni,
Melonie, Melonnie, Melony*

Melosa (Spanish) sweet; tender.

Melvina (Irish) armored chief.
See also Malvina.
*Melevine, Melva, Melveen,
Melvena, Melvene, Melvonna*

Melyne (Greek) a short form
of Melinda.
Melyn, Melynn, Melynne

Melyssa (Greek) a form of
Melissa.

Mena (German, Dutch)
strong. (Greek) a short form
of Philomena. History:
Menes is believed to be the
first king of Egypt.
Menah

Mendi (Basque) a form of
Mary.
Menda, Mendy

Meranda (Latin) a form of
Miranda.
*Merana, Merandah, Merandia,
Merannda*

Mérane (French) a form of
Mary.
Meraine, Merrane

Mercedes (Latin) reward, pay-
ment. (Spanish) merciful.
*Mercades, Mercadez, Mercadie,
Meceades, Merced, Mercede,
Mercedees, Mercedeez,
Mercedez, Mercedies, Mercedis,
Mersade, Mersades*

Mercia (English) a form of
Marcia. History: an ancient
British kingdom.

Mercy (English) compassion-
ate, merciful. See also Merry.
*Mercey, Merci, Mercie, Mercille,
Mersey*

Meredith (Welsh) protector of the sea.
Meredeth, Meredithe, Meredy, Meredyth, Meredythe, Meridath, Merideth, Meridie, Meridith, Merridie, Merridith, Merry

Meri (Finnish) sea. (Irish) a short form of Meriel.

Meriel (Irish) shining sea.
Meri, Merial, Meriol, Meryl

Merilyn (English) a combination of Merry + Lynn. See also Marilyn.
Merelyn, Merlyn, Merralyn, Merrelyn, Merrilyn

Merissa (Latin) a form of Marissa.
Merisa, Merisha

Merle (Latin, French) blackbird.
Merl, Merla, Merlina, Merline, Merola, Murle, Myrle, Myrleen, Myrlene, Myrline

Merry (English) cheerful, happy. A familiar form of Mercy, Meredith.
Merie, Merree, Merri, Merrie, Merrielle, Merrilee, Merrili, Merrilyn, Merris, Merrita

Meryl (German) famous. (Irish) shining sea. A form of Meriel, Muriel.
Meral, Merel, Merrall, Merrell, Merril, Merrile, Merrill, Merryl, Meryle, Meryll

Mesha (Hindi) another name for the zodiac sign Aries.
Meshal

Meta (German) a short form of Margaret.
Metta, Mette, Metti

Mhairie (Scottish) a form of Mary.
Mhaire, Mhairi, Mhari, Mhary

Mia (Italian) mine. A familiar form of Michaela, Michelle.
Mea, Meah, Miah

Micaela (Hebrew) a form of Michaela.
Macaela, Micaella, Micaila, Micala, Miceala

Micah (Hebrew) a short form of Michaela. Bible: one of the Old Testament prophets.
Meecah, Mica, Micha, Mika, Myca, Mycah

Micayla, Michayla (Hebrew) forms of Michaela.
Micayle, Micaylee, Michaylah

Michaela (Hebrew) who is like God?
Machaela, Maika, Makaela, Makaila, Makala, Makayla, Mia, Micaela, Micayla, Michael, Michaelann, Michala, Michayla, Michealia, Michaelina, Michaeline, Michaell, Michaella, Michaelyn, Michaila, Michal, Michala, Micheal, Micheala, Michelia, Michelina, Michelle, Michely, Michelyn, Micheyla,

Michaela *(cont.)*
Micheline, Micki, Miguela,
Mikaela, Mikala, Misha,
Mycala, Mychael, Mychal

Michala (Hebrew) a form of
Michaela.
Michalann, Michale, Michalene,
Michalin, Mchalina, Michalisha,
Michalla, Michalle, Michayla,
Michayle, Michela

Michele (Italian) a form of
Michaela.
Michaelle, Michal, Michela

Michelle (French) who is like
God? See also Shelley.
Machealle, Machele, Machell,
Machella, Machelle, Mechelle,
Meichelle, Meschell, Meshell,
Meshelle, Mia, Michel, Michéle,
Michell, Michella, Michellene,
Michellyn, Mischel, Mischelle,
Mishael, Mishaela, Mishayla,
Mishell, Mishelle, Mitchele,
Mitchelle

Michi (Japanese) righteous
way.
Miche, Michee, Michiko

Micki (American) a familiar
form of Michaela.
Mickee, Mickeeya, Mickia,
Mickie, Micky, Mickya, Miquia

Midori (Japanese) green.

Mieko (Japanese) prosperous.
Mieke

Mielikki (Finnish) pleasing.

Miette (French) small; sweet.

Migina (Omaha) new moon.

Mignon (French) dainty,
petite; graceful.
Mignonette, Minnionette,
Minnonette, Minyonette,
Minyonne

Miguela (Spanish) a form of
Michaela.
Micquel, Miguelina, Miguelita,
Miquel, Miquela, Miquella

Mika (Japanese) new moon.
(Russian) God's child.
(Native American) wise
racoon. (Hebrew) a form of
Micah. (Latin) a form of
Dominica.
Mikah, Mikka

Mikaela (Hebrew) a form of
Michaela.
Mekaela, Mekala, Mickael,
Mickaela, Mickala, Mickalla,
Mickeel, Mickell, Mickelle,
Mikael, Mikail, Mikaila, Mikal,
Mikalene, Mikalovna, Mikalyn,
Mikayla, Mikea, Mikeisha,
Mikeita, Mikel, Mikela, Mikele,
Mikell, Mikella, Mikesha,
Mikeya, Mikhaela, Mikie,
Mikiela, Mikkel, Mikyla,
Mykaela

Mikala (Hebrew) a form of
Michaela.
Mickala, Mikalah, Mikale,
Mikalea, Mikalee, Mikaleh

Mikayla (American) a form of
Mikaela.
*Mekayla, Mickayla, Mikala,
Mikayle, Mikyla*

Mikhaela (American) a form
of Mikaela.
*Mikhail, Mikhaila, Mikhala,
Mikhalea, Mikhayla, Mikhelle*

Miki (Japanese) flower stem.
*Mikia, Mikiala, Mikie, Mikita,
Mikiyo, Mikki, Mikkie,
Mikkiya, Mikko, Miko*

Mila (Russian) dear one.
(Italian, Slavic) a short form
of Camila, Ludmilla.
Milah, Milla

Milada (Czech) my love.
Mila, Milady

Milagros (Spanish) miracle.
*Mila, Milagritos, Milagro,
Milagrosa, Mirari*

Milana (Italian) from Milan,
Italy. (Russian) a form of
Melana.
*Milan, Milane, Milani,
Milanka, Milanna, Milanne*

Mildred (English) gentle
counselor.
*Mil, Mila, Mildrene, Mildrid,
Millie, Milly*

Milena (Greek, Hebrew,
Russian) a form of Ludmilla,
Magdalen, Melanie.
*Mila, Milène, Milenia, Milenny,
Milini, Millini*

Mileta (German) generous,
merciful.

Milia (German) industrious. A
short form of Amelia, Emily.
Mila, Milka, Milla, Milya

Miliani (Hawaiian) caress.
Milanni, Miliany

Mililani (Hawaiian) heavenly
caress.
Milliani

Milissa (Greek) a form of
Melissa.
Milessa, Milisa, Millisa, Millissa

Milka (Czech) a form of
Amelia.
Milica, Milika

Millicent (English) industri-
ous. (Greek) a form of
Melissa. See also Lissa,
Melisande.
*Melicent, Meliscent, Mellicent,
Mellisent, Melly, Milicent,
Milisent, Millie, Milliestone,
Millisent, Milly, Milzie, Missy*

Millie, Milly (English) familiar
forms of Amelia, Camille,
Emily, Kamila, Melissa,
Mildred, Millicent.
*Mili, Milla, Millee, Milley,
Millie, Mylie*

Mima (Burmese) woman.
Mimma

Mimi (French) a familiar form
of Miriam.

Mina (German) love. (Persian) blue sky. (Arabic) harbor. (Japanese) south. A short form of names ending in "mina."
Meena, Mena, Min

Minal (Native American) fruit.

Minda (Hindi) knowledge.

Mindy (Greek) a familiar form of Melinda.
Mindee, Mindi, Mindie, Mindyanne, Mindylee, Myndy

Mine (Japanese) peak; mountain range.
Mineko

Minerva (Latin) wise. Mythology: the goddess of wisdom.
Merva, Minivera, Minnie, Myna

Minette (French) faithful defender
Minnette, Minnita

Minka (Polish) a short form of Wilhelmina.

Minna (German) a short form of Wilhelmina.
Mina, Minka, Minnie, Minta

Minnie (American) a familiar form of Mina, Minerva, Minna, Wilhelmina.
Mini, Minie, Minne, Minni, Minny

Minowa (Native American) singer.
Minowah

Minta (English) Literature: originally coined by playwright Sir John Vanbrugh in his comedy *The Confederacy*.
Minty

Minya (Osage) older sister.

Mio (Japanese) three times as strong.

Mira (Latin) wonderful. (Spanish) look, gaze. A short form of Almira, Amira, Marabel, Mirabel, Miranda.
Mirae, Mirra, Mirah

Mirabel (Latin) beautiful.
Mira, Mirabell, Mirabella, Mirabelle, Mirable

Miracle (Latin) wonder, marvel.

Miranda (Latin) strange; wonderful; admirable. Literature: the heroine of Shakespeare's *The Tempest*. See also Randi.
Maranda, Marenda, Meranda, Mira, Miran, Miranada, Mirandia, Mirinda, Mirindé, Mironda, Mirranda, Muranda, Myranda

Mireille (Hebrew) God spoke. (Latin) wonderful.
Mireil, Mirel, Mirella, Mirelle, Mirelys, Mireya, Mireyda, Mirielle, Mirilla, Myrella, Myrilla

Mireya (Hebrew) a form of
Mireille.
Mireea, Miriah, Miryah

Miri (Gypsy) a short form of
Miriam.
Miria, Miriah

Miriam (Hebrew) bitter; sea of
bitterness. Bible: the original
form of Mary. See also
Macia, Mimi, Mitzi.
*Mairwen, Mariam, Maryam,
Miram, Mirham, Miri, Miriain,
Miriama, Miriame, Mirian,
Mirit, Mirjam, Mirjana,
Mirriam, Mirrian, Miryam,
Miryan, Myriam*

Misha (Russian) a form of
Michaela.
Mischa, Mishae

Missy (English) a familiar form
of Melissa, Millicent.
Missi, Missie

Misty (English) shrouded by
mist.
*Missty, Mistee, Mistey, Misti,
Mistie, Mistin, Mistina, Mistral,
Mistylynn, Mystee, Mysti,
Mystie*

Mitra (Hindi) Religion: god
of daylight. (Persian) angel.
Mita

Mituna (Moquelumnan) like a
fish wrapped up in leaves.

Mitzi (German) a form of
Mary, Miriam.
Mieze, Mitzee, Mitzie, Mitzy

Miwa (Japanese) wise eyes.
Miwako

Miya (Japanese) temple.
Miyah, Miyana, Miyanna

Miyo (Japanese) beautiful
generation.
Miyoko, Miyuko

Miyuki (Japanese) snow.

Moana (Hawaiian) ocean; fragrance.

Mocha (Arabic) chocolate-
flavored coffee.
Moka

Modesty (Latin) modest.
*Modesta, Modeste, Modestia,
Modestie, Modestina, Modestine,
Modestus*

Moesha (American) a short
form of Monisha.
Myesha

Mohala (Hawaiian) flowers in
bloom.
Moala

Moira (Irish) great. A form of
Mary. See also Maura.
*Moirae, Moirah, Moire, Moya,
Moyra, Moyrah*

Molara (Basque) a form of
Mary.

Mollie, Molly (Irish) familiar
forms of Mary.
*Moli, Molie, Moll, Mollee,
Molley, Molli, Mollissa*

Mona (Irish) noble. (Greek) a short form of Monica, Ramona, Rimona.
Moina, Monah, Mone, Monea, Monna, Moyna

Monet (French) Art: Claude Monet was a leading French impressionist remembered for his paintings of water lilies.
Monae, Monay, Monee

Monica (Greek) solitary. (Latin) advisor.
Mona, Monca, Monee, Monia, Monic, Monice, Monicia, Monicka, Monika, Monique, Monise, Monn, Monnica, Monnie, Monya

Monifa (Yoruba) I have my luck.

Monika (German) a form of Monica.
Moneka, Monieka, Monike, Monnika

Monique (French) a form of Monica.
Moneeke, Moneik, Moniqua, Moniquea, Moniquie, Munique

Monisha (American) a combination of Monica + Aisha.
Moesha, Moneisha, Monishia

Montana (Spanish) mountain. Geography: a U. S. state.
Montanna

Mora (Spanish) blueberry.
Morae, Morea, Moria, Morita

Morela (Polish) apricot.
Morelia, Morelle

Morena (Irish) a form of Maureen.

Morgan (Welsh) seashore. Literature: Morgan le Fay was the half-sister of King Arthur.
Morgana, Morgance, Morgane, Morganetta, Morganette, Morganica, Morgann, Morganna, Morganne, Morgen, Morghan, Morgyn, Morrigan

Morghan (Welsh) a form of Morgan.
Morghen, Morghin, Morghyn

Moriah (Hebrew) God is my teacher. (French) dark skinned. Bible: the mountain on which the Temple of Solomon was built. See also Mariah.
Moria, Moriel, Morit, Morria, Morriah

Morie (Japanese) bay.

Morowa (Akan) queen.

Morrisa (Latin) dark skinned; moor; marshland.
Morisa, Morissa, Morrissa

Moselle (Hebrew) drawn from the water. (French) a white wine.
Mozelle

Mosi (Swahili) first-born.

Moswen (Tswana) white.

Mouna (Arabic) wish, desire.
Moona, Moonia, Mounia,
Muna, Munia

Mrena (Slavic) white eyes.
Mren

Mumtaz (Arabic)
distinguished.

Mura (Japanese) village.

Muriel (Arabic) myrrh. (Irish)
shining sea. A form of Mary.
See also Meryl.
Merial, Meriel, Meriol, Merrial,
Merriel, Muire, Murial, Muriell,
Murielle

Musetta (French) little bag-
pipe.
Musette

Muslimah (Arabic) devout
believer.

Mya (Burmese) emerald.
(Italian) a form of Mia.
My, Myah, Myia, Myiah

Myesha (American) a form of
Moesha.
Myeisha, Myeshia, Myiesha,
Myisha

Mykaela, Mykayla (American)
forms of Mikaela.
Mykael, Mykaila, Mykal,
Mykala, Mykaleen, Mykel,
Mykela, Mykyla

Myla (English) merciful.

Mylene (Greek) dark.
Mylaine, Mylana, Mylee,
Myleen

Myra (Latin) fragrant
ointment.
Mayra, Myrena, Myria

Myranda (Latin) a form of
Miranda.
Myrandah, Myrandia,
Myrannda

Myriam (American) a form of
Miriam.
Myriame, Myryam

Myrna (Irish) beloved.
Merna, Mirna, Morna, Muirna

Myrtle (Greek) dark green
shrub.
Mertis, Mertle, Mirtle, Myrta,
Myrtia, Myrtias, Myrtice,
Myrtie, Myrtilla, Myrtis

N

Nabila (Arabic) born to nobility.
Nabeela, Nabiha, Nabilah

Nadda (Arabic) generous;
dewy.
Nada

Nadette (French) a short form
of Bernadette.

Nadia (French, Slavic) hopeful.
Nadea, Nadenka, Nadezhda, Nadiah, Nadie, Nadija, Nadijah, Nadine, Nadiya, Nadiyah, Nadja, Nadjae, Nadjah, Nadka, Nadusha, Nady, Nadya

Nadine (French, Slavic) a form of Nadia.
Nadean, Nadeana, Nadeen, Nadena, Nadene, Nadien, Nadin, Nadina, Nadyne, Naidene, Naidine

Nadira (Arabic) rare, precious.
Naadirah, Nadirah

Naeva (French) a form of Eve.
Nahvon

Nafuna (Luganda) born feet first.

Nagida (Hebrew) noble; prosperous.
Nagda, Nageeda

Nahid (Persian) Mythology: another name for Venus, the goddess of love and beauty.

Nahimana (Dakota) mystic.

Naida (Greek) water nymph.
Naiad, Naiya, Nayad, Nyad

Naila (Arabic) successful.
Nailah

Nairi (Armenian) land of rivers. History: a name for ancient Armenia.
Naira, Naire, Nayra

Naiya (Greek) a form of Naida.
Naia, Naiyana, Naja, Najah, Naya

Najam (Arabic) star.
Naja, Najma

Najila (Arabic) brilliant eyes.
Naja, Najah, Najia, Najja, Najla

Nakeisha (American) a combination of the prefix Na + Keisha.
Nakeesha, Nakesha, Nakeshea, Nakeshia, Nakeysha, Nakiesha, Nakisha, Nekeisha

Nakeita (American) a form of Nikita.
Nakeeta, Nakeitha, Nakeithra, Nakeitra, Nakeitress, Nakeitta, Nakeittia, Naketta, Nakieta, Nakitha, Nakitia, Nakitta, Nakyta

Nakia (Arabic) pure.
Nakea, Nakeia, Nakeya, Nakeyah, Nakeyia, Nakiah, Nakiaya, Nakiea, Nakiya, Nakiyah, Nekia

Nakita (American) a form of Nikita.
Nakkita, Naquita

Nalani (Hawaiian) calm as the heavens.
Nalanie, Nalany

Nami (Japanese) wave.
Namika, Namiko

Nan (German) a short form of Fernanda. (English) a form of Ann.
Nana, Nanice, Nanine, Nanna, Nanon

Nana (Hawaiian) spring.

Nanci (English) a form of Nancy.
Nancie, Nancsi, Nansi

Nancy (English) gracious. A familiar form of Nan.
Nainsi, Nance, Nancee, Nancey, Nanci, Nancine, Nancye, Nanette, Nanice, Nanncey, Nanncy, Nanouk, Nansee, Nansey, Nanuk

Nanette (French) a form of Nancy.
Nan, Nanete, Nannette, Nettie, Nineta, Ninete, Ninetta, Ninette, Nini, Ninita, Ninnetta, Ninnette, Nynette

Nani (Greek) charming. (Hawaiian) beautiful.
Nanni, Nannie, Nanny

Naomi (Hebrew) pleasant, beautiful. Bible: Ruth's mother-in-law.
Naoma, Naomia, Naomie, Naomy, Navit, Neoma, Neomi, Noami, Noemi, Noma, Nomi, Nyomi

Naomie (Hebrew) a form of Naomi.
Naome, Naomee, Noemie

Nara (Greek) happy. (English) north. (Japanese) oak.
Narah

Narcissa (Greek) daffodil. Mythology: Narcissus was the youth who fell in love with his own reflection.
Narcessa, Narcisa, Narcisse, Narcyssa, Narissa, Narkissa

Narelle (Australian) woman from the sea.
Narel

Nari (Japanese) thunder.
Narie, Nariko

Narmada (Hindi) pleasure giver.

Nashawna (American) a combination of the prefix Na + Shawna.
Nashan, Nashana, Nashanda, Nashaun, Nashauna, Nashaunda, Nashauwna, Nashawn, Nasheena, Nashounda, Nashuana

Nashota (Native American) double; second-born twin.

Nastasia (Greek) a form of Anastasia.
Nastasha, Nastashia, Nastasja, Nastassa, Nastassia, Nastassiya, Nastassja, Nastassya, Nastasya, Nastazia, Nastisija, Nastka, Nastusya, Nastya

Nasya (Hebrew) miracle.
Nasia, Nasyah

Nata (Sanskrit) dancer. (Latin) swimmer. (Native American) speaker; creator. (Polish, Russian) a form of Natalie. See also Nadia.
Natia, Natka, Natya

Natacha (Russian) a form of Natasha.
Natachia, Natacia, Naticha

Natalee, Natali (Latin) forms of Natalie.
Natale, Nataleh, Nataleigh, Nattlee

Natalia (Russian) a form of Natalie. See also Talia.
Nacia, Natala, Natalea, Nataliia, Natalija, Natalina, Nataliya, Nataliyah, Natalja, Natalka, Natallea, Natallia, Natalya, Nathalia, Natka

Natalie (Latin) born on Christmas day. See also Nata, Natasha, Noel, Talia.
Nat, Natalee, Natali, Natalia, Nataliee, Nataline, Natalle, Natallie, Nataly, Natelie, Nathalie, Nathaly, Natie, Natilie, Natlie, Nattalie, Nattilie

Nataline (Latin) a form of Natalie.
Natalene, Nataléne, Natalyn

Natalle (French) a form of Natalie.
Natale

Nataly (Latin) a form of Natalie.
Nathaly, Natally, Natallye

Natane (Arapaho) daughter.
Natanne

Natania (Hebrew) gift of God.
Natanya, Natée, Nathania, Nathenia, Netania, Nethania

Natara (Arabic) sacrifice.
Natori, Natoria

Natasha (Russian) a form of Natalie. See also Stacey, Tasha.
Nahtasha, Natacha, Natasa, Natascha, Natashah, Natashea, Natashenka, Natashia, Natashiea, Natashja, Natashka, Natasia, Natassia, Natassija, Natassja, Natasza, Natausha, Natawsha, Natesha, Nateshia, Nathasha, Nathassha, Natisha, Natishia, Natosha, Netasha, Notosha

Natesa (Hindi) cosmic dancer. Religion: another name for the Hindu god Shiva.
Natisa, Natissa

Nathalie, Nathaly (Latin) forms of Natalie.
Nathalee, Nathali, Nathalia, Nathalya

Natie (English) a familiar form of Natalie.
Nati, Natti, Nattie, Natty

Natosha (Russian) a form of
Natasha.
*Natoshia, Natoshya, Netosha,
Notosha*

Nava (Hebrew) beautiful;
pleasant.
Navah, Naveh, Navit

Nayely (Irish) a form of Neila.
*Naeyli, Nayelia, Nayelli,
Nayelly, Nayla*

Neala (Irish) a form of Neila.
*Nayela, Naylea, Naylia, Nealia,
Neela, Neelia, Neila*

Necha (Spanish) a form of
Agnes.
Necho

Neci (Hungarian) fiery,
intense.
Necia, Necie

Neda (Slavic) born on Sunday.
Nedah, Nedi, Nedia, Neida

Nedda (English) prosperous
guardian.
Neddi, Neddie, Neddy

Neely (Irish) a familiar form
of Neila, Nelia.
*Nealee, Nealie, Nealy, Neelee,
Neeley, Neeli, Neelie, Neili,
Neilie*

Neema (Swahili) born during
prosperous times.

Neena (Spanish) a form of
Nina.
Neenah, Nena

Neila (Irish) champion. See
also Neala, Neely.
*Nayely, Neilah, Neile, Neilia,
Neilla, Neille*

Nekeisha (American) a form
of Nakeisha.
*Nechesa, Neikeishia, Nekesha,
Nekeshia, Nekiesha, Nekisha,
Nekysha*

Nekia (Arabic) a form of
Nakia.
*Nekeya, Nekiya, Nekiyah,
Nekya, Nekiya*

Nelia (Spanish) yellow. (Latin)
a familiar form of Cornelia.
*Neelia, Neely, Neelya, Nela,
Neli, Nelka, Nila*

Nelle (Greek) stone.

Nellie, Nelly (English) familiar
forms of Cornelia, Eleanor,
Helen, Prunella.
*Nel, Neli, Nell, Nella, Nelley,
Nelli, Nellianne, Nellice, Nellis,
Nelma*

Nenet (Egyptian) born near
the sea. Mythology: Nunet
was the goddess of the sea.

Neola (Greek) youthful.
Neolla

Neona (Greek) new moon.

Nereida (Greek) a form of
Nerine.
Nereyda, Nereyida, Nerida

Nerine (Greek) sea nymph.
*Nereida, Nerina, Nerita,
Nerline*

Nerissa (Greek) sea nymph.
See also Rissa.
*Narice, Narissa, Nerice, Nerisa,
Nerisse, Nerrisa, Nerys, Neryssa*

Nessa (Scandinavian) promontory. (Greek) a short form of
Agnes. See also Nessie.
*Nesa, Nesha, Neshia, Nesiah,
Nessia, Nesta, Nevsa, Neysa,
Neysha, Neyshia*

Nessie (Greek) a familiar form
of Agnes, Nessa, Vanessa.
*Nese, Neshie, Nesho, Nesi,
Ness, Nessi, Nessy, Nest, Neys*

Neta (Hebrew) plant, shrub.
See also Nettie.
Netia, Netta, Nettia

Netis (Native American) trustworthy.

Nettie (French) a familiar
form of Annette, Nanette,
Antoinette.
*Neti, Netie, Netta, Netti, Netty,
Nety*

Neva (Spanish) snow. (English)
new. Geography: a river in
Russia.
*Neiva, Neve, Nevia, Neyva,
Nieve, Niva, Nivea, Nivia*

Nevada (Spanish) snow.
Geography: a western U. S.
state.
Neiva, Neva

Nevina (Irish) worshipper of
the saint.
*Neveen, Nevein, Nevena,
Neveyan, Nevin, Nivena*

Neylan (Turkish) fulfilled
wish.
Neya, Neyla

Neza (Slavic) a form of Agnes.

Nia (Irish) a familiar form of
Neila. Mythology: Nia Ben
Aur was a legendary Welsh
woman.
Neya, Niah, Niajia, Niya, Nya

Niabi (Osage) fawn.

Nichelle (American) a combination of Nicole + Michelle.
Culture: Nichelle Nichols was
the first African American
woman featured in a television
drama (*Star Trek*).
Nichele, Nichell, Nishelle

Nichole (French) a form of
Nicole.
*Nichol, Nichola, Nicholas,
Nicholle*

Nicki (French) a familiar form
of Nicole.
*Nicci, Nickey, Nickeya, Nickia,
Nickie, Nickiya, Nicky, Niki*

Nickole (French) a form of
Nicole.
Nickol

Nicola (Italian) a form of
Nicole.
Nacola, Necola, Nichola,

Nickola, Nicolea, Nicolla,
Nikkola, Nikola, Nikolia,
Nykola

Nicole (French) a form of
Nicholas. See also Colette,
Cosette, Nikita.
Nacole, Necole, Nica, Nichole,
Nicia, Nicki, Nickole, Nicol,
Nicola, Nicolette, Nicoli, Nicolie,
Nicoline, Nicolle, Nikayla,
Nikelle, Nikki, Niquole, Nocole,
Nycole

Nicolette (French) a form of
Nicole.
Nicholetta, Nicoletta, Nicollete,
Nicollette, Nikkolette, Nikoleta,
Nikoletta, Nikolette

Nicoline (French) a familiar
form of Nicole.
Nicholine, Nicholyn, Nicoleen,
Nicolene, Nicolina, Nicolyn,
Nicolyne, Nicolynn, Nicolynne,
Nikolene, Nikolina, Nikoline

Nicolle (French) a form of
Nicole.
Nicholle

Nida (Omaha) Mythology: an
elflike creature.
Nidda

Nidia (Latin) nest.
Nidi, Nidya

Niesha (American) pure.
(Scandinavian) a form of
Nissa.
Neisha, Neishia, Neissia,

Nesha, Neshia, Nesia, Nessia,
Niessia, Nisha, Nyesha

Nige (Latin) dark night.
Nigea, Nigela, Nija, Nijae,
Nijah

Nika (Russian) belonging to
God.
Nikka

Nikayla, Nikelle (American)
forms of Nicole.
Nikeille, Nikel, Nikela, Nikelie

Nike (Greek) victorious.
Mythology: the goddess of
victory.

Niki (Russian) a short form of
Nikita. (American) a familiar
form of Nicole.
Nikia, Nikiah

Nikita (Russian) victorious
people.
Nakeita, Nakita, Niki, Nikitah,
Nikitia, Nikitta, Nikki,
Nikkita, Niquita, Niquitta

Nikki (American) a familiar
form of Nicole, Nikita.
Nicki, Nikia, Nikkea, Nikkey,
Nikkia, Nikkiah, Nikkie,
Nikko, Nikky

Nikole (French) a form of
Nicole.
Nikkole, Nikkolie, Nikola,
Nikole, Nikolena, Nicolia,
Nikolina, Nikolle

Nila (Latin) Geography: the Nile River is in Africa. (Irish) a form of Neila.
Nilah, Nilesia, Nyla

Nili (Hebrew) Botany: a pea plant that yields indigo.

Nima (Hebrew) thread. (Arabic) blessing.
Nema, Niama, Nimali

Nina (Hebrew) a familiar form of Hannah. (Spanish) girl. (Native American) mighty. (Hebrew) a familiar form of Hannah.
Neena, Ninah, Ninacska, Ninja, Ninna, Ninon, Ninosca, Ninoshka

Ninon (French) a form of Nina.

Nirel (Hebrew) light of God.
Nirali, Nirelle

Nirveli (Hindi) water child.

Nisa (Arabic) woman.

Nisha (American) a form of Niesha, Nissa.
Niasha, Nishay

Nishi (Japanese) west.

Nissa (Hebrew) sign, emblem. (Scandinavian) friendly elf; brownie. See also Nyssa.
Nisha, Nisse, Nissie, Nissy

Nita (Hebrew) planter. (Choctaw) bear. (Spanish) a short form of Anita, Juanita.
Nitai, Nitha, Nithai, Nitika

Nitara (Hindi) deeply rooted.

Nitasha (American) a form of Natasha.
Nitasia, Niteisha, Nitisha, Nitishia

Nitsa (Greek) a form of Helen.

Nituna (Native American) daughter.

Nitza (Hebrew) flower bud.
Nitzah, Nitzana, Nitzanit, Niza, Nizah

Nixie (German) water sprite.

Niya (Irish) a form of Nia.
Niyah, Niyana, Niyia, Nyia

Nizana (Hebrew) a form of Nitza.
Nitzana, Nitzania, Zana

Noel (Latin) Christmas. See also Natalie.
Noël, Noela, Noelani, Noele, Noeleen, Noelene, Noelia, Noeline, Noelle, Noelyn, Noelynn, Nohely, Noleen, Novelenn, Novelia, Nowel, Noweleen, Nowell

Noelani (Hawaiian) beautiful one from heaven.
Noela

Noelle (French) Christmas.
Noell, Noella, Noelleen, Noelly, Noellyn

Noemi (Hebrew) a form of
Naomi.
*Noam, Noemie, Noemy,
Nohemi, Nomi*

Noemie (Hebrew) a form of
Noemi.

Noemy (Hebrew) a form of
Noemi.
Noamy

Noga (Hebrew) morning
light.

Nohely (Latin) a form of
Noel.
*Noeli, Noelie, Noely, Nohal,
Noheli*

Nokomis (Dakota) moon
daughter.

Nola (Latin) small bell. (Irish)
famous; noble. A short form
of Fionnula.
Nuala

Noleta (Latin) unwilling.
Nolita

Nollie (English) a familiar
form of Magnolia.
*Nolia, Nolle, Nolley, Nolli,
Nolly*

Noma (Hawaiian) a form of
Norma.

Nona (Latin) ninth.
*Nonah, Noni, Nonia, Nonie,
Nonna, Nonnah, Nonya*

Noor (Aramaic) a form of
Nura.
Noorie, Nour, Nur

Nora (Greek) light. A familiar
form of Eleanor, Honora,
Leonore.
Norah, Noreen

Noreen (Irish) a form of
Eleanor, Nora. (Latin) a
familiar form of Norma.
*Noorin, Noreena, Noreene,
Noren, Norena, Norene,
Norina, Norine, Nureen*

Norell (Scandinavian) from
the north.
*Narell, Narelle, Norela, Norelle,
Norely*

Nori (Japanese) law, tradition.
Noria, Norico, Noriko, Norita

Norma (Latin) rule, precept.
Noma, Noreen, Normi, Normie

Nova (Latin) new. A short
form of Novella, Novia.
(Hopi) butterfly chaser.
Astronomy: a star that
releases bright bursts of
energy.

Novella (Latin) newcomer.
Nova, Novela

Novia (Spanish) sweetheart.
Nova, Novka, Nuvia

Nu (Burmese) tender.
(Vietnamese) girl.
Nue

Nuala (Irish) a short form of
Fionnula.
Nola, Nula

Nuela (Spanish) a form of
Amelia.

Nuna (Native American) land.

Nunciata (Latin) messenger.
Nunzia

Nura (Aramaic) light.
*Noor, Noora, Noorah, Noura,
Nurah*

Nuria (Aramaic) the Lord's
light.
Nuri, Nuriel, Nurin

Nurita (Hebrew) Botany: a
flower with red and yellow
blossoms.
Nurit

Nuru (Swahili) daylight.

Nusi (Hungarian) a form of
Hannah.

Nuwa (Chinese) mother goddess. Mythology: another
name for Nü-gua, the creator
of mankind.

Nya (Irish) a form of Nia.
Nyaa, Nyah, Nyia

Nycole (French) a form of
Nicole.
Nychelle, Nycolette, Nycolle

Nydia (Latin) nest.
Nyda

Nyesha (American) a form of
Niesha.
Nyeisha, Nyeshia

Nyla (Latin, Irish) a form of
Nila.
Nylah

Nyoko (Japanese) gem, treasure.

Nyomi (Hebrew) a form of
Naomi.
Nyome, Nyomee, Nyomie

Nyree (Maori) sea.
Nyra, Nyrie

Nyssa (Greek) beginning. See
also Nissa.
*Nisha, Nissi, Nissy, Nyasia,
Nysa*

Nyusha (Russian) a form of
Agnes.
Nyushenka, Nyushka

Oba (Yoruba) chief, ruler.

Obelia (Greek) needle.

Oceana (Greek) ocean.
Mythology: Oceanus was the
god of the ocean.
*Ocean, Oceananna, Oceane,
Oceania, Oceanna, Oceanne,
Oceaonna, Oceon*

Octavia (Latin) eighth. See also Tavia.
Octabia, Octaviah, Octaviais, Octavice, Octavie, Octavienne, Octavio, Octavious, Octavise, Octavya, Octivia, Otavia, Ottavia

Odeda (Hebrew) strong; courageous.

Odele (Greek) melody, song.
Odelet, Odelette, Odell, Odelle

Odelia (Greek) ode; melodic. (Hebrew) I will praise God. (French) wealthy. See also Odetta.
Oda, Odeelia, Odeleya, Odelina, Odelinda, Odelyn, Odila, Odile, Odilia

Odella (English) wood hill.
Odela, Odelle, Odelyn

Odera (Hebrew) plough.

Odessa (Greek) odyssey, long voyage.
Adesha, Adeshia, Adessa, Adessia, Odessia

Odetta (German, French) a form of Odelia.
Oddetta, Odette

Odina (Algonquin) mountain.

Ofelia (Greek) a form of Ophelia.
Ofeelia, Ofilia

Ofira (Hebrew) gold.
Ofarrah, Ophira

Ofra (Hebrew) a form of Aphra.
Ofrat

Ogin (Native American) wild rose.

Ohanna (Hebrew) God's gracious gift.

Okalani (Hawaiian) heaven.
Okilani

Oki (Japanese) middle of the ocean.
Okie

Oksana (Latin) a form of Osanna.
Oksanna

Ola (Greek) a short form of Olesia.(Scandinavian) ancestor.

Olathe (Native American) beautiful.
Olathia

Oleda (Spanish) a form of Alida. See also Leda.
Oleta, Olida, Olita

Olena (Russian) a form of Helen.
Oleena, Olenka, Olenna, Olenya, Olya

Olesia (Greek) a form of Alexandra.
Cesya, Ola, Olecia, Oleesha, Oleishia, Olesha, Olesya, Olexa, Olice, Olicia, Olisha, Olishia, Ollicia

Oletha (Scandinavian) nimble.
Oleta, Yaletha

Olethea (Latin) truthful. See
also Alethea.
Oleta

Olga (Scandinavian) holy. See
also Helga, Olivia.
*Olenka, Olia, Olja, Ollya,
Olva, Olya*

Oliana (Polynesian) oleander.

Olina (Hawaiian) filled with
happiness.

Olinda (Latin) scented.
(Spanish) protector of prop-
erty. (Greek) a form of
Yolanda.

Olisa (Ibo) God.

Olive (Latin) olive tree.
Oliff, Oliffe, Olivet, Olivette

Olivia (Latin) a form of Olive.
(English) a form of Olga. See
also Liv, Livia.
*Alivia, Alyvia, Olevia, Oliva,
Olivea, Oliveia, Olivetta, Olivi,
Olivianne, Olivya, Oliwia,
Ollie, Olva, Olyvia*

Ollie (English) a familiar form
of Olivia.
Olla, Olly, Ollye

Olwen (Welsh) white
footprint.
*Olwenn, Olwin, Olwyn,
Olwyne, Olwynne*

Olympia (Greek) heavenly.
Olimpia, Olympe, Olympie

Olyvia (Latin) a form of
Olivia.

Oma (Hebrew) reverent.
(German) grandmother.
(Arabic) highest.

Omaira (Arabic) red.
*Omar, Omara, Omarah,
Omari, Omaria, Omarra*

Omega (Greek) last, final, end.
Linguistics: the last letter in
the Greek alphabet.

Ona (Latin, Irish) a form of
Oona, Una. (English) river.

Onatah (Iroquois) daughter of
the earth and the corn spirit.

Onawa (Native American)
wide awake.
Onaja, Onajah

Ondine (Latin) a form of
Undine.
Ondene, Ondina, Ondyne

Ondrea (Czech) a form of
Andrea.
*Ohndrea, Ohndreea, Ohndreya,
Ohndria, Ondraya, Ondreana,
Ondreea, Ondreya, Ondria,
Ondrianna, Ondriea*

Oneida (Native American)
eagerly awaited.
Onida, Onyda

Onella (Hungarian) a form of
Helen.

Onesha (American) a combination of Ondrea + Aisha.
Oneshia, Onesia, Onessa, Onessia, Onethia, Oniesha, Onisha

Oni (Yoruba) born on holy ground.
Onnie

Onora (Latin) a form of Honora.
Onoria, Onorine, Ornora

Oona (Latin, Irish) a form of Una.
Ona, Onna, Onnie, Oonagh, Oonie

Opa (Choctaw) owl. (German) grand-father.

Opal (Hindi) precious stone.
Opale, Opalina, Opaline

Ophelia (Greek) helper. Literature: Hamlet's love interest in the Shakespearean play *Hamlet*.
Filia, Ofelia, Ophélie, Ophilia, Phelia

Oprah (Hebrew) a form of Orpah.
Ophra, Ophrah, Opra

Ora (Latin) prayer. (Spanish) gold. (English) seacoast. (Greek) a form of Aura.
Orah, Orlice, Orra

Orabella (Latin) a form of Arabella.
Orabel, Orabela, Orabelle

Oralee (Hebrew) the Lord is my light. See also Yareli.
Areli, Orali, Oralit, Orelie, Orlee, Orli, Orly

Oralia (French) a form of Aurelia. See also Oriana.
Oralis, Oriel, Orielda, Orielle, Oriena, Orlena, Orlene

Orea (Greek) mountains.
Oreal, Oria, Oriah

Orela (Latin) announcement from the gods; oracle.
Oreal, Orella, Orelle, Oriel, Orielle

Orenda (Iroquois) magical power.

Oretha (Greek) a form of Aretha.
Oreta, Oretta, Orette

Oriana (Latin) dawn, sunrise. (Irish) golden.
Orane, Orania, Orelda, Orelle, Ori, Oria, Orian, Oriane, Orianna, Orieana, Oryan

Orina (Russian) a form of Irene.
Orya, Oryna

Orinda (Hebrew) pine tree. (Irish) light skinned, white.
Orenda

Orino (Japanese) worker's field.
Ori

Oriole (Latin) golden; black-and-orange bird.
Auriel, Oriel, Oriell, Oriella, Oriola

Orla (Irish) golden woman.
Orlagh, Orlie, Orly

Orlanda (German) famous throughout the land.
Orlandia, Orlantha, Orlenda, Orlinda

Orlenda (Russian) eagle.

Orli (Hebrew) light.
Orlice, Orlie, Orly

Ormanda (Latin) noble. (German) mariner.
Orma

Ornice (Hebrew) cedar tree. (Irish) pale; olive colored.
Orna, Ornah, Ornat, Ornette, Ornit

Orpah (Hebrew) runaway. See also Oprah.
Orpa, Orpha, Orphie

Orquidea (Spanish) orchid.
Orquidia

Orsa (Latin) a short form of Orseline. See also Ursa.
Orsaline, Orse, Orsel, Orselina, Orseline, Orsola

Ortensia (Italian) a form of Hortense.

Orva (French) golden; worthy. (English) brave friend.

Osanna (Latin) praise the Lord.
Oksana, Osana

Osen (Japanese) one thousand.

Oseye (Benin) merry.

Osma (English) divine protector.
Ozma

Otilie (Czech) lucky heroine.
Otila, Otilia, Otka, Ottili, Otylia

Ovia (Latin, Danish) egg.

Owena (Welsh) born to nobility; young warrior.

Oya (Moquelumnan) called forth.

Oz (Hebrew) strength.

Ozara (Hebrew) treasure, wealth.

P

Paca (Spanish) a short form of Pancha. See also Paka.

Padget (French) a form of Page.
Padgett, Paget, Pagett

Padma (Hindi) lotus.

Page (French) young assistant.
Padget, Pagen, Pagi, Payge

Paige (English) young child.
Payge

Paisley (Scottish) patterned fabric first made in Paisley, Scotland.
Paislay, Paislee, Paisleyann,

Paisleyanne, Paizlei, Paizleigh, Paizley, Pasley, Pazley

Paiton (English) warrior's town.
Paiten, Paityn, Paityne, Paiyton, Paten, Patton

Paka (Swahili) kitten. See also Paca.

Pakuna (Moquelumnan) deer bounding while running downhill.

Palila (Polynesian) bird.

Pallas (Greek) wise. Mythology: another name for Athena, the goddess of wisdom.

Palma (Latin) palm tree.
Pallma, Palmira

Palmira (Spanish) a form of Palma.
Pallmirah, Pallmyra, Palmer, Palmyra

Paloma (Spanish) dove. See also Aloma.
Palloma, Palometa, Palomita, Paluma, Peloma

Pamela (Greek) honey.
Pam, Pama, Pamala, Pamalla, Pamelia, Pamelina, Pamella, Pamila, Pamilla, Pammela, Pammi, Pammie, Pammy, Pamula

Pancha (Spanish) free; from France.
Paca, Panchita

Pandita (Hindi) scholar.

Pandora (Greek) all-gifted. Mythology: a woman who opened a box out of curiosity and released evil into the world. See also Dora.
Pandi, Pandorah, Pandorra, Pandorrah, Pandy, Panndora, Panndorah, Panndorra, Panndorrah

Pansy (Greek) flower; fragrant. (French) thoughtful.
Pansey, Pansie

Panthea (Greek) all the gods.
Pantheia, Pantheya

Panya (Swahili) mouse; tiny baby. (Russian) a familiar form of Stephanie.
Panyia

Panyin (Fante) older twin.

Paola (Italian) a form of Paula.
Paoli, Paolina

Papina (Moquelumnan) vine growing on an oak tree.

Paquita (Spanish) a form of Frances.
Paqua

Pari (Persian) fairy eagle.

Paris (French) Geography: the capital of France. Mythology: the Trojan prince who started the Trojan War by abducting Helen.
Parice, Paries, Parisa, Parise, Parish, Parisha, Pariss, Parissa, Parisse, Parris, Parys, Parysse

Parker (English) park keeper.
Park, Parke

Parris (French) a form of Paris.
Parrise, Parrish, Parrisha, Parrys, Parrysh

Parthenia (Greek) virginal.
Partheenia, Parthenie, Parthinia, Pathina

Parveneh (Persian) butterfly.

Pascale (French) born on Easter or Passover.
Pascalette, Pascaline, Pascalle, Paschale, Paskel

Pasha (Greek) sea.
Palasha, Pascha, Pasche, Pashae, Pashe, Pashel, Pashka, Pasia, Passia

Passion (Latin) passion.
Pashion, Pashonne, Pasion, Passionaé, Passionate, Passionette

Pasua (Swahili) born by cesarean section.

Pat (Latin) a short form of Patricia, Patsy.

Pati (Moquelumnan) fish baskets made of willow branches.

Patia (Gypsy, Spanish) leaf. (Latin, English) a familiar form of Patience, Patricia.

Patience (English) patient.
Paciencia, Patia, Patiance, Patient, Patince, Patishia

Patra (Greek, Latin) a form of Petra.

Patrice (French) a form of Patricia.
Patrease, Patrece, Patreece, Patreese, Patreice, Patriece, Patryce, Pattrice

Patricia (Latin) noblewoman. See also Payton, Peyton, Tricia, Trisha, Trissa.
Pat, Patia, Patresa, Patrica, Patrice, Patricea, Patriceia, Patrichea, Patriciana, Patricianna, Patricja, Patricka, Patrickia, Patrisha, Patrishia, Patrisia, Patrissa, Patrizia, Patrizzia, Patrycia, Patrycja, Patsy, Patty

Patsy (Latin) a familiar form of Patricia.
Pat, Patsey, Patsi

Patty (English) a familiar form of Patricia.
Patte, Pattee, Patti, Pattie

Paula (Latin) small. See also Pavla, Polly.
Paliki, Paola, Paulane, Paulann,

Paule, Paulette, Paulina,
Pauline, Paulla, Pavia

Paulette (Latin) a familiar
form of Paula.
Paulet, Paulett, Pauletta,
Paulita, Paullett, Paulletta,
Paullette

Paulina (Slavic) a form of
Paula.
Paulena, Paulene, Paulenia,
Pauliana, Paulianne, Paullena,
Paulyna, Pawlina, Polena,
Polina, Polinia

Pauline (French) a form of
Paula.
Pauleen, Paulene, Paulien,
Paulin, Paulyne, Paulynn,
Pouline

Pausha (Hindi) lunar month
of Capricorn.

Pavla (Czech, Russian) a form
of Paula.
Pavlina, Pavlinka

Paxton (Latin) peaceful town.
Paxtin, Paxtynn

Payge (English) a form of
Paige.

Payton (Irish) a form of
Patricia.
Paydon, Paytan, Payten, Paytin,
Paytn, Paytton

Paz (Spanish) peace.

Pazi (Ponca) yellow bird.

Pazia (Hebrew) golden.
Paz, Paza, Pazice, Pazit

Peace (English) peaceful.

Pearl (Latin) jewel.
Pearle, Pearleen, Pearlena,
Pearlene, Pearlette, Pearlina,
Pearline, Pearlisha, Pearlyn,
Perl, Perla, Perle, Perlette, Perlie,
Perline, Perlline

Peggy (Greek) a familiar form
of Margaret.
Peg, Pegeen, Pegg, Peggey, Peggi,
Peggie, Pegi

Peke (Hawaiian) a form of
Bertha.

Pela (Polish) a short form of
Penelope.
Pele

Pelagia (Greek) sea.
Pelage, Pelageia, Pelagie, Pelga,
Pelgia, Pellagia

Pelipa (Zuni) a form of
Philippa.

Pemba (Bambara) the power
that controls all life.

Penda (Swahili) loved.

Penelope (Greek) weaver.
Mythology: the clever and
loyal wife of Odysseus, a
Greek hero.
Pela, Pen, Penelopa, Penna,
Pennelope, Penny, Pinelopi

Peni (Carrier) mind.

Peninah (Hebrew) pearl.
*Penina, Peninit, Peninnah,
Penny*

Penny (Greek) a familiar form
of Penelope, Peninah.
*Penee, Peni, Penney, Penni,
Pennie*

Peony (Greek) flower.
Peonie

Pepita (Spanish) a familiar
form of Josephine.
Pepa, Pepi, Peppy, Peta

Pepper (Latin) condiment
from the pepper plant.

Perah (Hebrew) flower.

Perdita (Latin) lost. Literature:
a character in Shakespeare's
play *The Winter's Tale.*
Perdida, Perdy

Perfecta (Spanish) flawless.

Peri (Greek) mountain
dweller. (Persian) fairy or elf.
Perita

Perla (Latin) a form of Pearl.
Pearla

Perlie (Latin) a familiar form
of Pearl.
*Pearley, Pearlie, Pearly, Perley,
Perli, Perly, Purley, Purly*

Pernella (Greek, French) rock.
(Latin) a short form of
Petronella.
*Parnella, Pernel, Pernell,
Pernelle*

Perri (Greek, Latin) small
rock; traveler. (French) pear
tree. (Welsh) child of Harry.
(English) a form of Perry.
*Perre, Perrey, Perriann, Perrie,
Perrin, Perrine, Perry*

Persephone (Greek)
Mythology: the goddess of
the underworld.
*Persephanie, Persephany,
Persephonie*

Persis (Latin) from Persia.
Perssis, Persy

Peta (Blackfoot) golden eagle.

Petra (Greek, Latin) small
rock. A short form of
Petronella.
*Patra, Pet, Peta, Petena,
Peterina, Petraann, Petrice,
Petrina, Petrine, Petrova,
Petrovna, Pier, Pierce, Pietra*

Petronella (Greek) small rock.
(Latin) of the Roman clan
Petronius.
*Pernella, Peternella, Petra,
Petrona, Petronela, Petronella,
Petronelle, Petronia, Petronija,
Petronilla, Petronille*

Petula (Latin) seeker.
Petulah

Petunia (Native American)
flower.

Peyton (Irish) a form of
Patricia.
Peyden, Peydon, Peyten, Peytyn

Phaedra (Greek) bright.
Faydra, Phae, Phaidra, Phe, Phedre

Phallon (Irish) a form of Fallon.
Phalaine, Phalen, Phallan, Phallie, Phalon, Phalyn

Phebe (Greek) a form of Phoebe.
Pheba, Pheby

Pheodora (Greek, Russian) a form of Feodora.
Phedora, Phedorah, Pheodorah, Pheydora, Pheydorah

Philana (Greek) lover of mankind.
Phila, Philanna, Philene, Philiane, Philina, Philine

Philantha (Greek) lover of flowers.

Philicia (Latin) a form of Phylicia.
Philecia, Philesha, Philica, Philicha, Philycia

Philippa (Greek) lover of horses. See also Filippa.
Phil, Philipa, Philippe, Phillipina, Phillippine, Phillie, Philly, Pippa, Pippy

Philomena (Greek) love song; loved one. Bible: a first-century saint. See also Filomena, Mena.
Philoméne, Philomina

Phoebe (Greek) shining.
Phaebe, Phebe, Pheobe, Phoebey

Phylicia (Latin) fortunate; happy. (Greek) a form of Felicia.
Philicia, Phylecia, Phylesha, Phylesia, Phylica, Phylisha, Phylisia, Phylissa, Phyllecia, Phyllicia, Phyllisha, Phyllisia, Phyllissa, Phyllyza

Phyllida (Greek) a form of Phyllis.
Fillida, Philida, Phillida, Phillyda

Phyllis (Greek) green bough.
Filise, Fillys, Fyllis, Philis, Phillis, Philliss, Philys, Philyss, Phylis, Phyllida, Phyllis, Phylliss, Phyllys

Pia (Italian) devout.

Piedad (Spanish) devoted; pious.

Pier (French) a form of Petra.
Pierette, Pierrette, Pierra, Pierre

Pierce (English) a form of Petra.

Pilar (Spanish) pillar, column.
Peelar, Pilár, Pillar

Ping (Chinese) duckweed. (Vietnamese) peaceful.

Pinga (Eskimo) Mythology: the goddess of game and the hunt.

Piper (English) pipe player.

Pippa (English) a short form of Phillipa.

Pippi (French) rosy cheeked.
Pippen, Pippie, Pippin, Pippy

Pita (African) fourth daughter.

Placidia (Latin) serene.
Placida

Pleasance (French) pleasant.
Pleasence

Polla (Arabic) poppy.
Pola

Polly (Latin) a familiar form of
Paula.
*Paili, Pali, Pauli, Paulie, Pauly,
Poll, Pollee, Polley, Polli, Pollie*

Pollyam (Hindi) goddess of
the plague. Religion: the
Hindu name invoked to
ward off bad spirits.

Pollyanna (English) a combination of Polly + Anna.
Literature: an overly
optimistic heroine created by
Eleanor Porter.

Poloma (Choctaw) bow.

Pomona (Latin) apple.
Mythology: the goddess of
fruit and fruit trees.

Poni (African) second daughter.

Poppy (Latin) poppy flower.
Popi, Poppey, Poppi, Poppie

Pora, Poria (Hebrew) fruitful.

Porcha (Latin) a form of
Portia.
*Porchae, Porchai, Porche,
Porchia, Porcia*

Porscha, Porsche (German)
forms of Portia.
*Porcsha, Porcshe, Porschah,
Porché, Porschea, Porschia,
Pourche*

Porsha (Latin) a form of
Portia.
*Porshai, Porshay, Porshe,
Porshea, Porshia*

Portia (Latin) offering.
Literature: the heroine of
Shakespeare's play *The
Merchant of Venice*.
*Porcha, Porsca, Porsche,
Porsha, Portiea*

Precious (French) precious;
dear.
*Pracious, Preciouse, Precisha,
Prescious, Preshious, Presious*

Presley (English) priest's
meadow.
*Preslea, Preslee, Preslei, Presli,
Preslie, Presly, Preslye, Pressley,
Presslie, Pressly*

Prima (Latin) first, beginning;
first child.
*Prema, Primalia, Primetta,
Primina, Priminia*

Primavera (Italian, Spanish)
spring.

Primrose (English) primrose
flower.
Primula

Princess (English) daughter of
royalty.
*Princcess, Princes, Princesa,
Princessa, Princetta, Princie,
Princilla*

Priscilla (Latin) ancient.
*Cilla, Piri, Precila, Precilla,
Prescilla, Presilla, Pressilia,
Pricila, Pricilla, Pris, Prisca,
Priscela, Priscella, Priscila,
Priscilia, Priscill, Priscille,
Priscillia, Prisella, Prisila,
Prisilla, Prissila, Prissilla, Prissy,
Pryscylla, Prysilla*

Prissy (Latin) a familiar form
of Priscilla.
Prisi, Priss, Prissi, Prissie

Priya (Hindi) beloved; sweet
natured.
Pria

Procopia (Latin) declared
leader.

Promise (Latin) promise,
pledge.
*Promis, Promiss, Promys,
Promyse*

Pru (Latin) a short form of
Prudence.
Prue

Prudence (Latin) cautious;
discreet.
Pru, Prudencia, Prudens, Prudy

Prudy (Latin) a familiar form
of Prudence.
Prudee, Prudi, Prudie

Prunella (Latin) brown; little
plum. See also Nellie.
Prunela

Psyche (Greek) soul.
Mythology: a beautiful mor-
tal loved by Eros, the Greek
god of love.

Pua (Hawaiian) flower.

Pualani (Hawaiian) heavenly
flower.
Puni

Purity (English) purity.
Pura, Pureza, Purisima

Pyralis (Greek) fire.
Pyrene

Qadira (Arabic) powerful.
Kadira

Qamra (Arabic) moon.
Kamra

Qitarah (Arabic) fragrant.

Quaashie (Ewe) born on
Sunday.

Quadeisha (American) a combination of Qadira + Aisha.
Qudaisha, Quadaishia, Quadajah, Quadasha, Quadasia, Quadayshia, Quadaza, Quadejah, Quadesha, Quadeshia, Quadiasha, Quaesha

Quaneisha (American) a combination of the prefix Qu + Niesha.
Quaneasa, Quanece, Quanecia, Quaneice, Quanesha, Quanisha, Quansha, Quarnisha, Queisha, Qwanisha, Qynisha

Quanesha (American) a form of Quaneisha.
Quamesha, Quaneesha, Quaneshia, Quanesia, Quanessa, Quanessia, Quannesha, Quanneshia, Quannezia, Quayneshia, Quinesha

Quanika (American) a combination of the prefix Qu + Nika.
Quanikka, Quanikki, Quaniqua, Quanique, Quantenique, Quawanica, Queenika, Queenique

Quanisha (American) a form of Quaneisha.
Quaniesha, Quanishia, Quaynisha, Queenisha, Quenisha, Quenishia

Quartilla (Latin) fourth.
Quantilla

Qubilah (Arabic) agreeable.

Queen (English) queen. See also Quinn.
Queena, Queenie, Quenna

Queenie (English) a form of Queen.
Queenation, Queeneste, Queeny

Queisha (American) a short form of Quaneisha.
Qeysha, Queshia, Queysha

Quenby (Scandinavian) feminine.

Quenisha (American) a combination of Queen + Aisha.
Queneesha, Quenesha, Quennisha, Quensha, Quinesha, Quinisha

Quenna (English) a form of Queen.
Quenell, Quenessa

Querida (Spanish) dear; beloved.

Questa (French) searcher.

Queta (Spanish) a short form of names ending in "queta" or "quetta."
Quenetta, Quetta

Quiana (American) a combination of the prefix Qu + Anna.
Quian, Quianah, Quianda, Quiane, Quiani, Quianita, Quianna, Quianne, Quionna

Quinby (Scandinavian) queen's estate.

Quincy (Irish) fifth.
Quincee, Quincey, Quinci, Quincia, Quincie

Quinella (Latin) a form of Quintana.

Quinesha, Quinisha
(American) forms of Quenisha.
Quineshia, Quinessa, Quinessia, Quinisa, Quinishia, Quinnesha, Quinneshia, Quinnisha, Quneasha, Quonesha, Quonisha, Quonnisha

Quinetta (Latin) a form of Quintana.
Queenetta, Queenette, Quinette, Quinita, Quinnette

Quinn (German, English) queen. See also Queen.
Quin, Quinna, Quinne, Quynn

Quinshawna (American) a combination of Quinn + Shauna.
Quinshea

Quintana (Latin) fifth. (English) queen's lawn. See also Quinella, Quinetta.
Quinntina, Quinta, Quintanna, Quintara, Quintarah, Quintia, Quintila, Quintilla, Quintina, Quintona, Quintonice

Quintessa (Latin) essence. See also Tess.
Quintaysha, Quintesa, Quintesha, Quintessia,

Quintice, Quinticia, Quintisha, Quintosha

Quintrell (American) a combination of Quinn + Trella.
Quintela, Quintella, Quintrelle

Quiterie (Latin, French) tranquil.
Quita

Qwanisha (American) a form of Quaneisha.
Qwanechia, Qwanesha, Qwanessia, Qwantasha

R

Rabecca (Hebrew) a form of Rebecca.
Rabecka, Rabeca, Rabekah

Rabi (Arabic) breeze.
Rabia, Rabiah

Rachael (Hebrew) a form of Rachel.
Rachaele, Rachaell, Rachail, Rachalle

Racheal (Hebrew) a form of Rachel.

Rachel (Hebrew) female sheep. Bible: the second wife of Jacob. See also Lahela, Rae, Rochelle.
Racha, Rachael, Rachal, Racheal, Rachela, Rachelann, Rachele, Rachelle, Racquel, Raechel, Rahel, Rahela, Rahil, Raiche, Raquel, Rashel,

Rachel *(cont.)*
*Rashelle, Ray, Raycene,
Raychel, Raychelle, Rey, Ruchel*

Rachelle (French) a form of
Rachel. See also Shelley.
*Rachalle, Rachell, Rachella,
Raechell, Raechelle, Raeshelle,
Rashel, Rashele, Rashell,
Rashelle, Raychell, Rayshell,
Ruchelle*

Racquel (French) a form of
Rachel.
*Rackel, Racquell, Racquella,
Racquelle*

Radella (German) counselor.

Radeyah (Arabic) content,
satisfied.
*Radeeyah, Radhiya, Radiah,
Radiyah*

Radinka (Slavic) full of life;
happy, glad.

Radmilla (Slavic) worker for
the people.

Rae (English) doe. (Hebrew) a
short form of Rachel.
*Raeh, Raeneice, Raeneisha,
Raesha, Ray, Raye, Rayetta,
Rayette, Rayma, Rey*

Raeann (American) a combi-
nation of Rae + Ann. See
also Rayanne.
*Raea, Raean, Raeanna,
Raeannah, Raeona, Reanna,
Raeanne*

Raechel (Hebrew) a form of
Rachel.
*Raechael, Raechal, Raechele,
Raechell, Raechyl*

Raeden (Japanese) Mythology:
Raiden was the god of thun-
der and lightning.
Raeda, Raedeen

Raegan (Irish) a form of
Reagan.
*Raegen, Raegene, Raegine,
Raegyn*

Raelene (American) a combi-
nation of Rae + Lee.
*Rael, Raela, Raelani, Raele,
Raeleah, Raelee, Raeleen,
Raeleia, Raeleigh, Raeleigha,
Raelein, Raelene, Raelennia,
Raelesha, Raelin, Raelina,
Raelle, Raelyn, Raelynn*

Raelyn, Raelynn (American)
forms of Raelene.
Raelynda, Raelyne, Raelynne

Raena (German) a form of
Raina.
*Raenah, Raenia, Raenie,
Raenna, Raeonna, Raeyauna,
Raeyn, Raeyonna*

Raeven (English) a form of
Raven.
*Raevin, Raevion, Raevon,
Raevonna, Raevyn, Raevynne,
Raewyn, Raewynne, Raivan,
Raiven, Raivin, Raivyn*

Rafa (Arabic) happy; prosperous.

Rafaela (Hebrew) a form of
Raphaela.
Rafaelia, Rafaella

Ragan (Irish) a form of
Reagan.
*Ragean, Rageane, Rageen,
Ragen, Ragene, Rageni,
Ragenna, Raggan, Raygan,
Raygen, Raygene, Rayghan,
Raygin*

Ragine (English) a form of
Regina.
*Raegina, Ragin, Ragina,
Raginee*

Ragnild (Scandinavian) battle
counsel.
*Ragna, Ragnell, Ragnhild,
Rainell, Renilda, Renilde*

Raheem (Punjabi) compassionate God.
Raheema, Rahima

Ráidah (Arabic) leader.

Raina (German) mighty.
(English) a short form of
Regina. See also Rayna.
*Raeinna, Raena, Raheena,
Rain, Rainah, Rainai, Raine,
Rainea, Rainna, Reanna*

Rainbow (English) rainbow.
*Rainbeau, Rainbeaux, Rainbo,
Raynbow*

Raine (Latin) a short form of
Regina. A form of Raina,
Rane.
*Rainee, Rainey, Raini, Rainie,
Rainy, Reyne*

Raisa (Russian) a form of
Rose.
*Raisah, Raissa, Raiza, Raysa,
Rayza, Razia*

Raizel (Yiddish) a form of
Rose.
Rayzil, Razil, Reizel, Resel

Raja (Arabic) hopeful.
*Raia, Rajaah, Rajae, Rajah,
Rajai*

Raku (Japanese) pleasure.

Raleigh (Irish) a form of
Riley.
Ralea, Raleiah, Raley

Rama (Hebrew) lofty, exalted.
(Hindi) godlike. Religion: an
incarnation of the Hindu
god Vishnu.
Ramah

Raman (Spanish) a form of
Ramona.

Ramandeep (Sikh) covered by
the light of the Lord's love.

Ramla (Swahili) fortuneteller.
Ramlah

Ramona (Spanish) mighty;
wise protector. See also
Mona.
*Raman, Ramonda, Raymona,
Romona, Romonda*

Ramsey (English) ram's island.
*Ramsha, Ramsi, Ramsie,
Ramza*

Ran (Japanese) water lily.
(Scandinavian) destroyer.
Mythology: the Norse sea
goddess who destroys.

Rana (Sanskrit) royal. (Arabic)
gaze, look.
Rahna, Rahni, Rani

Ranait (Irish) graceful; prosperous.
Rane, Renny

Randall (English) protected.
*Randa, Randah, Randal,
Randalee, Randel, Randell,
Randelle, Randi, Randilee,
Randilynn, Randlyn, Randy,
Randyl*

Randi, Randy (English) famil-
iar forms of Miranda,
Randall.
*Rande, Randee, Randeen,
Randene, Randey, Randie,
Randii*

Rane (Scandinavian) queen.
Raine

Rani (Sanskrit) queen.
(Hebrew) joyful. A short
form of Kerani.
*Rahni, Ranee, Raney, Rania,
Ranie, Ranice, Ranique, Ranni,
Rannie*

Ranita (Hebrew) song; joyful.
*Ranata, Ranice, Ranit, Ranite,
Ranitta, Ronita*

Raniyah (Arabic) gazing.
Ranya, Ranyah

Rapa (Hawaiian) moonbeam.

Raphaela (Hebrew) healed by
God.
Rafaella, Raphaella, Raphaelle

Raphaelle (French) a form of
Raphaela.
Rafaelle, Raphael, Raphaele

Raquel (French) a form of
Rachel.
*Rakel, Rakhil, Rakhila,
Raqueal, Raquela, Raquella,
Raquelle, Rickelle, Rickquel,
Ricquel, Ricquelle, Rikell,
Rikelle, Rockell*

Rasha (Arabic) young gazelle.
*Rahshea, Rahshia; Rashae,
Rashai, Rashea, Rashi, Rashia*

Rashawna (American) a com-
bination of the prefix Ra +
Shawna.
*Rashana, Rashanae, Rashanah,
Rashanda, Rashane, Rashani,
Rashanna, Rashanta, Rashaun,
Rashauna, Rashaunda,
Rashaundra, Rashaune,
Rashawn, Rashawnda,
Rashawnna, Rashon, Rashona,
Rashonda, Rashunda*

Rashel, Rashelle (American)
forms of Rachel.
Rashele, Rashell, Rashella

Rashida (Swahili, Turkish)
righteous.
*Rahshea, Rahsheda, Rahsheita,
Rashdah, Rasheda, Rashedah,*

Rasheeda, Rasheedah, Rasheeta, Rasheida, Rashidah, Rashidi

Rashieka (Arabic) descended from royalty.
Rasheeka, Rasheika, Rasheka, Rashika, Rasika

Rasia (Greek) rose.

Ratana (Tai) crystal.
Ratania, Ratanya, Ratna, Rattan, Rattana

Ratri (Hindi) night. Religion: the goddess of the night.

Raula (French) wolf counselor.
Raoula, Raulla, Raulle

Raven (English) blackbird.
Raeven, Raveen, Raveena, Raveenn, Ravena, Ravene, Ravenn, Ravenna, Ravennah, Ravenne, Raveon, Ravin, Ravon, Ravyn, Rayven, Revena

Ravin (English) forms of Raven.
Ravi, Ravina, Ravine, Ravinne, Ravion,

Ravyn (English) a form of Raven.
Ravynn

Rawnie (Gypsy) fine lady.
Rawan, Rawna, Rhawnie

Raya (Hebrew) friend.
Raia, Raiah, Raiya, Ray, Rayah

Rayanne (American) a form of Raeann.
Rayane, Ray-Ann, Rayan, Rayana, Rayann, Rayanna, Rayeanna, Rayona, Rayonna, Reyan, Reyana, Reyann, Reyanna, Reyanne

Raychel, Raychelle (Hebrew) forms of Rachel.
Raychael, Raychele, Raychell, Raychil

Raylene (American) forms of Raylyn.
Ralina, Rayel, Rayele, Rayelle, Rayleana, Raylee, Rayleen, Rayleigh, Raylena, Raylin, Raylinn, Raylona, Raylyn, Raylynn, Raylynne

Raymonde (German) wise protector.
Rayma, Raymae, Raymie

Rayna (Scandinavian) mighty. (Yiddish) pure, clean. (English) king's advisor. (French) a familiar form of Lorraine. See also Raina.
Raynah, Rayne, Raynell, Raynelle, Raynette, Rayona, Rayonna, Reyna

Rayven (English) a form of Raven.
Rayvan, Rayvana, Rayvein, Rayvenne, Rayveona, Rayvin, Rayvon, Rayvonia

Rayya (Arabic) thirsty no longer.

Razi (Aramaic) secretive.
Rayzil, Rayzilee, Raz, Razia,
Raziah, Raziela, Razilee,
Razili

Raziya (Swahili) agreeable.

Rea (Greek) poppy flower.
Reah

Reagan (Irish) little ruler.
Reagen, Reaghan, Reagine

Reanna (German, English) a
form of Raina. (American) a
form of Raeann.
Reannah

Reanne (American) a form of
Raeann, Reanna.
Reana, Reane, Reann,
Reannan, Reanne, Reannen,
Reannon, Reeana

Reba (Hebrew) fourth-born
child. A short form of
Rebecca. See also Reva,
Riva.
Rabah, Reeba, Rheba

Rebeca (Hebrew) an alernate
form of Rebecca.
Rebbeca, Rebecah

Rebecca (Hebrew) tied,
bound. Bible: the wife of
Isaac. See also Becca, Becky.
Rabecca, Reba, Rebbecca,
Rebeca, Rebeccah, Rebeccea,
Rebeccka, Rebecha, Rebecka,
Rebeckah, Rebeckia, Rebecky,
Rebekah, Rebeque, Rebi,
Reveca, Riva, Rivka

Rebekah (Hebrew) a form of
Rebecca.
Rebeka, Rebekha, Rebekka,
Rebekkah, Rebekke, Revecca,
Reveka, Revekka, Rifka

Rebi (Hebrew) a familiar form
of Rebecca.
Rebbie, Rebe, Rebie, Reby, Ree,
Reebie

Reena (Greek) peaceful.
(English) a form of Rina.
(Hebrew) a form of Rinah.
Reen, Reenie, Rena, Reyna

Reet (Estonian) a form of
Margaret.
Reatha, Reta, Retha

Regan (Irish) a form of
Reagan.
Regane, Reghan

Reganne (Irish) a form of
Reagan.
Raegan, Ragan, Reagan, Regin

Reggie (English) a familiar
form of Regina.
Reggi, Reggy, Regi, Regia,
Regie

Regina (Latin) queen.
(English) king's advisor.
Geography: the capital of
Saskatchewan. See also Gina.
Ragine, Raina, Raine, Rega,
Regena, Regennia, Reggie,
Regiena, Regine, Reginia, Regis,
Reina, Rena

Regine (Latin) a form of
Regina.
Regin

Rei (Japanese) polite, well
behaved.
Reiko

Reilly (Irish) a form of Riley.
*Reilee, Reileigh, Reiley, Reili,
Reilley, Reily*

Reina (Spanish) a short form
of Regina. See also Reyna.
*Reinah, Reine, Reinette, Reinie,
Reinna, Reiny, Reiona, Renia,
Rina*

Rekha (Hindi) thin line.
Reka, Rekia, Rekiah, Rekiya

Remedios (Spanish) remedy.

Remi (French) from Rheims,
France.
Raymi, Remee, Remie, Remy

Remington (English) raven
estate.
Remmington

Ren (Japanese) arranger; water
lily; lotus.

Rena (Hebrew) song; joy. A
familiar form of Irene,
Regina, Renata, Sabrina,
Serena.
Reena, Rina, Rinna, Rinnah

Renae (French) a form of
Renée.
Renay

Renata (French) a form of
Renée.
*Ranata, Rena, Renada,
Renatta, Renita, Rennie,
Renyatta, Rinada, Rinata*

Rene (Greek) a short form of
Irene, Renée.
Reen, Reenie, Reney, Rennie

Renée (French) born again.
*Renae, Renata, Renay, Rene,
Renea, Reneigh, Renell,
Renelle, Renne*

Renita (French) a form of
Renata.
Reneeta, Renetta, Renitza

Rennie (English) a familiar
form of Renata.
Reni, Renie, Renni

Reseda (Spanish) fragrant
mignonette blossom.

Reshawna (American) a com-
bination of the prefix Re +
Shawna.
*Resaunna, Reshana,
Reshaunda, Reshawnda,
Reshawnna, Reshonda,
Reshonn, Reshonta*

Resi (German) a familiar form
of Theresa.
*Resia, Ressa, Resse, Ressie,
Reza, Rezka, Rezi*

Reta (African) shaken.
Reeta, Retta, Rheta, Rhetta

Reubena (Hebrew) behold a child.
Reubina, Reuvena, Rubena, Rubenia, Rubina, Rubine, Rubyna

Reva (Latin) revived. (Hebrew) rain; one-fourth. A form of Reba, Riva.
Ree, Reeva, Revia, Revida

Reveca, Reveka (Slavic) forms of Rebecca, Rebekah.
Reve, Revecca, Revekka, Rivka

Rexanne (American) queen.
Rexan, Rexana, Rexann, Rexanna

Reyhan (Turkish) sweet-smelling flower.

Reyna (Greek) peaceful. (English) a form of Reina.
Reyana, Reyanna, Reyni, Reynna

Reynalda (German) king's advisor.

Réz (Latin, Hungarian) copper-colored hair.

Reza (Czech) a form of Theresa.
Rezi, Rezka

Rhea (Greek) brook, stream. Mythology: the mother of Zeus.
Rheá, Rhéa, Rhealyn, Rheanna, Rhia, Rhianna

Rheanna, Rhianna (Greek) forms of Rhea.
Rheana, Rheann, Rheanne, Rhiana, Rhiauna

Rhian (Welsh) a short form of Rhiannon.
Rhianne, Rhyan, Rhyann, Rhyanne, Rian, Riane, Riann, Rianne, Riayn

Rhiannon (Welsh) witch; nymph; goddess.
Rheannan, Rheannin, Rheannon, Rheanon, Rhian, Rhianen, Rhianna, Rhiannan, Rhiannen, Rhianon, Rhianwen, Rhinnon, Rhyanna, Riana, Riannon, Rianon

Rhoda (Greek) from Rhodes, Greece.
Rhode, Rhodeia, Rhodie, Rhody, Roda, Rodi, Rodie, Rodina

Rhona (Scottish) powerful, mighty. (English) king's advisor.
Rhonae, Rhonnie

Rhonda (Welsh) grand.
Rhondene, Rhondiesha, Ronda, Ronelle, Ronnette

Ria (Spanish) river.
Riah

Riana, Rianna (Irish) short forms of Briana. (Arabic) forms of Rihana.
Reana, Reanna, Rhianna, Rhyanna, Riana, Rianah

Rica (Spanish) a short form of Erica, Frederica, Ricarda. See also Enrica, Sandrica, Terrica, Ulrica.
Ricca, Rieca, Riecka, Rieka, Rikka, Riqua, Rycca

Ricarda (Spanish) rich and
powerful ruler.
*Rica, Richanda, Richarda,
Richi, Ricki*

Richael (Irish) saint.

Richelle (German, French) a
form of Ricarda.
*Richel, Richela, Richele, Richell,
Richella, Richia*

Rickelle (American) a form of
Raquel.
Rickel, Rickela, Rickell

Ricki, Rikki (American) famil-
iar forms of Erica, Frederica,
Ricarda.
*Rica, Ricci, Riccy, Rici, Rickee,
Rickia, Rickie, Rickilee,
Rickina, Rickita, Ricky, Ricquie,
Riki, Rikia, Rikita, Rikka,
Rikke, Rikkia, Rikkie, Rikky,
Riko*

Ricquel (American) a form of
Raquel.
*Rickquell, Ricquelle, Rikell,
Rikelle*

Rida (Arabic) favored by God.

Rihana (Arabic) sweet basil.
*Rhiana, Rhianna, Riana,
Rianna*

Rika (Swedish) ruler.
Ricka

Rilee (Irish) a form of Riley.
Rielee, Rielle

Riley (Irish) valiant.
*Raleigh, Reilly, Rieley, Rielly,
Riely, Rilee, Rileigh, Rilie*

Rilla (German) small brook.

Rima (Arabic) white antelope.
*Reem, Reema, Reemah, Rema,
Remah, Rhymia, Rim, Ryma*

Rimona (Hebrew) pomegranate. See also Mona.

Rin (Japanese) park. Geography:
a Japanese village.
Rini, Rynn

Rina (English) a short form of
names ending in "rina."
(Hebrew) a form of Rena,
Rinah.
Reena, Rena

Rinah (Hebrew) joyful.
Rina

Riona (Irish) saint.

Risa (Latin) laughter.
Reesa, Resa

Risha (Hindi) born during the
lunar month of Taurus.
Rishah, Rishay

Rishona (Hebrew) first.
Rishina, Rishon

Rissa (Greek) a short form of
Nerissa.
Risa, Rissah, Ryssa, Ryssah

Rita (Sanskrit) brave; honest.
(Greek) a short form of
Margarita.
*Reatha, Reda, Reeta, Reida,
Reitha, Rheta, Riet, Ritah,
Ritamae, Ritamarie*

Ritsa (Greek) a familiar form
of Alexandra.
Ritsah, Ritsi, Ritsie, Ritsy

Riva (French) river bank.
(Hebrew) a short form of
Rebecca. See also Reba,
Reva.
Rivalee, Rivi, Rivvy

River (Latin, French) stream,
water.
*Rivana, Rivanna, Rivers,
Riviane*

Rivka (Hebrew) a short form
of Rebecca.
Rivca, Rivcah, Rivkah

Riza (Greek) a form of
Theresa.
Riesa, Rizus, Rizza

Roanna (American) a form of
Rosana.
*Ranna, Roana, Roanda,
Roanne*

Robbi, Robbie (English)
familiar forms of Roberta.
*Robby, Robbye, Robey, Robi,
Robia, Roby*

Roberta (English) famous
brilliance.
*Roba, Robbi, Robbie, Robena,
Robertena, Robertina*

Robin (English) robin. A form
of Roberta.
*Robann, Robbin, Robeen,
Roben, Robena, Robian,
Robina, Robine, Robinette,
Robinia, Robinn, Robinta,
Robyn*

Robinette (English) a familiar
form of Robin.
*Robernetta, Robinet, Robinett,
Robinita*

Robyn (English) a form of
Robin.
*Robbyn, Robbynn, Robyne,
Robynn, Robynne*

Rochelle (French) large stone.
(Hebrew) a form of Rachel.
See also Shelley.
*Reshelle, Roch, Rocheal,
Rochealle, Rochel, Rochele,
Rochell, Rochella, Rochette,
Rockelle, Roshele, Roshell,
Roshelle*

Rocio (Spanish) dewdrops.
Rocío

Roderica (German) famous
ruler.
*Rica, Rika, Rodericka,
Roderika, Rodreicka, Rodricka,
Rodrika*

Rodnae (English) island clearing.
Rodna, Rodnetta, Rodnicka

Rodneisha (American) a combination of Rodnae + Aisha.
Rodesha, Rodisha, Rodishah,

Rodnecia, Rodnesha,
Rodneshia, Rodneycia,
Rodneysha, Rodnisha

Rohana (Hindi) sandalwood.
(American) a combination of
Rose + Hannah.
Rochana, Rohena

Rohini (Hindi) woman.

Rolanda (German) famous
throughout the land.
Ralna, Rolande, Rolando,
Rolaunda, Roleesha, Rolene,
Rolinda, Rollande, Rolonda

Rolene (German) a form of
Rolanda.
Rolaine, Rolena, Rolleen,
Rollene

Roma (Latin) from Rome.
Romai, Rome, Romeise,
Romeka, Romelle, Romesha,
Rometta, Romia, Romilda,
Romilla, Romina, Romini,
Romma, Romonia

Romaine (French) from Rome.
Romana, Romanda, Romanelle,
Romania, Romanique, Romany,
Romayne, Romona, Romy

Romy (French) a familiar form
of Romaine. (English) a
familiar form of Rosemary.
Romi, Romie

Rona (Scandinavian) short
forms of Ronalda.
Rhona, Roana, Ronalda,
Ronna, Ronnae, Ronnay,
Ronne, Ronni, Ronsy

Ronaele (Greek) the name
Eleanor spelled backwards.
Ronalee, Ronni, Ronnie, Ronny

Ronda (Welsh) a form of
Rhonda.
Rondai, Rondesia, Rondi,
Rondie, Ronelle, Ronnette,
Ronni, Ronnie, Ronny

Rondelle (French) short poem.
Rhondelle, Rondel, Ronndelle

Roneisha (American) a com-
bination of Rhonda + Aisha.
Roneasha, Ronecia, Ronee,
Roneeka, Roneesha, Roneice,
Ronese, Ronesha, Roneshia,
Ronesia, Ronessa, Ronessia,
Ronichia, Ronicia, Roniesha,
Ronisha, Ronneisha, Ronnesa,
Ronnesha, Ronneshia, Ronni,
Ronnie, Ronniesha, Ronny

Ronelle (Welsh) a form of
Rhonda, Ronda.
Ranell, Ranelle, Ronel, Ronella,
Ronielle, Ronnella, Ronnelle

Ronisha (American) a form of
Roneisha.
Ronise, Ronnise, Ronnisha,
Ronnishia

Ronli (Hebrew) joyful.
Ronia, Ronice, Ronit, Ronlee,
Ronlie, Ronni, Ronnie, Ronny

Ronnette (Welsh) a familiar
form of Rhonda, Ronda.
Ronetta, Ronette, Ronit,
Ronita, Ronnetta, Ronni,
Ronnie, Ronny

Ronni, Ronnie, Ronny
(American) familiar forms of
Veronica and names begin-
ning with "Ron."
Rone, Ronee, Roni, Ronnee,
Ronney

Rori, Rory (Irish) famous brilliance; famous ruler.
Rorie

Ros, Roz (English) short forms
of Rosalind, Rosalyn.
Rozz, Rozzey, Rozzi, Rozzie,
Rozzy

Rosa (Italian, Spanish) a form
of Rose. History: Rosa Parks
inspired the American Civil
Rights movement by refusing
to give up her bus seat to a
white man in Montgomery,
Alabama. See also Charo,
Roza.

Rosabel (French) beautiful
rose.
Rosabelia, Rosabella, Rosabelle,
Rosebelle

Rosalba (Latin) white rose.
Rosalva, Roselba

Rosalie (English) a form of
Rosalind.
Rosalea, Rosalee, Rosaleen,
Rosaleigh, Rosalene, Rosalia,
Rosealee, Rosealie, Roselee,
Roseli, Roselia, Roselie, Roseley,
Rosely, Rosilee, Rosli, Rozali,
Rozália, Rozalie, Rozele

Rosalind (Spanish) fair rose.
Ros, Rosalie, Rosalinda,
Rosalinde, Rosalyn, Rosalynd,
Rosalynde, Roselind, Roselyn,
Rosie, Roz, Rozalind, Rozland

Rosalinda (Spanish) a form of
Rosalind.
Rosalina

Rosalyn (Spanish) a form of
Rosalind.
Ros, Rosaleen, Rosalin,
Rosaline, Rosalyne, Rosalynn,
Rosalynne, Rosilyn, Roslin,
Roslyn, Roslyne, Roslynn, Roz,
Rozalyn, Rozlyn

Rosamond (German) famous
guardian.
Rosamund, Rosamunda,
Rosemonde, Rozamond

Rosanna, Roseanna (English)
combinations of Rose + Anna.
Ranna, Roanna, Rosana,
Rosannah, Roseana,
Roseannah, Rosehanah,
Rosehannah, Rosie, Rossana,
Rossanna, Rozana, Rozanna

Rosanne, Roseanne (English)
combinations of Rose +
Ann.
Roanne, Rosan, Rosann,
Roseann, Rose Ann, Rose
Anne, Rossann, Rossanne,
Rozann, Rozanne

Rosario (Filipino, Spanish)
rosary.
Rosarah, Rosaria, Rosarie,
Rosary, Rosaura

Rose (Latin) rose. See also
Chalina, Raisa, Raizel, Roza.
*Rada, Rasia, Rasine, Rois,
Róise, Rosa, Rosea, Rosella,
Roselle, Roses, Rosetta, Rosie,
Rosina, Rosita, Rosse*

Roselani (Hawaiian) heavenly
rose.

Roselyn (Spanish) a form of
Rosalind.
*Roseleen, Roselene, Roselin,
Roseline, Roselyne, Roselynn,
Roselynne*

Rosemarie (English) a combi-
nation of Rose + Marie.
*Rosamaria, Rosamarie,
Rosemari, Rosemaria, Rose
Marie*

Rosemary (English) a combination of Rose + Mary.
Romi, Romy

Rosetta (Italian) a form of
Rose.
Roseta, Rosette

Roshan (Sanskrit) shining
light.

Roshawna (American) a com-
bination of Rose + Shawna.
*Roshan, Roshana, Roshanda,
Roshani, Roshann, Roshanna,
Roshanta, Roshaun, Roshauna,
Roshaunda, Roshawn,
Roshawnda, Roshawnna,
Roshona, Roshonda, Roshowna,
Roshunda*

Rosie (English) a familiar form
of Rosalind, Rosanna, Rose.
*Rosey, Rosi, Rosio, Rosse, Rosy,
Rozsi, Rozy*

Rosina (English) a familiar
form of Rose.
*Rosena, Rosenah, Rosene,
Rosheen, Rozena, Rozina*

Rosita (Spanish) a familiar
form of Rose.
*Roseeta, Roseta, Rozeta,
Rozita, Rozyte*

Roslyn (Scottish) a form of
Rossalyn.
*Roslin, Roslynn, Rosslyn,
Rosslynn*

Rossalyn (Scottish) cape;
promontory.
*Roslyn, Rosselyn, Rosylin,
Roszaliyn*

Rowan (English) tree with red
berries. (Welsh) a form of
Rowena.
Rowana

Rowena (Welsh) fair-haired.
(English) famous friend.
Literature: Ivanhoe's love
interest in Sir Walter Scott's
novel *Ivanhoe.*
*Ranna, Ronni, Row, Rowan,
Rowe, Roweena, Rowen,
Rowina*

Roxana, Roxanna (Persian)
forms of Roxann.
Rocsana, Roxannah

Roxann, Roxanne (Persian) sunrise. Literature: Roxanne is the heroine of Edmond Rostand's play *Cyrano de Bergerac*.
Rocxann, Roxan, Roxana, Roxane, Roxanna, Roxianne, Roxy

Roxy (Persian) a familiar form of Roxann.
Roxi, Roxie

Royale (English) royal.
Royal, Royalene, Royalle, Roylee, Roylene, Ryal, Ryale

Royanna (English) queenly, royal.
Roya

Roza (Slavic) a form of Rosa.
Roz, Rozalia, Roze, Rozel, Rozele, Rozell, Rozella, Rozelli, Rozia, Rozsa, Rozsi, Rozyte, Rozza, Rozzie

Rozene (Native American) rose blossom.
Rozena, Rozina, Rozine, Ruzena

Ruana (Hindi) stringed musical instrument.
Ruan, Ruon

Rubena (Hebrew) a form of Reubena.
Rubenia, Rubina, Rubine, Rubinia, Rubyn, Rubyna

Rubi (French) a form of Ruby.
Ruba, Rubbie, Rubee, Rubia, Rubie

Ruby (French) precious stone.
Rubby, Rubetta, Rubette, Rubey, Rubi, Rubiann, Rubyann, Rubye

Ruchi (Hindi) one who wishes to please.

Rudee (German) famous wolf.
Rudeline, Rudell, Rudella, Rudi, Rudie, Rudina, Rudy

Rudra (Hindi) seeds of the rudraksha plant.

Rue (German) famous. (French) street. (English) regretful; strong-scented herbs.
Ru, Ruey

Ruffina (Italian) redhead.
Rufeena, Rufeine, Rufina, Ruphyna

Rui (Japanese) affectionate.

Rukan (Arabic) steady; confident.

Rula (Latin, English) ruler.

Runa (Norwegian) secret; flowing.
Runna

Ruperta (Spanish) a form of Roberta.

Rupinder (Sanskrit) beautiful.

Ruri (Japanese) emerald.
Ruriko

Rusalka (Czech) wood nymph. (Russian) mermaid.

Russhell (French) redhead; fox colored.
Rushell, Rushelle, Russellynn, Russhelle

Rusti (English) redhead.
Russet, Rustie, Rusty

Ruth (Hebrew) friendship. Bible: daughter-in-law of Naomi.
Rutha, Ruthalma, Ruthe, Ruthella, Ruthetta, Ruthie, Ruthven

Ruthann (American) a combination of Ruth + Ann.
Ruthan, Ruthanna, Ruthannah, Ruthanne, Ruthina, Ruthine

Ruthie (Hebrew) a familiar form of Ruth.
Ruthey, Ruthi, Ruthy

Ruza (Czech) rose.
Ruzena, Ruzenka, Ruzha, Ruzsa

Ryan, Ryann (Irish) little ruler.
Raiann, Raianne, Rhyann, Riana, Riane, Ryana, Ryane, Ryanna, Ryanne, Rye, Ryen, Ryenne

Ryba (Czech) fish.

Rylee (Irish) valiant.
Rye, Ryelee, Rylea, Ryleigh, Ryley, Rylie, Rylina, Rylyn

Ryleigh, Rylie (Irish) forms of Rylee.
Ryelie, Ryli, Rylleigh, Ryllie

Ryley (Irish) a form of Rylee.
Ryeley, Rylly, Ryly

Ryo (Japanese) dragon.
Ryoko

S

Saarah (Arabic) princess.

Saba (Arabic) morning. (Greek) a form of Sheba.
Sabaah, Sabah, Sabba, Sabbah

Sabi (Arabic) young girl.

Sabina (Latin) History: the Sabine were a tribe in ancient Italy. See also Bina.
Sabeen, Sabena, Sabienne, Sabin, Sabine, Sabinka, Sabinna, Sabiny, Saby, Sabyne, Savina, Sebina, Sebinah

Sabiya (Arabic) morning; eastern wind.
Saba, Sabaya, Sabiyah

Sable (English) sable; sleek.
Sabel, Sabela, Sabella

Sabra (Hebrew) thorny cactus fruit. (Arabic) resting. History: a name for native-born Israelis, who were said to be hard on the outside and soft and sweet on the inside.
Sabera, Sabira, Sabrah, Sabre, Sabrea, Sabreah, Sabree, Sabreea, Sabri, Sabria, Sabriah, Sabriya, Sebra

Sabreena (English) a form of Sabrina.
Sabreen, Sabrena, Sabrene

Sabrina (Latin) boundary line. (English) princess. (Hebrew) a familiar form of Sabra. See also Bree, Brina, Rena, Zabrina.
Sabre, Sabreena, Salrinas, Sabrinah, Sabrine, Sabrinia, Sabrinna, Sabryna, Sebree, Sebrina, Subrina

Sabryna (English) a form of Sabrina.
Sabrynna

Sacha (Russian) a form of Sasha.
Sache, Sachia

Sachi (Japanese) blessed; lucky.
Saatchi, Sachie, Sachiko

Sada (Japanese) chaste. (English) a form of Sadie.
Sadá, Sadah, Sadako

Sade (Hebrew) a form of Chadee, Sarah, Shardae, Sharday.
Sáde, Sadé, Sadea, Sadee, Shaday

Sadella (American) a combination of Sade + Ella.
Sadelle, Sydel, Sydell, Sydella, Sydelle

Sadhana (Hindi) devoted.

Sadie (Hebrew) a familiar form of Sarah. See also Sada.
Saddie, Sadee, Sadey, Sadi, Sadiey, Sady, Sadye, Saide, Saidee, Saidey, Saidi, Saidia,
Saidie, Saidy, Sayde, Saydee, Seidy

Sadira (Persian) lotus tree. (Arabic) star.
Sadra

Sadiya (Arabic) lucky, fortunate.
Sadi, Sadia, Sadiah, Sadiyah, Sadiyyah, Sadya

Sadzi (Carrier) sunny disposition.

Saffron (English) Botany: a plant with purple or white flowers whose orange stigmas are used as a spice.
Safron

Safiya (Arabic) pure; serene; best friend.
Safa, Safeya, Saffa, Safia, Safiyah

Sagara (Hindi) ocean.

Sage (English) wise. Botany: an herb used as a seasoning.
Sagia, Saige, Salvia

Sahara (Arabic) desert; wilderness.
Sahar, Saharah, Sahari, Saheer, Saher, Sahira, Sahra, Sahrah

Sai (Japanese) talented.
Saiko

Saida (Hebrew) a form of Sarah. (Arabic) happy; fortunate.
Saidah

Saige (English) a form of Sage.

Saira (Hebrew) a form of Sara.
Sairah, Sairi

Sakaë (Japanese) prosperous.

Sakari (Hindi) sweet.
Sakkara

Saki (Japanese) cloak; rice wine.

Sakti (Hindi) energy, power.

Sakuna (Native American) bird.

Sakura (Japanese) cherry blossom; wealthy; prosperous.

Sala (Hindi) sala tree.
Religion: the sacred tree under which Buddha died.

Salali (Cherokee) squirrel.

Salama (Arabic) peaceful. See also Zulima.

Salena (French) a form of Salina.
Saleana, Saleen, Saleena, Salene, Salenna, Sallene

Salima (Arabic) safe and sound; healthy.
Saleema, Salema, Salim, Salimah, Salma

Salina (French) solemn, dignified.
Salena, Salin, Salinah, Salinda, Saline

Salliann (English) a combination of Sally + Ann.
Sallian, Sallianne, Sallyann, Sally-Ann, Sallyanne, Sally-Anne

Sally (English) princess.
History: Sally Ride, an American astronaut, became the first U. S. woman in space.
Sal, Salaid, Sallee, Salletta, Sallette, Salley, Salli, Sallie

Salome (Hebrew) peaceful.
History: Salome Alexandra was a ruler of ancient Judea. Bible: the niece of King Herod.
Saloma, Salomé, Salomey, Salomi

Salvadora (Spanish) savior.

Salvia (Spanish) healthy; saved. (Latin) a form of Sage.
Sallvia, Salviana, Salviane, Salvina, Salvine

Samala (Hebrew) asked of God.
Samale, Sammala

Samanta (Hebrew) a form of Samantha.
Samantah, Smanta

Samantha (Aramaic) listener. (Hebrew) told by God.
Sam, Samana, Samanath, Samanatha, Samanitha, Samanithia, Samanta, Samanth, Samanthe, Samanthi, Samanthia, Samatha, Sami, Sammanth, Sammantha, Semantha, Simantha, Smantha, Symantha

Samara (Latin) elm-tree seed.
Saimara, Samaira, Samar,
Samarah, Samari, Samaria,
Samariah, Samarie, Samarra,
Samarrea, Samary, Samera,
Sameria, Samira, Sammar,
Sammara, Samora

Samatha (Hebrew) a form of
Samantha.
Sammatha

Sameh (Hebrew) listener.
(Arabic) forgiving.
Samaiya, Samaya

Sami (Arabic) praised.
(Hebrew) a short form of
Samantha, Samuela.
Samia, Samiah, Samiha,
Samina, Sammey, Sammi,
Sammie, Sammijo, Sammy,
Sammyjo, Samya, Samye

Samira (Arabic) entertaining.
Samirah, Samire, Samiria,
Samirra, Samyra

Samone (Hebrew) a form of
Simone.
Samoan, Samoane, Samon,
Samona, Samoné, Samonia

Samuela (Hebrew) heard
God, asked of God.
Samala, Samelia, Samella,
Sami, Samielle, Samille,
Sammile, Samuelle

Samuelle (Hebrew) a form of
Samuela.
Samuella

Sana (Arabic) mountaintop;
splendid; brilliant.
Sanaa, Sanáa, Sanaah, Sane,
Sanah

Sancia (Spanish) holy, sacred.
Sanceska, Sancha, Sancharia,
Sanchia, Sancie, Santsia, Sanzia

Sandeep (Punjabi) enlightened.
Sandip

Sandi (Greek) a familiar form
of Sandra.
Sandee, Sandia, Sandie,
Sandiey, Sandine, Sanndie

Sandra (Greek) defender of
mankind. A short form of
Cassandra. History: Sandra
Day O'Connor was the first
woman appointed to the
U.S. Supreme Court. See also
Zandra.
Sahndra, Sandi, Sandira,
Sandrea, Sandria, Sandrica,
Sandy, Sanndra, Saundra

Sandrea (Greek) a form of
Sandra.
Sandreea, Sandreia, Sandrell,
Sandria, Sanndria

Sandrica (Greek) a form of
Sandra. See also Rica.
Sandricka, Sandrika

Sandrine (Greek) a form of
Alexandra.
Sandreana, Sandrene,
Sandrenna, Sandrianna,
Sandrina

Sandy (Greek) a familiar form of Cassandra, Sandra.
Sandya, Sandye

Sanne (Hebrew, Dutch) lily.
Sanea, Saneh, Sanna, Sanneen

Santana (Spanish) saint.
Santa, Santaniata, Santanna, Santanne, Santena, Santenna, Shantana

Santina (Spanish) little saint.
Santinia

Sanura (Swahili) kitten.
Sanora

Sanuye (Moquelumnan) red clouds at sunset.

Sanya (Sanskrit) born on Saturday.
Saneiya, Sania, Sanyia

Sanyu (Luganda) happiness.

Sapata (Native American) dancing bear.

Sapphira (Hebrew) a form of Sapphire.
Safira, Sapheria, Saphira, Saphyra, Sephira

Sapphire (Greek) blue gem-stone.
Saffire, Saphire, Saphyre, Sapphira

Sara (Hebrew) a form of Sarah.
Saira, Sarae, Saralee, Sarra, Sera

Sarah (Hebrew) princess. Bible: the wife of Abraham and mother of Isaac. See also Sadie, Saida, Sally, Saree, Sharai, Shari, Zara, Zarita. Sahra, Sara, Saraha, Sarahann, Sarahi, Sarai, Sarann, Saray, Sarha, Sariah, Sarina, Sarita, Sarolta, Sarotte, Sarrah, Sasa, Sayra, Sorcha.

Sarai, Saray (Hebrew) forms of Sarah.
Saraya

Saralyn (American) a combination of Sarah + Lynn.
Saralena, Saraly, Saralynn

Saree (Arabic) noble. (Hebrew) a familiar form of Sarah.
Sareeka, Sareka, Sari, Sarika, Sarka, Sarri, Sarrie, Sary

Sariah (Hebrew) forms of Sarah.
Saria, Sarie

Sarila (Turkish) waterfall.

Sarina (Hebrew) a familiar form of Sarah.
Sareen, Sareena, Saren, Sarena, Sarene, Sarenna, Sarin, Sarine, Sarinna, Sarinne

Sarita (Hebrew) a familiar form of Sarah.
Saretta, Sarette, Sarit, Saritia, Saritta

Sarolta (Hungarian) a form of Sarah.

Sarotte (French) a form of
Sarah.

Sarrah (Hebrew) a form of
Sarah.
Sarra

Sasa (Japanese) assistant.
(Hungarian) a form of Sarah,
Sasha.

Sasha (Russian) defender of
mankind. See also Zasha.
*Sacha, Sahsha, Sasa, Sascha,
Saschae, Sashae, Sashah, Sashai,
Sashana, Sashay, Sashea,
Sashel, Sashenka, Sashey, Sashi,
Sashia, Sashira, Sashsha,
Sashya, Sasjara, Sauscha,
Sausha, Shasha, Shashi,
Shashia*

Sass (Irish) Saxon.
Sassie, Sassoon, Sassy

Satara (American) a combina-
tion of Sarah + Tara.
*Sataria, Satarra, Sateriaa,
Saterra, Saterria*

Satin (French) smooth, shiny.
Satinder

Satinka (Native American)
sacred dancer.

Sato (Japanese) sugar.
Satu

Saundra (English) a form of
Sandra, Sondra.
*Saundee, Saundi, Saundie,
Saundy*

Saura (Hindi) sun worshiper.

Savana, Savanna (Spanish)
forms of Savannah.
*Saveena, Savhana, Savhanna,
Savina, Savine, Savona,
Savonna*

Savanah (Spanish) a form of
Savannah.
Savhannah

Savannah (Spanish) treeless
plain.
*Sahvannah, Savana, Savanah,
Savanha, Savanna, Savannha,
Savauna, Savonnah, Savonne,
Sevan, Sevanah, Sevanh,
Sevann, Sevanna, Svannah*

Sawa (Japanese) swamp.
(Moquelumnan) stone.

Sawyer (English) wood
worker.
Sawyar, Sawyor

Sayde, Saydee (Hebrew)
forms of Sadie.
Saydi, Saydia, Saydie, Saydy

Sayo (Japanese) born at night.

Sayra (Hebrew) a form of
Sarah.
Sayrah, Sayre, Sayri

Scarlett (English) bright red.
Literature: Scarlett O'Hara is
the heroine of Margaret
Mitchell's novel *Gone with the
Wind*.
*Scarlet, Scarlette, Scarlotte,
Skarlette*

Schyler (Dutch) sheltering.
*Schuyla, Schuyler, Schuylia,
Schylar*

Scotti (Scottish) from
Scotland.
Scota, Scotia, Scottie, Scotty

Seana, Seanna (Irish) forms
of Jane. See also Shauna,
Shawna.
*Seaana, Sean, Seane, Seann,
Seannae, Seannah, Seannalisa,
Seanté, Sianna, Sina*

Sebastiane (Greek) venerable.
(Latin) revered. (French) a
form of Sebastian (see Boys'
Names).
*Sebastene, Sebastia, Sebastian,
Sebastiana, Sebastien,
Sebastienne*

Seble (Ethiopian) autumn.

Sebrina (English) a form of
Sabrina.
*Sebrena, Sebrenna, Sebria,
Sebriana*

Secilia (Latin) a form of
Cecilia.
Saselia, Sasilia, Sesilia, Sileas

Secunda (Latin) second.

Seda (Armenian) forest
voices.

Sedna (Eskimo) well-fed.
Mythology: the goddess of
sea animals.

Seelia (English) a form of
Sheila.

Seema (Greek) sprout.
(Afghan) sky; profile.
Seemah, Sima, Simah

Sefa (Swiss) a familiar form of
Josefina.

Seirra (Irish) a form of Sierra.
Seiara, Seiarra, Seira, Seirria

Seki (Japanese) wonderful.
Seka

Sela (English) a short form of
Selena.
Seeley, Selah

Selam (Ethiopian) peaceful.

Selda (German) a short form
of Griselda. (Yiddish) a form
of Zelda.
Seldah, Selde, Sellda, Selldah

Selena (Greek) moon.
Mythology: Selene was the
goddess of the moon. See
also Celena.
*Saleena, Sela, Selana, Seleana,
Seleena, Selen, Selenah, Selene,
Séléné, Selenia, Selenna, Selina,
Sena, Syleena, Sylena*

Selene (Greek) a form of
Selena.
Seleni, Selenie, Seleny

Selia (Latin) a short form of
Cecilia.
Seel, Seil, Sela, Silia

Selima (Hebrew) peaceful.
Selema, Selemah, Selimah

Selina (Greek) a form of
Celina, Selena.
*Selie, Selin, Selinda, Seline,
Selinia, Selinka, Sellina, Selyna,
Selyne, Selynne, Sylina*

Selma (German) devine protector. (Irish) fair, just.
(Scandinavian) divinely protected. (Arabic) secure. See
also Zelma.
Sellma, Sellmah, Selmah

Sema (Turkish) heaven; divine
omen.
Semaj

Sen (Japanese) Mythology: a
magical forest elf that lives
for thousands of years.

Senalda (Spanish) sign.
Sena, Senda, Senna

Seneca (Iroquoian) a tribal
name.
*Senaka, Seneka, Senequa,
Senequae, Senequai, Seneque*

Septima (Latin) seventh.

Sequoia (Cherokee) giant
redwood tree.
*Seqoiyia, Seqouyia, Seqoya,
Sequoi, Sequoiah, Sequora,
Sequoya, Sequoyah, Sikoya*

Serafina (Hebrew) burning;
ardent. Bible: seraphim are an
order of angels.
*Sarafina, Serafine, Seraphe,
Seraphin, Seraphina, Seraphine,
Seraphita, Serapia, Serofina*

Serena (Latin) peaceful. See
also Rena.
*Sarina, Saryna, Seraina, Serana,
Sereen, Sereina, Seren, Serenah,
Serene, Serenea, Serenia,
Serenna, Serina, Serreana,
Serrena, Serrenna*

Serenity (Latin) peaceful.
*Serenidy, Serenitee, Serenitey,
Sereniti, Serenitiy, Serinity,
Serrennity*

Serilda (Greek) armed warrior woman.

Serina (Latin) a form of
Serena.
*Sereena, Serin, Serine, Serreena,
Serrin, Serrina, Seryna*

Sevilla (Spanish) from Seville.
Seville

Shaba (Spanish) rose.
Shabana, Shabina

Shada (Native American) pelican.
*Shadae, Shadea, Shadeana,
Shadee, Shadi, Shadia, Shadiah,
Shadie, Shadiya, Shaida*

Shaday (American) a form of
Sade.
*Shadai, Shadaia, Shadaya,
Shadayna, Shadei, Shadeziah,
Shaiday*

Shadrika (American) a combination of the prefix Sha +
Rika.
*Shadreeka, Shadreka, Shadrica,
Shadricka, Shadrieka*

Shae (Irish) a form of Shea.
Shaenel, Shaeya, Shai, Shaia

Shaelee (Irish) a form of Shea.
Shaeleigh, Shaeley, Shaelie, Shaely

Shaelyn (Irish) a form of Shea.
Shael, Shaelaine, Shaelan, Shaelanie, Shaelanna, Shaeleen, Shaelene, Shaelin, Shaeline, Shaelyne, Shaelynn, Shae-Lynn, Shaelynne

Shafira (Swahili) distinguished.
Shaffira

Shahar (Arabic) moonlit.
Shahara

Shahina (Arabic) falcon.
Shaheen, Shaheena, Shahi, Shahin

Shahla (Afghani) beautiful eyes.
Shaila, Shailah, Shalah

Shaianne (Cheyenne) a form of Cheyenne.
Shaeen, Shaeine, Shaian, Shaiana, Shaiandra, Shaiane, Shaiann, Shaianna

Shaila (Latin) a form of Sheila.
Shaela, Shaelea, Shaeyla, Shailah, Shailee, Shailey, Shaili, Shailie, Shailla, Shaily, Shailyn, Shailynn

Shaina (Yiddish) beautiful.
Shaena, Shainah, Shaine, Shainna, Shajna, Shanie, Shayna, Shayndel, Sheina, Sheindel

Shajuana (American) a combination of the prefix Sha + Juanita. See also Shawanna.
Shajuan, Shajuanda, Shajuanita, Shajuanna, Shajuanza

Shaka (Hindi) a form of Shakti. A short form of names beginning with "Shak." See also Chaka.
Shakah, Shakha

Shakarah (American) a combination of the prefix Sha + Kara.
Shacara, Shacari, Shaccara, Shaka, Shakari, Shakkara, Shikara

Shakayla (Arabic) a form of Shakila.
Shakaela, Shakail, Shakaila, Shakala

Shakeena (American) a combination of the prefix Sha + Keena.
Shaka, Shakeina, Shakeyna, Shakina, Shakyna

Shakeita (American) a combination of the prefix Sha + Keita. See also Shaqueita.
Shaka, Shakeeta, Shakeitha, Shakeithia, Shaketa, Shaketha, Shakethia, Shaketia, Shakita, Shakitra, Sheketa, Shekita, Shikita, Shikitha

Shakera (Arabic) a form of Shakira.
Chakeria, Shakeira, Shakeirra, Shakerah, Shakeria, Shakeriah, Shakeriay, Shakerra, Shakerri, Shakerria, Shakerya, Shakeryia, Shakeyra

Shakia (American) a combination of the prefix Sha + Kia.
Shakeeia, Shakeeyah, Shakeia, Shakeya, Shakiya, Shekeia, Shekia, Shekiah, Shikia

Shakila (Arabic) pretty.
Chakila, Shaka, Shakayla, Shakeela, Shakeena, Shakela, Shakelah, Shakilah, Shakyla, Shekila, Shekilla, Shikeela

Shakira (Arabic) thankful.
Shaakira, Shacora, Shaka, Shakeera, Shakeerah, Shakeeria, Shakera, Shakiera, Shakierra, Shakir, Shakirah, Shakirat, Shakirea, Shakirra, Shakora, Shakuria, Shakyra, Shaquira, Shekiera, Shekira, Shikira

Shakti (Hindi) energy, power. Religion: a form of the Hindu goddess Devi.
Sakti, Shaka, Sita

Shakyra (Arabic) a form of Shakira.
Shakyria

Shalana (American) a combination of the prefix Sha + Lana.
Shalaana, Shalain, Shalaina,

Shalaine, Shaland, Shalanda, Shalane, Shalann, Shalaun, Shalauna, Shalayna, Shalayne, Shalaynna, Shallan, Shelan, Shelanda

Shaleah (American) a combination of the prefix Sha + Leah.
Shalea, Shalee, Shaleea, Shalia, Shaliah

Shaleisha (American) a combination of the prefix Sha + Aisha.
Shalesha, Shalesia, Shalicia, Shalisha

Shalena (American) a combination of the prefix Sha + Lena.
Shaleana, Shaleen, Shaleena, Shalen, Shálena, Shalene, Shalené, Shalenna, Shalina, Shalinda, Shaline, Shalini, Shalinna, Shelayna, Shelayne, Shelena

Shalisa (American) a combination of the prefix Sha + Lisa.
Shalesa, Shalese, Shalessa, Shalice, Shalicia, Shaliece, Shalise, Shalisha, Shalishea, Shalisia, Shalissa, Shalisse, Shalyce, Shalys, Shalyse

Shalita (American) a combination of the prefix Sha + Lita.
Shaleta, Shaletta, Shalida, Shalitta

Shalona (American) a combination of the prefix Sha + Lona.
Shalon, Shalone, Shálonna, Shalonne

Shalonda (American) a combination of the prefix Sha + Ondine.
Shalonde, Shalondine, Shalondra, Shalondria

Shalyn (American) a combination of the prefix Sha + Lynn.
Shalin, Shalina, Shalinda, Shaline, Shalyna, Shalynda, Shalyne, Shalynn, Shalynne

Shamara (Arabic) ready for battle.
Shamar, Shamarah, Shamare, Shamarea, Shamaree, Shamari, Shamaria, Shamariah, Shamarra, Shamarri, Shammara, Shamora, Shamori, Shamorra, Shamorria, Shamorriah

Shameka (American) a combination of the prefix Sha + Meka.
Shameaka, Shameakah, Shameca, Shamecca, Shamecha, Shamecia, Shameika, Shameke, Shamekia

Shamika (American) a combination of the prefix Sha + Mika.
Shameeca, Shameeka, Shamica,
Shamicia, Shamicka, Shamieka, Shamikia

Shamira (Hebrew) precious stone.
Shamir, Shamiran, Shamiria, Shamyra

Shamiya (American) a combination of the prefix Sha + Mia.
Shamea, Shamia, Shamiah, Shamiyah, Shamyia, Shamyiah, Shamyne

Shana (Hebrew) God is gracious. (Irish) a form of Jane.
Shaana, Shan, Shanae, Shanda, Shandi, Shane, Shania, Shanna, Shannah, Shauna, Shawna

Shanae (Irish) a form of Shana.
Shanay, Shanea

Shanda (American) a form of Chanda, Shana.
Shandae, Shandah, Shandra, Shannda

Shandi (English) a familiar form of Shana.
Shandee, Shandeigh, Shandey, Shandice, Shandie

Shandra (American) a form of Shanda. See also Chandra.
Shandrea, Shandreka, Shandri, Shandria, Shandriah, Shandrice, Shandrie, Shandry

Shane (Irish) a form of Shana.
Shanea, Shaneah, Shanee, Shanée, Shanie

Shaneisha (American) a combination of the prefix Sha + Aisha.
Shanesha, Shaneshia, Shanessa, Shanisha, Shanissha

Shaneka (American) a form of Shanika.
Shanecka, Shaneeka, Shaneekah, Shaneequa, Shaneeque, Shaneika, Shaneikah, Shanekia, Shanequa, Shaneyka, Shonneka

Shanel, Shanell, Shanelle (American) forms of Chanel.
Schanel, Schanell, Shanella, Shanelly, Shannel, Shannell, Shannelle, Shenel, Shenela, Shenell, Shenelle, Shenelly, Shinelle, Shonelle, Shynelle

Shaneta (American) a combination of the prefix Sha + Neta.
Seanette, Shaneeta, Shanetha, Shanethis, Shanetta, Shanette, Shineta, Shonetta

Shani (Swahili) a form of Shany.

Shania (American) a form of Shana.
Shanasia, Shanaya, Shaniah, Shaniya, Shanya, Shenia

Shanice (American) a form of Janice. See also Chanise.
Chenise, Shanece, Shaneese, Shaneice, Shanese, Shanicea, Shaniece, Shanise, Shanneice, Shannice, Shanyce, Sheneice

Shanida (American) a combination of the prefix Sha + Ida.
Shaneeda, Shannida

Shanika (American) a combination of the prefix Sha + Nika.
Shaneka, Shanica, Shanicca, Shanicka, Shanieka, Shanike, Shanikia, Shanikka, Shanikqua, Shanikwa, Shaniqua, Shenika, Shineeca, Shonnika

Shaniqua (American) a form of Shanika.
Shaniqa, Shaniquah, Shanique, Shaniquia, Shaniquwa, Shaniqwa, Shenequa, Sheniqua, Shinequa, Shiniqua

Shanise (American) a form of Shanice.
Shanisa, Shanisha, Shanisia, Shanissa, Shanisse, Shineese

Shanita (American) a combination of the prefix Sha + Nita.
Shanitha, Shanitra, Shanitta, Shinita

Shanley (Irish) hero's child.
Shanlee, Shanleigh, Shanlie, Shanly

Shanna (Irish) a form of Shana, Shannon.
Shanea, Shannah, Shannea

Shannen (Irish) a form of Shannon.
Shanen, Shanena, Shanene

Shannon (Irish) small and wise.
Shanan, Shanadoah, Shann, Shanna, Shannan, Shanneen, Shannen, Shannie, Shannin, Shannyn, Shanon

Shanta, Shantae, Shante (French) forms of Chantal.
Shantai, Shantay, Shantaya, Shantaye, Shanté, Shantea, Shantee, Shantée, Shanteia

Shantal (American) a form of Shantel.
Shantall, Shontal

Shantana (American) a form of Santana.
Shantan, Shantanae, Shantanell, Shantanickia, Shantanika, Shantanna

Shantara (American) a combination of the prefix Sha + Tara.
Shantaria, Shantarra, Shantera, Shanteria, Shanterra, Shantira, Shontara, Shuntara

Shanteca (American) a combination of the prefix Sha + Teca.
Shantecca, Shanteka, Shantika, Shantikia

Shantel, Shantell (American) song.
Seantelle, Shanntell, Shanta, Shantal, Shantae, Shantale, Shante, Shanteal, Shanteil, Shantele, Shantella, Shantelle, Shantrell, Shantyl, Shantyle,

Shauntel, Shauntell, Shauntelle, Shauntrel, Shauntrell, Shauntrella, Shentel, Shentelle, Shontal, Shontalla, Shontalle, Shontel, Shontelle

Shanteria (American) a form of Shantara.
Shanterica, Shanterria, Shanterrie, Shantieria, Shantirea, Shonteria

Shantesa (American) a combination of the prefix Sha + Tess.
Shantese, Shantice, Shantise, Shantisha, Shontecia, Shontessia

Shantia (American) a combination of the prefix Sha + Tia.
Shanteya, Shanti, Shantida, Shantie, Shaunteya, Shauntia, Shontia

Shantille (American) a form of Chantilly.
Shanteil, Shantil, Shantilli, Shantillie, Shantilly, Shantyl, Shantyle

Shantina (American) a combination of the prefix Sha + Tina.
Shanteena, Shontina

Shantora (American) a combination of the prefix Sha + Tory.
Shantoia, Shantori, Shantoria, Shantory, Shantorya, Shantoya, Shanttoria

Shantrice (American) a combination of the prefix Sha + Trice. See also Chantrice.
Shantrece, Shantrecia, Shantreece, Shantreese, Shantrese, Shantress, Shantrezia, Shantricia, Shantriece, Shantris, Shantrisse, Shontrice

Shany (Swahili) marvelous, wonderful.
Shaney, Shannai, Shannea, Shanni, Shannia, Shannie, Shanny, Shanya

Shappa (Native American) red thunder.

Shaquanda (American) a combination of the prefix Sha + Wanda.
Shaquan, Shaquana, Shaquand, Shaquandey, Shaquandra, Shaquandria, Shaquanera, Shaquani, Shaquania, Shaquanna, Shaquanta, Shaquantae, Shaquantay, Shaquante, Shaquantia, Shaquona, Shaquonda, Shaquondra, Shaquondria

Shaqueita, Shaquita (American) forms of Shakeita.
Shaqueta, Shaquetta, Shaquette, Shaquitta, Shequida, Shequita, Shequittia

Shaquila, Shaquilla (American) forms of Shakila.
Shaquail, Shaquia, Shaquil, Shaquilah, Shaquile, Shaquill,
Shaquillah, Shaquille, Shaquillia, Shequela, Shequele, Shequila, Shquiyla

Shaquira (American) a form of Shakira.
Shaquirah, Shaquire, Shaquirra, Shaqura, Shaqurah, Shaquri

Shara (Hebrew) a short form of Sharon.
Shaara, Sharah, Sharal, Sharala, Sharalee, Sharlyn, Sharlynn, Sharra, Sharrah

Sharai (Hebrew) princess. See also Sharon.
Sharae, Sharaé, Sharah, Sharaiah, Sharay, Sharaya, Sharayah

Sharan (Hindi) protector.
Sharaine, Sharanda, Sharanjeet

Shardae, Sharday (Punjabi) charity. (Yoruba) honored by royalty. (Arabic) runaway. A form of Chardae.
Sade, Shadae, Sharda, Shar-Dae, Shardai, Shar-Day, Sharde, Shardea, Shardee, Shardée, Shardei, Shardeia, Shardey

Sharee (English) a form of Shari.
Shareen, Shareena, Sharine

Shari (French) beloved, dearest. (Hungarian) a form of Sarah. See also Sharita, Sheree, Sherry.
Shara, Share, Sharee, Sharia,

*Shariah, Sharian, Shariann,
Sharianne, Sharie, Sharra,
Sharree, Sharri, Sharrie, Sharry,
Shary*

Sharice (French) a form of
Cherice.
*Shareese, Sharesse, Sharese,
Sharica, Sharicka, Shariece,
Sharis, Sharise, Sharish, Shariss,
Sharissa, Sharisse, Sharyse*

Sharik (African) child of God.

Sharissa (American) a form of
Sharice.
*Sharesa, Sharessia, Sharisa,
Sharisha, Shereeza, Shericia,
Sherisa, Sherissa*

Sharita (French) a familiar form
of Shari. (American) a form of
Charity. See also Sherita.
Shareeta, Sharrita

Sharla (French) a short form
of Sharlene, Sharlotte.

Sharlene (French) little and
strong.
*Scharlane, Scharlene, Shar,
Sharla, Sharlaina, Sharlaine,
Sharlane, Sharlanna, Sharlee,
Sharleen, Sharleine, Sharlena,
Sharleyne, Sharline, Sharlyn,
Sharlyne, Sharlynn, Sharlynne,
Sherlean, Sherleen, Sherlene,
Sherline*

Sharlotte (American) a form
of Charlotte.
*Sharlet, Sharlett, Sharlott,
Sharlotta*

Sharma (American) a short
form of Sharmaine.
Sharmae, Sharme

Sharmaine (American) a form
of Charmaine.
*Sharma, Sharmain, Sharman,
Sharmane, Sharmanta,
Sharmayne, Sharmeen,
Sharmene, Sharmese, Sharmin,
Sharmine, Sharmon, Sharmyn*

Sharna (Hebrew) a form of
Sharon.
*Sharnae, Sharnay, Sharne,
Sharnea, Sharnease, Sharnee,
Sharneese, Sharnell, Sharnelle,
Sharnese, Sharnett, Sharnetta,
Sharnise*

Sharon (Hebrew) desert plain.
A form of Sharai.
*Shaaron, Shara, Sharai, Sharan,
Shareen, Sharen, Shari, Sharin,
Sharna, Sharonda, Sharone,
Sharran, Sharren, Sharrin,
Sharron, Sharrona, Sharyn,
Sharyon, Sheren, Sheron,
Sherryn*

Sharonda (Hebrew) a form of
Sharon.
*Sharronda, Sheronda,
Sherrhonda*

Sharrona (Hebrew) a form of
Sharon.
*Sharona, Sharone, Sharonia,
Sharonna, Sharony, Sharronne,
Sheron, Sherona, Sheronna,
Sherron, Sherronna, Sherronne,
Shirona*

Shatara (Hindi) umbrella.
(Arabic) good; industrious.
(American) a combination of
Sharon + Tara.
*Shatarea, Shatari, Shataria,
Shatarra, Shataura, Shateira,
Shatera, Shaterah, Shateria,
Shaterra, Shaterri, Shaterria,
Shatherian, Shatierra, Shatiria*

Shatoria (American) a combi-
nation of the prefix Sha +
Tory.
*Shatora, Shatorea, Shatori,
Shatorri, Shatorria, Shatory,
Shatorya, Shatoya*

Shauna (Hebrew) God is gra-
cious. (Irish) a form of
Shana. See also Seana, Shona.
*Shaun, Shaunah, Shaunda,
Shaune, Shaunee, Shauneen,
Shaunelle, Shaunette, Shauni,
Shaunice, Shaunicy, Shaunie,
Shaunika, Shaunisha, Shaunna,
Shaunnea, Shaunta, Shaunua,
Shaunya*

Shaunda (Irish) a form of
Shauna. See also Shanda,
Shawnda, Shonda.
*Shaundal, Shaundala,
Shaundel, Shaundela,
Shaundell, Shaundelle,
Shaundra, Shaundrea,
Shaundree, Shaundria,
Shaundrice*

Shaunta (Irish) a form of
Shauna. See also Shawnta,
Shonta.
Schunta, Shauntae, Shauntay,

*Shaunte, Shauntea, Shauntee,
Shauntée, Shaunteena,
Shauntei, Shauntia, Shauntier,
Shauntrel, Shauntrell,
Shauntrella*

Shavon (American) a form of
Shavonne.
*Schavon, Schevon, Shavan,
Shavana, Shavaun, Shavona,
Shavonda, Shavone, Shavonia,
Shivon*

Shavonne (American) a com-
bination of the prefix Sha +
Yvonne. See also Siobhan.
*Shavanna, Shavon, Shavondra,
Shavonn, Shavonna, Shavonni,
Shavonnia, Shavonnie,
Shavontae, Shavonte, Shavonté,
Shavoun, Shivaun, Shivawn,
Shivonne, Shyvon, Shyvonne*

Shawanna (American) a com-
bination of the prefix Sha +
Wanda. See also Shajuana,
Shawna.
*Shawan, Shawana, Shawanda,
Shawante, Shiwani*

Shawna (Hebrew) God is gra-
cious. (Irish) a form of Jane.
A form of Shana, Shauna.
See also Seana, Shona.
*Sawna, Shaw, Shawn, Shawnae,
Shawnai, Shawnea, Shawnee,
Shawneen, Shawneena,
Shawnell, Shawnette, Shawnna,
Shawnra, Shawnta, Sheona,
Siân, Siana, Sianna*

Shawnda (Irish) a form of
Shawna. See also Shanda,
Shaunda, Shonda.
*Shawndal, Shawndala,
Shawndan, Shawndel,
Shawndra, Shawndrea,
Shawndree, Shawndreel,
Shawndrell, Shawndria*

Shawnee (Irish) a form of
Shawna.
*Shawne, Shawneea, Shawney,
Shawni, Shawnie*

Shawnika (American) a com-
bination of Shawna + Nika.
*Shawnaka, Shawnequa,
Shawneika, Shawnicka*

Shawnta (Irish) a form of
Shawna. See also Shaunta,
Shonta.
*Shawntae, Shawntay, Shawnte,
Shawnté, Shawntee, Shawntell,
Shawntelle, Shawnteria,
Shawntia, Shawntil, Shawntile,
Shawntill, Shawntille,
Shawntina, Shawntish,
Shawntrese, Shawntriece*

Shay, Shaye (Irish) forms of
Shea.
*Shaya, Shayah, Shayda, Shayha,
Shayia, Shayla, Shey, Sheye*

Shayla (Irish) a form of Shay.
*Shaylagh, Shaylah, Shaylain,
Shaylan, Shaylea, Shayleah,
Shaylla, Shaylyn, Sheyla*

Shaylee (Irish) a form of Shea.
*Shaylei, Shayleigh, Shayley,
Shayli, Shaylie, Shayly, Shealy*

Shaylyn (Irish) a form of
Shea.
*Shaylin, Shaylina, Shaylinn,
Shaylynn, Shaylynne, Shealyn,
Sheylyn*

Shayna (Hebrew) beautiful.
*Shaynae, Shaynah, Shayne,
Shaynee, Shayney, Shayni,
Shaynie, Shaynna, Shaynne,
Shayny, Sheana, Sheanna*

Shea (Irish) fairy palace.
*Shae, Shay, Shaylee, Shaylyn,
Shealy, Shaelee, Shaelyn,
Shealyn, Sheann, Sheannon,
Sheanta, Sheaon, Shearra,
Sheatara, Sheaunna, Sheavon*

Sheba (Hebrew) a short form
of Bathsheba. Geography: an
ancient country of south
Arabia.
Saba, Sabah, Shebah, Sheeba

Sheena (Hebrew) God is gra-
cious. (Irish) a form of Jane.
*Sheenagh, Sheenah, Sheenan,
Sheeneal, Sheenika, Sheenna,
Sheina, Shena, Shiona*

Sheila (Latin) blind. (Irish) a
form of Cecelia. See also
Cheyla, Zelizi.
*Seelia, Seila, Selia, Shaila,
Sheela, Sheelagh, Sheelah,
Sheilagh, Sheilah, Sheileen,
Sheiletta, Sheilia, Sheillynn,
Sheilya, Shela, Shelagh, Shelah,
Shelia, Shiela, Shila, Shilah,
Shilea, Shyla*

Shelbi, Shelbie (English)
forms of Shelby.
Shelbbie, Shellbi, Shellbie

Shelby (English) ledge estate.
*Chelby, Schelby, Shel, Shelbe,
Shelbee, Shelbey, Shelbi, Shelbie,
Shelbye, Shellby*

Sheldon (English) farm on
the ledge.
*Sheldina, Sheldine, Sheldrina,
Sheldyn, Shelton*

Shelee (English) a form of
Shelley.
*Shelee, Sheleen, Shelena, Sheley,
Sheli, Shelia, Shelina, Shelinda,
Shelita*

Shelisa (American) a combi-
nation of Shelley + Lisa.
*Sheleza, Shelica, Shelicia,
Shelise, Shelisse, Sheliza*

Shelley, Shelly (English)
meadow on the ledge.
(French) familiar forms of
Michelle. See also Rochelle.
*Shelee, Shell, Shella, Shellaine,
Shellana, Shellany, Shellee,
Shellene, Shelli, Shellian,
Shelliann, Shellie, Shellina*

Shelsea (American) a form of
Chelsea.
*Shellsea, Shellsey, Shelsey,
Shelsie, Shelsy*

Shena (Irish) a form of
Sheena.
*Shenada, Shenae, Shenah,
Shenay, Shenda, Shene, Shenea,*

*Sheneda, Shenee, Sheneena,
Shenica, Shenika, Shenina,
Sheniqua, Shenita, Shenna,
Shennae, Shennah, Shenoa*

Shera (Aramaic) light.
*Sheera, Sheerah, Sherae, Sherah,
Sheralee, Sheralle, Sheralyn,
Sheralynn, Sheralynne, Sheray,
Sheraya*

Sheree (French) beloved, dearest.
*Scherie, Sheeree, Shere, Shereé,
Sherrelle, Shereen, Shereena*

Sherelle (French) a form of
Cherelle, Sheryl.
*Sherel, Sherell, Sheriel, Sherrel,
Sherrell, Sherrelle, Shirelle*

Sheri, Sherri (French) forms
of Sherry.
Sheria, Sheriah, Sherie, Sherrie

Sherian (American) a combination of Sheri + Ann.
Sherianne, Sherrina

Sherice (French) a form of
Cherice.
*Scherise, Sherece, Shereece,
Sherees, Shereese, Sherese,
Shericia, Sherise, Sherisse,
Sherrish, Sherryse, Sheryce*

Sheridan (Irish) wild.
*Sherida, Sheridane, Sherideen,
Sheriden, Sheridian, Sheridon,
Sherridan, Sherridon*

Sherika (Punjabi) relative.
(Arabic) easterner.
*Shereka, Sherica, Shericka,
Sherrica, Sherricka, Sherrika*

Sherissa (French) a form of Sherry, Sheryl.
Shereeza, Sheresa, Shericia, Sherrish

Sherita (French) a form of Sherry, Sheryl. See also Sharita.
Shereta, Sheretta, Sherette, Sherrita

Sherleen (French, English) a form of Sheryl, Shirley.
Sherileen, Sherlene, Sherlin, Sherlina, Sherline, Sherlyn, Sherlyne, Sherlynne, Shirlena, Shirlene, Shirlina, Shirlyn

Sherry (French) beloved, dearest. A familiar form of Sheryl. See also Sheree.
Sherey, Sheri, Sherissa, Sherrey, Sherri, Sherria, Sherriah, Sherrie, Sherye, Sheryy

Sheryl (French) beloved. A familiar form of Shirley. See also Sherry.
Sharel, Sharil, Sharilyn, Sharyl, Sharyll, Sheral, Sherell, Sheriel, Sheril, Sherill, Sherily, Sherilyn, Sherissa, Sherita, Sherleen, Sherral, Sherrelle, Sherril, Sherrill, Sherryl, Sherylly

Sherylyn (American) a combination of Sheryl + Lynn. See also Cherilyn.
Sharolin, Sharolyn, Sharyl-Lynn, Sheralyn, Sherilyn, Sherilynn, Sherilynne, Sherralyn, Sherralynn, Sherrilyn, Sherrilynn, Sherrilynne, Sherrylyn, Sherryn, Sherylanne

Shevonne (American) a combination of the prefix She + Yvonne.
Shevaun, Shevon, Shevonda, Shevone

Sheyenne (Cheyenne) a form of Cheyenne. See also Shyann, Shyanne.
Shayhan, Sheyan, Sheyane, Sheyann, Sheyanna, Sheyannah, Sheyanne, Sheyen, Sheyene, Shiante, Shyanne

Shianne (Cheyenne) a form of Cheyenne.
She, Shian, Shiana, Shianah, Shianda, Shiane, Shiann, Shianna, Shiannah, Shiany, Shieana, Shieann, Shieanne, Shiena, Shiene, Shienna

Shifra (Hebrew) beautiful.
Schifra, Shifrah

Shika (Japanese) gentle deer.
Shi, Shikah, Shikha

Shilo (Hebrew) God's gift. Bible: a sanctuary for the Israelites where the Ark of the Covenant was kept.
Shiloh

Shina (Japanese) virtuous, good; wealthy. (Chinese) a form of China.
Shinae, Shinay, Shine, Shinna

Shino (Japanese) bamboo stalk.

Shiquita (American) a form of Chiquita.
Shiquata, Shiquitta

Shira (Hebrew) song.
Shirah, Shiray, Shire, Shiree, Shiri, Shirit, Shyra

Shirlene (English) a form of Shirley.
Shirleen, Shirline, Shirlynn

Shirley (English) bright meadow. See also Sheryl.
Sherlee, Sherleen, Sherley, Sherli, Sherlie, Shir, Shirl, Shirlee, Shirlie, Shirly, Shirlly, Shurlee, Shurley

Shivani (Hindi) life and death.
Shiva, Shivana, Shivanie, Shivanna

Shizu (Japanese) silent.
Shizue, Shizuka, Shizuko, Shizuyo

Shona (Irish) a form of Jane. A form of Shana, Shauna, Shawna.
Shiona, Shonagh, Shonah, Shonalee, Shonda, Shone, Shonee, Shonette, Shoni, Shonie, Shonna, Shonnah, Shonta

Shonda (Irish) a form of Shona. See also Shanda, Shaunda, Shawnda.
Shondalette, Shondalyn, Shondel, Shondelle, Shondi,
Shondia, Shondie, Shondra, Shondreka, Shounda

Shonta (Irish) a form of Shona. See also Shaunta, Shawnta.
Shontá, Shontae, Shontai, Shontalea, Shontasia, Shontavia, Shontaviea, Shontay, Shontaya, Shonte, Shonté, Shontedra, Shontee, Shonteral, Shonti, Shontol, Shontoy, Shontrail, Shountáe

Shoshana (Hebrew) a form of Susan.
Shosha, Shoshan, Shoshanah, Shoshane, Shoshanha, Shoshann, Shoshanna, Shoshannah, Shoshauna, Shoshaunah, Shoshawna, Shoshona, Shoshone, Shoshonee, Shoshoney, Shoshoni, Shoushan, Shushana, Sosha, Soshana

Shu (Chinese) kind, gentle.

Shug (American) a short form of Sugar.

Shula (Arabic) flaming, bright.
Shulah

Shulamith (Hebrew) peaceful. See also Sula.
Shulamit, Sulamith

Shunta (Irish) a form of Shonta.
Shuntae, Shunté, Shuntel, Shuntell, Shuntelle, Shuntia

Shura (Russian) a form of Alexandra.
Schura, Shurah, Shuree,

Shureen, Shurelle, Shuritta,
Shurka, Shurlana

Shyann, Shyanne (Cheyenne)
forms of Cheyenne. See also
Sheyenne.
Shyan, Shyana, Shyandra,
Shyane, Shynee, Shyanna,
Shyannah, Shye, Shyene,
Shyenna, Shyenne

Shyla (English) a form of Sheila.
Shya, Shyah, Shylah, Shylan,
Shylayah, Shylana, Shylane,
Shyle, Shyleah, Shylee, Shyley,
Shyli, Shylia, Shylie, Shylo,
Shyloe, Shyloh, Shylon, Shylyn

Shyra (Hebrew) a form of
Shira.
Shyrae, Shyrah, Shyrai, Shyrie,
Shyro

Siara (Irish) a form of Sierra.
Siarah, Siarra, Siarrah, Sieara

Sianna (Irish) a form of
Seana.
Sian, Siana, Sianae, Sianai,
Sianey, Siannah, Sianne,
Sianni, Sianny, Siany

Sibeta (Moquelumnan) find-
ing a fish under a rock.

Sibley (English) sibling; friendly.
(Greek) a form of Sybil.
Sybley

Sidney (French) a form of
Sydney.
Sidne, Sidnee, Sidnei, Sidneya,
Sidni, Sidnie, Sidny, Sidnye

Sidonia (Hebrew) enticing.
Sydania, Syndonia

Sidonie (French) from Saint-
Denis, France. See also Sydney.
Sedona, Sidaine, Sidanni, Sidelle,
Sidoine, Sidona, Sidonae, Sidonia,
Sidony

Sidra (Latin) star child.
Sidrah, Sidras

Sienna (American) a form of
Ciana.
Seini, Siena

Siera (Irish) an alternte form
of Sierra.
Sierah, Sieria

Sierra (Irish) black. (Spanish)
saw toothed. Geography: any
rugged range of mountains
that, when viewed from a
distance, has a jagged profile.
See also Ciara.
Seara, Searria, Seera, Seirra,
Siara, Siearra, Siera, Sierrah,
Sierre, Sierrea, Sierriah, Syerra

Sigfreda (German) victorious
peace. See also Freda.
Sigfreida, Sigfrida, Sigfrieda,
Sigfryda

Sigmunda (German) victorious protector.
Sigmonda

Signe (Latin) sign, signal.
(Scandinavian) a short form
of Sigourney.
Sig, Signa, Signy, Singna,
Singne

Sigourney (English) victorious conquerer.
Signe, Sigournee, Sigourny

Sigrid (Scandinavian) victorious counselor.
Siegrid, Siegrida, Sigritt

Sihu (Native American) flower; bush.

Siko (African) crying baby.

Silvia (Latin) a form of Sylvia.
Silivia, Silva, Silvya

Simcha (Hebrew) joyful.

Simone (Hebrew) she heard. (French) a form of Simon (see Boys' Names).
Samone, Siminie, Simmi, Simmie, Simmona, Simmone, Simoane, Simona, Simonetta, Simonette, Simonia, Simonina, Simonne, Somone, Symone

Simran (Sikh) absorbed in God.
Simren, Simrin, Simrun

Sina (Irish) a form of Seana.
Seena, Sinai, Sinaia, Sinan, Sinay

Sinclaire (French) prayer.
Sinclair

Sindy (American) a form of Cindy.
Sinda, Sindal, Sindee, Sindi, Sindia, Sindie, Sinnedy, Synda, Syndal, Syndee, Syndey, Syndi, Syndia, Syndie, Syndy

Sinead (Irish) a form of Jane.
Seonaid, Sine, Sinéad

Siobhan (Irish) a form of Joan. See also Shavonne.
Shibahn, Shibani, Shibhan, Shioban, Shobana, Shobha, Shobhana, Siobahn, Siobhana, Siobhann, Siobhon, Siovaun, Siovhan

Sirena (Greek) enchanter. Mythology: Sirens were sea nymphs whose singing enchanted sailors and made them crash their ships into nearby rocks.
Sireena, Sirene, Sirine, Syrena, Syrenia, Syrenna, Syrina

Sisika (Native American) songbird.

Sissy (American) a familiar form of Cecelia.
Sisi, Sisie, Sissey, Sissie

Sita (Hindi) a form of Shakti.
Sitah, Sitarah, Sitha, Sithara

Siti (Swahili) respected woman.

Skye (Arabic) water giver. (Dutch) a short form of Skyler. Geography: an island in the Hebrides, Scotland.
Ski, Skie, Skii, Skky, Sky, Skya, Skyy

Skylar (Dutch) a form of Skyler.
Skyela, Skyelar, Skyla, Skylair, Skyylar

Skyler (Dutch) sheltering.
*Skila, Skilah, Skye, Skyeler,
Skyelur, Skyla, Skylar, Skylee,
Skylena, Skyli, Skylia, Skylie,
Skylin, Skyllar, Skylor, Skylyn,
Skylynn, Skylyr, Skyra*

Sloane (Irish) warrior.
Sloan, Sloanne

Socorro (Spanish) helper.

Sofia (Greek) a form of Sophia.
See also Zofia, Zsofia.
*Sofeea, Sofeeia, Soffi, Sofi, Soficita,
Sofie, Sofija, Sofiya, Sofka, Sofya*

Solada (Tai) listener.

Solana (Spanish) sunshine.
*Solande, Solanna, Soleil,
Solena, Soley, Solina, Solinda*

Solange (French) dignified.

Soledad (Spanish) solitary.
Sole, Soleda

Solenne (French) solemn, dig-
nified.
*Solaine, Solene, Soléne, Solenna,
Solina, Soline, Solonez, Souline,
Soulle*

Soma (Hindi) lunar.

Sommer (English) summer;
summoner. (Arabic) black.
See also Summer.
*Somara, Somer, Sommar,
Sommara, Sommers*

Sondra (Greek) defender of
mankind.
Saundra, Sondre, Sonndra, Sonndre

Sonia (Russian, Slavic) a form
of Sonya.
*Sonica, Sonida, Sonita, Sonna,
Sonni, Sonnia, Sonnie, Sonny*

Sonja (Scandinavian) a form
of Sonya.
Sonjae, Sonjia

Sonya (Greek) wise. (Russian,
Slavic) a form of Sophia.
*Sonia, Sonja, Sonnya, Sonyae,
Sunya*

Sook (Korean) pure.

Sopheary (Cambodian) beautiful girl.

Sophia (Greek) wise. See also
Sonya, Zofia.
Sofia, Sophie

Sophie (Greek) a familiar form
of Sophia. See also Zocha.
Sophey, Sophi, Sophy

Sophronia (Greek) wise; sensible.
Soffrona, Sofronia

Sora (Native American)
chirping songbird.

Soraya (Persian) princess.
Suraya

Sorrel (French) reddish
brown. Botany: a plant
whose leaves are used as salad
greens.

Soso (Native American) tree
squirrel dining on pine nuts;
chubby-cheeked baby.

Souzan (Persian) burning fire.
Sousan, Souzanne

Spencer (English) dispenser of
provisions.
Spenser

Speranza (Italian) a form of
Esperanza.
Speranca

Spring (English) springtime.
Spryng

Stacey, Stacy (Greek) resur-
rection. (Irish) a short form
of Anastasia, Eustacia,
Natasha.
*Stace, Stacee, Staceyan,
Staceyann, Staicy, Stasey,
Stasya, Stayce, Staycee, Staci,
Steacy*

Staci, Stacie (Greek) forms of
Stacey.
Stacci, Stacia, Stayci

Stacia (English) a short form
of Anastasia.
Stasia, Staysha

Starla (English) a form of
Starr.
Starrla

Starleen (English) a form of
Starr.
*Starleena, Starlena, Starlene,
Starlin, Starlyn, Starlynn, Starrlen*

Starley (English) a familiar
form of Starr.
Starle, Starlee, Staly

Starling (English) bird.

Starr (English) star.
*Star, Staria, Starisha, Starla,
Starleen, Starlet, Starlette,
Starley, Starlight, Starre, Starri,
Starria, Starrika, Starrsha,
Starsha, Starshanna, Startish*

Stasya (Greek) a familiar form
of Anastasia. (Russian) a form
of Stacey.
*Stasa, Stasha, Stashia, Stasia,
Stasja, Staska*

Stefani, Steffani (Greek)
forms of Stephanie.
*Stafani, Stefanni, Steffane,
Steffanee, Stefini, Stefoni*

Stefanie (Greek) a form of
Stephanie.
*Stafanie, Staffany, Stefane,
Stefanee, Stefaney, Stefania,
Stefanié, Stefanija, Stefannie,
Stefcia, Stefenie, Steffanie, Steffi,
Stefinie, Stefka*

Stefany, Steffany (Greek)
forms of Stephanie.
Stefanny, Stefanya, Steffaney

Steffi (Greek) a familiar form
of Stefanie, Stephanie.
*Stefa, Stefcia, Steffee, Steffie,
Steffy, Stefi, Stefka, Stefy,
Stepha, Stephi, Stephie, Stephy*

Stella (Latin) star. (French) a
familiar form of Estelle.
Steile, Stellina

Stepania (Russian) a form of
Stephanie.
Stepa, Stepahny, Stepanida,

Stepanie, Stepanyda, Stepfanie, Stephana

Stephani (Greek) a form of Stephanie.
Stephania, Stephanni

Stephanie (Greek) crowned. See also Estefani, Estephanie, Panya, Stevie, Zephania.
Stamatios, Stefani, Stefanie, Stefany, Steffie, Stepania, Stephaija, Stephaine, Stephanas, Stephane, Stephanee, Stephani, Stephanida, Stéphanie, Stephanine, Stephann, Stephannie, Stephany, Stephene, Stephenie, Stephianie, Stephney, Stesha, Steshka, Stevanee

Stephany (Greek) a form of Stephanie.
Stephaney, Stephanye

Stephene (Greek) a form of Stephanie.
Stephina, Stephine, Stephyne

Stephenie (Greek) a form of Stephanie.
Stephena, Stephenee, Stepheney, Stepheni, Stephenny, Stepheny, Stephine, Stephinie

Stephney (Greek) a form of Stephanie.
Stephne, Stephni, Stephnie, Stephny

Sterling (English) valuable; silver penny.

Stevie (Greek) a familiar form of Stephanie.
Steva, Stevana, Stevanee, Stevee, Stevena, Stevey, Stevi, Stevy, Stevye

Stina (German) a short form of Christina.
Steena, Stena, Stine, Stinna

Stockard (English) stockyard.

Stormie (English) a form of Stormy.
Stormee, Stormi, Stormii

Stormy (English) impetuous by nature.
Storm, Storme, Stormey, Stormie, Stormm

Suchin (Tai) beautiful thought.

Sue (Hebrew) a short form of Susan, Susanna.

Sueann, Sueanna (American) combinations of Sue + Ann, Sue + Anna.
Suann, Suanna, Suannah, Suanne, Sueanne

Suela (Spanish) consolation.
Suelita

Sugar (American) sweet as sugar.
Shug

Sugi (Japanese) cedar tree.

Suke (Hawaiian) a form of Susan.

Sukey (Hawaiian) a familiar form of Susan.
Suka, Sukee, Suki, Sukie, Suky

Sukhdeep (Sikh) light of peace and bliss.
Sukhdip

Suki (Japanese) loved one. (Moquelumnan) eagle-eyed.
Sukie

Sula (Icelandic) large sea bird. (Greek, Hebrew) a short form of Shulamith, Ursula. Suletu (Moquelumnan) soaring bird.

Sulia (Latin) a form of Julia.
Suliana

Sulwen (Welsh) bright as the sun.

Sumalee (Tai) beautiful flower.

Sumati (Hindi) unity.

Sumaya (American) a combination of Sue + Maya.
Sumayah, Sumayya, Sumayyah

Sumi (Japanese) elegant, refined.
Sumiko

Summer (English) summertime. See also Sommer.
Sumer, Summar, Summerann, Summerbreeze, Summerhaze, Summerine, Summerlee, Summerlin, Summerlyn, Summerlynn, Summers, Sumrah, Summyr, Sumyr

Sun (Korean) obedient.
Suncance, Sundee, Sundeep, Sundi, Sundip, Sundrenea, Sunta, Sunya

Sunee (Tai) good.
Suni

Sun-Hi (Korean) good; joyful.

Suni (Zuni) native; member of our tribe.
Sunita, Sunitha, Suniti, Sunne, Sunni, Sunnie, Sunnilei

Sunki (Hopi) swift.
Sunkia

Sunny (English) bright, cheerful.
Sunni, Sunnie

Sunshine (English) sunshine.
Sunshyn, Sunshyne

Surata (Pakistani) blessed joy.

Suri (Todas) pointy nose.
Suree, Surena, Surenia

Surya (Sanskrit) Mythology: a sun god.
Suria, Suriya, Surra

Susammi (French) a combination of Susan + Aimee.
Suzami, Suzamie, Suzamy

Susan (Hebrew) lily. See also Shoshana, Sukey, Zsa Zsa, Zusa.
Sawsan, Siusan, Sosan, Sosana, Sue, Suesan, Sueva, Suisan, Suke, Susana, Susann, Susanna, Suse, Susen, Susette,

*Susie, Suson, Suzan, Suzanna,
Suzannah, Suzanne, Suzette*

Susana (Hebrew) a form of
Susan.
Susanah, Susane

Susanna, Susannah (Hebrew)
forms of Susan. See also
Xuxa, Zanna, Zsuzsanna.
*Sonel, Sosana, Sue, Suesanna,
Susana, Susanah, Susanka,
Susette, Susie, Suzanna*

Suse (Hawaiian) a form of
Susan.

Susette (French) a familiar
form of Susan, Susanna.
Susetta

Susie, Suzie (American)
familiar forms of Susan,
Susanna.
*Suse, Susey, Susi, Sussi, Sussy,
Susy, Suze, Suzi, Suzy, Suzzie*

Suzanna, Suzannah (Hebrew)
forms of Susan.
Suzana, Suzenna, Suzzanna

Suzanne (English) a form of
Susan.
*Susanne, Suszanne, Suzane,
Suzann, Suzzane, Suzzann,
Suzzanne*

Suzette (French) a form of
Susan.
Suzetta, Suzzette

Suzu (Japanese) little bell.
Suzue, Suzuko

Suzuki (Japanese) bell tree.

Svetlana (Russian) bright light.
Sveta, Svetochka

Syá (Chinese) summer.

Sybella (English) a form of
Sybil.
*Sebila, Sibbella, Sibeal, Sibel,
Sibell, Sibella, Sibelle, Sibilla,
Sibylla, Sybel, Sybelle, Sybila,
Sybilla*

Sybil (Greek) prophet.
Mythology: sibyls were ora-
cles who relayed the mes-
sages of the gods. See also
Cybele, Sibley.
*Sib, Sibbel, Sibbie, Sibbill, Sibby,
Sibeal, Sibel, Sibyl, Sibylle,
Sibylline, Sybella, Sybille, Syble*

Sydnee (French) a form of
Sydney.
Sydne, Sydnea, Sydnei

Sydney (French) from Saint-
Denis, France. See also
Sidonie.
*Cidney, Cydney, Sidney, Sy,
Syd, Sydel, Sydelle, Sydna,
Sydnee, Sydni, Sydnie, Sydny,
Sydnye, Syndona, Syndonah*

Sydni, Sydnie (French) forms
of Sydney.

Sying (Chinese) star.

Sylvana (Latin) forest.
*Silvaine, Silvana, Silvanna,
Silviane, Sylva, Sylvaine,
Sylvanah, Sylvania, Sylvanna,
Sylvie, Sylvina, Sylvinnia,
Sylvonah, Sylvonia, Sylvonna*

Sylvia (Latin) forest. Literature: Sylvia Plath was a well-known American poet. See also Silvia, Xylia.
Sylvette, Sylvie, Sylwia

Sylvianne (American) a combination of Sylvia + Anne.
Sylvian

Sylvie (Latin) a familiar form of Sylvia.
Silvi, Silvie, Silvy, Sylvi

Symone (Hebrew) a form of Simone.
Symmeon, Symmone, Symona, Symoné, Symonne

Symphony (Greek) symphony, harmonious sound.
Symfoni, Symphanie, Symphany, Symphanée, Symphoni, Symphoni

Syreeta (Hindi) good traditions. (Arabic) companion.
Syretta, Syrrita

T

Tabatha (Greek, Aramaic) a form of Tabitha.
Tabathe, Tabathia, Tabbatha

Tabby (English) a familiar form of Tabitha.
Tabbi

Tabia (Swahili) talented.
Tabea

Tabetha (Greek, Aramaic) a form of Tabitha.

Tabina (Arabic) follower of Muhammad.

Tabitha (Greek, Aramaic) gazelle.
Tabatha, Tabbee, Tabbetha, Tabbey, Tabbi, Tabbie, Tabbitha, Tabby, Tabetha, Tabiatha, Tabita, Tabithia, Tabotha, Tabtha, Tabytha

Tabytha (Greek, Aramaic) a form of Tabitha.
Tabbytha

Tacey (English) a familiar form of Tacita.
Tace, Tacee, Taci, Tacy, Tacye

Taci (Zuni) washtub. (English) a form of Tacey.
Tacia, Taciana, Tacie

Tacita (Latin) silent.
Tacey

Tadita (Omaha) runner.
Tadeta, Tadra

Taelor (English) a form of Taylor.
Taelar, Taeler, Taellor, Taelore, Taelyr

Taesha (Latin) a form of Tisha. (American) a combination of the prefix Ta + Aisha.
Tadasha, Taeshayla, Taeshia, Taheisha, Tahisha, Taiesha,

Taisha, Taishae, Teasha, Teashia,
Teisha, Tesha

Taffy (Welsh) beloved.
Taffia, Taffine, Taffye, Tafia,
Tafisa, Tafoya

Tahira (Arabic) virginal, pure.
Taheera, Taheerah, Tahera,
Tahere, Taheria, Taherri, Tahiara,
Tahirah, Tahireh

Tahlia (Greek, Hebrew) a
form of Talia.
Tahleah, Tahleia

Tailor (English) a form of
Taylor.
Tailar, Tailer, Taillor, Tailyr

Taima (Native American) clash
of thunder.
Taimi, Taimia, Taimy

Taipa (Moquelumnan) flying
quail.
Taite (English) cheerful.
Tate, Tayte, Tayten

Taja (Hindi) crown.
Taiajára, Taija, Tajae, Tajah,
Tahai, Tehya, Teja, Tejah, Tejal

Taka (Japanese) honored.

Takala (Hopi) corn tassel.

Takara (Japanese) treasure.
Takarah, Takaria, Takarra, Takra

Takayla (American) a combi-
nation of the prefix Ta +
Kayla.
Takayler, Takeyli

Takeisha (American) a combi-
nation of the prefix Ta +
Keisha.
Takecia, Takesha, Takeshia,
Takesia, Takisha, Takishea,
Takishia, Tekeesha, Tekeisha,
Tekeshi, Tekeysia, Tekisha,
Tikesha, Tikisha, Tokesia, Tykeisha

Takenya (Hebrew) animal
horn. (Moquelumnan) fal-
con. (American) a combination of the prefix Ta +
Kenya.
Takenia, Takenja

Takeria (American) a form of
Takira.
Takera, Takeri, Takerian, Takerra,
Takerria, Takierria, Takoria

Taki (Japanese) waterfall.
Tiki

Takia (Arabic) worshiper.
Takeia, Takeiyah, Takeya,
Takeyah, Takhiya, Takiah,
Takija, Takiya, Takiyah, Takkia,
Takya, Takyah, Takyia, Taqiyya,
Taquaia, Taquaya, Taquiia,
Tekeiya, Tekeiyah, Tekeyia,
Tekiya, Tekiyah, Tikia, Tykeia,
Tykia

Takila (American) a form of
Tequila.
Takayla, Takeila, Takela, Takelia,
Takella, Takeyla, Takiela,
Takilah, Takilla, Takilya, Takyla,
Takylia, Tatakyla, Tehilla,
Tekeila, Tekela, Tekelia, Tekilaa,
Tekilia, Tekilla, Tekilyah, Tekla

Takira (American) a combination of the prefix Ta + Kira. *Takara, Takarra, Takeara, Takeera, Takeira, Takeirah, Takera, Takiara, Takiera, Takierah, Takierra, Takirah, Takiria, Takirra, Takora, Takyra, Takyrra, Taquera, Taquira, Tekeria, Tikara, Tikira, Tykera*

Tala (Native American) stalking wolf.

Talasi (Hopi) corn tassel. *Talasea, Talasia*

Taleah (American) a form of Talia. *Talaya, Talayah, Talayia, Talea, Taleana, Taleea, Taleéi, Talei, Taleia, Taleiya, Tylea, Tyleah, Tylee*

Taleisha (American) a combination of Talia + Aisha. *Taileisha, Taleise, Talesha, Talicia, Taliesha, Talisa, Talisha, Talysha, Telisha, Tilisha, Tyleasha, Tyleisha, Tylicia, Tylisha, Tylishia*

Talena (American) a combination of the prefix Ta + Lena. *Talayna, Talihna, Taline, Tallenia, Talná, Tilena, Tilene, Tylena*

Talesha (American) a form of Taleisha. *Taleesha, Talesa, Talese, Taleshia, Talesia, Tallese, Tallesia, Tylesha, Tyleshia, Tylesia*

Talia (Greek) blooming. (Hebrew) dew from heaven. (Latin, French) birthday. A short form of Natalie. See also Thalia. *Tahlia, Taleah, Taliah, Taliatha, Taliea, Taliyah, Talley, Tallia, Tallya, Talya, Tylia*

Talina (American) a combination of Talia + Lina. *Talin, Talinda, Taline, Tallyn, Talyn, Talynn, Tylina, Tyline*

Talisa (English) a form of Tallis. *Talisha, Talishia, Talisia, Talissa, Talysa, Talysha, Talysia, Talyssa*

Talitha (Arabic) young girl. *Taleetha, Taletha, Talethia, Taliatha, Talita, Talithia, Taliya, Telita, Tiletha*

Taliyah (Greek) a form of Talia. *Taleya, Taleyah, Talieya, Talliyah, Talya, Talyah, Talyia*

Talley (French) a familiar form of Talia. *Tali, Talle, Tallie, Tally, Taly, Talye*

Tallis (French, English) forest. *Talice, Talisa, Talise, Tallys*

Tallulah (Choctaw) leaping water. *Tallou, Talula*

Tam (Vietnamese) heart.

Tama (Japanese) jewel.
Tamaa, Tamah, Tamaiah, Tamala, Tema

Tamaka (Japanese) bracelet.
Tamaki, Tamako, Timaka

Tamar (Hebrew) a short form of Tamara. (Russian) History: a twelfth-century Georgian queen. (Hebrew) a short form of Tamara.
Tamer, Tamor, Tamour

Tamara (Hebrew) palm tree. See also Tammy.
Tamar, Tamará, Tamarae, Tamarah, Tamaria, Tamarin, Tamarla, Tamarra, Tamarria, Tamarrian, Tamarsha, Tamary, Tamera, Tamira, Tamma, Tammara, Tamora, Tamoya, Tamra, Tamura, Tamyra, Temara, Temarian, Thama, Thamar, Thamara, Thamarra, Timara, Tomara, Tymara

Tamassa (Hebrew) a form of Thomasina.
Tamasin, Tamasine, Tamsen, Tamsin, Tamzen, Tamzin

Tameka (Aramaic) twin.
Tameca, Tamecia, Tamecka, Tameeka, Tamekia, Tamiecka, Tamieka, Temeka, Timeeka, Timeka, Tomeka, Tomekia, Trameika, Tymeka, Tymmeeka, Tymmeka

Tamera (Hebrew) a form of Tamara.
Tamer, Tamerai, Tameran,
Tameria, Tamerra, Tammera, Thamer, Timera

Tamesha (American) a combination of the prefix Ta + Mesha.
Tameesha, Tameisha, Tameshia, Tameshkia, Tameshya, Tamisha, Tamishia, Tamnesha, Temisha, Timesha, Timisha, Tomesha, Tomiese, Tomise, Tomisha, Tramesha, Tramisha, Tymesha

Tamika (Japanese) a form of Tamiko.
Tamica, Tamieka, Tamikah, Tamikia, Tamikka, Tammika, Tamyka, Timika, Timikia, Tomika, Tymika, Tymmicka

Tamiko (Japanese) child of the people.
Tami, Tamika, Tamike, Tamiqua, Tamiyo, Tammiko

Tamila (American) a combination of the prefix Ta + Mila.
Tamala, Tamela, Tamelia, Tamilla, Tamille, Tamillia, Tamilya

Tamira (Hebrew) a form of Tamara.
Tamir, Tamirae, Tamirah, Tamiria, Tamirra, Tamyra, Tamyria, Tamyrra

Tammi, Tammie (English) forms of Tammy.
Tameia, Tami, Tamia, Tamiah, Tamie, Tamijo, Tamiya

Tammy (English) twin. (Hebrew) a familiar form of Tamara.
Tamilyn, Tamlyn, Tammee, Tammey, Tammi, Tammie, Tamy, Tamya

Tamra (Hebrew) a short form of Tamara.
Tammra, Tamrah

Tamsin (English) a short form of Thomasina.

Tana (Slavic) a short form of Tanya.
Taina, Tanae, Tanaeah, Tanah, Tanairi, Tanairy, Tanalia, Tanara, Tanavia, Tanaya, Tanaz, Tanna, Tannah

Tandy (English) team.
Tanda, Tandalaya, Tandi, Tandie, Tandis, Tandra, Tandrea, Tandria

Taneisha, Tanesha
(American) combinations of the prefix Ta + Nesha.
Tahniesha, Taineshia, Tanasha, Tanashia, Tanaysia, Taneasha, Taneesha, Taneshea, Taneshia, Taneshya, Tanesia, Tanesian, Tanessa, Tanessia, Taniesha, Tannesha, Tanneshia, Tanniecia, Tanniesha, Tantashea

Taneya (Russian, Slavic) a form of Tanya.
Tanea, Taneah, Tanee, Taneé, Taneia

Tangia (American) a combination of the prefix Ta + Angela.
Tangela, Tangi, Tangie, Tanja, Tanji, Tanjia, Tanjie

Tani (Japanese) valley. (Slavic) stand of glory. A familiar form of Tania.
Tahnee, Tahni, Tahnie, Tanee, Taney, Tanie, Tany

Tania (Russian, Slavic) fairy queen.
Taneea, Tani, Taniah, Tanija, Tanika, Tanis, Taniya, Tannia, Tannis, Tanniya, Tannya, Tarnia

Taniel (American) a combination of Tania + Danielle.
Taniele, Tanielle, Teniel, Teniele, Tenielle

Tanika (American) a form of Tania.
Tanikka, Tanikqua, Taniqua, Tanique, Tannica, Tianeka, Tianika

Tanis, Tannis (Slavic) forms of Tania, Tanya.
Tanas, Tanese, Taniese, Tanise, Tanisia, Tanka, Tannese, Tanniece, Tanniese, Tannis, Tannise, Tannus, Tannyce, Tenice, Tenise, Tenyse, Tiannis, Tonise, Tranice, Tranise, Tynice, Tyniece, Tyniese, Tynise

Tanisha (American) a combination of the prefix Ta + Nisha.
Tahniscia, Tahnisha, Tanasha, Tanashea, Tanicha, Taniesha, Tanish, Tanishah, Tanishia, Tanitia, Tannicia, Tannisha, Tenisha, Tenishka, Tinisha, Tonisha, Tonnisha, Tynisha

Tanissa (American) a combination of the prefix Tania + Nissa.
Tanesa, Tanisa, Tannesa, Tannisa, Tennessa, Tranissa

Tanita (American) a combination of the prefix Ta + Nita.
Taneta, Tanetta, Tanitra, Tanitta, Teneta, Tenetta, Tenita, Tenitta, Tyneta, Tynetta, Tynette, Tynita, Tynitra, Tynitta

Tanith (Phoenician) Mythology: Tanit is the goddess of love.
Tanitha

Tanner (English) leather worker, tanner.
Tannor

Tansy (Greek) immortal. (Latin) tenacious, persistent.
Tancy, Tansee, Tansey, Tanshay, Tanzey

Tanya (Russian, Slavic) fairy queen.
Tahnee, Tahnya, Tana, Tanaya, Taneya, Tania, Tanis, Taniya, Tanka, Tannis, Tannya, Tanoya, Tany, Tanyia, Taunya, Tawnya, Thanya

Tao (Chinese, Vietnamese) peach.

Tara (Aramaic) throw; carry. (Irish) rocky hill. (Arabic) a measurement.
Taira, Tairra, Taraea, Tarah, Taráh, Tarai, Taralee, Tarali, Tarasa, Tarasha, Taraya, Tarha, Tari, Tarra, Taryn, Tayra, Tehra

Taraneh (Persian) melody.

Taree (Japanese) arching branch.
Tarea, Tareya, Tari, Taria

Tari (Irish) a familiar form of Tara.
Taria, Tarika, Tarila, Tarilyn, Tarin, Tarina, Tarita

Tarissa (American) a combination of Tara + Rissa.
Taris, Tarisa, Tarise, Tarisha

Tarra (Irish) a form of Tara.
Tarrah

Taryn (Irish) a form of Tara.
Taran, Tareen, Tareena, Taren, Tarene, Tarin, Tarina, Tarren, Tarrena, Tarrin, Tarrina, Tarron, Tarryn, Taryna

Tasarla (Gypsy) dawn.

Tasha (Greek) born on Christmas day. (Russian) a short form of Natasha. See also Tashi, Tosha.
Tacha, Tachiana, Tahsha, Tasenka, Tashae, Tashana, Tashay, Tashe, Tashee, Tasheka, Tashka, Tasia, Taska, Taysha, Thasha, Tiaisha, Tysha

Tashana (American) a combination of the prefix Ta + Shana.
Tashan, Tashanda, Tashani, Tashanika, Tashanna, Tashiana, Tashianna, Tashina, Tishana, Tishani, Tishanna, Tishanne, Toshanna, Toshanti, Tyshana

Tashara (American) a combination of the prefix Ta + Shara.
Tashar, Tasharah, Tasharia, Tasharna, Tasharra, Tashera, Tasherey, Tasheri, Tasherra, Tashira, Tashirah

Tashawna (American) a combination of the prefix Ta + Shawna.
Tashauna, Tashauni, Tashaunie, Tashaunna, Tashawanna, Tashawn, Tashawnda, Tashawnna, Tashawnnia, Tashonda, Tashondra, Tiashauna, Tishawn, Tishunda, Tishunta, Toshauna, Toshawna, Tyshauna, Tyshawna

Tasheena (American) a combination of the prefix Ta + Sheena.
Tasheana, Tasheeana, Tasheeni, Tashena, Tashenna, Tashennia, Tasheona, Tashina, Tisheena, Tosheena, Tysheana, Tysheena, Tyshyna

Tashelle (American) a combination of the prefix Ta + Shelley.
Tachell, Tashell, Techell, Techelle, Teshell, Teshelle, Tochell, Tochelle, Toshelle, Tychell, Tychelle, Tyshell, Tyshelle

Tashi (Hausa) a bird in flight. (Slavic) a form of Tasha.
Tashia, Tashie, Tashika, Tashima, Tashiya

Tasia (Slavic) a familiar form of Tasha.
Tachia, Tashea, Tasiya, Tassi, Tassia, Tassiana, Tassie, Tasya

Tassos (Greek) a form of Theresa.

Tata (Russian) a familiar form of Tatiana.
Tate, Tatia

Tate (English) a short form of Tatum. A form of Taite, Tata.

Tatiana (Slavic) fairy queen. See also Tanya, Tiana.
Tata, Tatania, Tatanya, Tateana, Tati, Tatia, Tatianna, Tatie, Tatihana, Tatiyana, Tatjana, Tatyana, Tiatiana

Tatianna (Slavic) a form of Tatiana.
Taitiann, Taitianna, Tateanna, Tateonna, Tationna

Tatiyana (Slavic) a form of Tatiana.
Tateyana, Tatiayana, Tatiyanna, Tatiyona, Tatiyonna

Tatum (English) cheerful.
Tate, Tatumn

Tatyana (Slavic) a form of Tatiana.
Tatyanah, Tatyani, Tatyanna, Tatyannah, Tatyona, Tatyonna

Taura (Latin) bull. Astrology: Taurus is a sign of the zodiac.
Taurae, Tauria, Taurina

Tauri (English) a form of Tory.
Taure, Taurie, Taury

Tavia (Latin) a short form of
Octavia. See also Tawia.
*Taiva, Tauvia, Tava, Tavah,
Tavita*

Tavie (Scottish) twin.
Tavey, Tavi

Tawanna (American) a combi-
nation of the prefix Ta +
Wanda.
*Taiwana, Taiwanna, Taquana,
Taquanna, Tawan, Tawana,
Tawanda, Tawanne, Tequana,
Tequanna, Tequawna, Tewanna,
Tewauna, Tiquana, Tiwanna,
Tiwena, Towanda, Towanna,
Tywania, Tywanna*

Tawia (African) born after
twins. (Polish) a form of
Tavia.

Tawni (English) a form of
Tawny.
*Tauni, Taunia, Tawnia, Tawnie,
Tawnnie, Tiawni*

Tawny (Gypsy) little one.
(English) brownish yellow,
tan.
*Tahnee, Tany, Tauna, Tauné,
Taunisha, Tawnee, Tawnesha,
Tawney, Tawni, Tawnyell,
Tiawna*

Tawnya (American) a combination of Tawny + Tonya.
Tawna

Taya, Taye (English) short
forms of Taylor.
*Tay, Tayah, Tayana, Tayiah,
Tayna, Tayra, Taysha, Taysia,
Tayva, Tayvonne, Teya, Teyanna,
Teyona, Teyuna, Tiaya, Tiya,
Tiyah, Tiyana, Tye*

Tayla (English) a short form of
Taylor.
*Taylah, Tayleah, Taylee, Tayleigh,
Taylie, Teila*

Taylar (English) a form of
Taylor.
*Talar, Tayla, Taylah, Taylare,
Tayllar*

Tayler (English) a form of Taylor.
Tayller

Taylor (English) tailor.
*Taelor, Tailor, Taiylor, Talor,
Talora, Taya, Taye, Tayla, Taylar,
Tayler, Tayllor, Tayllore, Tayloir,
Taylorann, Taylore, Taylorr,
Taylour, Taylur, Teylor*

Tazu (Japanese) stork; longevity.
Taz, Tazi, Tazia

Teagan (Welsh) beautiful,
attractive.
*Taegen, Teage, Teagen, Teaghan,
Teaghanne, Teaghen, Teagin,
Teague, Teegan, Teeghan, Tegan,
Tegwen, Teigan, Tejan, Tiegan,
Tigan, Tijan, Tijana*

Teaira (Latin) a form of Tiara.
*Teairra, Teairre, Teairria, Teara,
Tearah, Teareya, Teari, Tearia,
Teariea, Tearra, Tearria*

Teal (English) river duck; blue green.
Teala, Teale, Tealia, Tealisha

Teanna (American) a combination of the prefix Te + Anna. A form of Tiana.
Tean, Teana, Teanah, Teann, Teannah, Teanne, Teaunna, Teena, Teuana

Teca (Hungarian) a form of Theresa.
Techa, Teka, Tica, Tika

Tecla (Greek) God's fame.
Tekla, Theckla

Teddi (Greek) a familiar form of Theodora.
Tedde, Teddey, Teddie, Teddy, Tedi, Tediah, Tedy

Tedra (Greek) a short form of Theodora.
Teddra, Teddreya, Tedera, Teedra, Teidra

Tegan (Welsh) a form of Teagan.
Tega, Tegen, Teggan, Teghan, Tegin, Tegyn, Teigen

Telisha (American) a form of Taleisha.
Teleesha, Teleisia, Telesa, Telesha, Teleshia, Telesia, Telicia, Telisa, Telishia, Telisia, Telissa, Telisse, Tellisa, Tellisha, Telsa, Telysa

Temira (Hebrew) tall.
Temora, Timora

Tempest (French) stormy.
Tempesta, Tempeste, Tempestt, Tempist, Tempistt, Tempress, Tempteste

Tenesha, Tenisha (American) combinations of the prefix Te + Niesha. Tenecia, Teneesha, Teneisha, Teneshia, Tenesia, Tenessa, Teneusa, Teniesha, Tenishia*

Tennille (American) a combination of the prefix Te + Nellie.
Taniel, Tanille, Teneal, Teneil, Teneille, Teniel, Tenille, Tenneal, Tenneill, Tenneille, Tennia, Tennie, Tennielle, Tennile, Tineal, Tiniel, Tonielle, Tonille

Teodora (Czech) a form of Theodora.
Teadora

Teona, Teonna (Greek) forms of Tiana, Tianna.
Teon, Teoni, Teonia, Teonie, Teonney, Teonnia, Teonnie

Tequila (Spanish) a kind of liquor. See also Takila.
Taquela, Taquella, Taquila, Taquilla, Tequilia, Tequilla, Tiquila, Tiquilia

Tera, Terra (Latin) earth. (Japanese) swift arrow. (American) forms of Tara.
Terah, Terai, Teria, Terrae, Terrah, Terria, Tierra

Teralyn (American) a combination of Terri + Lynn.
Taralyn, Teralyn, Teralynn, Terralin, Terralyn

Teresa (Greek) a form of Theresa. See also Tressa.
Taresa, Taressa, Tarissa, Terasa, Tercza, Tereasa, Tereatha, Terese, Teresea, Teresha, Teresia, Teresina, Teresita, Tereska, Tereson, Teressa, Teretha, Tereza, Terezia, Terezie, Terezilya, Terezinha, Terezka, Terezsa, Terisa, Terisha, Teriza, Terrasa, Terresa, Terresha, Terresia, Terressa, Terrosina, Tersa, Tersea, Teruska, Terza, Teté, Tyresa, Tyresia

Terese (Greek) a form of Teresa.
Tarese, Taress, Taris, Tarise, Tereece, Tereese, Teress, Terez, Teris, Terrise

Teri (Greek) reaper. A familiar form of Theresa.
Terie

Terrelle (Greek) a form of Theresa.
Tarrell, Teral, Terall, Terel, Terell, Teriel, Terral, Terrall, Terrell, Terrella, Terriel, Terriell, Terrielle, Terrill, Terryelle, Terryl, Terryll, Terrylle, Teryl, Tyrell, Tyrelle

Terrene (Latin) smooth.
Tareena, Tarena, Teran, Teranee, Tereena, Terena, Terencia, Terene, Terenia, Terentia, Terina, Terran,

Terren, Terrena, Terrin, Terrina, Terron, Terrosina, Terryn, Terun, Teryn, Teryna, Terynn, Tyreen, Tyrene

Terri (Greek) reaper. A familiar form of Theresa.
Terree, Terria, Terrie

Terriann (American) a combination of Terri + Ann.
Teran, Terian, Teriann, Terianne, Teriyan, Terria, Terrian, Terrianne, Terryann

Terrianna (American) a combination of Terri + Anna.
Teriana, Terianna, Terriana, Terriauna, Terrina, Terriona, Terrionna, Terriyana, Terriyanna, Terryana, Terryauna, Tyrina

Terrica (American) a combination of Terri + Erica. See also Rica.
Tereka, Terica, Tericka, Terika, Terreka, Terricka, Terrika, Tyrica, Tyricka, Tyrika, Tyrikka, Tyronica

Terry (Greek) a short form of Theresa.
Tere, Teree, Terelle, Terene, Teri, Terie, Terrey, Terri, Terrie, Terrye, Tery

Terry-Lynn (American) a combination of Terry + Lynn.
Terelyn, Terelynn, Terri-Lynn, Terrilynn, Terrylynn

Tertia (Latin) third.
Tercia, Tercina, Tercine, Terecena, Tersia, Terza

Tess (Greek) a short form of Quintessa, Theresa.
Tes, Tese

Tessa (Greek) reaper.
Tesa, Tesah, Tesha, Tesia, Tessah, Tessia, Tezia

Tessie (Greek) a familiar form of Theresa.
Tesi, Tessey, Tessi, Tessy, Tezi

Tetsu (Japanese) strong as iron.

Tetty (English) a familiar form of Elizabeth.

Tevy (Cambodian) angel.
Teva

Teylor (English) a form of Taylor.
Teighlor, Teylar

Thaddea (Greek) courageous. (Latin) praiser.
Thada, Thadda

Thalassa (Greek) sea, ocean.

Thalia (Greek) a form of Talia. Mythology: the Muse of comedy.
Thaleia, Thalie, Thalya

Thana (Arabic) happy occasion.
Thaina, Thania, Thanie

Thanh (Vietnamese) bright blue. (Punjabi) good place.
Thantra, Thanya

Thao (Vietnamese) respectful of parents.

Thea (Greek) goddess. A short form of Althea.
Theo

Thelma (Greek) willful.
Thelmalina

Thema (African) queen.

Theodora (Greek) gift of God. See also Dora, Dorothy, Feodora.
Taedra, Teddi, Tedra, Teodora, Teodory, Teodosia, Theda, Thedorsha, Thedrica, Theo, Theodore, Theodoria, Theodorian, Theodosia, Theodra

Theone (Greek) gift of God.
Theondra, Theoni, Theonie

Theophania (Greek) God's appearance. See also Tiffany.
Theo, Theophanie

Theophila (Greek) loved by God.
Theo

Theresa (Greek) reaper. See also Resi, Reza, Riza, Tassos, Teca, Terrelle, Tracey, Tracy, Zilya.
Teresa, Teri, Terri, Terry, Tersea, Tess, Tessa, Tessie, Theresia, Theresina, Theresita, Theressa, Thereza, Therisa, Therissie, Thersa, Thersea, Tresha, Tressa, Trice

Therese (Greek) a form of
Theresa.
*Terese, Thérèse, Theresia,
Theressa, Therra, Therressa,
Thersa*

Theta (Greek) Linguistics: a
letter in the Greek alphabet.

Thetis (Greek) disposed.
Mythology: the mother of
Achilles.

Thi (Vietnamese) poem.
Thia, Thy, Thya

Thirza (Hebrew) pleasant.
*Therza, Thirsa, Thirzah,
Thursa, Thurza, Thyrza,
Tirshka, Tirza*

Thomasina (Hebrew) twin.
See also Tamassa.
*Tamsin, Thomasa, Thomasia,
Thomasin, Thomasine,
Thomazine, Thomencia,
Thomethia, Thomisha,
Thomsina, Toma, Tomasa,
Tomasina, Tomasine, Tomina,
Tommie, Tommina*

Thora (Scandinavian) thunder.
*Thordia, Thordis, Thorri, Thyra,
Tyra*

Thuy (Vietnamese) gentle.

Tia (Greek) princess. (Spanish)
aunt.
*Téa, Teah, Teeya, Teia, Ti,
Tiakeisha, Tialeigh, Tiamarie,
Tianda, Tiandria, Tiante, Tiia,
Tiye, Tyja*

Tiana, Tianna (Greek)
princess. (Latin) short forms
of Tatiana.
*Teana, Teanna, Tiahna, Tianah,
Tiane, Tianea, Tianee, Tiani,
Tiann, Tiannah, Tianne, Tianni,
Tiaon, Tiauna, Tiena, Tiona,
Tionna, Tiyana*

Tiara (Latin) crowned.
*Teair, Teaira, Teara, Téare, Tearia,
Tearria, Teearia, Teira, Teirra,
Tiaira, Tiare, Tiarea, Tiareah,
Tiari, Tiaria, Tiarra, Tiera,
Tierra, Tyara*

Tiarra (Latin) a form of Tiara.
Tiairra, Tiarrah, Tyarra

Tiauna (Greek) a form of
Tiana.
Tiaunah, Tiaunia, Tiaunna

Tiberia (Latin) Geography: the
Tiber River in Italy.
Tib, Tibbie, Tibby

Tichina (American) a combi-
nation of the prefix Ti +
China.
Tichian, Tichin, Tichinia

Tida (Tai) daughter.
Tiera, Tierra (Latin) forms of
Tiara.
*Tieara, Tiéra, Tierah, Tierre,
Tierrea, Tierria*

Tierney (Irish) noble.
*Tieranae, Tierani, Tieranie,
Tieranni, Tierany, Tiernan,
Tiernee, Tierny*

Tiff (Latin) a short form of
Tiffani, Tiffanie, Tiffany.

Tiffani, Tiffanie (Latin) forms
of Tiffany.
*Tephanie, Tifanee, Tifani,
Tifanie, Tiff, Tiffanee, Tiffayne,
Tiffeni, Tiffenie, Tiffennie,
Tiffiani, Tiffianie, Tiffine, Tiffini,
Tiffinie, Tiffni, Tiffy, Tiffynie,
Tifni*

Tiffany (Latin) trinity. (Greek)
a short form of Theophania.
See also Tyfany.
*Taffanay, Taffany, Tifaney, Tifany,
Tiff, Tiffaney, Tiffani, Tiffanie,
Tiffanny, Tiffeney, Tiffiany,
Tiffiney, Tiffiny, Tiffnay, Tiffney,
Tiffny, Tiffy, Tiphanie, Triffany*

Tiffy (Latin) a familiar form
of Tiffani, Tiffany.
Tiffey, Tiffi, Tiffie

Tijuana (Spanish) Geography:
a border town in Mexico.
*Tajuana, Tajuanna, Thejuana,
Tiajuana, Tiajuanna, Tiawanna*

Tilda (German) a short form
of Matilda.
Tilde, Tildie, Tildy, Tylda, Tyldy

Tillie (German) a familiar
form of Matilda.
*Tilia, Tilley, Tilli, Tillia, Tilly,
Tillye*

Timi (English) a familiar form
of Timothea.
Timia, Timie, Timmi, Timmie

Timothea (English) honoring
God.
Thea, Timi

Tina (Spanish, American) a
short form of Augustine,
Martina, Christina, Valentina.
*Teanna, Teena, Teina, Tena,
Tenae, Tinai, Tine, Tinea, Tinia,
Tiniah, Tinna, Tinnia, Tyna,
Tynka*

Tinble (English) sound bells
make.
Tynble

Tinesha (American) a combi-
nation of the prefix Ti +
Niesha.
*Timnesha, Tinecia, Tineisha,
Tinesa, Tineshia, Tinessa,
Tinisha, Tinsia*

Tinisha (American) a form of
Tenisha.
*Tiniesha, Tinieshia, Tinishia,
Tinishya*

Tiona, Tionna (American)
forms of Tiana.
*Teona, Teonna, Tionda, Tiondra,
Tiondre, Tioné, Tionette, Tioni,
Tionia, Tionie, Tionja, Tionnah,
Tionne, Tionya, Tyonna*

Tiphanie (Latin) a form of
Tiffany.
Tiphanee, Tiphani, Tiphany

Tiponya (Native American)
great horned owl.
Tipper

Tipper (Irish) water pourer.
(Native American) a short
form of Tiponya.

Tira (Hindi) arrow.
Tirah, Tirea, Tirena

Tirtha (Hindi) ford.

Tirza (Hebrew) pleasant.
*Thersa, Thirza, Tierza, Tirsa,
Tirzah, Tirzha, Tyrzah*

Tisa (Swahili) ninth-born.
Tisah, Tysa, Tyssa

Tish (Latin) a short form of
Tisha.

Tisha (Latin) joy. A short form
of Leticia.
*Taesha, Tesha, Teisha, Tiesha,
Tieshia, Tish, Tishal, Tishia,
Tysha, Tyshia*

Tita (Greek) giant. (Spanish) a
short form of names ending
in "tita." A form of Titus (see
Boys' Names).

Titania (Greek) giant.
Mythology: the Titans were a
race of giants.
*Tania, Teata, Titanna, Titanya,
Titiana, Tiziana, Tytan, Tytania,
Tytiana*

Titiana (Greek) a form of
Titania.
*Titianay, Titiania, Titianna,
Titiayana, Titionia, Titiyana,
Titiyanna, Tityana*

Tivona (Hebrew) nature lover.

Tiwa (Zuni) onion.

Tiyana (Greek) a form of
Tiana.
*Tiyan, Tiyani, Tiyania,
Tiyanna, Tiyonna*

Tobi (Hebrew) God is good.
*Tobe, Tobee, Tobey, Tobie, Tobit,
Toby, Tobye, Tova, Tovah, Tove,
Tovi, Tybi, Tybie*

Tocarra (American) a combination of the prefix To + Cara.
Tocara, Toccara

Toinette (French) a short
form of Antoinette.
*Toinetta, Tola, Tonetta, Tonette,
Toni, Toniette, Twanette*

Toki (Japanese) hopeful.
Toko, Tokoya, Tokyo

Tola (Polish) a form of Toinette.
Tolsia

Tomi (Japanese) rich.
Tomie, Tomiju

Tommie (Hebrew) a short
form of Thomasina.
*Tomme, Tommi, Tommia,
Tommy*

Tomo (Japanese) intelligent.
Tomoko

Tonesha (American) a combi-
nation of the prefix To +
Niesha.
*Toneisha, Toneisheia, Tonesha,
Tonesia, Toniece, Tonisha,
Tonneshia*

Toni (Greek) flourishing. (Latin) praiseworthy.
Tonee, Toney, Tonia, Tonie, Toniee, Tonni, Tonnie, Tony, Tonye

Tonia (Latin, Slavic) a form of Toni, Tonya.
Tonea, Toniah, Toniea, Tonja, Tonje, Tonna, Tonni, Tonnia, Tonnie, Tonnja

Tonisha (American) a form of Toneisha.
Toniesha, Tonisa, Tonise, Tonisia, Tonnisha

Tonya (Slavic) fairy queen.
Tonia, Tonnya, Tonyea, Tonyetta, Tonyia

Topaz (Latin) golden yellow gem.

Topsy (English) on top. Literature: a slave in Harriet Beecher Stowe's novel *Uncle Tom's Cabin*.
Toppsy, Topsey, Topsie

Tora (Japanese) tiger.

Tori (Japanese) bird. (English) a form of Tory.
Toria, Toriana, Torie, Torri, Torrie, Torrita

Toria (English) a form of Tori, Tory.
Toriah, Torria

Toriana (English) a form of Tori.
Torian, Toriane, Toriann, Torianna, Torianne, Toriauna, Torin, Torina, Torine, Torinne, Torion, Torionna, Torionne, Toriyanna, Torrina

Torie, Torrie (English) forms of Tori.
Tore, Toree, Torei, Torre, Torree

Torilyn (English) a combination of Tori + Lynn.
Torilynn, Torrilyn, Torrilynn

Torri (English) a form of Tori.

Tory (English) victorious. (Latin) a short form of Victoria.
Tauri, Torey, Tori, Torrey, Torreya, Torry, Torrye, Torya, Torye, Toya

Tosha (Punjabi) armaments. (Polish) a familiar form of Antonia. (Russian) a form of Tasha.
Toshea, Toshia, Toshiea, Toshke, Tosia, Toska

Toshi (Japanese) mirror image.
Toshie, Toshiko, Toshikyo

Toski (Hopi) squashed bug.

Totsi (Hopi) moccasins.

Tottie (English) a familiar form of Charlotte.
Tota, Totti, Totty

Tovah (Hebrew) good.
Tova, Tovia

Toya (Spanish) a form of Tory.
Toia, Toyanika, Toyanna, Toyea, Toylea, Toyleah, Toylenn, Toylin, Toylyn

Tracey (Greek) a familiar form of Theresa. (Latin) warrior.
Trace, Tracee, Tracell, Traci, Tracie, Tracy, Traice, Trasey, Treesy

Traci, Tracie (Latin) forms of Tracey.
Tracia, Tracilee, Tracilyn, Tracilynn, Tracina, Traeci

Tracy (Greek) a familiar form of Theresa. (Latin) warrior.
Treacy

Tralena (Latin) a combination of Tracy + Lena.
Traleen, Tralene, Tralin, Tralinda, Tralyn, Tralynn, Tralynne

Tranesha (American) a combination of the prefix Tra + Niesha.
Traneice, Traneis, Traneise, Traneisha, Tranese, Traneshia, Tranice, Traniece, Traniesha, Tranisha, Tranishia

Trashawn (American) a combination of the prefix Tra + Shawn.
Trashan, Trashana, Trashauna, Trashon, Trayshauna

Trava (Czech) spring grasses.

Treasure (Latin) treasure, wealth; valuable.
Treasa, Treasur, Treasuré, Treasury

Trella (Spanish) a familiar form of Estelle.

Tresha (Greek) a form of Theresa.
Trescha, Trescia, Treshana, Treshia

Tressa (Greek) a short form of Theresa. See also Teresa.
Treaser, Tresa, Tresca, Trese, Treska, Tressia, Tressie, Trez, Treza, Trisa

Trevina (Irish) prudent. (Welsh) homestead.
Treva, Trevanna, Trevena, Trevenia, Treveon, Trevia, Treviana, Trevien, Trevin, Trevona

Trevona (Irish) a form of Trevina.
Trevion, Trevon, Trevonia, Trevonna, Trevonne, Trevonye

Triana (Latin) third. (Greek) a form of Trina.
Tria, Triann, Trianna, Trianne

Trice (Greek) a short form of Theresa.
Treece

Tricia (Latin) a form of Trisha.
Trica, Tricha, Trichelle, Tricina, Trickia

Trilby (English) soft hat.
Tribi, Trilbie, Trillby

Trina (Greek) pure.
Treena, Treina, Trenna, Triana, Trinia, Trinchen, Trind, Trinda, Trine, Trinette, Trini, Trinica, Trinice, Triniece, Trinika, Trinique, Trinisa, Tryna

Trini (Greek) a form of Trina.
Trinia, Trinie

Trinity (Latin) triad. Religion:
the Father, the Son, and the
Holy Spirit.
*Trinita, Trinite, Trinitee, Triniti,
Trinnette, Trinty*

Trish (Latin) a short form of
Beatrice, Trisha.
Trishell, Trishelle

Trisha (Latin) noblewoman.
(Hindi) thirsty. See also
Tricia.
*Treasha, Trish, Trishann,
Trishanna, Trishanne, Trishara,
Trishia, Trishna, Trissha, Trycia*

Trissa (Latin) a familiar form
of Patricia.
*Trisa, Trisanne, Trisia, Trisina,
Trissi, Trissie, Trissy, Tryssa*

Trista (Latin) a short form of
Tristen.
*Trisatal, Tristess, Tristia, Trysta,
Trystia*

Tristan (Latin) bold.
*Trista, Tristane, Tristanni,
Tristany, Tristen, Tristian,
Tristiana, Tristin, Triston,
Trystan, Trystyn*

Tristen (Latin) a form of
Tristan.
Tristene, Trysten

Tristin (Latin) a form of
Tristan.
*Tristina, Tristine, Tristinye,
Tristn, Trystin*

Triston, Trystyn (Latin) forms
of Tristan.
Tristony, Trystyn

Trixie (American) a familiar
form of Beatrice.
*Tris, Trissie, Trissina, Trix, Trixi,
Trixy*

Troya (Irish) foot soldier.
Troi, Troia, Troiana, Troiya, Troy

Trudel (Dutch) a form of
Trudy.

Trudy (German) a familiar
form of Gertrude.
*Truda, Trude, Trudel, Trudessa,
Trudey, Trudi, Trudie*

Trycia (Latin) a form of Trisha.

Tryna (Greek) a form of Trina.
Tryane, Tryanna, Trynee

Tryne (Dutch) pure.
Trine

Tsigana (Hungarian) a form
of Zigana.
Tsigane, Tzigana, Tzigane

Tu (Chinese) jade.

Tuesday (English) born on the
third day of the week.
*Tuesdae, Tuesdea, Tuesdee,
Tuesdey, Tusdai*

Tula (Hindi) born in the lunar
month of Capricorn.
Tulah, Tulla, Tullah, Tuula

Tullia (Irish) peaceful, quiet.
Tulia, Tulliah

Tulsi (Hindi) basil, a sacred
Hindi herb.
Tulsia

Turquoise (French) blue-
green semi-precious stone.
*Turkois, Turkoise, Turkoys,
Turkoyse*

Tusa (Zuni) prairie dog.

Tuyen (Vietnamese) angel.

Tuyet (Vietnamese) snow.

Twyla (English) woven of
double thread.
Twila, Twilla

Tyanna (American) a combina-
tion of the prefix Ty + Anna.
*Tya, Tyana, Tyann, Tyannah,
Tyanne, Tyannia*

Tyeisha (American) a form of
Tyesha.
*Tyeesha, Tyeishia, Tyieshia,
Tyisha, Tyishea, Tyishia*

Tyesha (American) a combina-
tion of Ty + Aisha.
*Tyasha, Tyashia, Tyasia, Tyasiah,
Tyeisha, Tyeshia, Tyeyshia, Tyisha*

Tyfany (American) a short
form of Tiffany.
*Tyfani, Tyfanny, Tyffani,
Tyffanni, Tyffany, Tyffini,
Typhanie, Typhany*

Tykeisha (American) a form
of Takeisha.
*Tkeesha, Tykeisa, Tykeishia,
Tykesha, Tykeshia, Tykeysha,
Tykeza, Tykisha*

Tykera (American) a form of
Takira.
*Tykeira, Tykeirah, Tykereiah,
Tykeria, Tykeriah, Tykerria,
Tykiera, Tykierra, Tykira,
Tykiria, Tykirra*

Tyler (English) tailor.
Tyller, Tylor

Tyna (Czech) a short form of
Kristina.
Tynae, Tynea, Tynia

Tyne (English) river.
*Tine, Tyna, Tynelle, Tynessa,
Tynetta*

Tynesha (American) a combi-
nation of Ty + Niesha.
*Tynaise, Tynece, Tyneicia, Tynesa,
Tynesha, Tyneshia, Tynessia,
Tyniesha, Tynisha, Tyseisha*

Tynisha (American) a form of
Tynesha.
*Tyneisha, Tyneisia, Tynisa,
Tynise, Tynishi*

Tyra (Scandinavian) battler.
Mythology: Tyr was the god
of war. A form of Thora.
(Hindi) a form of Tira.
Tyraa, Tyrah, Tyran, Tyree, Tyria

Tyshanna (American) a com-
bination of Ty + Shawna.
*Tyshana, Tyshanae, Tyshane,
Tyshaun, Tyshaunda, Tyshawn,
Tyshawna, Tyshawnah,
Tyshawnda, Tyshawnna,
Tysheann, Tysheanna, Tyshonia,
Tyshonna, Tyshonya*

Tytiana (Greek) a form of
Titania.
*Tytana, Tytanna, Tyteana,
Tyteanna, Tytianna, Tytianni,
Tytionna, Tytiyana, Tytiyanna,
Tytyana, Tytyauna*

U

U (Korean) gentle.

Udele (English) prosperous.
Uda, Udella, Udelle, Yudelle

Ula (Irish) sea jewel.
(Scandinavian) wealthy.
(Spanish) a short form of
Eulalia.
Uli, Ulla

Ulani (Polynesian) cheerful.
Ulana, Ulane

Ulima (Arabic) astute; wise.
Ullima

Ulla (German, Swedish) willful. (Latin) a short form of
Ursula. Ulli

Ulrica (German) wolf ruler;
ruler of all. See also Rica.
*Ulka, Ullrica, Ullricka, Ullrika,
Ulrika, Ulrike*

Ultima (Latin) last, endmost,
farthest.

Ululani (Hawaiian) heavenly
inspiration.

Ulva (German) wolf.

Uma (Hindi) mother.
Religion: another name for
the Hindu goddess Devi.

Umay (Turkish) hopeful.
Umai

Umeko (Japanese) plum-blos-
som child; patient.
Ume, Umeyo

Una (Latin) one; united.
(Hopi) good memory. (Irish)
a form of Agnes. See also
Oona.
Unna, Uny

Undine (Latin) little wave.
Mythology: the undines were
water spirits. See also
Ondine.
Undeen, Undene

Unice (English) a form of
Eunice.

Unika (American) a form of
Unique.
*Unica, Unicka, Unik, Unikqua,
Unikue*

Unique (Latin) only one.
*Unika, Uniqia, Uniqua,
Uniquia*

Unity (English) unity.
Uinita, Unita, Unitee

Unn (Norwegian) she who is
loved.

Unna (German) woman.

Urania (Greek) heavenly.
Mythology: the Muse of
astronomy.
*Urainia, Uranie, Uraniya,
Uranya*

Urbana (Latin) city dweller.
Urbanah, Urbanna

Urika (Omaha) useful to
everyone.
Ureka

Urit (Hebrew) bright.
Urice

Ursa (Greek) a short form of
Ursula. (Latin) a form of
Orsa.
Ursey, Ursi, Ursie, Ursy

Ursula (Greek) little bear. See
also Sula, Ulla, Vorsila.
*Irsaline, Ursa, Ursala, Ursel,
Ursela, Ursella, Ursely, Ursilla,
Ursillane, Ursola, Ursule,
Ursulina, Ursuline, Urszula,
Urszuli, Urzula*

Usha (Hindi) sunrise.

Ushi (Chinese) ox. Astrology: a
sign of the Chinese zodiac.

Uta (German) rich. (Japanese)
poem.
Utako

Utina (Native American)
woman of my country.
Utahna, Utona, Utonna

V

Vail (English) valley.
Vale, Vayle

Val (Latin) a short form of
Valentina, Valerie.

Vala (German) singled out.
Valla

Valarie (Latin) a form of
Valerie.
*Valarae, Valaree, Valarey, Valari,
Valaria, Vallarie*

Valda (German) famous ruler.
Valida, Velda

Valencia (Spanish) strong.
Geography: a region in east-
ern Spain.
*Valecia, Valence, Valenica,
Valentia, Valenzia*

Valene (Latin) a short form of
Valentina.
*Valaine, Valean, Valeda, Valeen,
Valen, Valena, Valeney, Valien,
Valina, Valine, Vallan, Vallen*

Valentina (Latin) strong.
History: Valentina Tereshkova,
a Soviet cosmonaut, was the
first woman in space. See also
Tina, Valene, Valli.
*Val, Valantina, Vale, Valenteen,
Valentena, Valentijn, Valentin,
Valentine, Valiaka, Valtina,
Valyn, Valynn*

Valera (Russian) a form of
Valerie. See also Lera.

Valeria (Latin) a form of
Valerie.
*Valaria, Valeriana, Valeriane,
Veleria*

Valerie (Latin) strong.
*Vairy, Val, Valarie, Vale, Valera,
Valeree, Valeri, Valeria, Valérie,
Valery, Valka, Valleree, Valleri,
Vallerie, Valli, Vallirie, Valora,
Valorie, Valry, Valya, Velerie,
Waleria*

Valery (Latin) a form of
Valerie.
Valerye, Vallary, Vallery

Valeska (Slavic) glorious ruler.
*Valesca, Valese, Valeshia,
Valeshka, Valezka, Valisha*

Valli (Latin) a familiar form of
Valentina, Valerie. Botany: a
plant native to India.
Vallie, Vally

Valma (Finnish) loyal defender.

Valonia (Latin) shadow valley.
Vallon, Valona

Valora (Latin) a form of Valerie.
Valoria, Valorya, Velora

Valorie (Latin) a form of
Valerie.
Vallori, Vallory, Valori, Valory

Vanda (German) a form of
Wanda.
*Vandana, Vandella, Vandetta,
Vandi, Vannda*

Vanesa (Greek) a form of
Vanessa.
*Vanesha, Vaneshah, Vanesia,
Vanisa*

Vanessa (Greek) butterfly.
Literature: a name invented
by Jonathan Swift as a nick-
name for Esther Vanhomrigh.
See also Nessie.
*Van, Vanassa, Vanesa, Vaneshia,
Vanesse, Vanessia, Vanessica,
Vanetta, Vaneza, Vaniece,
Vaniessa, Vanija, Vanika,
Vanissa, Vanita, Vanna, Vannesa,
Vannessa, Vanni, Vannie, Vanny,
Varnessa, Venessa*

Vanetta (English) a form of
Vanessa.
*Vaneta, Vanita, Vanneta,
Vannetta, Vannita, Venetta*

Vania, Vanya (Russian) famil-
iar forms of Anna.
*Vanija, Vanina, Vaniya, Vanja,
Vanka, Vannia*

Vanity (English) vain.
Vaniti, Vanitty

Vanna (Cambodian) golden.
(Greek) a short form of
Vanessa.
*Vana, Vanae, Vanelly, Vannah,
Vannalee, Vannaleigh, Vannie,
Vanny*

Vannesa, Vannessa (Greek)
forms of Vanessa.
Vannesha, Vanneza

Vanora (Welsh) white wave.
Vannora

Vantrice (American) a combination of the prefix Van +
Trice.
*Vantrece, Vantricia, Vantrisa,
Vantrissa*

Varda (Hebrew) rose.
*Vadit, Vardia, Vardice, Vardina,
Vardis, Vardit*

Varvara (Slavic) a form of
Barbara.
*Vara, Varenka, Varina, Varinka,
Varya, Varyusha, Vava, Vavka*

Vashti (Persian) lovely. Bible:
the wife of Ahasuerus, king
of Persia.
Vashtee, Vashtie, Vashty

Veanna (American) a combination of the prefix Ve +
Anna.
Veeana, Veena, Veenaya, Veeona

Veda (Sanskrit) sacred lore;
knowledge. Religion: the
Vedas are the sacred writings
of Hinduism.
*Vedad, Vedis, Veeda, Veida,
Veleda, Vida*

Vedette (Italian) sentry; scout.
(French) movie star.
Vedetta

Vega (Arabic) falling star.

Velda (German) a form of
Valda.

Velika (Slavic) great,
wondrous.

Velma (German) a familiar
form of Vilhelmina.
Valma, Vellma, Vilma, Vilna

Velvet (English) velvety.

Venecia (Italian) from Venice,
Italy.
*Vanecia, Vanetia, Veneise, Venesa,
Venesha, Venesher, Venesse,
Venessia, Venetia, Venette,
Venezia, Venice, Venicia, Veniece,
Veniesa, Venise, Venisha,
Venishia, Venita, Venitia, Venize,
Vennesa, Vennice, Vennisa,
Vennise, Vonitia, Vonizia*

Venessa (Latin) a form of
Vanessa.
*Veneese, Venesa, Venese,
Veneshia, Venesia, Venisa,
Venissa, Vennessa*

Venus (Latin) love. Mythology:
the goddess of love and
beauty.
Venis, Venusa, Venusina, Vinny

Vera (Latin) true. (Slavic) faith.
A short form of Elvera,
Veronica. See also Verena,
Wera.
*Vara, Veera, Veira, Veradis,
Verasha, Vere, Verka, Verla,
Viera, Vira*

Verbena (Latin) sacred plants.
Verbeena, Verbina

Verda (Latin) young, fresh.
  Verdi, Verdie, Viridiana, Viridis

Verdad (Spanish) truthful.

Verena (Latin) truthful. A
  familiar form of Vera, Verna.
  *Verene, Verenis, Vereniz, Verina,
  Verine, Verinka, Veroshka,
  Verunka, Verusya, Virna*

Verenice (Latin) a form of
  Veronica.
  Verenis, Verenise, Vereniz

Verity (Latin) truthful.
  Verita, Veritie

Verlene (Latin) a combination
  of Veronica + Lena.
  *Verleen, Verlena, Verlin, Verlina,
  Verlinda, Verline, Verlyn*

Verna (Latin) springtime.
  (French) a familiar form of
  Laverne. See also Verena,
  Wera.
  *Verasha, Verla, Verne, Vernetia,
  Vernetta, Vernette, Vernia,
  Vernice, Vernita, Verusya, Viera,
  Virida, Virna, Virnell*

Vernice (Latin) a form of
  Bernice, Verna.
  *Vernese, Vernesha, Verneshia,
  Vernessa, Vernica, Vernicca,
  Verniece, Vernika, Vernique,
  Vernis, Vernise, Vernisha,
  Vernisheia, Vernissia*

Veronica (Latin) true image.
  See also Ronni, Weronika.
  *Varonica, Vera, Veranique,
  Verenice, Verhonica, Verinica,*
  *Verohnica, Veron, Verona, Verone,
  Veronic, Véronic, Veronice,
  Veronika, Veronique, Véronique,
  Veronne, Veronnica, Veruszhka,
  Vironica, Vron, Vronica*

Veronika (Latin) a form of
  Veronica.
  *Varonika, Veronick, Véronick,
  Veronik, Veronike, Veronka,
  Veronkia, Veruka*

Veronique, Véronique
  (French) forms of Veronica.
  Vespera (Latin) evening star.

Vesta (Latin) keeper of the
  house. Mythology: the goddess of the home.
  Vessy, Vest, Vesteria

Veta (Slavic) a familiar form of
  Elizabeth.
  Veeta, Vita

Vi (Latin, French) a short form
  of Viola, Violet.
  Vye

Vianca (Spanish) a form of
  Bianca.
  Vianeca, Vianica

Vianey (American) a familiar
  form of Vianna.
  Vianney, Viany

Vianna (American) a combination of Vi + Anna.
  Viana, Vianey, Viann, Vianne

Vica (Hungarian) a form of
  Eve.

Vicki, Vickie (Latin) familiar forms of Victoria.
Vic, Vicci, Vicke, Vickee, Vickiana, Vickilyn, Vickki, Vicky, Vika, Viki, Vikie, Vikki, Vikky

Vicky (Latin) a familiar form of Victoria.
Viccy, Vickey, Viky, Vikkey, Vikky

Victoria (Latin) victorious. See also Tory, Wicktoria, Wisia.
Vicki, Vicky, Victoire, Victoriana, Victorianna, Victorie, Victorina, Victorine, Victoriya, Victorria, Victorriah, Victory, Victorya, Viktoria, Vitoria, Vyctoria

Vida (Sanskrit) a form of Veda. (Hebrew) a short form of Davida.
Vidamarie

Vidonia (Portuguese) branch of a vine.
Vedonia, Vidonya

Vienna (Latin) Geography: the capital of Austria.
Veena, Vena, Venna, Vienette, Vienne, Vina

Viktoria (Latin) a form of Victoria.
Viktorie, Viktorija, Viktorina, Viktorine, Viktorka

Vilhelmina (German) a form of Wilhelmina.
Velma, Vilhelmine, Vilma

Villette (French) small town.
Vietta

Vilma (German) a short form of Vilhemina.

Vina (Hindi) Mythology: a musical instrument played by the Hindu goddess of wisdom. (Spanish) vineyard. (Hebrew) a short form of Davina. (English) a short form of Alvina. See also Lavina.
Veena, Vena, Viña, Vinesha, Vinessa, Vinia, Viniece, Vinique, Vinisha, Viñita, Vinna, Vinni, Vinnie, Vinny, Vinora, Vyna

Vincentia (Latin) victor, conqueror.
Vicenta, Vincenta, Vincentena, Vincentina, Vincentine, Vincenza, Vincy, Vinnie

Viñita (Spanish) a form of Vina.
Viñeet, Viñeeta, Viñetta, Viñette, Viñitha, Viñta, Viñti, Viñtia, Vyñetta, Vyñette

Viola (Latin) violet; stringed instrument in the violin family. Literature: the heroine of Shakespeare's play *Twelfth Night*.
Vi, Violaine, Violanta, Violante, Viole, Violeine

Violet (French) Botany: a plant with purplish blue flowers.
Vi, Violeta, Violette, Vyolet, Vyoletta, Vyolette

Violeta (French) a form of
Violet.
Violetta

Virgilia (Latin) rod bearer, staff
bearer.
Virgillia

Virginia (Latin) pure, virginal.
Literature: Virginia Woolf was
a well-known British writer.
See also Gina, Ginger, Ginny,
Jinny.
*Verginia, Verginya, Virge, Virgen,
Virgenia, Virgenya, Virgie,
Virgine, Virginie, Virginië,
Virginio, Virginnia, Virgy,
Virjeana*

Virginie (French) a form of
Virginia.

Viridiana (Latin) a form of
Viridis.

Viridis (Latin) green.
Virdis, Virida, Viridia, Viridiana

Virtue (Latin) virtuous.

Vita (Latin) life.
*Veeta, Veta, Vitaliana, Vitalina,
Vitel, Vitella, Vitia, Vitka, Vitke*

Vitoria (Spanish) a form of
Victoria.
Vittoria

Viv (Latin) a short form of
Vivian.

Viva (Latin) a short form of
Aviva, Vivian.
Vica, Vivan, Vivva

Viveca (Scandinavian) a form
of Vivian.
*Viv, Vivecca, Vivecka, Viveka,
Vivica, Vivieca, Vyveca*

Vivian (Latin) full of life.
*Vevay, Vevey, Viv, Viva, Viveca,
Vivee, Vivi, Vivia, Viviana,
Viviane, Viviann, Vivianne,
Vivie, Vivien, Vivienne, Vivina,
Vivion, Vivyan, Vivyann,
Vivyanne, Vyvyan, Vyvyann,
Vyvyanne*

Viviana (Latin) a form of
Vivian.
*Viv, Vivianna, Vivyana,
Vyvyana*

Vondra (Czech) loving
woman.
Vonda, Vondrea

Voneisha (American) a combination of Yvonne + Aisha.
Voneishia, Vonesha, Voneshia

Vonna (French) a form of
Yvonne.
Vona

Vonny (French) a familiar
form of Yvonne.
Vonney, Vonni, Vonnie

Vontricia (American) a com-
bination of Yvonne + Tricia.
*Vontrece, Vontrese, Vontrice,
Vontriece*

Vorsila (Greek) a form of
Ursula.
*Vorsilla, Vorsula, Vorsulla,
Vorsyla*

W

Wadd (Arabic) beloved.

Waheeda (Arabic) one and only.

Wainani (Hawaiian) beautiful water.

Wakana (Japanese) plant.

Wakanda (Dakota) magical power.
Wakenda

Wakeisha (American) a combination of the prefix Wa + Keisha.
Wakeishia, Wakesha, Wakeshia, Wakesia

Walad (Arabic) newborn.
Waladah, Walidah

Walda (German) powerful; famous.
Waldina, Waldine, Walida, Wallda, Welda

Waleria (Polish) a form of Valerie.
Wala

Walker (English) cloth; walker.
Wallker

Wallis (English) from Wales.
Wallie, Walliss, Wally, Wallys

Wanda (German) wanderer. See also Wendy.
Vanda, Wahnda, Wandah, Wandely, Wandie, Wandis, Wandja, Wandzia, Wannda, Wonda, Wonnda

Wandie (German) a familiar form of Wanda.
Wandi, Wandy

Waneta (Native American) charger. See also Juanita.
Waneeta, Wanita, Wanite, Wanneta, Waunita, Wonita, Wonnita, Wynita

Wanetta (English) pale face.
Wanette, Wannetta, Wannette

Wanika (Hawaiian) a form of Juanita.
Wanicka

Warda (German) guardian.
Wardah, Wardeh, Wardena, Wardenia, Wardia, Wardine

Washi (Japanese) eagle.

Wattan (Japanese) homeland.

Wauna (Moquelumnan) snow geese honking.
Waunakee

Wava (Slavic) a form of Barbara.

Waverly (English) quaking aspen-tree meadow.
Waverley, Waverli, Wavierlee

Waynesha (American) a combination of Waynette + Niesha.
Wayneesha, Wayneisha, Waynie, Waynisha

Waynette (English) wagon
maker.
*Waynel, Waynelle, Waynetta,
Waynlyn*

Weeko (Dakota) pretty girl.

Wehilani (Hawaiian) heavenly
adornment.

Wenda (Welsh) a form of
Wendy.
Wendaine, Wendayne

Wendelle (English) wanderer.
*Wendaline, Wendall, Wendalyn,
Wendeline, Wendella,
Wendelline, Wendelly*

Wendi (Welsh) a form of
Wendy.
Wendie

Wendy (Welsh) white; light
skinned. A familiar form of
Gwendolyn, Wanda.
*Wenda, Wende, Wendee,
Wendey, Wendi, Wendye,
Wuendy*

Wera (Polish) a form of Vera.
See also Verna.
Wiera, Wiercia, Wierka

Weronika (Polish) a form of
Veronica.
Weronikra

Wesisa (Musoga) foolish.

Weslee (English) western
meadow.
*Weslea, Wesleigh, Weslene,
Wesley, Wesli, Weslia, Weslie,
Weslyn*

Whitley (English) white field.
*Whitely, Whitlee, Whitleigh,
Whitlie, Whittley*

Whitney (English) white island.
*Whiteney, Whitne, Whitné,
Whitnee, Whitneigh, Whitnie,
Whitny, Whitnye, Whytne,
Whytney, Witney*

Whitnie (English) a form of
Whitney.
*Whitani, Whitnei, Whitni,
Whytni, Whytnie*

Whittney (English) a form of
Whitney.
*Whittaney, Whittanie, Whittany,
Whitteny, Whittnay, Whittnee,
Whittney, Whittni, Whittnie*

Whoopi (English) happy;
excited.
Whoopie, Whoopy

Wicktoria (Polish) a form of
Victoria.
Wicktorja, Wiktoria, Wiktorja

Wilda (German) untamed.
(English) willow.
Willda, Wylda

Wileen (English) a short form
of Wilhelmina.
Wilene, Willeen, Willene

Wilhelmina (German) a form
of Wilhelm (see Boys'
Names). See also Billie,
Guillerma, Helma, Minka,
Minna, Minnie.
*Vilhelmina, Wileen, Wilhelmine,
Willa, Willamina, Willamine,*

*Willemina, Willette, Williamina,
Willie, Willmina, Willmine,
Wilma, Wimina*

Wilikinia (Hawaiian) a form of
Virginia.

Willa (German) a short form
of Wilhelmina.
Willabella, Willette, Williabelle

Willette (English) a familiar
form of Wilhelmina, Willa.
*Wiletta, Wilette, Willetta,
Williette*

Willie (English) a familiar
form of Wilhelmina.
*Willi, Willina, Willisha,
Willishia, Willy*

Willow (English) willow tree.
Willough

Wilma (German) a short form
of Wilhelmina.
*Williemae, Wilmanie, Wilmayra,
Wilmetta, Wilmette, Wilmina,
Wilmyne, Wylma*

Wilona (English) desired.
Willona, Willone, Wilone

Win (German) a short form of
Winifred. See also Edwina.
Wyn

Winda (Swahili) hunter.

Windy (English) windy.
*Windee, Windey, Windi,
Windie, Wyndee, Wyndy*

Winema (Moquelumnan)
woman chief.

Winifred (German) peaceful
friend. (Welsh) a form of
Guinevere. See also Freddi,
Una, Winnie.
*Win, Winafred, Winefred,
Winefride, Winfreda, Winfrieda,
Winiefrida, Winifrid, Winifryd,
Winnafred, Winnefred,
Winniefred, Winnifred,
Winnifrid, Wynafred, Wynifred,
Wynnifred*

Winna (African) friend.
Winnah

Winnie (English) a familiar
form of Edwina, Gwyneth,
Winnifred, Winona, Wynne.
History: Winnie Mandela
kept the anti-apartheid
movement alive in South
Africa while her then-hus-
band, Nelson Mandela, was
imprisoned. Literature: the
lovable bear in A. A. Milne's
children's story *Winnie-the-
Pooh.*
*Wina, Winne, Winney, Winni,
Winny, Wynnie*

Winola (German) charming
friend.
Wynola

Winona (Lakota) oldest
daughter.
*Wanona, Wenona, Wenonah,
Winnie, Winonah, Wynonna*

Winter (English) winter.
Wintr, Wynter

Wira (Polish) a form of Elvira.
Wiria, Wirke

Wisia (Polish) a form of
Victoria.
Wicia, Wikta

Wren (English) wren, songbird.

Wyanet (Native American)
legendary beauty.
Wyaneta, Wyanita, Wynette

Wynne (Welsh) white, light
skinned. A short form of
Blodwyn, Guinivere,
Gwyneth.
Winnie, Wyn, Wynn

Wynonna (Lakota) a form of
Winona.
Wynnona, Wynona

Wynter (English) a form of
Winter.
Wynteria

Wyoming (Native American)
Geography: a western U.S.
state.
Wy, Wye, Wyoh, Wyomia

Xandra (Greek) a form of
Zandra. (Spanish) a short
form of Alexandra.
Xander, Xandrea, Xandria

Xanthe (Greek) yellow, blond.
See also Zanthe.
*Xanne, Xantha, Xanthia,
Xanthippe*

Xanthippe (Greek) a form of
Xanthe. History: Socrates's
wife.
Xantippie

Xaviera (Basque) owner of the
new house. (Arabic) bright.
See also Javiera, Zaviera.
*Xavia, Xaviére, Xavyera,
Xiveria*

Xela (Quiché) my mountain
home.

Xena (Greek) a form of
Xenia.

Xenia (Greek) hospitable. See
also Zena, Zina.
*Xeenia, Xena, Xenea, Xenya,
Xinia*

Xiang (Chinese) fragrant.

Xiomara (Teutonic) glorious
forest.
Xiomaris, Xiomayra

Xiu Mei (Chinese) beautiful
plum.

Xochitl (Aztec) place of many
flowers.
*Xochil, Xochilt, Xochilth,
Xochiti*

Xuan (Vietnamese) spring.

Xuxa (Portuguese) a familiar
form of Susanna.

Xylia (Greek) a form of Sylvia.
Xylina, Xylona

Y

Yachne (Hebrew) hospitable.

Yadira (Hebrew) friend.
Yadirah, Yadirha, Yadyra

Yael (Hebrew) strength of
God. See also Jael.
Yaeli, Yaella, Yeala

Yaffa (Hebrew) beautiful. See
also Jaffa.
Yafeal, Yaffit, Yafit

Yahaira (Hebrew) a form of
Yakira.
Yahara, Yahayra, Yahira

Yajaira (Hebrew) a form of
Yakira.
Yahaira, Yajara, Yajayra, Yajhaira

Yakira (Hebrew) precious;
dear.
Yahaira, Yajaira

Yalanda (Greek) a form of
Yolanda.
Yalando, Yalonda, Ylana, Ylanda

Yalena (Greek, Russian) a
form of Helen. See also
Lena, Yelena.

Yaletha (American) a form of
Oletha.
Yelitsa

Yamary (American) a combi-
nation of the prefix Ya +
Mary.
*Yamairy, Yamarie, Yamaris,
Yamayra*

Yamelia (American) a form of
Amelia.
Yameily, Yamelya, Yamelys

Yamila (Arabic) a form of
Jamila.
*Yamela, Yamely, Yamil, Yamile,
Yamilet, Yamiley, Yamilla, Yamille*

Yaminah (Arabic) right,
proper.
*Yamina, Yamini, Yemina,
Yeminah, Yemini*

Yamka (Hopi) blossom.

Yamuna (Hindi) sacred river.

Yana (Slavic) a form of Jana.
*Yanae, Yanah, Yanay, Yanaye,
Yanesi, Yanet, Yaneth, Yaney,
Yani, Yanik, Yanina, Yanis,
Yanisha, Yanitza, Yanixia,
Yanna, Yannah, Yanni, Yannica,
Yannick, Yannina*

Yanaba (Navajo) brave.

Yaneli (American) a combina-
tion of the prefix Ya +
Nellie.
*Yanela, Yanelis, Yaneliz, Yanelle,
Yanelli, Yanely, Yanelys*

Yanet (American) a form of
Janet.
*Yanete, Yaneth, Yanethe, Yanette,
Yannet, Yanneth, Yannette*

Yáng (Chinese) sun.

Yareli (American) a form of Oralee.
Yarely, Yaresly

Yarina (Slavic) a form of Irene.
Yaryna

Yaritza (American) a combination of Yana + Ritsa.
Yaritsa, Yaritsa

Yarkona (Hebrew) green.

Yarmilla (Slavic) market trader.

Yashira (Afghan) humble; takes it easy. (Arabic) wealthy.

Yasmeen (Persian) a form of Yasmin.
Yasemeen, Yasemin, Yasmeena, Yasmen, Yasmene, Yasmeni, Yasmenne, Yassmeen, Yassmen

Yasmin, Yasmine (Persian) jasmine flower.
Yashmine, Yasiman, Yasimine, Yasma, Yasmain, Yasmaine, Yasmina, Yasminda, Yasmon, Yasmyn, Yazmin, Yesmean, Yesmeen, Yesmin, Yesmina, Yesmine, Yesmyn

Yasu (Japanese) resting, calm.
Yasuko, Yasuyo

Yazmin (Persian) a form of Yasmin.
Yazmeen, Yazmen, Yazmene, Yazmina, Yazmine, Yazmyn,
Yazmyne, Yazzmien, Yazzmine, Yazzmine, Yazzmyn

Yecenia (Arabic) a form of Yesenia.

Yehudit (Hebrew) a form of Judith.
Yudit, Yudita, Yuta

Yei (Japanese) flourishing.

Yeira (Hebrew) light.

Yekaterina (Russian) a form of Katherine.

Yelena (Russian) a form of Helen, Jelena. See also Lena, Yalena.
Yeleana, Yelen, Yelenna, Yelenne, Yelina, Ylena, Ylenia, Ylenna

Yelisabeta (Russian) a form of Elizabeth.
Yelizaveta

Yemena (Arabic) from Yemen.
Yemina

Yen (Chinese) yearning; desirous.
Yeni, Yenih, Yenny

Yenene (Native American) shaman.

Yenifer (Welsh) a form of Jennifer.
Yenefer, Yennifer

Yeo (Korean) mild.
Yee

Yepa (Native American) snow girl.

Yesenia (Arabic) flower.
Yasenya, Yecenia, Yesinia, Yesnia, Yessenia

Yesica (Hebrew) a form of Jessica.
Yesika, Yesiko

Yessenia (Arabic) a form of Yesenia.
Yessena, Yessenya, Yissenia

Yessica (Hebrew) a form of Jessica.
Yessika, Yesyka

Yetta (English) a short form of Henrietta.
Yette, Yitta, Yitty

Yeva (Ukrainian) a form of Eve.

Yiesha (Arabic, Swahili) a form of Aisha.
Yiasha

Yín (Chinese) silver.

Ynez (Spanish) a form of Agnes. See also Inez.
Ynes, Ynesita

Yoanna (Hebrew) a form of Joanna.
Yoana, Yohana, Yohanka, Yohanna, Yohannah

Yocelin, Yocelyn (Latin) forms of Jocelyn.
Yoceline, Yocelyne, Yuceli

Yoi (Japanese) born in the evening.

Yoki (Hopi) bluebird.
Yokie

Yoko (Japanese) good girl.
Yo

Yolie (Greek) a familiar form of Yolanda.
Yola, Yoley, Yoli, Yoly

Yolanda (Greek) violet flower. See also Iolanthe, Jolanda, Olinda.
Yalanda, Yolie, Yolaine, Yolana, Yoland, Yolande, Yolane, Yolanna, Yolantha, Yolanthe, Yolette, Yolonda, Yorlanda, Youlanda, Yulanda, Yulonda

Yoluta (Native American) summer flower.

Yomara (American) a combination of Yolanda + Tamara.
Yomaira, Yomarie, Yomira

Yon (Burmese) rabbit. (Korean) lotus blossom.
Yona, Yonna

Yoné (Japanese) wealth; rice.

Yonina (Hebrew) a form of Jonina.
Yona, Yonah

Yonita (Hebrew) a form of Jonita.
Yonat, Yonati, Yonit

Yoomee (Coos) star.
Yoome

Yordana (Basque) descendant. See also Jordana.

Yori (Japanese) reliable.
Yoriko, Yoriyo

Yoselin (Latin) a form of
Jocelyn.
*Yoseline, Yoselyn, Yosselin,
Yosseline, Yosselyn*

Yosepha (Hebrew) a form of
Josephine.
Yosefa, Yosifa, Yuseffa

Yoshi (Japanese) good; respectful.
Yoshie, Yoshiko, Yoshiyo

Yovela (Hebrew) joyful heart;
rejoicer.

Ysabel (Spanish) a form of
Isabel.
*Ysabell, Ysabella, Ysabelle, Ysbel,
Ysbella, Ysobel*

Ysanne (American) a combination of Ysabel + Ann.
Ysande, Ysann, Ysanna

Yseult (German) ice rule.
(Irish) fair; light skinned.
(Welsh) a form of Isolde.
Yseulte, Ysolt

Yuana (Spanish) a form of
Juana.
Yuan, Yuanna

Yudelle (English) a form of
Udele.
Yudela, Yudell, Yudella

Yudita (Russian) a form of
Judith.
Yudit, Yudith, Yuditt

Yuki (Japanese) snow.
Yukie, Yukiko, Yukiyo

Yulene (Basque) a form of
Julia.
Yuleen

Yulia (Russian) a form of Julia.
*Yula, Yulenka, Yulinka, Yulka,
Yulya*

Yuliana (Spanish) a form of
Juliana.
Yulenia, Yuliani

Yuri (Japanese) lily.
Yuree, Yuriko, Yuriyo

Yvanna (Slavic) a form of
Ivana.
Yvan, Yvana, Yvannia

Yvette (French) a familiar
form of Yvonne. See also
Evette, Ivette.
*Yavette, Yevett, Yevette, Yevetta,
Yvet, Yveta, Yvett, Yvetta*

Yvonne (French) young
archer. (Scandinavian) yew
wood; bow wood. See also
Evonne, Ivonne, Vonna,
Vonny, Yvette.
*Yavanda, Yavanna, Yavanne,
Yavonda, Yavonna, Yavonne,
Yveline, Yvon, Yvone, Yvonna,
Yvonnah, Yvonnia, Yvonnie,
Yvonny*

Z

Zabrina (American) a form of Sabrina.
Zabreena, Zabrinia, Zabrinna, Zabryna

Zacharie (Hebrew) God remembered.
Zacari, Zacceaus, Zacchaea, Zachary, Zachoia, Zackaria, Zackeisha, Zackeria, Zakaria, Zakaya, Zakeshia, Zakiah, Zakiria, Zakiya, Zakiyah, Zechari

Zachary (Hebrew) a form of Zacharie.
Zackery, Zakary

Zada (Arabic) fortunate, prosperous.
Zaida, Zayda, Zayeda

Zafina (Arabic) victorious.

Zafirah (Arabic) successful; victorious.

Zahar (Hebrew) daybreak; dawn.
Zahara, Zaharra, Zahera, Zahira, Zahirah, Zeeherah

Zahavah (Hebrew) golden.
Zachava, Zachavah, Zechava, Zechavah, Zehava, Zehavi, Zehavit, Zeheva, Zehuva

Zahra (Swahili) flower. (Arabic) white.
Zahara, Zahraa, Zahrah, Zahreh, Zahria

Zaira (Hebrew) a form of Zara.
Zaire, Zairea, Zirrea

Zakia (Swahili) smart. (Arabic) chaste.
Zakea, Zakeia, Zakiah, Zakiya

Zakira (Hebrew) a form of Zacharie.
Zaakira, Zakiera, Zakierra, Zakir, Zakirah, Zakiria, Zakiriya, Zykarah, Zykera, Zykeria, Zykerria, Zykira, Zykuria

Zakiya (Arabic) a form of Zakia.
Zakeya, Zakeyia, Zakiyaa, Zakiyah, Zakiyya, Zakiyyah, Zakkiyya, Zakkiyyah, Zakkyyah

Zalika (Swahili) born to royalty.
Zuleika

Zaltana (Native American) high mountain.

Zandra (Greek) a form of Sandra.
Zahndra, Zandrea, Zandria, Zandy, Zanndra, Zondra

Zaneta (Spanish) a form of Jane.
Zanita, Zanitra

Zanna (Spanish) a form of Jane. (English) a short form of Susanna.
Zaina, Zainah, Zainna, Zana, Zanae, Zanah, Zanella, Zanette, Zannah, Zannette, Zannia, Zannie

Zanthe (Greek) a form of Xanthe.
Zanth, Zantha

Zara (Hebrew) a form of Sarah, Zora.
Zaira, Zarah, Zarea, Zaree, Zareea, Zareen, Zareena, Zareh, Zareya, Zari, Zaria, Zariya, Zarria

Zarifa (Arabic) successful.

Zarita (Spanish) a form of Sarah.

Zasha (Russian) a form of Sasha.
Zascha, Zashenka, Zashka, Zasho

Zaviera (Spanish) a form of Xaviera.
Zavera, Zavirah

Zawati (Swahili) gift.

Zayit (Hebrew) olive.

Zaynah (Arabic) beautiful.
Zayn, Zayna

Zea (Latin) grain.

Zelda (Yiddish) gray haired. (German) a short form of Griselda. See also Selda.
Zelde, Zella, Zellda

Zelene (English) sunshine.
Zeleen, Zelena, Zeline

Zelia (Spanish) sunshine.
Zele, Zelene, Zelie, Zélie, Zelina

Zelizi (Basque) a form of Sheila.

Zelma (German) a form of Selma.

Zemirah (Hebrew) song of joy.

Zena (Greek) a form of Xenia. (Ethiopian) news. (Persian) woman. See also Zina.
Zanae, Zanah, Zeena, Zeenat, Zeenet, Zeenia, Zeenya, Zein, Zeina, Zenah, Zenana, Zenea, Zenia, Zenna, Zennah, Zennia, Zenya

Zenaida (Greek) white-winged dove.
Zenaide, Zenaïde, Zenayda, Zenochka

Zenda (Persian) sacred; feminine.

Zenobia (Greek) sign, symbol. History: a queen who ruled the city of Palmyra in ancient Syria.
Zeba, Zeeba, Zenobie, Zenovia

Zephania, Zephanie (Greek) forms of Stephanie.
Zepania, Zephanas, Zephany

Zephyr (Greek) west wind.
*Zefiryn, Zephra, Zephria,
Zephyer, Zephyrine*

Zera (Hebrew) seeds.
Zerah, Zeriah

Zerdali (Turkish) wild apricot.

Zerlina (Latin, Spanish) beautiful dawn. Music: a character in Mozart's opera *Don Giovanni.*
Zerla, Zerlinda

Zerrin (Turkish) golden.
Zerren

Zeta (English) rose.
Linguistics: a letter in the Greek alphabet.
Zayit, Zetana, Zetta

Zetta (Portuguese) rose.

Zhana, Zhane (Slavic) forms of Jane.
*Zhanae, Zhanay, Zhanaya,
Zhané, Zhanea, Zhanee,
Zhaney, Zhani, Zhaniah,
Zhanna*

Zhen (Chinese) chaste.

Zia (Latin) grain. (Arabic) light.
Zea

Zigana (Hungarian) gypsy girl. See also Tsigana.
Zigane

Zihna (Hopi) one who spins tops.

Zilla (Hebrew) shadow.
Zila, Zillah, Zylla

Zilpah (Hebrew) dignified.
Bible: Jacob's wife.
Zilpha, Zylpha

Zilya (Russian) a form of Theresa.

Zimra (Hebrew) song of praise.
*Zamora, Zemira, Zemora,
Zimria*

Zina (African) secret spirit.
(English) hospitable. (Greek) a form of Zena.
Zinah, Zine

Zinnia (Latin) Botany: a plant with beautiful, rayed, colorful flowers.
Zinia, Zinny, Zinnya, Zinya

Zipporah (Hebrew) bird.
Bible: Moses' wife.
*Zipora, Ziporah, Zipporia,
Ziproh*

Zita (Spanish) rose. (Arabic) mistress. A short form of names ending in "sita" or "zita."
Zeeta, Zyta, Zytka

Ziva (Hebrew) bright; radiant.
Zeeva, Ziv, Zivanka, Zivi, Zivit

Zizi (Hungarian) a familiar form of Elizabeth.
Zsi Zsi

Zocha (Polish) a form of Sophie.

Zoe (Greek) life.
*Zoé, Zoë, Zoee, Zoelie, Zoeline,
Zoelle, Zoey, Zoi, Zoie, Zowe,
Zowey, Zowie, Zoya*

Zoey (Greek) a form of Zoe.
Zooey

Zofia (Slavic) a form of
Sophia. See also Sofia.
Zofka, Zsofia

Zohar (Hebrew) shining, brilliant.
Zoheret

Zohra (Hebrew) blossom.

Zohreh (Persian) happy.
Zahreh, Zohrah

Zola (Italian) piece of earth.
Zoela, Zoila

Zona (Latin) belt, sash.
Zonia

Zondra (Greek) a form of
Zandra.
Zohndra

Zora (Slavic) aurora; dawn.
See also Zara.
*Zorah, Zorana, Zoreen,
Zoreena, Zorna, Zorra, Zorrah,
Zorya*

Zorina (Slavic) golden.
*Zorana, Zori, Zorie, Zorine,
Zorna, Zory*

Zoya (Slavic) a form of Zoe.
*Zoia, Zoyara, Zoyechka,
Zoyenka, Zoyya*

Zsa Zsa (Hungarian) a familiar form of Susan.
Zhazha

Zsofia (Hungarian) a form of
Sofia.
Zofia, Zsofi, Zsofika

Zsuzsanna (Hungarian) a
form of Susanna.
*Zsuska, Zsuzsa, Zsuzsi,
Zsuzsika, Zsuzska*

Zudora (Sanskrit) laborer.

Zuleika (Arabic) brilliant.
*Zeleeka, Zul, Zulay, Zulekha,
Zuleyka*

Zulima (Arabic) a form of
Salama.
*Zuleima, Zulema, Zulemah,
Zulimah*

Zurafa (Arabic) lovely.
Ziraf, Zuruf

Zuri (Basque) white; light
skinned. (Swahili) beautiful.
Zuria, Zurie, Zurisha, Zury

Zusa (Czech, Polish) a form of
Susan.
*Zuzana, Zuzanka, Zuzia,
Zuzka, Zuzu*

Zuwena (Swahili) good.
Zwena

Zytka (Polish) rose.

Boys

Aakash (Hindi) a form of Akash.

Aaron (Hebrew) enlightened. (Arabic) messenger. Bible: the brother of Moses and the first high priest. See also Ron.
Aahron, Aaran, Aaren, Aareon, Aarin, Aaronn, Aarron, Aaryn, Aeron, Aharon, Ahran, Ahren, Aranne, Arek, Aren, Ari, Arin, Aron, Aronek, Aronne, Aronos, Arran, Arron

Aban (Persian) Mythology: a figure associated with water and the arts.

Abasi (Swahili) stern.

Abbey (Hebrew) a familiar form of Abe.
Abey, Abbie, Abby

Abbott (Hebrew) father; abbot.
Ab, Abba, Abbah, Abbán, Abbé, Abbot, Abott

Abbud (Arabic) devoted.

Abdirahman (Arabic) a form of Abdulrahman.
Abdirehman

Abdul (Arabic) servant.
Abdal, Abdeel, Abdel, Abdoul, Abdual, Abdull, Abul

Abdulaziz (Arabic) servant of the Mighty.
Abdelazim, Abdelaziz, Abdulazaz, Abdulazeez

Abdullah (Arabic) servant of Allah.
Abdalah, Abdalla, Abdallah, Abduala, Abdualla, Abduallah, Abdulah, Abdulahi, Abdulha, Abdulla, Abdullahi

Abdulrahman (Arabic) servant of the Merciful.
Abdelrahim, Abdelrahman, Abdirahman, Abdolrahem, Abdularahman, Abdurrahman, Abdurram

Abe (Hebrew) a short form of Abel, Abraham.

Abel (Hebrew) breath. (Assyrian) meadow. (German) a short form of Abelard. Bible: Adam and Eve's second son.
Abe, Abele, Abell, Able, Adal, Avel

Abelard (German) noble; resolute.
Ab, Abalard, Abel, Abelardo, Abelhard, Abilard, Adalard, Adelard

Abi (Turkish) older brother.

Abiah (Hebrew) God is my father.
Abia, Abiel, Abija, Abijah, Abisha, Abishai, Aviya, Aviyah

Abie (Hebrew) a familiar form of Abraham.

Abiel (Hebrew) a form of Abiah.

Abir (Hebrew) strong.

Abisha (Hebrew) gift of God.
Abijah, Abishai

Abner (Hebrew) father of light. Bible: the commander of Saul's army.
Ab, Avner, Ebner

Abraham (Hebrew) father of many nations. Bible: the first Hebrew patriarch. See also Avram, Bram, Ibrahim.
Abarran, Abe, Aberham, Abey, Abhiram, Abie, Abrahaim, Abrahame, Abrahamo, Abrahan, Abrahán, Abraheem, Abrahem, Abrahim, Abrahm, Abram, Abramo, Abrán, Abrao, Arram, Avram

Abrahan (Spanish) a form of Abraham.
Abrahon

Abram (Hebrew) a short form of Abraham. See also Bram.
Abramo, Abrams, Avram

Absalom (Hebrew) father of peace. Bible: the rebellious third son of King David. See also Avshalom, Axel.
Absalaam, Absalon, Abselon, Absolum

Acar (Turkish) bright.

Ace (Latin) unity.
Acer, Acey, Acie

Achilles (Greek) Mythology: a hero of the Trojan War. Literature: the hero of Homer's epic poem *Iliad*.
Achill, Achille, Achillea, Achillios, Akil, Akili, Akilles

Ackerley (English) meadow of oak trees.
Accerley, Ackerlea, Ackerleigh, Ackersley, Acklea, Ackleigh, Ackley, Acklie

Acton (English) oak-tree settlement.

Adahy (Cherokee) in the woods.

Adair (Scottish) oak-tree ford.
Adaire, Adare

Adam (Phoenician) man; mankind. (Hebrew) earth; man of the red earth. Bible: the first man created by God. See also Adamson, Addison, Damek, Keddy, Macadam.
Ad, Adama, Adamec, Adamo, Adão, Adas, Addam, Addams, Addis, Addy, Adem, Adham, Adhamh, Adné, Adok, Adomas

Adamec (Czech) a form of Adam.
Adamek, Adamik, Adamka, Adamko, Adamok

Adamson (Hebrew) son of Adam.
Adams, Adamsson, Addamson

Adan (Irish) a form of Aidan.
Aden, Adian, Adin

Adar (Syrian) ruler; prince.
(Hebrew) noble; exalted.
Addar

Adarius (American) a combi-
nation of Adam + Darius.
*Adareus, Adarias, Adarrius,
Adarro, Adarruis, Adaruis,
Adauris*

Addison (English) son of
Adam.
*Addis, Addisen, Addisun,
Addyson, Adison, Adisson,
Adyson*

Addy (Hebrew) a familiar
form of Adam, Adlai.
(German) a familiar form of
Adelard.
Addey, Addi, Addie, Ade, Adi

Ade (Yoruba) royal.

Adelard (German) noble;
courageous.
*Adal, Adalar, Adalard, Addy,
Adel, Adél, Adelar*

Aden (Arabic) Geography: a
region in southern Yemen.
(Irish) a form of Aidan,
Aiden.

Adham (Arabic) black.

Adil (Arabic) just; wise.
Adeel, Adeele

Adin (Hebrew) pleasant.

Adir (Hebrew) majestic; noble.
Adeer

Adiv (Hebrew) pleasant; gentle.
Adeev

Adlai (Hebrew) my ornament.
Ad, Addy, Adley

Adler (German) eagle.
Ad, Addler, Adlar

Adli (Turkish) just; wise.

Admon (Hebrew) peony.

Adnan (Arabic) pleasant.
Adnaan

Adney (English) noble's island.
Adny

Adolf (German) noble wolf.
History: Adolf Hitler's
German army was defeated
in World War II. See also
Dolf.
Ad, Adolfo, Adolfus, Adolph

Adolfo (Spanish) a form of
Adolf.
Adolpho

Adolph (German) a form of
Adolf.
*Adolphe, Adolpho, Adolphus,
Adulphus*

Adom (Akan) help from God.

Adon (Hebrew) Lord. (Greek)
a short form of Adonis.

Adonis (Greek) highly attractive. Mythology: the attrac-

tive youth loved by
Aphrodite.
Adon, Adonnis, Adonys

Adri (Indo-Pakistani) rock.
Adrey

Adrian (Greek) rich. (Latin)
dark. (Swedish) a short form
of Hadrian.
*Adarian, Ade, Adorjan, Adrain,
Adreian, Adreyan, Adri,
Adriaan, Adriane, Adriann,
Adrianne, Adriano, Adriean,
Adrien, Adrik, Adrion, Adrionn,
Adrionne, Adron, Adryan,
Adryn, Adryon*

Adriano (Italian) a form of
Adrian.
Adrianno

Adriel (Hebrew) member of
God's flock.
Adrial

Adrien (French) a form of
Adrian.
Adriene, Adrienne

Adrik (Russian) a form of
Adrian.
Adric

Aeneas (Greek) praised.
(Scottish) a form of Angus.
Literature: the Trojan hero of
Vergil's epic poem *Aeneid*.
See also Eneas.

Afram (African) Geography: a
river in Ghana, Africa.

Afton (English) from Afton,
England.
Affton

Agamemnon (Greek) resolute.
Mythology: the king of
Mycenae who led the
Greeks in the Trojan War.

Agni (Hindi) Religion: the
Hindu fire god.

Agu (Ibo) leopard.

Agustin (Latin) a form of
Augustine.
*Agostino, Agoston, Aguistin,
Agustine, Agustis, Agusto,
Agustus*

Ahab (Hebrew) father's
brother. Literature: the cap-
tain of the Pequod in
Herman Melville's novel
Moby-Dick.

Ahanu (Native American)
laughter.

Ahdik (Native American) cari-
bou; reindeer.

Ahearn (Scottish) lord of the
horses. (English) heron.
*Ahearne, Aherin, Ahern,
Aherne, Hearn*

Ahir (Turkish) last.

Ahmad (Arabic) most highly
praised. See also Muhammad.
*Achmad, Achmed, Ahamad,
Ahamada, Ahamed, Ahmaad,
Ahmaud, Amad, Amahd, Amed*

Ahmed (Swahili) praiseworthy.

Ahsan (Arabic) charitable.

Aidan (Irish) fiery.
Adan, Aden, Aiden, Aydan,
Ayden, Aydin

Aiden, Ayden (Irish) a form
of Aidan.
Aden, Aidon, Aidyn, Aydean

Aiken (English) made of oak.
Aicken, Aikin, Ayken, Aykin

Aimery (French) a form of
Emery.
Aime, Aimerey, Aimeric, Amerey,
Aymeric, Aymery

Aimon (French) house. (Irish)
a form of Eamon.

Aindrea (Irish) a form of
Andrew.
Aindreas

Ainsley (Scottish) my own
meadow.
Ainsleigh, Ainslie, Ansley,
Aynslee, Aynsley, Aynslie

Aizik (Russian) a form of
Isaac.

Ajala (Yoruba) potter.

Ajay (Punjabi) victorious;
undefeatable. (American) a
combination of the initials A.
+ J.
Aj, Aja, Ajae, Ajai, Ajaye, Ajaz,
Ajé, Ajee, Ajit

Ajit (Sanskrit) unconquerable.
Ajeet, Ajith

Akar (Turkish) flowing stream.
Akara

Akash (Hindi) sky.
Aakash, Akasha, Akshay

Akbar (Arabic) great.

Akecheta (Sioux) warrior.

Akeem, Akim (Hebrew) short
forms of Joachim.
Achim, Ackeem, Ackim,
Ahkieme, Akeam, Akee, Akiem,
Akima, Arkeem

Akemi (Japanese) dawn.

Akil (Arabic) intelligent.
(Greek) a form of Achilles.
Ahkeel, Akeel, Akeil, Akeyla,
Akhil, Akiel, Akila, Akilah,
Akile, Akili

Akins (Yoruba) brave.

Akira (Japanese) intelligent.
Akihito, Akio, Akiyo

Akiva (Hebrew) a form of
Jacob.
Akiba, Kiva

Akmal (Arabic) perfect.

Aksel (Norwegian) father of
peace.
Aksell

Akshay (American) a form of
Akash.
Akshaj, Akshaya

Akshat (Sanskrit) uninjurable.

Akule (Native American) he
looks up.

Al (Irish) a short form of Alan, Albert, Alexander.

Aladdin (Arabic) height of faith. Literature: the hero of a story in the *Arabian Nights*.
Ala, Alaa, Alaaddin, Aladean, Aladin, Aladino

Alain (French) a form of Alan.
Alaen, Alainn, Alayn, Allain

Alaire (French) joyful.

Alam (Arabic) universe.

Alan (Irish) handsome; peaceful.
Ailan, Ailin, Al, Alaan, Alain, Alair, Aland, Alande, Alando, Alani, Alann, Alano, Alanson, Alante, Alao, Allan, Allen, Alon, Alun

Alaric (German) ruler of all. See also Ulrich.
Alarick, Alarico, Alarik, Aleric, Allaric, Allarick, Alric, Alrick, Alrik

Alastair (Scottish) a form of Alexander.
Alaisdair, Alaistair, Alaister, Alasdair, Alasteir, Alaster, Alastor, Aleister, Alester, Alistair, Allaistar, Allastair, Allaster, Allastir, Allysdair, Alystair

Alban (Latin) from Alba, Italy.
Albain, Albany, Albean, Albein, Alby, Auban, Auben

Albern (German) noble; courageous.

Albert (German, French) noble and bright. See also Elbert, Ulbrecht.
Adelbert, Ailbert, Al, Albertik, Alberto, Alberts, Albie, Albrecht, Alby, Alvertos, Aubert

Alberto (Italian) a form of Albert.
Berto

Albie, Alby (German, French) familiar forms of Albert.
Albee, Albi

Albin (Latin) a form of Alvin.
Alben, Albeno, Albinek, Albino, Albins, Albinson, Alby, Auben

Albion (Latin) white cliffs. Geography: a reference to the white cliffs in Dover, England.

Alcandor (Greek) manly; strong.

Alcott (English) old cottage.
Alcot, Alkot, Alkott, Allcot, Allcott, Allkot, Allkott

Aldair (German, English) a form of Alder.
Aldahir, Aldayr

Alden (English) old; wise protector.
Aldan, Aldean, Aldin, Aldous, Elden

Alder (German, English) alder tree.
Aldair

Aldo (Italian) old; elder.
(German) a short form of
Aldous.

Aldous (German) a form of
Alden.
Aldis, Aldo, Aldon, Aldus, Elden

Aldred (English) old; wise
counselor.
Alldred, Eldred

Aldrich (English) wise.
*Aldric, Aldrick, Aldridge,
Aldrige, Aldritch, Alldric,
Alldrich, Alldrick, Alldridge,
Eldridge*

Aldwin (English) old friend.
Aldwyn, Eldwin

Alec, Alek (Greek) short
forms of Alexander.
Aleck, Alekko, Elek

Alejándro (Spanish) a form of
Alexander.
Alejándra, Aléjo, Alexjándro

Aleksandar, Aleksander
(Greek) forms of Alexander.
*Aleksandor, Aleksandr,
Aleksandras, Aleksandur*

Aleksei (Russian) a short form
of Alexander.
*Aleks, Aleksey, Aleksi, Aleksis,
Aleksy, Alexei, Alexey*

Alekzander, Alexzander
(Greek) forms of Alexander.
*Alekxander, Alekxzander,
Alexkzandr, Alexzandr,
Alexzandyr*

Alem (Arabic) wise.

Aleric (German) a form of
Alaric.
Alerick, Alleric, Allerick

Aleron (Latin) winged.

Alessandro (Italian) a form of
Alexander.
Alessand, Allessandro

Alex (Greek) a short form of
Alexander.
Alax, Alix, Allax, Allex, Elek

Alexander (Greek) defender
of mankind. History:
Alexander the Great was the
conqueror of the civilized
world. See also Alastair,
Alistair, Iskander, Jando, Leks,
Lex, Lexus, Macallister,
Oleksandr, Olés, Sander,
Sándor, Sandro, Sandy, Sasha,
Xan, Xander, Zander, Zindel.
*Al, Alec, Alecsandar, Alejándro,
Alek, Alekos, Aleksandar,
Aleksander, Aleksei, Alekzander,
Alessandro, Alex, Alexandar,
Alexandor, Alexandr, Alexandre,
Alexandro, Alexandros, Alexi,
Alexis, Alexxander, Alexzander,
Alic, Alick, Alisander, Alixander*

Alexandre (French) a form of
Alexander.

Alexandro (Greek) a form of
Alexander.
*Alexandras, Alexandros,
Alexandru*

Alexi (Russian) a form of
Aleksei. (Greek) a short form
of Alexander.
*Alexe, Alexee, Alexey, Alexie,
Alexio, Alexy*

Alexis (Greek) a short form of
Alexander.
*Alexei, Alexes, Alexey, Alexios,
Alexius, Alexiz, Alexsis,
Alexsus, Alexus*

Alfie (English) a familiar form
of Alfred.
Alfy

Alfonso (Italian, Spanish) a
form of Alphonse.
*Affonso, Alfons, Alfonse,
Alfonsus, Alfonza, Alfonzo,
Alfonzus*

Alford (English) old river ford.

Alfred (English) elf counselor;
wise counselor. See also
Fred.
*Ailfrid, Ailfryd, Alf, Alfeo, Alfie,
Alfredo, Alured*

Alfredo (Italian, Spanish) a
form of Alfred.
Alfrido

Alger (German) noble spearman. (English) a short form
of Algernon. See also Elger.
Algar, Allgar

Algernon (English) bearded,
wearing a moustache.
*Algenon, Alger, Algie, Algin,
Algon*

Algie (English) a familiar form
of Algernon.
Algee, Algia, Algy

Algis (German) spear.

Ali (Arabic) greatest. (Swahili)
exalted.
Aly

Alic (Greek) a short form of
Alexander.
Alick, Aliek, Alik, Aliko

Alim (Arabic) scholar. (Arabic)
a form of Alem.

Alisander (Greek) a form of
Alexander.
*Alissander, Alissandre, Alsandair,
Alsandare, Alsander*

Alistair (English) a form of
Alexander.
*Alisdair, Alistaire, Alistar, Alister,
Allistair, Allistar, Allister, Allistir,
Alstair*

Alixander (Greek) a form of
Alexander.
*Alixandre, Alixandru,
Alixzander*

Allan (Irish) a form of Alan.
Allayne

Allard (English) noble, brave.
Alard, Ellard

Allen (Irish) a form of Alan.
*Alen, Alley, Alleyn, Alleyne,
Allie, Allin, Allon, Allyn*

Almon (Hebrew) widower.

Alois (German) a short form of Aloysius.
Aloys

Aloisio (Spanish) a form of Louis.

Alok (Sanskrit) victorious cry.

Alon (Hebrew) oak.

Alonso, Alonzo (Spanish) forms of Alphonse.
Alano, Alanzo, Alon, Alonza, Elonzo, Lon, Lonnie, Lonso, Lonzo

Aloysius (German) a form of Louis.
Alaois, Alois, Aloisius, Aloisio

Alphonse (German) noble and eager.
Alf, Alfie, Alfonso, Alonzo, Alphons, Alphonsa, Alphonso, Alphonsus, Alphonza, Alphonzus, Fonzie

Alphonso (Italian) a form of Alphonse.
Alphanso, Alphonzo, Fonso

Alpin (Irish) attractive.
Alpine

Alroy (Spanish) king.

Alston (English) noble's settlement.
Allston, Alstun

Altair (Greek) star. (Arabic) flying.

Altman (German) old man.
Altmann, Atman

Alton (English) old town.
Alten

Alva (Hebrew) sublime.
Alvah

Alvan (German) a form of Alvin.
Alvand

Alvar (English) army of elves.
Alvara

Alvaro (Spanish) just; wise.

Alvern (Latin) spring.
Elvern

Alvin (Latin) white; light skinned. (German) friend to all; noble friend; friend of elves. See also Albin, Elvin.
Aloin, Aluin, Aluino, Alvan, Alven, Alvie, Alvino, Alvy, Alvyn, Alwin, Elwin

Alvis (Scandinavian) all-knowing.

Alwin (German) a form of Alvin.
Ailwyn, Alwyn, Alwynn, Aylwin

Amadeo (Italian) a form of Amadeus.

Amadeus (Latin) loves God. Music: Wolfgang Amadeus Mozart was a famous eighteenth-century Austrian composer.
Amad, Amadeaus, Amadée, Amadeo, Amadei, Amadio, Amadis, Amado, Amador,

Amadou, Amando, Amedeo,
Amodaos

Amal (Hebrew) worker.
(Arabic) hopeful.

Amandeep (Punjabi) light of
peace.
Amandip, Amanjit, Amanjot,
Amanpreet

Amando (French) a form of
Amadeus.
Amand, Amandio, Amaniel,
Amato

Amani (Arabic) believer.
(Yoruba) strength; builder.
Amanee

Amar (Punjabi) immortal.
(Arabic) builder.
Amare, Amaree, Amari, Amario,
Amaris, Amarjit, Amaro,
Amarpreet, Amarri, Ammar,
Ammer

Amato (French) loved.
Amatto

Ambar (Sanskrit) sky.
Amber

Ambrose (Greek) immortal.
Ambie, Ambroise, Ambros,
Ambrosi, Ambrosio, Ambrosius,
Ambrus, Amby

Ameer (Hebrew) a form of
Amir.
Ameir, Amer, Amere

Amerigo (Teutonic) industrious. History: Amerigo
Vespucci was the Italian
explorer for whom America
is named.
Americo, Americus

Ames (French) friend.

Amicus (English, Latin)
beloved friend.
Amico

Amiel (Hebrew) God of my
people.
Ammiel

Amin (Hebrew, Arabic) trustworthy; honest. (Hindi) faithful.
Amine

Amir (Hebrew) proclaimed.
(Punjabi) wealthy; king's
minister. (Arabic) prince.
Aamer, Aamir, Ameer, Amire,
Amiri

Amish (Sanskrit) honest.

Amit (Punjabi) unfriendly.
(Arabic) highly praised.
Amitan, Amreet

Ammon (Egyptian) hidden.
Mythology: the ancient god
associated with reproduction.
Amman

Amol (Hindi) priceless, valuable.
Amul

Amon (Hebrew) trustworthy;
faithful.

Amory (German) a form of
Emory.
Amery, Amor

Amos (Hebrew) burdened,
troubled. Bible: an Old
Testament prophet.
Amose

Amram (Hebrew) mighty
nation.
Amarien, Amran, Amren

Amrit (Sanskrit) nectar.
(Punjabi, Arabic) a form of
Amit.

An (Chinese, Vietnamese)
peaceful.
Ana

Anand (Hindi) blissful.
Ananda, Anant, Ananth

Anastasius (Greek) resurrec-
tion.
*Anas, Anastacio, Anastacios,
Anastagio, Anastas, Anastase,
Anastasi, Anastasio, Anastasios,
Anastice, Anastisis, Anaztáz,
Athanasius*

Anatole (Greek) east.
*Anatol, Anatoley, Anatoli,
Anatolijus, Anatolio, Anatoliy,
Anatoly, Anitoly*

Anchali (Taos) painter.

Anders (Swedish) a form of
Andrew.
Ander

Anderson (Swedish) son of
Andrew.
Andersen

Andonios (Greek) a form of
Anthony.
Andoni, Andonis, Andonny

Andor (Hungarian) a form of
Andrew.

András (Hungarian) a form of
Andrew.
*Andraes, Andri, Andris, Andrius,
Andriy, Aundras, Aundreas*

Andre, André (French) forms
of Andrew.
*Andra, Andrae, Andrecito,
Andree, Andrei, Aundre, Aundré*

Andrea (Greek) a form of
Andrew.
Andrean, Andreani, Andrian

Andreas (Greek) a form of
Andrew.
Andres, Andries

Andrei (Bulgarian, Romanian,
Russian) a form of Andrew.
*Andreian, Andrej, Andrey,
Andreyan, Andrie, Aundrei*

Andres (Spanish) a form of
Andrew.
Andras, Andrés, Andrez

Andrew (Greek) strong;
manly; courageous. Bible:
one of the Twelve Apostles.
See also Bandi, Drew, Endre,
Evangelos, Kendrew, Ondro.
Aindrea, Anders, Andery,

Andonis, Andor, András, Andre, André, Andrea, Andreas, Andrei, Andres, Andrews, Andru, Andrue, Andrus, Andy, Anker, Anndra, Antal, Audrew

Andros (Polish) sea. Mythology: the god of the sea.
Andris, Andrius, Andrus

Andy (Greek) a short form of Andrew.
Andino, Andis, Andje

Aneurin (Welsh) honorable; gold. See also Nye.
Aneirin

Anfernee (Greek) a form of Anthony.
Anferney, Anfernie, Anferny, Anfranee, Anfrene, Anfrenee, Anpherne

Angel (Greek) angel. (Latin) messenger. See also Gotzon.
Ange, Angell, Angelo, Angie, Angy

Angelo (Italian) a form of Angel.
Angeleo, Angelito, Angello, Angelos, Anglo

Angus (Scottish) exceptional; outstanding. Mythology: Angus Og was the Celtic god of youth, love, and beauty. See also Ennis, Gus.
Aeneas, Aonghas

Anh (Vietnamese) peace; safety.

Anibal (Phoenician) a form of Hannibal.

Anil (Hindi) wind god.
Aneel, Anel, Aniel, Aniello

Anka (Turkish) phoenix.

Anker (Danish) a form of Andrew.
Ankur

Annan (Scottish) brook. (Swahili) fourth-born son.

Annas (Greek) gift from God.
Anis, Anish, Anna, Annais

Anno (German) a familiar form of Johann.

Anoki (Native American) actor.

Ansel (French) follower of a nobleman.
Ancell, Ansa, Ansell

Anselm (German) divine protector. See also Elmo.
Anse, Anselme, Anselmi, Anselmo

Ansis (Latvian) a form of Janis.

Ansley (Scottish) a form of Ainsley.
Anslea, Anslee, Ansleigh, Anslie, Ansly, Ansy

Anson (German) divine. (English) Anne's son.
Ansun

Antal (Hungarian) a form of Anthony.
Antek, Anti, Antos

Antares (Greek) giant, red star. Astronomy: the brightest star in the constellation Scorpio.
Antar, Antario, Antarious, Antarius, Antarr, Antarus

Antavas (Lithuanian) a form of Anthony.
Antae, Antaeus, Antavious, Antavius, Ante, Anteo

Anthany (Latin, Greek) a form of Anthony.
Antanee, Antanie, Antenee, Anthan, Antheny, Anthine, Anthney

Anthonie (Latin, Greek) a form of Anthony.
Anthone, Anthonee, Anthoni, Anthonia

Anthony (Latin) praiseworthy. (Greek) flourishing. See also Tony.
Anathony, Andonios, Andor, András, Anothony, Antal, Antavas, Anfernee, Anthany, Anthawn, Anthey, Anthian, Anthino, Anthone, Anthoney, Anthonie, Anthonio, Anthonu, Anthonysha, Anthoy, Anthyoine, Anthyonny, Antione, Antjuan, Antoine, Anton, Antonio, Antony, Antwan, Antwon

Antione (French) a form of Anthony.
Antion, Antionio, Antionne, Antiono

Antjuan (Spanish) a form of Anthony.
Antajuan, Anthjuan, Antuan, Antuane

Antoan (Vietnamese) safe, secure.

Antoine (French) a form of Anthony.
Anntoin, Anthoine, Antoiné, Antoinne, Atoine

Anton (Slavic) a form of Anthony.
Anthon, Antone, Antonn, Antonne, Antons, Antos

Antonio (Italian) a form of Anthony. See also Tino, Tonio.
Anthonio, Antinio, Antoinio, Antoino, Antonello, Antoneo, Antonin, Antonín, Antonino, Antonnio, Antonios, Antonius, Antonyia, Antonyio, Antonyo

Antony (Latin) a form of Anthony.
Antin, Antini, Antius, Antoney, Antoni, Antonie, Antonin, Antonios, Antonius, Antonyia, Antonyio, Antonyo, Anty

Antti (Finnish) manly.
Anthey, Anthi, Anti

Antwan (Arabic) a form of Anthony.
Antaw, Antawan, Antawn, Anthawn, Antowan, Antowaun, Antowine, Antowne, Antowyn, Antuwan, Antwain, Antwaina, Antwaine, Antwainn, Antwaion, Antwane, Antwann, Antwanne, Antwarn, Antwaun, Antwen, Antwian, Antwine, Antwuan, Antwun, Antwyné

Antwon (Arabic) a form of Anthony.
Antown, Antuwon, Antwion, Antwione, Antwoan, Antwoin, Antwoine, Antwone, Antwonn, Antwonne, Antwoun, Antwyon, Antwyone, Antyon, Antyonne, Antywon

Anwar (Arabic) luminous.
Anour, Anouar, Anwi

Apiatan (Kiowa) wooden lance.

Apollo (Greek) manly. Mythology: the god of prophecy, healing, music, poetry, and light. See also Polo.
Apolinar, Apolinario, Apollos, Apolo, Apolonio, Appollo

Aquila (Latin, Spanish) eagle.
Acquilla, Aquil, Aquilas, Aquileo, Aquiles, Aquilino, Aquilla, Aquille, Aquillino

Araldo (Spanish) a form of Harold.
Aralodo, Aralt, Aroldo, Arry

Aram (Syrian) high, exalted.
Ara, Aramia, Arra, Arram

Aramis (French) Literature: one of the title characters in Alexandre Dumas's novel *The Three Musketeers.*
Airamis, Aramith, Aramys

Aran (Tai) forest. (Danish) a form of Aren. (Hebrew, Scottish) a form of Arran.

Archer (English) bowman.
Archie

Archibald (German) bold. See also Arkady.
Arch, Archaimbaud, Archambault, Archibaldo, Archibold, Archie

Archie (German, English) a familiar form of Archer, Archibald.
Archy

Ardal (Irish) a form of Arnold.
Ardale

Ardell (Latin) eager; industrious.
Ardel

Arden (Latin) ardent; fiery.
Ard, Ardan, Ardene, Ardian, Ardie, Ardin, Ardn, Arduino

Ardon (Hebrew) bronzed.

Aren (Danish) eagle; ruler. (Hebrew, Arabic) a form of Aaron.

Aretino (Greek, Italian) victorious.

Argus (Danish) watchful, vigilant.
Agos

Ari (Hebrew) a short form of Ariel. (Greek) a short form of Aristotle.
Aria, Arias, Arie, Arieh, Arih, Arij, Ario, Arri, Ary, Arye

Arian (Greek) a form of Arion.
Ariana, Ariane, Ariann, Arianne, Arrian, Aryan

Aric (German) a form of Richard. (Scandinavian) a form of Eric.
Aaric, Arec, Areck, Arich, Arick, Ariek, Arik, Arrek, Arric, Arrick, Arrik, Aryk

Ariel (Hebrew) lion of God. Bible: another name for Jerusalem. Literature: the name of a sprite in the Shakespearean play *The Tempest.*
Airel, Arel, Areli, Ari, Ariell, Ariya, Ariyel, Arrial, Arriel

Aries (Latin) ram. Astrology: the first sign of the zodiac.
Ares, Arie, Ariez

Arif (Arabic) knowledgeable.
Areef

Arion (Greek) enchanted. (Hebrew) melodious.
Arian, Arien, Ario, Arione, Aryon

Aristides (Greek) son of the best.
Aris, Aristedes, Aristeed, Aristide, Aristides, Aristidis

Aristotle (Greek) best; wise. History: a third-century B.C. philosopher who tutored Alexander the Great.
Ari, Aris, Aristito, Aristo, Aristokles, Aristotelis

Arjun (Hindi) white; milk colored.
Arjen, Arjin, Arju, Arjuna, Arjune

Arkady (Russian) a form of Archibald.
Arcadio, Arkadi, Arkadij, Arkadiy

Arkin (Norwegian) son of the eternal king.
Aricin, Arkeen, Arkyn

Arledge (English) lake with the hares.
Arlidge, Arlledge

Arlen (Irish) pledge.
Arlan, Arland, Arlend, Arlin, Arlinn, Arlyn, Arlynn

Arley (English) a short form of Harley.
Arleigh, Arlie, Arly

Arlo (Spanish) barberry. (English) fortified hill. A form of Harlow. (German) a form of Charles.

Arman (Persian) desire, goal.
Armaan, Armahn, Armaine

Armand (Latin, German) a form of Herman. See also Mandek.
Armad, Arman, Armanda, Armando, Armands, Armanno, Armaude, Armenta, Armond

Armando (Spanish) a form of Armand.
Armondo

Armani (Hungarian) sly. (Hebrew) a form of Armon.
Arman, Armann, Armoni, Armonie, Armonio, Armonni, Armony

Armon (Hebrew) high fortress, stronghold.
Armani, Armen, Armin, Armino, Armonn, Armons

Armstrong (English) strong arm. History: astronaut Neil Armstrong was the commander of Apollo 11 and the first person to walk on the moon.

Arnaud (French) a form of Arnold.
Arnauld, Arnault, Arnoll

Arne (German) a form of Arnold.
Arna, Arnay, Arnel, Arnele, Arnell, Arnelle

Arnette (English) little eagle.
Arnat, Arnet, Arnett, Arnetta, Arnot, Arnott

Arnie (German) a familiar form of Arnold.
Arney, Arni, Arnny, Arny

Arno (German) a short form of Arnold. (Czech) a short form of Ernest.
Arnou, Arnoux

Arnold (German) eagle ruler.
Ardal, Arnald, Arnaldo, Arnaud, Arne, Arnie, Arno, Arnol, Arnoldas, Arnoldo, Arnoll, Arndt, Arnulfo

Arnon (Hebrew) rushing river.
Arnan

Arnulfo (German) a form of Arnold.

Aron, Arron (Hebrew) forms of Aaron. (Danish) forms of Aren.
Arrion

Aroon (Tai) dawn.

Arran (Scottish) island dweller. Geography: an island off the west coast of Scotland. (Hebrew) a form of Aaron.
Arren, Arrin, Arryn, Aryn

Arrigo (Italian) a form of Harry.
Alrigo, Arrighetto

Arrio (Spanish) warlike.
Ario, Arrow, Arryo, Aryo

Arsenio (Greek) masculine; virile. History: Saint Arsenius was a teacher in the Roman Empire.
Arsen, Arsène, Arsenius, Arseny, Arsinio

Arsha (Persian) venerable.

Art (English) a short form of Arthur.

Artemus (Greek) gift of Artemis. Mythology: Artemis was the goddess of the hunt and the moon.
Artemas, Artemio, Artemis, Artimas, Artimis, Artimus

Arthur (Irish) noble; lofty hill. (Scottish) bear. (English) rock. (Icelandic) follower of Thor. See also Turi.
Art, Artair, Artek, Arth, Arther, Arthor, Artie, Artor, Arturo, Artus, Aurthar, Aurther, Aurthur

Artie (English) a familiar form of Arthur.
Arte, Artian, Artis, Arty, Atty

Arturo (Italian) a form of Arthur.
Arthuro, Artur

Arun (Cambodian, Hindi) sun.
Aruns

Arundel (English) eagle valley.

Arve (Norwegian) heir, inheritor.

Arvel (Welsh) wept over.
Arval, Arvell, Arvelle

Arvid (Hebrew) wanderer. (Norwegian) eagle tree. See also Ravid.
Arv, Arvad, Arve, Arvie, Arvind, Arvinder, Arvydas

Arvin (German) friend of the people; friend of the army.
Arv, Arvie, Arvind, Arvinder, Arvon, Arvy

Aryeh (Hebrew) lion.

Asa (Hebrew) physician, healer. (Yoruba) falcon.
Asaa, Ase

Asád (Arabic) lion.
Asaad, Asad, Asid, Assad, Azad

Asadel (Arabic) prosperous.
Asadour, Asadul, Asael

Ascot (English) eastern cottage; style of necktie. Geography: a village near London and the site of the Royal Ascot horseraces.

Asgard (Scandinavian) court of the gods.

Ash (Hebrew) ash tree.
Ashby

Ashanti (Swahili) from a tribe in West Africa.
Ashan, Ashani, Ashante, Ashantee, Ashaunte

Ashby (Scandinavian) ash-tree farm. (Hebrew) a form of Ash.
Ashbey

Asher (Hebrew) happy; blessed.
Ashar, Ashor, Ashur

Ashford (English) ash-tree ford.
Ash, Ashtin

Ashley (English) ash-tree meadow.
Ash, Asheley, Ashelie, Ashely, Ashlan, Ashlee, Ashleigh, Ashlen, Ashlie, Ashlin, Ashling, Ashlinn, Ashlone, Ashly, Ashlyn, Ashlynn, Aslan

Ashon (Swahili) seventh-born son.

Ashton (English) ash-tree settlement.
Ashtan, Ashten, Ashtian, Ashtin, Ashtion, Ashtonn, Ashtun, Ashtyn

Ashur (Swahili) Mythology: the principal Assyrian deity.

Ashwani (Hindi) first. Religion: the first of the twenty-seven galaxies revolving around the moon.
Ashwan

Ashwin (Hindi) star.

Asiel (Hebrew) created by God.

Asker (Turkish) soldier.

Aspen (English) aspen tree.

Aston (English) eastern town.
Asten, Astin

Aswad (Arabic) dark skinned, black.

Ata (Fante) twin.

Atek (Polish) a form of Tanek.

Athan (Greek) immortal.

Atherton (English) town by a spring.

Atid (Tai) sun.

Atif (Arabic) caring.
Ateef, Atef

Atlas (Greek) lifted; carried. Mythology: Atlas was forced by Zeus to carry the heavens on his shoulders as a punishment for his share of the war of the Titans.

Atley (English) meadow.
Atlea, Atlee, Atleigh, Atli, Attley

Attila (Gothic) little father. History: the Hun leader who invaded the Roman Empire.
Atalik, Atila, Atilio, Atilla, Atiya, Attal, Attilio

Atwater (English) at the water's edge.

Atwell (English) at the well.

Atwood (English) at the forest.

Atworth (English) at the farmstead.

Auberon (German) a form of Oberon.
Auberron, Aubrey

Aubrey (German) noble; bear-like. (French) a familiar form of Auberon. See also Avery.
Aubary, Aube, Aubery, Aubie, Aubré, Aubree, Aubreii, Aubrie, Aubry, Aubury

Auburn (Latin) reddish brown.

Auden (English) old friend.

Audie (German) noble; strong. (English) a familiar form of Edward.
Audi, Audiel, Audley, Audy

Audon (French) old; rich.
Audelon

Audrey (English) noble strength.
Audra, Audre, Audrea, Audrius, Audry

Audric (English) wise ruler.
Audrick, Audrik

Audun (Scandinavian) deserted, desolate.

Augie (Latin) a familiar form of August.
Auggie, Augy

August (Latin) a short form of Augustine, Augustus.
Agosto, Augie, Auguste, Augusto

Augustine (Latin) majestic. Religion: Saint Augustine was the first archbishop of Canterbury. See also Austin, Gus, Tino.
August, Agustin, Augustin,

Augustinas, Augustino, Austen, Austin, Auston, Austyn

Augustus (Latin) majestic; venerable. History: an honorary title given to the first Roman emperor, Octavius Caesar.
August

Aukai (Hawaiian) seafarer.

Aundre (Greek) a form of Andre.
Aundrae, Aundray, Aundrea, Aundrey, Aundry

Aurek (Polish) golden haired.

Aurelio (Latin) a short form of Aurelius.
Aurel, Aurele, Aureli, Aurellio

Aurelius (Latin) golden. History: Marcus Aurelius was a second-century A.D. philosopher and emperor of Rome.
Arelian, Areliano, Aurèle, Aureliano, Aurelien, Aurélien, Aurelio, Aurey, Auriel, Aury

Aurick (German) protecting ruler.
Auric

Austen, Auston, Austyn (Latin) short forms of Augustine.
Austan, Austun, Austyne

Austin (Latin) a short form of Augustine.
Astin, Austine, Oistin, Ostin

Avel (Greek) breath.

Avent (French) born during Advent.
Aventin, Aventino

Averill (French) born in April.
Ave, Averel, Averell, Averiel, Averil, Averyl, Averyll, Avrel, Avrell, Avrill, Avryll

Avery (English) a form of Aubrey.
Avary, Aveary, Avere, Averee, Averey, Averi, Averie, Avrey, Avry

Avi (Hebrew) God is my father.
Avian, Avidan, Avidor, Aviel, Avion

Aviv (Hebrew) youth; springtime.

Avner (Hebrew) a form of Abner.
Avneet, Avniel

Avram (Hebrew) a form of Abraham, Abram.
Arram, Avraam, Avraham, Avrahom, Avrohom, Avrom, Avrum

Avshalom (Hebrew) father of peace. See also Absalom.
Avsalom

Awan (Native American) somebody.

Axel (Latin) axe. (German) small oak tree; source of life. (Scandinavian) a form of Absalom.
Aksel, Ax, Axe, Axell, Axil, Axill, Axl, Axle, Axyle

Aydin (Turkish) intelligent.

Ayers (English) heir to a fortune.

Ayinde (Yoruba) we gave praise and he came.

Aylmer (English) a form of Elmer.
Aillmer, Ailmer, Allmer, Ayllmer

Aymil (Greek) a form of Emil.

Aymon (French) a form of Raymond.

Ayo (Yoruba) happiness.

Azad (Turkish) free.

Azeem (Arabic) a form of Azim.
Aseem, Asim

Azi (Nigerian) youth.

Azim (Arabic) defender.
Azeem

Aziz (Arabic) strong.

Azizi (Swahili) precious.

Azriel (Hebrew) God is my aid.

Azuriah (Hebrew) aided by God.
Azaria, Azariah, Azuria

B

Baden (German) bather.
Baeden, Bayden, Baydon

Bahir (Arabic) brilliant, dazzling.

Bahram (Persian) ancient king.

Bailey (French) bailiff, steward.
Bail, Bailee, Bailie, Bailio, Baillie, Baily, Bailye, Baley, Bayley

Bain (Irish) a short form of Bainbridge.
Baine, Bayne, Baynn

Bainbridge (Irish) fair bridge.
Bain, Baynbridge, Bayne, Baynebridge

Baird (Irish) traveling minstrel, bard; poet.
Bairde, Bard

Bakari (Swahili) noble promise.
Bacari, Baccari, Bakarie

Baker (English) baker. See also Baxter.
Bakir, Bakory, Bakr

Bal (Sanskrit) child born with lots of hair.

Balasi (Basque) flat footed.

Balbo (Latin) stammerer.
Bailby, Balbi, Ballbo

Baldemar (German) bold; famous.
Baldemer, Baldomero, Baumar, Baumer

Balder (Scandinavian) bald. Mythology: the Norse god of light, summer, purity, and innocence.
Baldier, Baldur, Baudier

Baldric (German) brave ruler.
Baldrick, Baudric

Baldwin (German) bold friend.
Bald, Baldovino, Balduin, Baldwinn, Baldwyn, Baldwynn, Balldwin, Baudoin

Balfour (Scottish) pastureland.
Balfor, Balfore

Balin (Hindi) mighty soldier.
Bali, Baylen, Baylin, Baylon, Valin

Ballard (German) brave; strong.
Balard

Balraj (Hindi) strongest.

Baltazar (Greek) a form of Balthasar.
Baltasar

Balthasar (Greek) God save the king. Bible: one of the three wise men who bore gifts for the infant Jesus.
Badassare, Baldassare, Baltazar,

Balthasaar, Balthazar,
Balthazzar, Baltsaros, Belshazar,
Belshazzar, Boldizsár

Bancroft (English) bean field.
Ban, Bancrofft, Bank, Bankroft,
Banky, Binky

Bandi (Hungarian) a form of
Andrew.
Bandit

Bane (Hawaiian) a form of
Bartholomew.

Banner (Scottish, English) flag
bearer.
Bannor, Banny

Banning (Irish) small and fair.
Bannie, Banny

Barak (Hebrew) lightning
bolt. Bible: the valiant warrior who helped Deborah.
Barrak

Baran (Russian) ram.
Baren

Barasa (Kikuyu) meeting
place.

Barclay (Scottish, English)
birch-tree meadow.
Bar, Barcley, Barklay, Barkley,
Barklie, Barrclay, Berkeley

Bard (Irish) a form of Baird.
Bar, Barde, Bardia, Bardiya,
Barr

Bardolf (German) bright wolf.
Bardo, Bardolph, Bardou,
Bardoul, Bardulf, Bardulph

Bardrick (Teutonic) axe ruler.
Bardric, Bardrik

Baris (Turkish) peaceful.

Barker (English) lumberjack;
advertiser at a carnival.

Barlow (English) bare hillside.
Barlowe, Barrlow, Barrlowe

Barnabas (Greek, Hebrew,
Aramaic, Latin) son of the
missionary. Bible: Christian
apostle and companion of
Paul on his first missionary
journey.
Bane, Barna, Barnaba,
Barnabus, Barnaby, Barnebas,
Barnebus, Barney

Barnaby (English) a form of
Barnabas.
Barnabe, Barnabé, Barnabee,
Barnabey, Barnabi, Barnabie,
Bernabé, Burnaby

Barnard (French) a form of
Bernard.
Barn, Barnard, Barnhard,
Barnhardo

Barnes (English) bear; son of
Barnett.

Barnett (English) nobleman;
leader.
Barn, Barnet, Barney, Baronet,
Baronett, Barrie, Barron, Barry

Barney (English) a familiar
form of Barnabas, Barnett.
Barnie, Barny

Barnum (German) barn; storage place. (English) baron's home.
Barnham

Baron (German, English) nobleman, baron.
Baaron, Barion, Baronie, Barrin, Barrion, Barron, Baryn, Bayron, Berron

Barrett (German) strong as a bear.
Bar, Baret, Barrat, Barret, Barretta, Barrette, Barry, Berrett, Berrit

Barric (English) grain farm.
Barrick, Beric, Berric, Berrick, Berrik

Barrington (English) fenced town. Geography: a town in England.

Barry (Welsh) son of Harry. (Irish) spear, marksman. (French) gate, fence.
Baris, Barri, Barrie, Barris, Bary

Bart (Hebrew) a short form of Bartholomew, Barton.
Barrt, Bartel, Bartie, Barty

Bartholomew (Hebrew) son of Talmaí. Bible: one of the Twelve Apostles. See also Jerney, Parlan, Parthalán.
Balta, Bane, Bart, Bartek, Barth, Barthel, Barthelemy, Barthélemy, Barthélmy, Bartho, Bartholo, Bartholomaus, Bartholome, Bartholomeo, Bartholomeus, Bartholomieu, Bartimous, Bartlet, Barto, Bartolome, Bartolomé, Bartolomeo, Bartolomeð, Bartolommeo, Bartome, Bartz, Bat

Bartlet (English) a form of Bartholomew.
Bartlett, Bartley

Barto (Spanish) a form of Bartholomew.
Bardo, Bardol, Bartol, Bartoli, Bartolo, Bartos

Barton (English) barley town; Bart's town.
Barrton, Bart

Bartram (English) a form of Bertram.
Barthram

Baruch (Hebrew) blessed.
Boruch

Basam (Arabic) smiling.
Basem, Basim, Bassam

Basil (Greek, Latin) royal, kingly. Religion: a saint and founder of monasteries. Botany: an herb often used in cooking. See also Vasilis, Wasili.
Bas, Basal, Base, Baseal, Basel, Basle, Basile, Basilio, Basilios, Basilius, Bassel, Bazek, Bazel, Bazil, Bazyli

Basir (Turkish) intelligent, discerning.
Bashar, Basheer, Bashir, Bashiyr, Bechir, Bhasheer

Bassett (English) little person.
Basett, Basit, Basset, Bassit

Bastien (German) a short form of Sebastian.
Baste, Bastiaan, Bastian, Bastion

Bat (English) a short form of Bartholomew.

Baul (Gypsy) snail.

Bavol (Gypsy) wind; air.

Baxter (English) a form of Baker.
Bax, Baxie, Baxty, Baxy

Bay (Vietnamese) seventh son. (French) chestnut brown color; evergreen tree. (English) howler.

Bayard (English) reddish brown hair.
Baiardo, Bay, Bayardo, Bayerd, Bayrd

Bayley (French) a form of Bailey.
Baylee, Bayleigh, Baylie, Bayly

Beacan (Irish) small.
Beacán, Becan

Beacher (English) beech trees.
Beach, Beachy, Beech, Beecher, Beechy

Beagan (Irish) small.
Beagen, Beagin

Beale (French) a form of Beau.
Beal, Beall, Bealle, Beals

Beaman (English) beekeeper.
Beamann, Beamen, Beeman, Beman

Beamer (English) trumpet player.

Beasley (English) field of peas.

Beattie (Latin) blessed; happy; bringer of joy.
Beatie, Beatty, Beaty

Beau (French) handsome.
Beale, Beaux, Bo

Beaufort (French) beautiful fort.

Beaumont (French) beautiful mountain.

Beauregard (French) handsome; beautiful; well regarded.

Beaver (English) beaver.
Beav, Beavo, Beve, Bevo

Bebe (Spanish) baby.

Beck (English, Scandinavian) brook.
Beckett

Bede (English) prayer. Religion: the patron saint of lectors.

Bela (Czech) white.
(Hungarian) bright.
Béla, Belaal, Belal, Belall,
Belay, Bellal

Belden (French, English)
pretty valley.
Beldin, Beldon, Bellden, Belldon

Belen (Greek) arrow.

Bell (French) handsome.
(English) bell ringer.

Bellamy (French) beautiful
friend.
Belamy, Bell, Bellamey, Bellamie

Bello (African) helper or pro-
moter of Islam.

Belmiro (Portuguese) good-
looking; attractive.

Bem (Tiv) peace.
Behm

Ben (Hebrew) a short form of
Benjamin.
Behn, Benio, Benn, Benne,
Benno

Ben-ami (Hebrew) son of my
people.
Baram, Barami

Benedict (Latin) blessed. See
also Venedictos, Venya.
Benci, Bendick, Bendict,
Bendino, Bendix, Bendrick,
Benedetto, Benedick, Benedicto,
Benedictus, Benedikt, Bengt,
Benito, Benoit

Benedikt (German, Slavic) a
form of Benedict.
Bendek, Bendik, Benedek,
Benedik

Bengt (Scandinavian) a form
of Benedict.
Beng, Benke, Bent

Beniam (Ethiopian) a form of
Benjamin.
Beneyam, Beniamin, Beniamino

Benito (Italian) a form of
Benedict. History: Benito
Mussolini led Italy during
World War II.
Benedo, Benino, Benno, Beno,
Betto, Beto

Benjamen (Hebrew) a form
of Benjamin.
Benejamen, Benjermen,
Benjjmen

Benjamin (Hebrew) son of
my right hand. See also
Peniamina, Veniamin.
Behnjamin, Bejamin,
Bemjiman, Ben, Benejaminas,
Bengamin, Beniam, Benja,
Benjahmin, Benjaim, Benjam,
Benjamaim, Benjaman,
Benjamen, Benjamine,
Benjaminn, Benjamino,
Benjamon, Benjamyn,
Benjamynn, Benjemin,
Benjermain, Benjermin, Benji,
Benjie, Benjiman, Benjy,
Benkamin, Bennjamin, Benny,
Benyamin, Benyamino,
Binyamin, Mincho

Benjiman (Hebrew) a form of Benjamin.
Benjimen, Benjimin, Benjimon, Benjmain

Benjiro (Japanese) enjoys peace.

Bennett (Latin) little blessed one.
Benet, Benett, Bennet, Benette, Bennete, Bennette

Benny (Hebrew) a familiar form of Benjamin.
Bennie

Beno (Hebrew) son. (Mwera) band member.

Benoit (French) a form of Benedict.
Benott

Benoni (Hebrew) son of my sorrow. Bible: Ben-oni was the son of Jacob and Rachel.
Ben-Oni

Benson (Hebrew) son of Ben. A short form of Ben Zion.
Bensan, Bensen, Benssen, Bensson

Bentley (English) moor; coarse grass meadow.
Bent, Bentlea, Bentlee, Bentlie, Lee

Benton (English) Ben's town; town on the moors.
Bent

Benzi (Hebrew) a familiar form of Ben Zion.

Ben Zion (Hebrew) son of Zion.
Benson, Benzi

Beppe (Italian) a form of Joseph.
Beppy

Ber (English) boundary. (Yiddish) bear.

Beredei (Russian) a form of Hubert.
Berdry, Berdy, Beredej, Beredy

Berg (German) mountain.
Berdj, Berge, Bergh, Berje

Bergen (German, Scandinavian) hill dweller.
Bergin, Birgin

Berger (French) shepherd.

Bergren (Scandinavian) mountain stream.
Berg

Berk (Turkish) solid, rugged.

Berkeley (English) a form of Barclay.
Berk, Berkely, Berkie, Berkley, Berklie, Berkly, Berky

Berl (German) a form of Burl.
Berle, Berlie, Berlin, Berlyn

Berlyn (German) boundary line. See also Burl.
Berlin, Burlin

Bern (German) a short form of Bernard.
Berne

Bernal (German) strong as a bear.
Bernald, Bernaldo, Bernel, Bernhald, Bernhold, Bernold

Bernard (German) brave as a bear. See also Bjorn.
Barnard, Bear, Bearnard, Benek, Ber, Berend, Bern, Bernabé, Bernadas, Bernardel, Bernardin, Bernardo, Bernardus, Bernardyn, Bernarr, Bernat, Bernek, Bernal, Bernel, Bernerd, Berngards, Bernhard, Bernhards, Bernhardt, Bernie, Bjorn, Burnard

Bernardo (Spanish) a form of Bernard.
Barnardino, Barnardo, Barnhardo, Benardo, Bernardino, Bernhardo, Berno, Burnardo, Nardo

Bernie (German) a familiar form of Bernard.
Berney, Berni, Berny, Birney, Birnie, Birny, Burney

Berry (English) berry; grape.
Berrie

Bersh (Gypsy) one year.

Bert (German, English) bright, shining. A short form of Berthold, Berton, Bertram, Bertrand, Egbert, Filbert.
Bertie, Bertus, Birt, Burt

Berthold (German) bright; illustrious; brilliant ruler.
Bert, Berthoud, Bertold, Bertolde

Bertie (English) a familiar form of Bert, Egbert.
Berty, Birt, Birtie, Birty

Bertín (Spanish) distinguished friend.
Berti

Berto (Spanish) a short form of Alberto.

Berton (English) bright settlement; fortified town.
Bert

Bertram (German) bright; illustrious. (English) bright raven. See also Bartram.
Beltran, Beltrán, Beltrano, Bert, Berton, Bertrae, Bertraim, Bertraum, Bertron

Bertrand (German) bright shield.
Bert, Bertran, Bertrando, Bertranno

Berwyn (Welsh) white head.
Berwin, Berwynn, Berwynne

Bevan (Welsh) son of Evan.
Beavan, Beaven, Beavin, Bev, Beve, Beven, Bevin, Bevo, Bevon

Beverly (English) beaver meadow.
Beverlea, Beverleigh, Beverley, Beverlie

Bevis (French) from Beauvais, France; bull.
Beauvais, Bevys

Bhagwandas (Hindi) servant of God.

Bickford (English) axe-man's ford.

Bienvenido (Filipino) welcome.

Bijan (Persian) ancient hero.
Bihjan, Bijann, Bijhan, Bijhon, Bijon

Bilal (Arabic) chosen.
Bila, Bilaal, Bilale, Bile, Bilel, Billaal, Billal

Bill (German) a short form of William.
Bil, Billee, Billijo, Billye, Byll, Will

Billy (German) a familiar form of Bill, William.
Bille, Billey, Billie, Billy, Bily, Willie

Binah (Hebrew) understanding; wise.
Bina

Bing (German) kettle-shaped hollow.

Binh (Vietnamese) peaceful.

Binkentios (Greek) a form of Vincent.

Binky (English) a familiar form of Bancroft, Vincent.
Bink, Binkentios, Binkie

Birch (English) white; shining; birch tree.
Birk, Burch

Birger (Norwegian) rescued.

Birkey (English) island with birch trees.
Birk, Birkie, Birky

Birkitt (English) birch-tree coast.
Birk, Birket, Birkit, Burket, Burkett, Burkitt

Birley (English) meadow with the cow barn.
Birlee, Birlie, Birly

Birney (English) island with a brook.
Birne, Birnie, Birny, Burney, Burnie, Burny

Birtle (English) hill with birds.

Bishop (Greek) overseer. (English) bishop.
Bish, Bishup

Bjorn (Scandinavian) a form of Bernard.
Bjarne

Blackburn (Scottish) black brook.

Blade (English) knife, sword.
Bladen, Bladon, Bladyn, Blae, Blaed, Blayde

Bladimir (Russian) a form of Vladimir.
Bladimer

Blaine (Irish) thin, lean. (English) river source.
Blain, Blane, Blayne

Blair (Irish) plain, field.
(Welsh) place.
Blaire, Blare, Blayr, Blayre

Blaise, Blaize (French) forms
of Blaze.
*Ballas, Balyse, Blais, Blaisot,
Blas, Blase, Blasi, Blasien,
Blasius, Blass, Blaz, Blaze,
Blayz, Blayze, Blayzz*

Blake (English) attractive;
dark.
*Blaik, Blaike, Blakely,
Blakeman, Blakey, Blayke*

Blakely (English) dark
meadow.
*Blakelee, Blakeleigh, Blakeley,
Blakelie, Blakelin, Blakelyn,
Blakeny, Blakley, Blakney*

Blanco (Spanish) light
skinned; white; blond.

Blane (Irish) a form of Blaine.
Blaney, Blanne

Blayne (Irish) a form of
Blaine.
Blayn, Blayney

Blaze (Latin) stammerer.
(English) flame; trail mark
made on a tree.
*Balázs, Biaggio, Biagio, Blaise,
Blaize, Blazen, Blazer*

Bliss (English) blissful; joyful.

Bly (Native American) high.

Blythe (English) carefree;
merry, joyful.
Blithe, Blyth

Bo (English) a form of Beau,
Beauregard. (German) a form
of Bogart.
Boe

Boaz (Hebrew) swift; strong.
Bo, Boas, Booz, Bos, Boz

Bob (English) a short form of
Robert.
Bobb, Bobby, Bobek, Rob

Bobby (English) a familiar
form of Bob, Robert.
*Bobbey, Bobbi, Bobbie, Bobbye,
Boby*

Bobek (Czech) a form of
Bob, Robert.

Boden (Scandinavian) shel-
tered. (French) messenger,
herald.
*Bodie, Bodin, Bodine, Bodyne,
Boe*

Bodie (Scandinavian) a famil-
iar form of Boden.
*Boddie, Bode, Bodee, Bodey,
Bodhi, Bodi, Boedee, Boedi,
Boedy*

Bodil (Norwegian) mighty
ruler.

Bodua (Akan) animal's tail.

Bogart (German) strong as a
bow. (Irish, Welsh) bog,
marshland.
Bo, Bogey, Bogie, Bogy

Bohdan (Ukrainian) a form of Donald.
Bogdan, Bogdashka, Bogdon, Bohden, Bohdon

Bonaro (Italian, Spanish) friend.
Bona, Bonar

Bonaventure (Italian) good luck.

Bond (English) tiller of the soil.
Bondie, Bondon, Bonds, Bondy

Boniface (Latin) do-gooder.
Bonifacio, Bonifacius, Bonifacy

Booker (English) bookmaker; book lover; Bible lover.
Bookie, Books, Booky

Boone (Latin, French) good. History: Daniel Boone was an American pioneer.
Bon, Bone, Bonne, Boonie, Boony

Booth (English) hut. (Scandinavian) temporary dwelling.
Boot, Boote, Boothe

Borak (Arabic) lightning. Mythology: the horse that carried Muhammed to seventh heaven.

Borden (French) cottage. (English) valley of the boar; boar's den.
Bord, Bordie, Bordy

Borg (Scandinavian) castle.

Boris (Slavic) battler, warrior. Religion: the patron saint of Moscow, princes, and Russia.
Boriss, Borja, Borris, Borya, Boryenka, Borys

Borka (Russian) fighter.
Borkinka

Boseda (Tiv) born on Saturday.

Bosley (English) grove of trees.

Botan (Japanese) blossom, bud.

Bourey (Cambodian) country.

Bourne (Latin, French) boundary. (English) brook, stream.

Boutros (Arabic) a form of Peter.

Bowen (Welsh) son of Owen.
Bow, Bowe, Bowie

Bowie (Irish) yellow haired. History: James Bowie was an American-born Mexican colonist who died during the defense of the Alamo.
Bow, Bowen

Boyce (French) woods, forest.
Boice, Boise, Boy, Boycey, Boycie

Boyd (Scottish) yellow haired.
Boid, Boyde

Brad (English) a short form of Bradford, Bradley.
Bradd, Brade

Bradburn (English) broad stream.

Braden (English) broad valley.
Bradan, Bradden, Bradeon, Bradin, Bradine, Bradyn, Braeden, Braiden, Brayden, Bredan, Bredon

Bradford (English) broad river crossing.
Brad, Braddford, Ford

Bradlee (English) a form of Bradley.
Bradlea, Bradleigh, Bradlie

Bradley (English) broad meadow.
Brad, Braddly, Bradlay, Bradlee, Bradly, Bradlyn, Bradney

Bradly (English) a form of Bradley.

Bradon (English) broad hill.
Braedon, Braidon, Braydon

Bradshaw (English) broad forest.

Brady (Irish) spirited. (English) broad island.
Bradey, Bradi, Bradie, Bradye, Braidy

Bradyn (English) a form of Braden.
Bradynne, Breidyn

Braeden, Braiden (English) forms of Braden.
Braedan, Braedin, Braedyn, Braidyn

Braedon (English) a form of Bradon.
Breadon

Bragi (Scandinavian) poet. Mythology: the god of poetry, eloquence, and song.
Brage

Braham (Hindi) creator.
Braheem, Braheim, Brahiem, Brahima, Brahm

Brainard (English) bold raven; prince.
Brainerd

Bram (Scottish) bramble, brushwood. (Hebrew) a short form of Abraham, Abram.
Brame, Bramm, Bramdon

Bramwell (English) bramble spring.
Brammel, Brammell, Bramwel, Bramwyll

Branch (Latin) paw; claw; tree branch.

Brand (English) firebrand; sword. A short form of Brandon.
Brandall, Brande, Brandel, Brandell, Brander, Brandley, Brandol, Brandt, Brandy, Brann

Brandeis (Czech) dweller on a burned clearing.
Brandis

Branden (English) beacon valley.
Brandden, Brandene, Brandin, Brandine, Brandyn, Breandan

Brandon (English) beacon hill.
Bran, Brand, Brandan, Branddon, Brandone, Brandonn, Brandyn, Branndan, Branndon, Brannon, Breandon, Brendon

Brandt (English) a form of Brant. .

Brandy (Dutch) brandy. (English) a familiar form of Brand.
Branddy, Brandey, Brandi, Brandie

Brandyn (English) a form of Branden, Brandon.
Brandynn

Brannon (Irish) a form of Brandon.
Branen, Brannan, Brannen, Branon

Branson (English) son of Brandon, Brant. A form of Bronson.
Bransen, Bransin, Brantson

Brant (English) proud.
Brandt, Brannt, Brante, Brantley, Branton

Brantley (English) a form of Brant.
Brantlie, Brantly, Brentlee, Brentley, Brently

Braulio (Italian) a form of Brawley.
Brauli, Brauliuo

Brawley (English) meadow on the hillside.
Braulio, Brawlee, Brawly

Braxton (English) Brock's town.
Brax, Braxdon, Braxston, Braxten, Braxtin, Braxxton

Brayan (Irish, Scottish) a form of Brian.
Brayn, Brayon

Brayden (English) a form of Braden.
Braydan, Braydn, Bradyn, Breydan, Breyden, Brydan, Bryden

Braydon (English) a form of Bradon.
Braydoon, Brydon, Breydon

Breck (Irish) freckled.
Brec, Breckan, Brecken, Breckie, Breckin, Breckke, Breckyn, Brek, Brexton

Brede (Scandinavian) iceberg, glacier.

Brencis (Latvian) a form of Lawrence.
Brence

Brendan (Irish) little raven. (English) sword.
Breandan, Bren, Brenden, Brendis, Brendon, Brendyn, Brenn, Brennan, Brennen, Brenndan, Brenyan, Bryn

Brenden (Irish) a form of
Brendan.
*Bren, Brendene, Brendin,
Brendine, Brennden*

Brendon (English) a form of
Brandon. (Irish, English) a
form of Brendan.
Brenndon

Brennan, Brennen (English,
Irish) forms of Brendan.
*Bren, Brenan, Brenen, Brenin,
Brenn, Brenna, Brennann,
Brenner, Brennin, Brennon,
Brennor, Brennyn, Brenon*

Brent (English) a short form
of Brenton.
Brendt, Brente, Brentson, Brentt

Brenton (English) steep hill.
*Brent, Brentan, Brenten,
Brentin, Brentten, Brentton,
Brentyn*

Bret, Brett (Scottish) from
Great Britain. See also
Britton.
*Bhrett, Braten, Braton, Brayton,
Bretin, Bretley, Bretlin, Breton,
Brettan, Brette, Bretten, Bretton,
Brit, Britt*

Brewster (English) brewer.
Brew, Brewer, Bruwster

Breyon (Irish, Scottish) a form
of Brian.
Breon, Breyan

Brian (Irish, Scottish) strong;
virtuous; honorable. History:
Brian Boru was an eleventh-

century Irish king and
national hero. See also
Palaina.
*Brayan, Breyon, Briana, Briann,
Brianna, Brianne, Briano,
Briant, Briante, Briaun,
Briayan, Brien, Brience, Brient,
Brin, Briny, Brion, Bryan,
Bryen*

Briar (French) heather.
Brier, Brierly, Bryar, Bryer, Bryor

Brice (Welsh) alert; ambitious.
(English) son of Rice.
Bricen, Briceton, Bryce

Brick (English) bridge.
*Bricker, Bricklen, Brickman,
Brik*

Bridger (English) bridge
builder.
*Bridd, Bridge, Bridgeley,
Bridgely*

Brigham (English) covered
bridge. (French) troops,
brigade.
Brig, Brigg, Briggs, Brighton

Brighton (English) bright
town.
*Breighton, Bright, Brightin,
Bryton*

Brion (Irish, Scottish) a form
of Brian.
Brieon, Brione, Brionn, Brionne

Brit, Britt (Scottish) forms of
Bret, Brett. See also Britton.
Brit, Brityce

Britton (Scottish) from Great Britain. See also Bret, Brett, Brit, Britt.
Britain, Briten, Britian, Britin, Briton, Brittain, Brittan, Britten, Brittian, Brittin, Britton

Brock (English) badger.
Broc, Brocke, Brockett, Brockie, Brockley, Brockton, Brocky, Brok, Broque

Brod (English) a short form of Broderick.
Brode, Broden

Broderick (Welsh) son of the famous ruler. (English) broad ridge. See also Roderick.
Brod, Broddie, Brodderick, Brodderrick, Broddy, Broderic, Broderrick, Brodrick,

Brodie (Irish) a form of Brody.
Brodi, Broedi

Brodrick (Welsh, English) a form of Broderick.
Broddrick, Brodric, Brodryck

Brody (Irish) ditch; canal builder.
Brodee, Broden, Brodey, Brodie, Broedy

Brogan (Irish) a heavy work shoe.
Brogen, Broghan, Broghen

Bromley (English) brushwood meadow.

Bron (Afrikaans) source.

Bronislaw (Polish) weapon of glory.

Bronson (English) son of Brown.
Bransen, Bransin, Branson, Bron, Bronnie, Bronnson, Bronny, Bronsan, Bronsen, Bronsin, Bronsonn, Bronsson, Bronsun, Bronsyn, Brunson

Brook (English) brook, stream.
Brooke, Brooker, Brookin, Brooklyn

Brooks (English) son of Brook.
Brookes, Broox

Brown (English) brown; bear.

Bruce (French) brushwood thicket; woods.
Brucey, Brucy, Brue, Bruis

Bruno (German, Italian) brown haired; brown skinned.
Brunon, Bruns

Bryan (Irish) a form of Brian.
Brayan, Bryann, Bryant, Bryen

Bryant (Irish) a form of Bryan.
Bryent

Bryce (Welsh) a form of Brice.
Brycen, Bryceton, Bryson, Bryston

Bryon (German) cottage.
(English) bear.
*Bryeon, Bryn, Bryne, Brynn,
Brynne, Bryone*

Bryson (Welsh) son of Brice.
Brysan, Brysen, Brysun, Brysyn

Bryton (English) a form of
Brighton.
*Brayten, Brayton, Breyton,
Bryeton, Brytan, Bryten, Brytin,
Brytten, Brytton*

Bubba (German) a boy.
Babba, Babe, Bebba

Buck (German, English) male
deer.
*Buckie, Buckley, Buckner,
Bucko, Bucky*

Buckley (English) deer
meadow.
Bucklea, Bucklee

Buckminster (English)
preacher.

Bud (English) herald, messenger.
Budd, Buddy

Buddy (American) a familiar
form of Bud.
Budde, Buddey, Buddie

Buell (German) hill dweller.
(English) bull.

Buford (English) ford near the
castle.
Burford

Burgess (English) town
dweller; shopkeeper.
*Burg, Burges, Burgh, Burgiss,
Burr*

Burian (Ukrainian) lives near
weeds.

Burke (German, French)
fortress, castle.
*Berk, Berke, Birk, Bourke,
Burk, Burkley*

Burl (English) cup bearer;
wine servant; knot in a tree.
(German) a short form of
Berlyn
Berl, Burley, Burlie, Byrle

Burleigh (English) meadow
with knotted tree trunks.
*Burlee, Burley, Burlie, Byrleigh,
Byrlee*

Burne (English) brook.
*Beirne, Burn, Burnell, Burnett,
Burney, Byrn, Byrne*

Burney (English) island with a
brook. A familiar form of
Rayburn.

Burr (Swedish) youth.
(English) prickly plant.

Burris (English) town dweller.

Burt (English) a form of Bert.
A short form of Burton.
Burrt, Burtt, Burty

Burton (English) fortified
town.
Berton, Burt

Busby (Scottish) village in the thicket; tall military hat made of fur.
Busbee, Buzby, Buzz

Buster (American) hitter, puncher.

Butch (American) a short form of Butcher.

Butcher (English) butcher.
Butch

Buzz (Scottish) a short form of Busby.
Buzzy

Byford (English) by the ford.

Byram (English) cattle yard.

Byrd (English) birdlike.
Bird, Birdie, Byrdie

Byrne (English) a form of Burne.
Byrn, Byrnes

Byron (French) cottage. (English) barn.
Beyren, Beyron, Biren, Biron, Buiron, Byram, Byran, Byrann, Byren, Byrom, Byrone

C

Cable (French, English) rope maker.
Cabell

Cadao (Vietnamese) folksong.

Cadby (English) warrior's settlement.

Caddock (Welsh) eager for war.

Cade (Welsh) a short form of Cadell.
Cady

Cadell (Welsh) battler.
Cade, Cadel, Cedell

Caden (American) a form of Kadin.
Cadan, Caddon, Cadian, Cadien, Cadin, Cadon, Cadyn, Caeden, Caedon, Caid, Caiden, Cayden

Cadmus (Greek) from the east. Mythology: a Phoenician prince who founded Thebes and introduced writing to the Greeks.

Caelan (Scottish) a form of Nicholas.
Cael, Caelon, Caelyn, Cailan, Cailean, Caillan, Cailun, Cailyn, Calan, Calen, Caleon, Caley, Calin, Callan, Callon, Callyn, Calon, Calyn, Caylan, Cayley

Caesar (Latin) long-haired. History: a title for Roman emperors. See also Kaiser, Kesar, Sarito.
Caesarae, Caesear, Caeser, Caezar, Caseare, Ceasar, Cesar, Ceseare, Cezar, Cézar, Czar, Seasar

Cahil (Turkish) young, naive.

Cai (Welsh) a form of Gaius.
Caio, Caius, Caw

Cain (Hebrew) spear; gatherer. Bible: Adam and Eve's oldest son. See also Kabil, Kane, Kayne.
Cainaen, Cainan, Caine, Cainen, Caineth, Cayn, Cayne

Cairn (Welsh) landmark made of a mound of stones.
Cairne, Carn, Carne

Cairo (Arabic) Geography: the capital of Egypt.
Kairo

Cal (Latin) a short form of Calvert, Calvin.

Calder (Welsh, English) brook, stream.

Caldwell (English) cold well.

Cale (Hebrew) a short form of Caleb.

Caleb (Hebrew) dog; faithful. (Arabic) bold, brave. Bible: one of the twelve spies sent by Moses. See also Kaleb, Kayleb.
Caeleb, Calab, Calabe, Cale, Caley, Calib, Calieb, Callob,

Calob, Calyb, Cayleb, Caylebb, Caylib, Caylob

Calen, Calin (Scottish) forms of Caelan.
Caelen, Caelin, Caellin, Cailen, Cailin, Caillin, Calean, Callen, Caylin

Caley (Irish) a familiar form of Caleb.
Calee, Caleigh

Calhoun (Irish) narrow woods. (Scottish) warrior.
Colhoun, Colhoune, Colquhoun

Callahan (Irish) descendant of Ceallachen.
Calahan, Callaghan

Callum (Irish) dove.
Callam, Calum, Calym

Calvert (English) calf herder.
Cal, Calbert, Calvirt

Calvin (Latin) bald. See also Kalvin, Vinny.
Cal, Calv, Calvien, Calvon, Calvyn

Cam (Gypsy) beloved. (Scottish) a short form of Cameron. (Latin, French, Scottish) a short form of Campbell.
Camm, Cammie, Cammy, Camy

Camaron (Scottish) a form of Cameron.
Camar, Camari, Camaran, Camaren

Camden (Scottish) winding valley.
Kamden

Cameron (Scottish) crooked nose. See also Kameron.
Cam, Camaron, Cameran, Cameren, Camerin, Cameroun, Camerron, Camerson, Camerun, Cameryn, Camiren, Camiron, Cammeron, Camron

Camille (French) young ceremonial attendant.
Camile

Camilo (Latin) child born to freedom; noble.
Camiel, Camillo, Camillus

Campbell (Latin, French) beautiful field. (Scottish) crooked mouth.
Cam, Camp, Campy

Camron (Scottish) a short form of Cameron.
Camren, Cammrin, Cammron, Camran, Cameron, Camrin, Camryn, Camrynn

Canaan (French) a form of Cannon. History: an ancient region between the Jordan River and the Mediterranean.
Canan, Canen, Caynan

Candide (Latin) pure; sincere.
Candid, Candido, Candonino

Cannon (French) church official; large gun. See also Kannon.
Canaan, Cannan, Cannen, Cannin, Canning, Canon

Canute (Latin) white haired. (Scandinavian) knot. History: a Danish king who became king of England after 1016. See also Knute.
Cnut, Cnute

Cappi (Gypsy) good fortune.

Car (Irish) a short form of Carney.

Carey (Greek) pure. (Welsh) castle; rocky island. See also Karey.
Care, Caree, Cari, Carre, Carree, Carrie, Cary

Carl (German, English) a short form of Carlton. A form of Charles. See also Carroll, Kale, Kalle, Karl, Karlen, Karol.
Carle, Carles, Carless, Carlis, Carll, Carlo, Carlos, Carlson, Carlston, Carlus, Carolos

Carlin (Irish) little champion.
Carlan, Carlen, Carley, Carlie, Carling, Carlino, Carly

Carlisle (English) Carl's island.
Carlyle, Carlysle

Carlito (Spanish) a familiar form of Carlos.
Carlitos

Carlo (Italian) a form of Carl, Charles.
Carolo

Carlos (Spanish) a form of Carl, Charles.
Carlito

Carlton (English) Carl's town.
Carl, Carleton, Carllton, Carlston, Carltonn, Carltton, Charlton

Carmel (Hebrew) vineyard, garden. See also Carmine.
Carmello, Carmelo, Karmel

Carmichael (Scottish) follower of Michael.

Carmine (Latin) song; crimson. (Italian) a form of Carmel.
Carmain, Carmaine, Carman, Carmen, Carmon

Carnelius (Greek, Latin) a form of Cornelius.
Carnealius, Carneilius, Carnellius, Carnilious

Carnell (English) defender of the castle. (French) a form of Cornell.

Carney (Irish) victorious. (Scottish) fighter. See also Kearney.
Car, Carny, Karney

Carr (Scandinavian) marsh. See also Kerr.
Karr

Carrick (Irish) rock.
Carooq, Carricko

Carrington (Welsh) rocky town.

Carroll (Irish) champion. (German) a form of Carl.
Carel, Carell, Cariel, Cariell, Carol, Carole, Carolo, Carols, Carollan, Carolus, Carrol, Cary, Caryl

Carson (English) son of Carr.
Carsen, Carsino, Carrson, Karson

Carsten (Greek) a form of Karsten.
Carston

Carter (English) cart driver.
Cart

Cartwright (English) cart builder.

Carvell (French, English) village on the marsh.
Carvel, Carvelle, Carvellius

Carver (English) wood-carver; sculptor.

Cary (Welsh) a form of Carey. (German, Irish) a form of Carroll.
Carray, Carry

Case (Irish) a short form of
Casey. (English) a short form
of Casimir.

Casey (Irish) brave.
*Case, Casie, Casy, Cayse,
Caysey, Kacey, Kasey*

Cash (Latin) vain. (Slavic) a
short form of Casimir.
Cashe

Casimir (Slavic) peacemaker.
*Cachi, Cas, Case, Cash,
Cashemere, Cashi, Cashmeire,
Cashmere, Casimere, Casimire,
Casimiro, Castimer, Kasimir,
Kazio*

Casper (Persian) treasurer.
(German) imperial. See also
Gaspar, Jasper, Kasper.
Caspar, Cass

Cass (Irish, Persian) a short
form of Casper, Cassidy.

Cassidy (Irish) clever; curly
haired. See also Kazio.
*Casidy, Cass, Cassady, Cassie,
Kassidy*

Cassie (Irish) a familiar form
of Cassidy.
*Casi, Casie, Casio, Cassey,
Cassy, Casy*

Cassius (Latin, French) box;
protective cover.
Cassia, Cassio, Cazzie

Castle (Latin) castle.
Cassle, Castel

Castor (Greek) beaver.
Astrology: one of the twins
in the constellation Gemini.
Mythology: one of the
patron saints of mariners.
Caster, Caston

Cater (English) caterer.

Cato (Latin) knowledgeable,
wise.
Caton, Catón

Cavan (Irish) handsome. See
also Kevin.
Caven, Cavin, Cavan, Cawoun

Cayden (American) a form of
Caden.
Cayde, Caydin

Caylan (Scottish) a form of
Caelan.
Caylans, Caylen, Caylon

Cazzie (American) a familiar
form of Cassius.
Caz, Cazz, Cazzy

Ceasar (Latin) a form of Caesar.
Ceaser

Cecil (Latin) blind.
*Cece, Cecile, Cecilio, Cecilius,
Cecill, Celio, Siseal*

Cedric (English) battle chief-
tain. See also Kedrick, Rick.
*Cad, Caddaric, Ced, Cederic,
Cedrec, Cédric, Cedrick,
Cedryche, Sedric*

Cedrick (English) a form of Cedric.
Ceddrick, Cederick, Cederrick, Cedirick, Cedrik

Ceejay (American) a combination of the initials C. + J.
Cejay, C.J.

Cemal (Arabic) attractive.

Cephas (Latin) small rock. Bible: the term used by Jesus to describe Peter.
Cepheus, Cephus

Cerdic (Welsh) beloved.
Caradoc, Caradog, Ceredig, Ceretic

Cerek (Polish) lordly. (Greek) a form of Cyril.

Cesar (Spanish) a form of Caesar.
Casar, César, Cesare, Cesareo, Cesario, Cesaro, Cessar

Cestmir (Czech) fortress.

Cezar (Slavic) a form of Caesar.
Cézar, Cezary, Cezek, Chezrae, Sezar

Chace (French) a form of Chase.
Chayce

Chad (English) warrior. A short form of Chadwick. Geography: a country in north-central Africa.
Ceadd, Chaad, Chadd, Chaddie, Chaddy, Chade,
Chadleigh, Chadler, Chadley, Chadlin, Chadlyn, Chadmen, Chado, Chadron, Chady

Chadrick (German) mighty warrior.
Chaddrick, Chaderic, Chaderick, Chadrack, Chadric

Chadwick (English) warrior's town.
Chad, Chaddwick, Chadvic, Chadwyck

Chago (Spanish) a form of Jacob.
Chango, Chanti

Chaim (Hebrew) life. See also Hyman.
Chai, Chaimek, Haim, Khaim

Chaise (French) a form of Chase.
Chais, Chaisen, Chaison

Chal (Gypsy) boy; son.
Chalie, Chalin

Chalmers (Scottish) son of the lord.
Chalmer, Chalmr, Chamar, Chamarr

Cham (Vietnamese) hard worker.
Chams

Chan (Sanskrit) shining. (English) a form of Chauncey. (Spanish) a form of Juan.
Chann, Chano, Chayo

Chanan (Hebrew) cloud.

Chico (Spanish) boy.

Chik (Gypsy) earth.

Chike (Ibo) God's power.

Chiko (Japanese) arrow; pledge.

Chilo (Spanish) a familiar form of Francisco.

Chilton (English) farm by the spring.
Chil, Chill, Chillton, Chilt

Chim (Vietnamese) bird.

Chinua (Ibo) God's blessing.
Chino, Chinou

Chioke (Ibo) gift of God.

Chip (English) a familiar form of Charles.
Chipman, Chipper

Chiram (Hebrew) exalted; noble.

Chris (Greek) a short form of Christian, Christopher. See also Kris.
Chriss, Christ, Chrys, Cris, Crist

Christain (Greek) a form of Christian.
Christai, Christan, Christane, Christaun, Christein

Christian (Greek) follower of Christ; anointed. See also Jaan, Kerstan, Khristian, Kit, Krister, Kristian, Krystian.
Chretien, Chris, Christa, Christain, Christé, Christen, Christensen, Christiaan, Christiana, Christiane, Christiann, Christianna, Christianno, Christiano, Christianos, Christien, Christin, Christino, Christion, Christon, Christos, Christyan, Christyon, Chritian, Chrystian, Cristian, Crystek

Christien (Greek) a form of Christian.
Christienne, Christinne, Chrystien

Christofer (Greek) a form of Christopher.
Christafer, Christafur, Christefor, Christerfer, Christifer, Christoffer, Christofher, Christofper, Chrystofer

Christoff (Russian) a form of Christopher.
Chrisof, Christif, Christof, Cristofe

Christophe (French) a form of Christopher.
Christoph

Christopher (Greek) Christ-bearer. Religion: the patron saint of travelers. See also Cristopher, Kester, Kit, Kristopher, Risto, Stoffel, Tobal, Topher.
Chris, Chrisopherson, Christapher, Christepher, Christerpher, Christhoper, Christipher, Christobal, Christofer, Christoff, Christoforo, Christoher, Christopehr, Christoper, Christophe,

Christopher *(cont.)*
Christopherr, Christophor,
Christophoros, Christophr,
Christophre, Christophyer,
Christophyr, Christorpher,
Christos, Christovao, Christpher,
Christphere, Christphor,
Christpor, Christrpher,
Chrystopher, Cristobal

Christophoros (Greek) a
form of Christopher.
Christoforo, Christoforos,
Christophor, Christophorus,
Christphor, Cristoforo,
Cristopher

Christos (Greek) a form of
Christopher. See also
Khristos.

Chucho (Hebrew) a familiar
form of Jesus.

Chuck (American) a familiar
form of Charles.
Chuckey, Chuckie, Chucky

Chui (Swahili) leopard.

Chul (Korean) firm.

Chuma (Ibo) having many
beads, wealthy. (Swahili) iron.

Chuminga (Spanish) a familiar
form of Dominic.
Chumin

Chumo (Spanish) a familiar
form of Thomas.

Chun (Chinese) spring.

Chung (Chinese) intelligent.
Chungo, Chuong

Churchill (English) church on
the hill. History: Sir Winston
Churchill served as British
prime minister and won a
Nobel Prize for literature.

Cian (Irish) ancient.
Céin, Cianán, Kian

Cicero (Latin) chickpea.
History: a famous Roman
orator, philosopher, and
statesman.
Cicerón

Cid (Spanish) lord. History:
title for Rodrigo Díaz de
Vivar, an eleventh-century
Spanish soldier and national
hero.
Cyd

Ciqala (Dakota) little.

Cirrillo (Italian) a form of Cyril.
Cirilio, Cirillo, Cirilo, Ciro

Cisco (Spanish) a short form
of Francisco.

Clancy (Irish) redheaded
fighter.
Clancey, Claney

Clare (Latin) a short form of
Clarence.
Clair, Clarey, Clary

Clarence (Latin) clear; victori-
ous.
Clarance, Clare, Clarrance,
Clarrence, Clearence

Clark (French) cleric; scholar.
Clarke, Clerc, Clerk

Claude (Latin, French) lame.
*Claud, Claudan, Claudel,
Claudell, Claudey, Claudi,
Claudian, Claudianus, Claudie,
Claudien, Claudin, Claudio,
Claudis, Claudius, Claudy*

Claudio (Italian) a form of
Claude.

Claus (German) a short form
of Nicholas. See also Klaus.
Claas, Claes, Clause

Clay (English) clay pit. A short
form of Clayborne, Clayton.
Klay

Clayborne (English) brook
near the clay pit.
*Claibern, Claiborn, Claiborne,
Claibrone, Clay, Claybon,
Clayborn, Claybourn,
Claybourne, Clayburn,
Clebourn*

Clayton (English) town built
on clay.
*Clay, Clayten, Cleighton,
Cleyton, Clyton, Klayton*

Cleary (Irish) learned.

Cleavon (English) cliff.
*Clavin, Clavion, Clavon,
Clavone, Clayvon, Claywon,
Clévon, Clevonn, Clyvon*

Clem (Latin) a short form of
Clement.
Cleme, Clemmy, Clim

Clement (Latin) merciful.
Bible: a coworker of Paul.
See also Klement, Menz.
*Clem, Clemens, Clément,
Clemente, Clementius,
Clemmons*

Clemente (Italian, Spanish) a
form of Clement.
Clemento, Clemenza

Cleon (Greek) famous.
Kleon

Cletus (Greek) illustrious.
History: a Roman pope and
martyr.
*Cleatus, Cledis, Cleotis, Clete,
Cletis*

Cleveland (English) land of
cliffs.
*Cleaveland, Cleavland,
Cleavon, Cleve, Clevelend,
Clevelynn, Clevey, Clevie,
Clevon*

Cliff (English) a short form of
Clifford, Clifton.
*Clif, Clift, Clive, Clyff, Clyph,
Kliff*

Clifford (English) cliff at the
river crossing.
Cliff, Cliford, Clyfford, Klifford

Clifton (English) cliff town.
*Cliff, Cliffton, Clift, Cliften,
Clyfton*

Clint (English) a short form of
Clinton.
Klint

Clinton (English) hill town.
*Clenten, Clint, Clinten,
Clintion, Clintton, Clynton,
Klinton*

Clive (English) a form of Cliff.
*Cleve, Clivans, Clivens, Clyve,
Klyve*

Clovis (German) famous soldier. See also Louis.

Cluny (Irish) meadow.

Clyde (Welsh) warm.
(Scottish) Geography: a river
in Scotland.
Cly, Clywd, Klyde

Coby (Hebrew) a familiar
form of Jacob.
*Cob, Cobby, Cobe, Cobey, Cobi,
Cobia, Cobie*

Cochise (Apache) hardwood.
History: a famous Chiricahua
Apache leader.

Coco (French) a familiar form
of Jacques.
Coko, Koko

Codey (English) a form of
Cody.
Coday

Codi, Codie (English) forms
of Cody.
Coadi, Codea

Cody (English) cushion.
History: William "Buffalo
Bill" Cody was an American
frontier scout who toured
America and Europe with
his Wild West show. See also
Kody.
*Coady, Coddy, Code, Codee,
Codell, Codey, Codi, Codiak,
Codie, Coedy*

Coffie (Ewe) born on Friday.

Cola (Italian) a familiar form
of Nicholas, Nicola.
Colas

Colar (French) a form of
Nicholas.

Colbert (English) famous seafarer.
Cole, Colt, Colvert, Culbert

Colby (English) dark; dark
haired.
*Colbey, Colbi, Colbie, Colbin,
Colebee, Coleby, Collby, Kolby*

Cole (Latin) cabbage farmer.
(English) a short form of
Coleman.
Colet, Coley, Colie, Kole

Coleman (Latin) cabbage
farmer. (English) coal miner.
*Cole, Colemann, Colm,
Colman, Koleman*

Colin (Irish) young cub.
(Greek) a short form of
Nicholas.
*Cailean, Colan, Cole, Colen,
Coleon, Colinn, Collin, Colyn,
Kolin*

Colley (English) black haired;
swarthy.
Colee, Collie, Collis

Collier (English) miner.
Colier, Collayer, Collie, Collyer, Colyer

Collin (Scottish) a form of Colin, Collins.
Collan, Collen, Collian, Collon, Collyn

Collins (Greek) son of Colin. (Irish) holly.
Collin, Collis

Colson (Greek, English) son of Nicholas.
Colsen, Coulson

Colt (English) young horse; frisky. A short form of Colter, Colton.
Colte

Colten (English) a form of Colton.

Colter (English) herd of colts.
Colt

Colton (English) coal town.
Colt, Coltan, Colten, Coltin, Coltinn, Coltn, Coltrane, Colttan, Coltton, Coltun, Coltyn, Coltyne, Kolton

Columba (Latin) dove.
Coim, Colum, Columbia, Columbus

Colwyn (Welsh) Geography: a river in Wales.
Colwin, Colwinn

Coman (Arabic) noble. (Irish) bent.
Comán

Conall (Irish) high, mighty.
Conal, Connal, Connel, Connell, Connelly, Connolly

Conan (Irish) praised; exalted. (Scottish) wise.
Conant, Conary, Connen, Connie, Connon, Connor, Conon

Conary (Irish) a form of Conan.
Conaire

Conlan (Irish) hero.
Conlen, Conley, Conlin, Conlyn

Conner (Irish) a form of Connor.
Connar, Connary, Conneer, Connery, Konner

Connie (English, Irish) a familiar form of Conan, Conrad, Constantine, Conway.
Con, Conn, Conney, Conny

Connor (Scottish) wise. (Irish) a form of Conan.
Conner, Connoer, Connory, Connyr, Conor, Konner, Konnor

Conor (Irish) a form of Connor.
Conar, Coner, Conour, Konner

Conrad (German) brave counselor.
Connie, Conrade, Conrado, Corrado, Konrad

Conroy (Irish) wise.
Conry, Roy

Constant (Latin) a short form of Constantine.

Constantine (Latin) firm, constant. History: Constantine the Great was the Roman emperor who adopted the Christian faith. See also Dinos, Konstantin, Stancio.
Connie, Constadine, Constandine, Constandios, Constanstine, Constant, Constantin, Constantino, Constantinos, Constantios, Costa

Conway (Irish) hound of the plain.
Connie, Conwy

Cook (English) cook.
Cooke

Cooper (English) barrel maker. See also Keiffer.
Coop, Couper

Corbett (Latin) raven.
Corbbitt, Corbet, Corbette, Corbit, Corbitt

Corbin (Latin) raven.
Corban, Corben, Corbey, Corbie, Corbon, Corby, Corbyn, Korbin

Corcoran (Irish) ruddy.

Cordaro (Spanish) a form of Cordero.
Coradaro, Cordairo, Cordara, Cordarel, Cordarell, Cordarelle, Cordareo, Cordarin, Cordario, Cordarion, Cordarious, Cordarius, Cordarrel, Cordarrell, Cordarris, Cordarrius, Cordarro, Cordarrol, Cordarus, Cordarryl, Cordaryal, Corddarro, Corrdarl

Cordell (French) rope maker.
Cord, Cordae, Cordale, Corday, Cordeal, Cordeil, Cordel, Cordele, Cordelle, Cordie, Cordy, Kordell

Cordero (Spanish) little lamb.
Cordaro, Cordeal, Cordeara, Cordearo, Cordeiro, Cordelro, Corder, Cordera, Corderall, Corderias, Corderious, Corderral, Corderro, Corderryn, Corderun, Corderus, Cordiaro, Cordierre, Cordy, Corrderio

Corey (Irish) hollow. See also Korey, Kory.
Core, Coreaa, Coree, Cori, Corian, Corie, Corio, Correy, Corria, Corrie, Corry, Corrye, Cory

Cormac (Irish) raven's son. History: a third-century king of Ireland who was a great lawmaker.
Cormack, Cormick

Cornelius (Greek) cornel tree. (Latin) horn colored. See also Kornel, Kornelius, Nelek.
Carnelius, Conny, Cornealous, Corneili, Corneilius, Corneilus, Corneliaus, Cornelious, Cornelias, Cornelis, Corneliu,

Cornell, Cornellious, Cornellis,
Cornellius, Cornelous,
Corneluis, Cornelus, Corney,
Cornie, Cornielius, Corniellus,
Corny, Cournelius, Cournelyous,
Nelius, Nellie

Cornell (French) a form of
Cornelius.
Carnell, Cornall, Corneil,
Cornel, Cornelio, Corney,
Cornie, Corny, Nellie

Cornwallis (English) from
Cornwall.

Corrado (Italian) a form of
Conrad.
Carrado

Corrigan (Irish) spearman.
Carrigan, Carrigen, Corrigon,
Corrigun, Korrigan

Corrin (Irish) spear carrier.
Corin, Corion

Corry (Latin) a form of
Corey.

Cort (German) bold.
(Scandinavian) short.
(English) a short form of
Courtney.
Corte, Cortie, Corty, Kort

Cortez (Spanish) conqueror.
History: Hernando Cortés
was a Spanish conquistador
who conquered Aztec
Mexico.
Cartez, Cortes, Cortis, Cortize,
Courtes, Courtez, Curtez,
Kortez

Corwin (English) heart's com-
panion; heart's delight.
Corwinn, Corwyn, Corwynn,
Corwynne

Cory (Latin) a form of Corey.
(French) a familiar form of
Cornell. (Greek) a short
form of Corydon.
Corye

Corydon (Greek) helmet, crest.
Coridon, Corradino, Cory,
Coryden, Coryell

Cosgrove (Irish) victor, champion.

Cosmo (Greek) orderly; har-
monious; universe.
Cos, Cosimo, Cosme, Cosmé,
Cozmo, Kosmo

Costa (Greek) a short form of
Constantine.
Costandinos, Costantinos,
Costas, Costes

Coty (French) slope, hillside.
Cote, Cotee, Cotey, Coti, Cotie,
Cotty, Cotye

Courtland (English) court's
land.
Court, Courtlan, Courtlana,
Courtlandt, Courtlin,
Courtlind, Courtlon, Courtlyn,
Kourtland

Courtney (English) court.
Cort, Cortnay, Cortne, Cortney,
Court, Courten, Courtenay,
Courteney, Courtnay, Courtnee,
Curt, Kortney

Cowan (Irish) hillside hollow.
*Coe, Coven, Covin, Cowen,
Cowey, Cowie*

Coy (English) woods.
Coye, Coyie, Coyt

Coyle (Irish) leader in battle.

Coyne (French) modest.
Coyan

Craddock (Welsh) love.
Caradoc, Caradog

Craig (Irish, Scottish) crag;
steep rock.
*Crag, Craige, Craigen, Craigery,
Craigh, Craigon, Creag, Creg,
Cregan, Cregg, Creig, Creigh,
Criag, Kraig*

Crandall (English) crane's val-
ley.
*Cran, Crandal, Crandel,
Crandell, Crendal*

Crawford (English) ford
where crows fly.
Craw, Crow, Ford

Creed (Latin) belief.
Creedon

Creighton (English) town
near the rocks.
*Cray, Crayton, Creighm,
Creight, Creighto, Crichton*

Crepin (French) a form of
Crispin.

Crispin (Latin) curly haired.
Crepin, Cris, Crispian,

*Crispien, Crispino, Crispo,
Krispin*

Cristian (Greek) a form of
Christian.
*Crétien, Cristean, Cristhian,
Cristiano, Cristien, Cristino,
Cristle, Criston, Cristos, Cristy,
Cristyan, Crystek, Crystian*

Cristobal (Greek) a form of
Christopher.
Cristóbal, Cristoval, Cristovao

Cristoforo (Italian) a form of
Christopher.
Cristofor

Cristopher (Greek) a form of
Christopher.
*Cristaph, Cristhofer, Cristifer,
Cristofer, Cristoph, Cristophe,
Crystapher, Crystifer*

Crofton (Irish) town with
cottages.

Cromwell (English) crooked
spring, winding spring.

Crosby (Scandinavian) shrine
of the cross.
Crosbey, Crosbie, Cross

Crosley (English) meadow of
the cross.
Cross

Crowther (English) fiddler.

Cruz (Portuguese, Spanish)
cross.
Cruze, Kruz

Crystek (Polish) a form of Christian.

Cullen (Irish) handsome.
Cull, Cullan, Cullie, Cullin

Culley (Irish) woods.
Cullie, Cully

Culver (English) dove.
Colver, Cull, Cullie, Cully

Cunningham (Irish) village of the milk pail.

Curran (Irish) hero.
Curan, Curon, Curr, Curren, Currey, Curri, Currie, Currin, Curry

Currito (Spanish) a form of Curtis.
Curcio

Curt (Latin) a short form of Courtney, Curtis. See also Kurt.

Curtis (Latin) enclosure. (French) courteous. See also Kurtis.
Curio, Currito, Curt, Curtice, Curtiss, Curtus

Cuthbert (English) brilliant.

Cutler (English) knife maker.
Cut, Cuttie, Cutty

Cy (Persian) a short form of Cyrus.

Cyle (Irish) a form of Kyle.

Cyprian (Latin) from the island of Cyprus.
Ciprian, Cipriano, Ciprien, Cyprien

Cyrano (Greek) from Cyrene, an ancient city in North Africa. Literature: *Cyrano de Bergerac* is a play by Edmond Rostand about a great guardsman and poet whose large nose prevented him from pursuing the woman he loved.

Cyril (Greek) lordly. See also Kiril.
Cerek, Cerel, Cyrell, Ceril, Ciril, Cirillo, Cirrillo, Cyra, Cyrel, Cyrell, Cyrelle, Cyrill, Cyrille, Cyrillus, Syrell, Syril

Cyrus (Persian) sun. Historical: Cyrus the Great was a king in ancient Persia. See also Kir.
Ciro, Cy, Cyress, Cyris, Cyriss, Cyruss, Syris, Syrus

D

Dabi (Basque) a form of David.

Dabir (Arabic) tutor.

Dacey (Latin) from Dacia, an area now in Romania. (Irish) southerner.
Dace, Dache, Dacian, Dacias, Dacio, Dacy, Daicey, Daicy

Dada (Yoruba) curly haired.
Dadi

Daegel (English) from Daegel,
England.

Daelen (English) a form of
Dale.
*Daelan, Daelin, Daelon,
Daelyn, Daelyne*

Daemon (Greek) a form of
Damian. (Greek, Latin) a
form of Damon.
*Daemean, Daemeon, Daemien,
Daemin, Daemion, Daemyen*

Daequan (American) a form
of Daquan.
*Daequane, Daequon, Daequone,
Daeqwan*

Daeshawn (American) a com-
bination of the prefix Da +
Shawn.
*Daesean, Daeshaun, Daeshon,
Daeshun, Daisean, Daishaun,
Daishawn, Daishon, Daishoun*

Daevon (American) a form of
Davon.
*Daevion, Daevohn, Daevonne,
Daevonte, Daevontey*

Dafydd (Welsh) a form of
David.
Dafyd

Dag (Scandinavian) day; bright.
*Daeg, Daegan, Dagen, Dagny,
Deegan*

Dagan (Hebrew) corn; grain.
*Daegan, Daegon, Dagen,
Dageon, Dagon*

Dagwood (English) shining
forest.

Dai (Japanese) big.

Daimian (Greek) a form of
Damian.
*Daiman, Daimean, Daimen,
Daimeon, Daimeyon, Daimien,
Daimin, Daimion, Daimyan*

Daimon (Greek, Latin) a form
of Damon.
Daimone

Daiquan (American) a form
of Dajuan.
*Daekwaun, Daekwon, Daiqone,
Daiqua, Daiquane, Daiquawn,
Daiquon, Daiqwan, Daiqwon*

Daivon (American) a form of
Davon.
*Daivain, Daivion, Daivonn,
Daivonte, Daiwan*

Dajon (American) a form of
Dajuan.
*Dajean, Dajiawn, Dajin,
Dajion, Dajn, Dajohn, Dajonae*

Dajuan (American) a combi-
nation of the prefix Da +
Juan. See also Dejuan.
*Daejon, Daejuan, Daiquan,
Dajon, Da Jon, Da-Juan,
Dajwan, Dajwoun, Dakuan,
Dakwan, Dawan, Dawaun,
Dawawn, Dawon, Dawoyan,*

Dijuan, Diuan, Dujuan,
D'Juan, D'juan, Dwaun

Dakarai (Shona) happy.
Dakairi, Dakar, Dakaraia,
Dakari, Dakarri

Dakoda (Dakota) a form of
Dakota.
Dacoda, Dacodah, Dakodah,
Dakodas

Dakota (Dakota) friend; part-
ner; tribal name.
Dac, Dack, Dackota, Dacota,
DaCota, Dak, Dakcota,
Dakkota, Dakoata, Dakoda,
Dakotah, Dakotha, Dakotta,
Dekota

Dakotah (Dakota) a form of
Dakota.
Dakottah

Daksh (Hindi) efficient.

Dalal (Sanskrit) broker.

Dalbert (English) bright, shining. See also Delbert.

Dale (English) dale, valley.
Dael, Daelen, Dal, Dalen,
Daley, Dalibor, Dallan, Dallin,
Dallyn, Daly, Dayl, Dayle

Dalen (English) a form of Dale.
Dailin, Dalaan, Dalan, Dalane,
Daleon, Dalian, Dalibor, Dalione,
Dallan, Dalon, Daylan, Daylen,
Daylin, Daylon

Daley (Irish) assembly. (English)
a familiar form of Dale.
Daily, Daly, Dawley

Dallan (English) a form of Dale.
Dallen, Dallon

Dallas (Scottish) valley of
the water; resting place.
Geography: a town in
Scotland; a city in Texas.
Dal, Dalieass, Dall, Dalles,
Dallis, Dalys, Dellis

Dallin, Dallyn (English) pride's
people.
Dalin, Dalyn

Dalston (English) Daegel's
place.
Dalis, Dallon

Dalton (English) town in the
valley.
Dal, Dalaton, Dallton, Dalt,
Daltan, Dalten, Daltin, Daltyn,
Daulton, Delton

Dalvin (English) a form of
Delvin.
Dalven, Dalvon, Dalvyn

Dalziel (Scottish) small field.

Damar (American) a short
form of Damarcus, Damario.
Damare, Damari, Damarre,
Damauri

Damarcus (American) a com-
bination of the prefix Da +
Marcus.
Damacus, Damar, Damarco,
Damarcue, Damarick, Damark,
Damarkco, Damarkis, Damarko,
Damarkus, Damarques,
Damarquez, Damarquis,
Damarrco

Damario (Greek) gentle.
(American) a combination of
the prefix Da + Mario.
Damar, Damarea, Damareus,
Damaria, Damarie, Damarino,
Damarion, Damarious,
Damaris, Damarius, Damarrea,
Damarrion, Damarrious,
Damarrius, Damaryo, Dameris,
Damerius

Damek (Slavic) a form of
Adam.
Damick, Damicke

Dameon (Greek) a form of
Damian.
Damein, Dameion, Dameone

Dametrius (Greek) a form of
Demetrius.
Dametri, Dametries,
Dametrious, Damitri, Damitric,
Damitrie, Damitrious,
Damitrius

Damian (Greek) tamer;
soother.
Daemon, Daimian, Damaiaon,
Damaian, Damaien, Damain,
Damaine, Damaion, Damani,
Damanni, Damaun, Damayon,
Dame, Damean, Dameon,
Damián, Damiane, Damiann,
Damiano, Damianos, Damien,
Damion, Damiyan, Damján,
Damyan, Daymian, Dema,
Demyan

Damien (Greek) a form of
Damian. Religion: Father
Damien ministered to the
leper colony on the
Hawaiian island Molokai.
Daemien, Daimien, Damie,
Damienne, Damyen

Damion (Greek) a form of
Damian.
Damieon, Damiion, Damin,
Damine, Damionne, Damiyon,
Dammion, Damyon

Damon (Greek) constant,
loyal. (Latin) spirit, demon.
Daemen, Daemon, Daemond,
Daimon, Daman, Damen,
Damond, Damone, Damoni,
Damonn, Damonni, Damonta,
Damontae, Damonte,
Damontez, Damontis, Damyn,
Daymon, Daymond

Dan (Vietnamese) yes. (Hebrew)
a short form of Daniel.
Dahn, Danh, Danne

Dana (Scandinavian) from
Denmark.
Dain, Daina, Dayna

Dandin (Hindi) holy man.

Dandré (French) a combina-
tion of the prefix De +
André.
D'André, Dandrae, D'andrea,
Dandras, Dandray, Dandre,
Dondrea

Dane (English) from
Denmark. See also Halden.
Dain, Daine, Danie, Dayne,
Dhane

Danek (Polish) a form of
Daniel.

Danforth (English) a form of
Daniel.

Danial (Hebrew) a form of
Daniel.
*Danal, Daneal, Danieal,
Daniyal, Dannial*

Danick, Dannick (Slavic)
familiar forms of Daniel.
*Danek, Danieko, Danik,
Danika, Danyck*

Daniel (Hebrew) God is my
judge. Bible: a Hebrew
prophet. See also Danno,
Kanaiela.
*Dacso, Dainel, Dan, Daneel,
Daneil, Danek, Danel,
Danforth, Danial, Danick,
Dániel, Daniël, Daniele,
Danielius, Daniell, Daniels,
Danielson, Danilo, Daniyel,
Dan'l, Dannel, Dannick,
Danniel, Dannil, Danno,
Danny, Dano, Danukas, Dany,
Danyel, Danyell, Daoud, Dasco,
Dayne, Deniel, Doneal, Doniel,
Donois, Dusan, Nelo*

Daniele (Hebrew) a form of
Daniel.
Danile, Danniele

Danilo (Slavic) a form of
Daniel.
*Danielo, Danil, Danila,
Danilka, Danylo*

Danior (Gypsy) born with
teeth.

Danladi (Hausa) born on
Sunday.

Danno (Hebrew) a familiar
form of Daniel. (Japanese)
gathering in the meadow.
(Hebrew) a familiar form of
Daniel.
Dannon, Dano

Dannon (American) a form of
Danno.
*Daenan, Daenen, Dainon,
Danaan, Danen, Danon*

Danny, Dany (Hebrew) famil-
iar forms of Daniel.
*Daney, Dani, Dannee, Danney,
Danni, Dannie, Dannye*

Dano (Czech) a form of
Daniel.
Danko, Danno

Dante, Danté (Latin) lasting,
enduring.
*Danatay, Danaté, Dant,
Dantae, Dantay, Dantee,
Dauntay, Dauntaye, Daunté,
Dauntrae, Deante, Dontae,
Donté*

Dantrell (American) a combi-
nation of Dante + Darell.
*Dantrel, Dantrey, Dantril,
Dantyrell, Dontrell*

Danyel (Hebrew) a form of
Daniel.
Danya, Danyal, Danyale,
Danyele, Danyell, Danyiel,
Danyl, Danyle, Danylets,
Danylo, Donyell

Daoud (Arabic) a form of
David.
Daudi, Daudy, Dauod, Dawud

Daquan (American) a combi-
nation of the prefix Da +
Quan.
Daequan, Daqon, Daquain,
Daquaine, Da'quan,
Daquandre, Daquandrey,
Daquane, Daquann,
Daquantae, Daquante,
Daquarius, Daquaun,
Daquawn, Daquin, Daquon,
Daquone, Daquwon, Daqwain,
Daqwan, Daqwane, Daqwann,
Daqwon, Daqwone, Dayquan,
Dequain, Dequan, Dequann,
Dequaun

Dar (Hebrew) pearl.

Dara (Cambodian) stars.

Daran (Irish) a form of Darren.
Darann, Darawn, Darian,
Darran, Dayran, Deran

Darby (Irish) free. (English)
deer park.
Dar, Darb, Darbee, Darbey,
Darbie, Derby

Darcy (Irish) dark. (French)
from Arcy, France.
Dar, Daray, D'Aray, Darce,

Darcee, Darcel, Darcey, Darcio,
D'Arcy, Darsey, Darsy

Dareh (Persian) wealthy.

Darell (English) a form of
Darrell.
Darall, Daralle, Dareal, Darel,
Darelle, Darral, Darrall

Daren (Hausa) born at night.
(Irish, English) a form of
Darren.
Dare, Dayren, Dheren

Darian, Darrian (Irish) forms
of Darren.
Daryan

Darick (German) a form of
Derek.
Darek, Daric, Darico, Darieck,
Dariek, Darik, Daryk

Darien, Darrien (Irish) forms
of Darren.

Darin (Irish) a form of
Darren.
Daryn, Darynn, Dayrin,
Dearin, Dharin

Dario (Spanish) affluent.

Darion Darrion (Irish) forms
of Darren.
Daryeon, Daryon

Darius (Greek) wealthy.
Dairus, Dare, Darieus,
Darioush, Dariuse, Dariush,
Dariuss, Dariusz, Darrius

Darnell (English) hidden place.
Dar, Darn, Darnall, Darneal, Darneil, Darnel, Darnelle, Darnyell, Darnyll

Daron (Irish) a form of Darren.
Daeron, Dairon, Darone, Daronn, Darroun, Dayron, Dearon, Dharon, Diron

Darrell (French) darling, beloved; grove of oak trees.
Dare, Darel, Darell, Darral, Darrel, Darrill, Darrol, Darryl, Derrell

Darren (Irish) great. (English) small; rocky hill.
Daran, Dare, Daren, Darian, Darien, Darin, Darion, Daron, Darran, Darrian, Darrien, Darrience, Darrin, Darrion, Darron, Darryn, Darun, Daryn, Dearron, Deren, Dereon, Derren, Derron

Darrick (German) a form of Derek.
Darrec, Darrek, Darric, Darrik, Darryk

Darrin (Irish) a form of Darren.

Darrion (Irish) a form of Darren.
Dairean, Dairion, Darian, Darien, Darion, Darrian, Darrien, Darrione, Darriyun, Derrian, Derrion

Darrius (Greek) a form of Darius.
Darreus, Darrias, Darrious, Darris, Darriuss, Darrus, Darryus, Derrious, Derris, Derrius

Darron (Irish) a form of Darren.
Darriun, Darroun

Darryl (French) darling, beloved; grove of oak trees. A form of Darrell.
Dahrll, Darryle, Darryll, Daryl, Daryle, Daryll, Derryl

Darshan (Hindi) god; godlike. Religion: another name for the Hindu god Shiva.
Darshaun, Darshon

Darton (English) deer town.
Dartel, Dartrel

Darwin (English) dear friend. History: Charles Darwin was the British naturalist who established the theory of evolution.
Darvin, Darvon, Darwyn, Derwin, Derwynn, Durwin

Daryl (French) a form of Darryl.
Darel, Daril, Darl, Darly, Daryell, Daryle, Daryll, Darylle, Daroyl

Dasan (Pomo) leader of the bird clan.
Dassan

Dashawn (American) a combination of the prefix Da + Shawn.
Dasean, Dashan, Dashane, Dashante, Dashaun, Dashaunte, Dashean, Dashon, Dashonnie, Dashonte, Dashuan, Dashun, Dashwan, Dayshawn

Dauid (Swahili) a form of David.

Daulton (English) a form of Dalton.

Davante (American) a form of Davonte.
Davanta, Davantay, Davinte

Davaris (American) a combination of Dave + Darius.
Davario, Davarious, Davarius, Davarrius, Davarus

Dave (Hebrew) a short form of David, Davis.

Davey (Hebrew) a familiar form of David.
Davee, Davi, Davie, Davy

David (Hebrew) beloved. Bible: the second king of Israel. See also Dov, Havika, Kawika, Taaveti, Taffy, Tevel.
Dabi, Daevid, Dafydd, Dai, Daivid, Daoud, Dauid, Dav, Dave, Daved, Daveed, Daven, Davey, Davidde, Davide, Davidek, Davido, Davon, Davoud, Davyd, Dawid, Dawit, Dawud, Dayvid, Dodya, Dov

Davin (Scandinavian) brilliant Finn.
Daevin, Davion, Davon, Davyn, Dawan, Dawin, Dawine, Dayvon, Deavan, Deaven

Davion (American) a form of Davin.
Davione, Davionne, Daviyon, Davyon, Deaveon

Davis (Welsh) son of David.
Dave, Davidson, Davies, Davison

Davon (American) a form of Davin.
Daevon, Daivon, Davon, Davone, Davonn, Davonne, Deavon, Deavone, Devon

Davonte (American) a combination of Davon + the suffix Te.
Davante, Davonnte, Davonta, Davontae, Davontah, Davontai, Davontay, Davontaye, Davontea, Davontee, Davonti

Dawan (American) a form of Davin.
Dawann, Dawante, Dawaun, Dawayne, Dawon, Dawone, Dawoon, Dawyne, Dawyun

Dawit (Ethiopian) a form of David.

Dawson (English) son of David.
Dawsyn

Dax (French, English) water.
Daylon (American) a form of
Dillon.
Daylan, Daylen, Daylin,
Daylun, Daylyn

Daymian (Greek) a form of
Damian.
Daymayne, Daymen, Daymeon,
Daymiane, Daymien, Daymin,
Dayminn, Daymion, Daymn

Dayne (Scandinavian) a form
of Dane.
Dayn

Dayquan (American) a form
of Daquan.
Dayquain, Dayquawane,
Dayquin, Dayqwan

Dayshawn (American) a form
of Dashawn.
Daysean, Daysen, Dayshaun,
Dayshon, Dayson

Dayton (English) day town;
bright, sunny town.
Daeton, Daiton, Daythan,
Daython, Daytona, Daytonn,
Deyton

Dayvon (American) a form of
Davin.
Dayven, Dayveon, Dayvin,
Dayvion, Dayvonn

De (Chinese) virtuous.

Deacon (Greek) one who
serves.
Deke

Dean (French) leader.
(English) valley. See also
Dino.
Deane, Deen, Dene, Deyn,
Deyne

Deandre (French) a combina-
tion of the prefix De +
André.
D'andre, D'andré, D'André,
D'andrea, Deandra, Deandrae,
Déandre, Deandré, De André,
Deandrea, De Andrea,
Deandres, Deandrey,
Deaundera, Deaundra,
Deaundray, Deaundre, De
Aundre, Deaundrey, Deaundry,
Deondre, Diandre, Dondre

Deangelo (Italian) a combina-
tion of the prefix De +
Angelo.
Dang, Dangelo, D'Angelo,
Danglo, Deaengelo, Deangelio,
Deangello, Déangelo, De Angelo,
Deangilio, Deangleo, Deanglo,
Deangulo, Diangelo, Di'angelo

Deante (Latin) a form of
Dante.
Deanta, Deantai, Deantay,
Deanté, De Anté, Deanteé,
Deaunta, Diantae, Diante,
Diantey

Deanthony (Italian) a combi-
nation of the prefix De +
Anthony.
D'anthony, Danton, Dianthony

Dearborn (English) deer brook.
Dearbourn, Dearburne, Deaurburn, Deerborn

Decarlos (Spanish) a combination of the prefix De + Carlos.
Dacarlos, Decarlo, Di'carlos

Decha (Tai) strong.

Decimus (Latin) tenth.

Declan (Irish) man of prayer. Religion: Saint Declan was a fifth-century Irish bishop.
Deklan

Dedrick (German) ruler of the people. See also Derek, Theodoric.
Deadrick, Deddrick, Dederick, Dedrek, Dedreko, Dedric, Dedrix, Dedrrick, Deedrick, Diedrich, Diedrick, Dietrich, Detrick

Deems (English) judge's child.

Deion (Greek) a form of Dion.
Deione, Deionta, Deionte

Dejuan (American) a combination of the prefix De + Juan. See also Dajuan.
Dejan, Dejon, Dejuane, Dejun, Dewan, Dewaun, Dewon, Dijaun, Djuan, D'Juan, Dujuan, Dujuane, D'Won

Dekel (Hebrew, Arabic) palm tree, date tree.

Dekota (Dakota) a form of Dakota.
Decoda, Dekoda, Dekodda, Dekotes

Del (English) a short form of Delbert, Delvin, Delwin.

Delaney (Irish) descendant of the challenger.
Delaine, Delainey, Delainy, Delan, Delane, Delanny, Delany

Delano (French) nut tree. (Irish) dark.
Delanio, Delayno, Dellano

Delbert (English) bright as day. See also Dalbert.
Bert, Del, Dilbert

Delfino (Latin) dolphin.
Delfine

Délì (Chinese) virtuous.

Dell (English) small valley. A short form of Udell.

Delling (Scandinavian) scintillating.

Delmar (Latin) sea.
Dalmar, Dalmer, Delmare, Delmario, Delmarr, Delmer, Delmor, Delmore

Delon (American) a form of Dillon.
Deloin, Delone, Deloni, Delonne

Delroy (French) belonging to the king. See also Elroy, Leroy.
Delray, Delree, Delroi

Delshawn (American) a combination of Del + Shawn.
Delsean, Delshon, Delsin, Delson

Delsin (Native American) he is so.
Delsy

Delton (English) a form of Dalton.
Delten, Deltyn

Delvin (English) proud friend; friend from the valley.
Dalvin, Del, Delavan, Delvian, Delvon, Delvyn, Delwin

Delwin (English) a form of Delvin.
Dalwin, Dalwyn, Del, Dellwin, Dellwyn, Delwyn, Delwynn

Deman (Dutch) man.

Demarco (Italian) a combination of the prefix De + Marco.
Damarco, Demarcco, Demarceo, Demarcio, Demarkco, Demarkeo, Demarko, Demarquo, D'Marco

Demarcus (American) a combination of the prefix De + Marcus.
Damarcius, Damarcus, Demarces, Demarcis, Demarcius, Demarcos, Demarcuse, Demarkes, Demarkis, Demarkos, Demarkus, Demarqus, D'Marcus

Demario (Italian) a combination of the prefix De + Mario.
Demarea, Demaree, Demareo, Demari, Demaria, Demariea, Demarion, Demarreio, Demariez, Demarious, Demaris, Demariuz, Demarrio, Demerio, Demerrio

Demarius (American) a combination of the prefix De + Marius.

Demarquis (American) a combination of the prefix De + Marquis.
Demarques, Demarquez, Demarqui

Dembe (Luganda) peaceful.
Damba

Demetri, Demitri (Greek) short forms of Demetrius.
Dametri, Damitré, Demeter, Demetre, Demetrea, Demetriel, Demitre, Demitrie, Domotor

Demetris (Greek) a short form of Demetrius.
Demeatric, Demeatrice, Demeatris, Demetres, Demetress, Demetric, Demetrice, Demetrick, Demetrics, Demetricus, Demetrik, Demitrez, Demitries, Demitris

Demetrius (Greek) lover of the earth. Mythology: a follower of Demeter, the goddess of the harvest. See also Dimitri, Mimis, Mitsos.
Dametrius, Demeitrius, Demeterious, Demetreus, Demetri, Demetrias, Demetrio, Demetrios, Demetrious, Demetris, Demetriu, Demetrium, Demetrois, Demetruis, Demetrus, Demitirus, Demitri, Demitrias, Demitriu, Demitrius, Demitrus, Demtrius, Demtrus, Dimitri, Dimitrios, Dimitrius, Dmetrius, Dymek

Demichael (American) a combination of the prefix De + Michael.
Dumichael

Demond (Irish) a short form of Desmond.
Demonde, Demonds, Demone, Dumonde

Demont (French) mountain.
Démont, Demonta, Demontae, Demontay, Demontaz, Demonte, Demontez, Demontre

Demorris (American) a combination of the prefix De + Morris.
Demoris, DeMorris, Demorus

Demos (Greek) people.
Demas, Demosthenes

Demothi (Native American) talks while walking.

Dempsey (Irish) proud.
Demp, Demps, Dempsie, Dempsy

Dempster (English) one who judges.
Demster

Denby (Scandinavian) Geography: a Danish village.
Danby, Den, Denbey, Denney, Dennie, Denny

Denham (English) village in the valley.

Denholm (Scottish) Geography: a town in Scotland.

Denis (Greek) a form of Dennis.
Denise, Deniz

Denley (English) meadow; valley.
Denlie, Denly

Denman (English) man from the valley.

Dennis (Greek) Mythology: a follower of Dionysus, the god of wine. See also Dion, Nicho.
Den, Dénes, Denies, Denis, Deniz, Dennes, Dennet, Dennez, Denny, Dennys, Denya, Denys, Deon, Dinis

Dennison (English) son of Dennis. See also Dyson, Tennyson.
Den, Denison, Denisson, Dennyson

Denny (Greek) a familiar form of Dennis.
Den, Denney, Dennie, Deny

Denton (English) happy home.
Dent, Denten, Dentin

Denver (English) green valley. Geography: the capital of Colorado.

Denzel (Cornish) a form of Denzil.
Danzel, Danzell, Dennzel, Denzal, Denzale, Denzall, Denzell, Denzelle, Denzle, Denzsel

Denzell (Cornish) Geography: a location in Cornwall, England.
Dennzil, Dennzyl, Denzel, Denzial, Denziel, Denzil, Denzill, Denzyel, Denzyl, Donzell

Deon (Greek) a form of Dennis. See also Dion.
Deion, Deone, Deonn, Deonno

Deondre (French) a form of Deandre.
Deiondray, Deiondre, Deondra, Deondrae, Deondray, Deondré, Deondrea, Deondree, Deondrei, Deondrey, Diondra, Diondrae, Diondre, Diondrey

Deontae (American) a combination of the prefix De + Dontae.
Deonta, Deontai, Deontay, Deontaye, Deonte, Deonté, Deontea, Deonteya, Deonteye, Deontia, Deontre, Dionte

Deonte, Deonté (American) forms of Deontae.
D'Ante, Deante, Deontée, Deontie

Deontre (American) forms of Deontae.
Deontrae, Deontrais, Deontray, Deontrea, Deontrey, Deontrez, Deontreze, Deontrus

Dequan (American) a combination of the prefix De + Quan.
Dequain, Dequane, Dequann, Dequante, Dequantez, Dequantis, Dequaun, Dequavius, Dequawn, Dequian, Dequin, Dequine, Dequinn, Dequion, Dequoin, Dequon, Deqwan, Deqwon, Deqwone

Dereck, Derick (German) forms of Derek.
Derekk, Dericka, Derico, Deriek, Derique, Deryck, Deryk, Deryke, Detrek

Derek (German) a short form of Theodoric. See also Dedrick, Dirk.
Darek, Darick, Darrick, Derak, Dereck, Derecke, Derele, Deric, Derick, Derik, Derk, Derke, Derrek, Derrick, Deryek

Deric, Derik (German) forms of Derek.
Deriek, Derikk

Dermot (Irish) free from envy.
(English) free. (Hebrew) a
short form of Jeremiah. See
also Kermit.
Der, Dermod, Dermott,
Diarmid, Diarmuid

Deron (Hebrew) bird; free-
dom. (American) a combina-
tion of the prefix De + Ron.
Daaron, Daron, Da-Ron,
Darone, Darron, Dayron,
Dereon, Deronn, Deronne,
Derrin, Derrion, Derron,
Derronn, Derronne, Derryn,
Diron, Duron, Durron, Dyron

Deror (Hebrew) lover of freedom.
Derori, Derorie

Derrek (German) a form of
Derek.
Derrec, Derreck

Derrell (French) a form of
Darrell.
Derel, Derele, Derell, Derelle,
Derrel, Dérrell, Derriel, Derril,
Derrill, Deryl, Deryll

Derren (Irish, English) a form
of Darren.
Deren, Derran, Derraun,
Derreon, Derrian, Derrien,
Derrin, Derrion, Derron,
Derryn, Deryan, Deryn, Deryon

Derrick (German) ruler of the
people. A form of Derek.
Derric, Derrik, Derryck, Derryk

Derry (Irish) redhead.
Geography: a city in
Northern Ireland.
Darrie, Darry, Derri, Derrie,
Derrye, Dery

Derryl (French) a form of
Darryl.
Deryl, Deryll

Derward (English) deer keeper.

Derwin (English) a form of
Darwin.
Derwyn

Desean (American) a combi-
nation of the prefix De +
Sean.
Dasean, D'Sean, Dusean

Deshane (American) a com-
bination of the prefix De +
Shane.
Deshan, Deshayne

Deshaun (American) a com-
bination of the prefix De +
Shaun.
Deshan, Deshane, Deshann,
Deshaon, Deshaune, D'shaun,
D'Shaun, Dushaun

Deshawn (American) a com-
bination of the prefix De +
Shawn.
Dashaun, Dashawn,
Deshauwn, Deshawan,
Deshawon, Deshon, D'shawn,
D'Shawn, Dushan, Dushawn

Deshea (American) a combination of the prefix De + Shea.
Deshay

Déshì (Chinese) virtuous.

Deshon (American) a form of Deshawn.
Deshondre, Deshone, Deshonn, Deshonte, Deshun, Deshunn

Desiderio (Spanish) desired.

Desmond (Irish) from south Munster.
Demond, Des, Desi, Desimon, Desman, Desmand, Desmane, Desmen, Desmine, Desmon, Desmound, Desmund, Desmyn, Dezmon, Dezmond

Destin (French) destiny, fate.
Destan, Desten, Destine, Deston, Destry, Destyn

Destry (American) a form of Destin.
Destrey, Destrie

Detrick (German) a form of Dedrick.
Detrek, Detric, Detrich, Detrik, Detrix

Devan (Irish) a form of Devin.
Devaan, Devain, Devane, Devann, Devean, Devun, Diwan

Devante (American) a combination of Devan + the suffix Te.
Devanta, Devantae, Devantay, Devanté, Devantée, Devantez, Devanty, Devaughntae, Devaughnte, Devaunte, Deventae, Deventay, Devente, Divante

Devaughn (American) a form of Devin.
Devaugh, Devaun

Devayne (American) a form of Dewayne.
Devain, Devaine, Devan, Devane, Devayn, Devein, Deveion

Deven (Hindi) for God. (Irish) a form of Devin.
Deaven, Deiven, Devein, Devenn, Devven, Diven

Deverell (English) riverbank.

Devin (Irish) poet.
Deavin, Deivin, Dev, Devan, Devaughn, Deven, Devlyn, Devon, Devvin, Devy, Devyn, Dyvon

Devine (Latin) divine. (Irish) ox.
Davon, Devinn, Devon, Devyn, Devyne, Dewine

Devlin (Irish) brave, fierce.
Dev, Devlan, Devland, Devlen, Devlon, Devlyn

Devon (Irish) a form of Devin.
Deavon, Deivon, Deivone, Deivonne, Deveon, Deveone, Devion, Devoen, Devohn, Devonae, Devone, Devoni, Devonio, Devonn, Devonne, Devontaine, Devvon, Devvonne, Dewon, Dewone, Divon, Diwon

Devonta (American) a combination of Devon + the suffix Ta.
Deveonta, Devonnta, Devonntae, Devontae, Devontai, Devontay, Devontaye

Devonte (American) a combination of Devon + the suffix Te.
Deveonte, Devionte, Devonté, Devontea, Devontee, Devonti, Devontia, Devontre

Devyn (Irish) a form of Devin.
Devyin, Devynn, Devynne

Dewayne (Irish) a form of Dwayne. (American) a combination of the prefix De + Wayne.
Deuwayne, Devayne, Dewain, Dewaine, Dewan, Dewane, Dewaun, Dewaune, Dewayen, Dewean, Dewon, Dewune

Dewei (Chinese) highly virtuous.

Dewey (Welsh) prized.
Dew, Dewi, Dewie

DeWitt (Flemish) blond.
Dewitt, Dwight, Wit

Dexter (Latin) dexterous, adroit. (English) fabric dyer.
Daxter, Decca, Deck, Decka, Dekka, Dex, Dextar, Dextor, Dextrel, Dextron

Dezmon, Dezmond (Irish) forms of Desmond.
Dezman, Dezmand, Dezmen, Dezmin

Diamond (English) brilliant gem; bright guardian.
Diaman, Diamanta, Diamante, Diamend, Diamenn, Diamont, Diamonta, Diamonte, Diamund, Dimond, Dimonta, Dimontae, Dimonte

Dick (German) a short form of Frederick, Richard.
Dic, Dicken, Dickens, Dickie, Dickon, Dicky, Dik

Dickran (Armenian) History: an ancient Armenian king.
Dicran, Dikran

Dickson (English) son of Dick.
Dickenson, Dickerson, Dikerson, Diksan

Didi (Hebrew) a familiar form of Jedidiah, Yedidyah.

Didier (French) desired, longed for.

Diedrich (German) a form of Dedrick, Dietrich.
Didrich, Didrick, Didrik, Diederick

Diego (Spanish) a form of Jacob, James.
Iago, Diaz, Jago

Dietbald (German) a form of
Theobald.
Dietbalt, Dietbolt

Dieter (German) army of the
people.
Deiter

Dietrich (German) a form of
Dedrick.
*Deitrich, Deitrick, Deke,
Diedrich, Dietrick, Dierck,
Dieter, Dieterich, Dieterick,
Dietz*

Digby (Irish) ditch town; dike
town.

Dillan (Irish) a form of Dillon.
Dilan, Dillian, Dilun, Dilyan

Dillon (Irish) loyal, faithful.
See also Dylan.
*Daylon, Delon, Dil, Dill,
Dillan, Dillen, Dillie, Dillin,
Dillion, Dilly, Dillyn, Dilon,
Dilyn, Dilynn*

Dilwyn (Welsh) shady place.
Dillwyn

Dima (Russian) a familiar
form of Vladimir.
Dimka

Dimitri (Russian) a form of
Demetrius.
*Dimetra, Dimetri, Dimetric,
Dimetrie, Dimitr, Dimitric,
Dimitrie, Dimitrik, Dimitris,
Dimitry, Dimmy, Dmitri,
Dymitr, Dymitry*

Dimitrios (Greek) a form of
Demetrius.
*Dhimitrios, Dimitrius, Dimos,
Dmitrios*

Dimitrius (Greek) a form of
Demetrius.
*Dimetrius, Dimitricus,
Dimitrius, Dimetrus, Dmitrius*

Dingbang (Chinese) protector
of the country.

Dinh (Vietnamese) calm,
peaceful.
Din

Dino (German) little sword.
(Italian) a form of Dean.
Deano

Dinos (Greek) a familiar form
of Constantine, Konstantin.

Dinsmore (Irish) fortified hill.
Dinnie, Dinny, Dinse

Diogenes (Greek) honest.
History: an ancient philosopher who searched with a
lantern in daylight for an
honest man.
Diogenese

Dion (Greek) a short form of
Dennis, Dionysus.
*Deion, Deon, Dio, Dione,
Dionigi, Dionis, Dionn,
Dionne, Diontae, Dionte,
Diontray*

Dionte (American) a form of Deontae.
Diante, Dionta, Diontae, Diontay, Diontaye, Dionté, Diontea

Dionysus (Greek) celebration. Mythology: the god of wine.
Dion, Dionesios, Dionicio, Dionisio, Dionisios, Dionusios, Dionysios, Dionysius, Dunixi

Diquan (American) a combination of the prefix Di + Quan.
Diqawan, Diqawn, Diquane

Dirk (German) a short form of Derek, Theodoric.
Derk, Dirck, Dirke, Durc, Durk, Dyrk

Dixon (English) son of Dick.
Dickson, Dix

Dmitri (Russian) a form of Dimitri.
Dmetriy, Dmitiri, Dmitri, Dmitrik, Dmitriy

Doane (English) low, rolling hills.
Doan

Dob (English) a familiar form of Robert.
Dobie

Dobry (Polish) good.

Doherty (Irish) harmful.
Docherty, Dougherty, Douherty

Dolan (Irish) dark haired.
Dolin, Dolyn

Dolf, Dolph (German) short forms of Adolf, Adolph, Rudolf, Rudolph.
Dolfe, Dolfi, Dolphe, Dolphus

Dom (Latin) a short form of Dominic.
Dome, Domó

Domenic (Latin) an alternate form of Dominic.
Domanick, Domenick

Domenico (Italian) a form of Dominic.
Domenic, Domicio, Dominico, Menico

Domingo (Spanish) born on Sunday. See also Mingo.
Demingo, Domingos

Dominic (Latin) belonging to the Lord. See also Chuminga.
Deco, Demenico, Dom, Domanic, Domeka, Domenic, Domenico, Domini, Dominie, Dominik, Dominique, Dominitric, Dominy, Domminic, Domnenique, Domokos, Domonic, Nick

Dominick (Latin) a form of Dominic.
Domiku, Domineck, Dominick, Dominicke, Dominiek, Dominik, Dominnick, Dominyck, Domminick, Dommonick, Domnick, Domokos, Domonick, Donek, Dumin

Dominik (Latin) an alternte
form of Dominic.
*Domenik, Dominiko, Dominyk,
Domonik*

Dominique (French) a form
of Dominic.
*Domeniq, Domeniqu,
Domenique, Domenque,
Dominiqu, Dominque,
Dominiqueia, Domnenique,
Domnique, Domoniqu,
Domonique, Domunique*

Domokos (Hungarian) a form
of Dominic.
*Dedo, Dome, Domek, Domok,
Domonkos*

Don (Scottish) a short form of
Donald. See also Kona.
Donn

Donahue (Irish) dark warrior.
Donohoe, Donohue

Donal (Irish) a form of
Donald.

Donald (Scottish) world
leader; proud ruler. See also
Bohdan, Tauno.
*Don, Donal, Dónal, Donaldo,
Donall, Donalt, Donát,
Donaugh, Donnie*

Donatien (French) gift.
Donathan, Donathon

Donato (Italian) gift.
*Dodek, Donatello, Donati,
Donatien, Donatus*

Donavan (Irish) a form of
Donovan.
*Donaven, Donavin, Donavon,
Donavyn*

Dondre (French) a form of
Deandre.
*Dondra, Dondrae, Dondray,
Dondré, Dondrea*

Dong (Vietnamese) easterner.
Duong

Donkor (Akan) humble.

Donnell (Irish) brave; dark.
*Doneal, Donel, Donele, Donell,
Donelle, Donnel, Donnele,
Donnelly, Doniel, Donielle,
Donnel, Donnelle, Donniel,
Donyel, Donyell*

Donnelly (Irish) a form of
Donnell.
Donelly, Donlee, Donley

Donnie, Donny (Irish) familiar forms of Donald.

Donovan (Irish) dark warrior.
*Dohnovan, Donavan, Donevan,
Donevon, Donivan, Donnivan,
Donnovan, Donnoven,
Donoven, Donovin, Donovon,
Donvan*

Dontae, Donté (American)
forms of Dante.
*Donta, Dontai, Dontao,
Dontate, Dontavious,
Dontavius, Dontay, Dontaye,
Dontea, Dontee, Dontez*

Dontrell (American) a form of Dantrell.
Dontral, Dontrall, Dontray, Dontre, Dontreal, Dontrel, Dontrelle, Dontriel, Dontriell

Donzell (Cornish) a form of Denzell.
Donzeil, Donzel, Donzelle, Donzello

Dooley (Irish) dark hero.
Dooly

Dor (Hebrew) generation.

Doran (Greek, Hebrew) gift. (Irish) stranger; exile.
Dore, Dorin, Dorran, Doron, Dorren, Dory

Dorian (Greek) from Doris, Greece. See also Isidore.
Dore, Dorey, Dorie, Dorien, Dorin, Dorion, Dorján, Doron, Dorrian, Dorrien, Dorrin, Dorrion, Dorron, Dorryen, Dory

Dorrell (Scottish) king's doorkeeper. See also Durell.
Dorrel, Dorrelle

Dotan (Hebrew) law.
Dothan

Doug (Scottish) a short form of Dougal, Douglas.
Dougie, Dougy, Dugey, Dugie, Dugy

Dougal (Scottish) dark stranger. See also Doyle.
Doug, Dougall, Dugal, Dugald, Dugall, Dughall

Douglas (Scottish) dark river, dark stream. See also Koukalaka.
Doug, Douglass, Dougles, Dugaid, Dughlas

Dov (Yiddish) bear. (Hebrew) a familiar form of David.
Dovid, Dovidas, Dowid

Dovev (Hebrew) whisper.

Dow (Irish) dark haired.

Doyle (Irish) a form of Dougal.
Doy, Doyal, Doyel

Drago (Italian) a form of Drake.

Drake (English) dragon; owner of the inn with the dragon trademark.
Drago

Draper (English) fabric maker.
Dray, Draypr

Draven (American) a combination of the letter D + Raven.
Dravian, Dravin, Dravion, Dravon, Dravone, Dravyn, Drayven, Drevon

Dreng (Norwegian) hired hand; brave.

Dreshawn (American) a combination of Drew + Shawn.
Dreshaun, Dreshon, Dreshown

Drevon (American) a form of Draven.
Drevan, Drevaun, Dreven, Drevin, Drevion, Drevone

Drew (Welsh) wise. (English) a short form of Andrew.
Drewe, Dru

Dru (English) a form of Drew.
Druan, Drud, Drue, Drugi, Drui

Drummond (Scottish) druid's mountain.
Drummund, Drumond, Drumund

Drury (French) loving. Geography: Drury Lane is a street in London's theater district.

Dryden (English) dry valley.
Dry

Duane (Irish) a form of Dwayne.
Deune, Duain, Duaine, Duana

Duarte (Portuguese) rich guard. See also Edward.

Duc (Vietnamese) moral.
Duoc, Duy

Dudd (English) a short form of Dudley.
Dud, Dudde, Duddy

Dudley (English) common field.
Dudd, Dudly

Duer (Scottish) heroic.

Duff (Scottish) dark.
Duffey, Duffie, Duffy

Dugan (Irish) dark.
Doogan, Dougan, Douggan, Duggan

Duke (French) leader; duke.
Dukey, Dukie, Duky

Dukker (Gypsy) fortuneteller.

Dulani (Nguni) cutting.

Dumaka (Ibo) helping hand.

Duman (Turkish) misty, smoky.

Duncan (Scottish) brown warrior. Literature: King Duncan was Macbeth's victim in Shakespeare's play *Macbeth*.
Dunc, Dunn

Dunham (Scottish) brown.

Dunixi (Basque) a form of Dionysus.

Dunley (English) hilly meadow.

Dunlop (Scottish) muddy hill.

Dunmore (Scottish) fortress on the hill.

Dunn (Scottish) a short form of Duncan.
Dun, Dune, Dunne

Dunstan (English) brownstone
fortress.
Dun, Dunston

Dunton (English) hill town.

Dur (Hebrew) stacked up.
(English) a short form of
Durwin.

Durand (Latin) a form of
Durant.

Durant (Latin) enduring.
*Duran, Durance, Durand,
Durante, Durontae, Durrant*

Durell (Scottish, English)
king's doorkeeper. See also
Dorrell.
*Durel, Durial, Durreil, Durrell,
Durrelle*

Durko (Czech) a form of
George.

Durriken (Gypsy)
fortuneteller.

Durril (Gypsy) gooseberry.
Durrel, Durrell

Durward (English) gatekeeper.
Dur, Ward

Durwin (English) a form of
Darwin.

Dushawn (American) a com-
bination of the prefix Du +
Shawn.
*Dusan, Dusean, Dushan,
Dushane, Dushaun, Dushon,
Dushun*

Dustin (German) valiant
fighter. (English) brown rock
quarry.
*Dust, Dustain, Dustan, Dusten,
Dustie, Dustine, Dustion,
Duston, Dusty, Dustyn,
Dustynn*

Dusty (English) a familiar
form of Dustin.
Dustyn (English) a form of
Dustin.

Dutch (Dutch) from the
Netherlands; from Germany.

Duval (French) a combination
of the prefix Du + Val.
Duvall, Duveuil

Dwaun (American) a form of
Dajuan.
*Dwan, Dwaunn, Dwawn,
Dwon, Dwuann*

Dwayne (Irish) dark. See also
Dewayne.
*Dawayne, Dawyne, Duane,
Duwain, Duwan, Duwane,
Duwayn, Duwayne, Dwain,
Dwaine, Dwan, Dwane,
Dwyane, Dywan, Dywane,
Dywayne, Dywone*

Dwight (English) a form of
DeWitt.

Dyami (Native American)
soaring eagle.

Dyer (English) fabric dyer.

Dyke (English) dike; ditch.
Dike

Dylan (Welsh) sea. See also
Dillon.
Dylane, Dylann, Dylen,
Dylian, Dylin, Dyllan, Dyllen,
Dyllian, Dyllin, Dyllyn, Dylon,
Dylyn

Dylon (Welsh) a form of
Dylan.
Dyllion, Dyllon

Dyre (Norwegian) dear heart.

Dyson (English) a short form
of Dennison.
Dysen, Dysonn

E

Ea (Irish) a form of Hugh.

Eachan (Irish) horseman.

Eagan (Irish) very mighty.
Egan, Egon

Eamon (Irish) a form of
Edmond, Edmund.
Aimon, Eammon, Eamonn

Ean (English) a form of Ian.
Eaen, Eann, Eayon, Eion, Eon,
Eyan, Eyon

Earl (Irish) pledge. (English)
nobleman.
Airle, Earld, Earle, Earlie,
Earlson, Early, Eorl, Erl, Erle,
Errol

Earnest (English) a form of
Ernest.
Earn, Earnesto, Earnie, Eranest

Easton (English) eastern town.
Eason, Easten, Eastin, Eastton

Eaton (English) estate on the
river.
Eatton, Eton, Eyton

Eb (Hebrew) a short form of
Ebenezer.
Ebb, Ebbie, Ebby

Eben (Hebrew) rock.
Eban, Ebin, Ebon

Ebenezer (Hebrew) founda-
tion stone. Literature:
Ebenezer Scrooge is a
miserly character in Charles
Dickens's *A Christmas Carol.*
Eb, Ebbaneza, Eben, Ebeneezer,
Ebeneser, Ebenezar, Eveneser

Eberhard (German) coura-
geous as a boar. See also
Everett.
Eber, Ebere, Eberardo, Eberhardt,
Evard, Everard, Everardo,
Everhardt, Everhart

Ebner (English) a form of
Abner.

Ebo (Fante) born on Tuesday.

Ed (English) a short form of
Edgar, Edsel, Edward.
Edd

Edan (Scottish) fire.
Edain

Edbert (English) wealthy;
bright.
Ediberto

Eddie (English) a familiar
form of Edgar, Edsel,
Edward.
Eddee, Eddy, Edi, Edie

Eddy (English) a form of
Eddie.
Eddye, Edy

Edel (German) noble.
Adel, Edell, Edelmar, Edelweiss

Eden (Hebrew) delightful.
Bible: the garden that was
first home to Adam and Eve.
*Eaden, Eadin, Edan, Edenson,
Edin, Edyn, Eiden*

Eder (Hebrew) flock.
Ederick, Edir

Edgar (English) successful
spearman. See also Garek,
Gerik, Medgar.
*Ed, Eddie, Edek, Edgard,
Edgardo, Edgars*

Edgardo (Spanish) a form of
Edgar.

Edison (English) son of
Edward.
Eddison, Edisen, Edson

Edmond (English) a form of
Edmund.
*Eamon, Edmon, Edmonde,
Edmondo, Edmondson, Esmond*

Edmund (English) prosperous
protector.
*Eadmund, Eamon, Edmand,
Edmaund, Edmond, Edmun,
Edmundo, Edmunds*

Edmundo (Spanish) a form of
Edmund.
Edmando, Mundo

Edo (Czech) a form of
Edward.

Edoardo (Italian) a form of
Edward.

Edorta (Basque) a form of
Edward.

Edouard (French) a form of
Edward.
Édoard, Édouard

Edric (English) prosperous
ruler.
*Eddric, Eddrick, Ederick, Edrek,
Edrice, Edrick, Edrico*

Edsel (English) rich man's
house.
Ed, Eddie, Edsell

Edson (English) a short form
of Edison.
Eddson, Edsen

Eduardo (Spanish) a form of
Edward.
Estuardo, Estvardo

Edur (Basque) snow.

Edward (English) prosperous
guardian. See also Audie,
Duarte, Ekewaka, Ned, Ted,

Teddy.
Ed, Eddie, Edik, Edko, Edo, Edoardo, Edorta, Édouard, Eduard, Eduardo, Edus, Edvard, Edvardo, Edwardo, Edwards, Edwy, Edzio, Ekewaka, Etzio, Ewart

Edwin (English) prosperous friend. See also Ned, Ted.
Eadwinn, Edik, Edlin, Eduino, Edwan, Edwen, Edwon, Edwyn

Efrain (Hebrew) fruitful.
Efran, Efrane, Efrayin, Efren, Efrian, Eifraine

Efrat (Hebrew) honored.

Efrem (Hebrew) a short form of Ephraim.
Efe, Efraim, Efrim, Efrum

Efren (Hebrew) a form of Efrain, Ephraim.

Egan (Irish) ardent, fiery.
Egann, Egen, Egon

Egbert (English) bright sword. See also Bert, Bertie.

Egerton (English) Edgar's town.
Edgarton, Edgartown, Edgerton, Egeton

Egil (Norwegian) awe inspiring.
Eigil

Eginhard (German) power of the sword.
Eginhardt, Einhard, Einhardt, Enno

Egon (German) formidable.

Egor (Russian) a form of George. See also Igor, Yegor.

Ehren (German) honorable.

Eikki (Finnish) ever powerful.

Einar (Scandinavian) individualist.
Ejnar, Inar

Eion (Irish) a form of Ean, Ian.
Eann, Eian, Ein, Eine, Einn

Eitan (Hebrew) a form of Ethan.
Eita, Eithan, Eiton

Ejau (Ateso) we have received.

Ekewaka (Hawaiian) a form of Edward.

Ekon (Nigerian) strong.

Elam (Hebrew) highlands.

Elan (Hebrew) tree. (Native American) friendly.
Elann

Elbert (English) a form of Albert.
Elberto

Elchanan (Hebrew) a form of John.
Elchan, Elchonon, Elhanan, Elhannan

Elden (English) a form of Alden, Aldous.
Eldan, Eldin

Elder (English) dweller near the elder trees.

Eldon (English) holy hill.

Eldred (English) a form of Aldred.
Eldrid

Eldridge (English) a form of Aldrich.
El, Eldred, Eldredge, Eldrege, Eldrid, Eldrige, Elric

Eldwin (English) a form of Aldwin.
Eldwinn, Eldwyn, Eldwynn

Eleazar (Hebrew) God has helped. See also Lazarus.
Elazar, Elazaro, Eleasar, Eléazar, Eliazar, Eliezer

Elek (Hungarian) a form of Alec, Alex.
Elec, Elic, Elik

Elger (German) a form of Alger.
Elger, Ellgar, Ellger

Elgin (English) noble; white.
Elgan, Elgen

Eli (Hebrew) uplifted. A short form of Elijah, Elisha. Bible: the high priest who trained the prophet Samuel. See also Elliot.
Elie, Elier, Ellie, Eloi, Eloy, Ely

Elia (Zuni) a short form of Elijah.
Eliah, Elio, Eliya, Elya

Elian (English) a form of Elijah. See also Trevelyan.
Elion

Elias (Greek) a form of Elijah.
Elia, Eliasz, Elice, Eliyas, Ellias, Ellice, Ellis, Elyas, Elyes

Eliazar (Hebrew) a form of Eleazar.
Eliasar, Eliazer, Elizar, Elizardo

Elie (Hebrew) a form of Eli.

Eliezer (Hebrew) a form of Eleazar.
Elieser

Elihu (Hebrew) a short form of Eliyahu.
Elih, Eliu, Ellihu

Elijah (Hebrew) a form of Eliyahu. Bible: a Hebrew prophet. See also Eli, Elisha, Elliot, Ilias, Ilya.
El, Elia, Elian, Elias, Elija, Elijha, Elijiah, Elijio, Elijuah, Elijuo, Elisjsha, Eliya, Eliyah, Ellis

Elika (Hawaiian) a form of Eric.

Eliseo (Hebrew) a form of Elisha.
Elisee, Elisée, Elisei, Elisiah, Elisio

Elisha (Hebrew) God is my salvation. Bible: a Hebrew prophet, successor to Elijah. See also Eli, Elijah.
Elijsha, Eliseo, Elish, Elishah,

Elisher, Elishia, Elishua, Elysha, Lisha

Eliyahu (Hebrew) the Lord is my God.
Eliyahou, Elihu

Elkan (Hebrew) God is jealous.
Elkana, Elkanah, Elkin, Elkins

Elki (Moquelumnan) hanging over the top.

Ellard (German) sacred; brave.
Allard, Ellerd

Ellery (English) from a surname derived from the name Hilary.
Ellary, Ellerey

Elliot, Elliott (English) forms of Eli, Elijah.
Elio, Eliot, Eliott, Eliud, Eliut, Elliotte, Elyot, Elyott

Ellis (English) a form of Elias.
Elis

Ellison (English) son of Ellis.
Elison, Ellson, Ellyson, Elson

Ellsworth (English) nobleman's estate.
Ellswerth, Elsworth

Elman (German) like an elm tree.
Elmen

Elmer (English) noble; famous.
Aylmer, Elemér, Ellmer, Elmir, Elmo

Elmo (Greek) lovable, friendly. (Italian) guardian. (Latin) a familiar form of Anselm. (English) a form of Elmer.

Elmore (English) moor where the elm trees grow.

Elonzo (Spanish) a form of Alonzo.
Elon, Élon, Elonso

Eloy (Latin) chosen.
Eloi

Elrad (Hebrew) God rules.
Rad, Radd

Elroy (French) a form of Delroy, Leroy.
Elroi

Elsdon (English) nobleman's hill.

Elston (English) noble's town.
Ellston

Elsu (Native American) swooping, soaring falcon.

Elsworth (English) noble's estate.

Elton (English) old town.
Alton, Eldon, Ellton, Elthon, Eltonia

Elvern (Latin) a form of Alvern.
Elver, Elverne

Elvin (English) a form of Alvin.
El, Elvyn, Elwin, Elwyn, Elwynn

Elvio (Spanish) light skinned; blond.

Elvis (Scandinavian) wise.
El, Elviz, Elvys

Elvy (English) elfin warrior.

Elwell (English) old well.

Elwood (English) old forest. See also Wood, Woody.

Ely (Hebrew) a form of Eli. Geography: a region of England with extensive drained fens.
Elya, Elyie

Eman (Czech) a form of Emmanuel.
Emaney, Emani

Emanuel (Hebrew) a form of Emmanuel.
Emaniel, Emannual, Emannuel, Emanual, Emanueal, Emanuele, Emanuell, Emanuell, Emanuelle

Emerson (German, English) son of Emery.
Emmerson, Emreson

Emery (German) industrious leader.
Aimery, Emari, Emarri, Emeri, Emerich, Emerio, Emmerich, Emmerie, Emmery, Emmo, Emory, Emrick, Emry, Inre, Imrich

Emil (Latin) flatterer. (German) industrious. See also Milko, Milo.
Aymil, Emiel, Émile, Emilek,

Emiliano, Emilio, Emill, Emils, Emilyan, Emlyn

Émile (French) a form of Emil.
Emiel, Emile, Emille

Emiliano (Italian) a form of Emil.
Emilian, Emilion

Emilien (Latin) friendly; industrious.

Emilio (Italian, Spanish) a form of Emil.
Emielio, Emileo, Emilio, Emilios, Emillio, Emilo

Emlyn (Welsh) waterfall.
Emelen, Emlen, Emlin

Emmanuel (Hebrew) God is with us. See also Immanuel, Maco, Mango, Manuel.
Eman, Emanuel, Emanuell, Emek, Emmahnuel, Emmanel, Emmaneuol, Emmanle, Emmanual, Emmanueal, Emmanuele, Emmanuell, Emmanuelle, Emmanuil, Enmanuel

Emmett (German) industrious; strong. (English) ant. History: Robert Emmett was an Irish patriot.
Em, Emet, Emett, Emitt, Emmet, Emmette, Emmitt, Emmot, Emmott, Emmy

Emmitt (German, English) a form of Emmett.
Emmit

Emory (German) a form of
Emery.
Amory, Emmory, Emorye

Emre (Turkish) brother.
Emra, Emrah, Emreson

Emrick (German) a form of
Emery.
*Emeric, Emerick, Emric,
Emrique, Emryk*

Enapay (Sioux) brave appearance; he appears.

Endre (Hungarian) a form of
Andrew.
Ender

Eneas (Greek) a form of
Aeneas.
Eneias, Enné

Engelbert (German) bright as
an angel. See also Ingelbert.
Bert, Englebert

Enli (Dene) that dog over
there.

Ennis (Greek) mine. (Scottish)
a form of Angus.
Eni, Enni

Enoch (Hebrew) dedicated,
consecrated. Bible: the father
of Methuselah.
Enoc, Enock, Enok

Enos (Hebrew) man.
Enosh

Enric (Romanian) a form of
Henry.
Enrica

Enrick (Spanish) a form of
Henry.
Enricky

Enrico (Italian) a form of
Henry.
Enzio, Enzo, Rico

Enrikos (Greek) a form of
Henry.

Enrique (Spanish) a form of
Henry. See also Quiqui.
*Enrigué, Enriqué, Enriquez,
Enrrique*

Enver (Turkish) bright; handsome.

Enyeto (Native American)
walks like a bear.

Enzi (Swahili) powerful.

Eoin (Welsh) a form of Evan.

Ephraim (Hebrew) fruitful.
Bible: the second son of
Joseph.
*Efraim, Efrayim, Efrem, Efren,
Ephraen, Ephrain, Ephram,
Ephrem, Ephriam*

Erasmus (Greek) lovable.
Érasme, Erasmo, Rasmus

Erastus (Greek) beloved.
Éraste, Erastious, Ras, Rastus

Erbert (German) a short form
of Herbert.
Ebert, Erberto

Ercole (Italian) splendid gift.

Erek (Scandinavian) a form of Eric.
Erec

Erhard (German) strong; resolute.
Erhardt, Erhart

Eriberto (Italian) a form of Herbert.
Erberto, Heriberto

Eric (Scandinavian) ruler of all. (English) brave ruler. (German) a short form of Frederick. History: Eric the Red was a Norwegian explorer who founded Greenland's first colony.
Aric, Ehrich, Elika, Erek, Éric, Erica, Ericc, Erich, Erick, Erico, Erik, Erikur, Erric, Eryc, Rick

Erich (Czech, German) a form of Eric.

Erick (English) a form of Eric.
Errick, Eryck

Erickson (English) son of Eric.
Erickzon, Erics, Ericson, Ericsson, Erikson, Erikzzon, Eriqson

Erik (Scandinavian) a form of Eric.
Erek, Erike, Eriks, Erikur, Errick, Errik, Eryk

Erikur (Icelandic) a form of Eric, Erik.

Erin (Irish) peaceful. History: an ancient name for Ireland.
Erine, Erinn, Erino, Eron, Errin, Eryn, Erynn

Erland (English) nobleman's land.
Erlend

Erling (English) nobleman's son.

Ermanno (Italian) a form of Herman.
Erman

Ermano (Spanish) a form of Herman.
Ermin, Ermine, Erminio, Ermon

Ernest (English) earnest, sincere. See also Arno.
Earnest, Ernestino, Ernesto, Ernestus, Ernie, Erno, Ernst

Ernesto (Spanish) a form of Ernest.
Ernester, Neto

Ernie (English) a familiar form of Ernest.
Earnie, Erney, Erny

Erno (Hungarian) a form of Ernest.
Ernö

Ernst (German) a form of Ernest.
Erns

Erol (Turkish) strong, courageous.
Eroll

Eron (Irish) a form of Erin.
Erran, Erren, Errion, Erron

Errando (Basque) bold.

Errol (Latin) wanderer.
(English) a form of Earl.
Erol, Erold, Erroll, Erryl

Erroman (Basque) from Rome.

Erskine (Scottish) high cliff.
(English) from Ireland.
Ersin, Erskin, Kinny

Ervin, Erwin (English) sea
friend. Forms of Irving,
Irwin.
*Earvin, Erv, Erven, Ervyn,
Erwan, Erwinek, Erwinn,
Erwyn, Erwynn*

Ervine (English) a form of
Irving.
*Erv, Ervin, Ervince, Erving,
Ervins*

Esau (Hebrew) rough; hairy.
Bible: Jacob's twin brother.
Esaw

Esequiel (Hebrew) a form of
Ezekiel.

Eshkol (Hebrew) grape clusters.

Eskil (Norwegian) god vessel.

Esmond (English) rich protector.

Espen (Danish) bear of the gods.

Essien (Ochi) sixth-born son.

Este (Italian) east.
Estes

Estéban (Spanish) a form of
Stephen.
*Estabon, Esteben, Estefan,
Estefano, Estefen, Estephan,
Estephen*

Estebe (Basque) a form of
Stephen.

Estevan (Spanish) a form of
Stephen.
Esteven, Estevon, Estiven

Estevao (Spanish) a form of
Stephen.
Estevez

Ethan (Hebrew) strong; firm.
*Eathan, Eathen, Eathon,
Eeathen, Eitan, Etan, Ethaen,
Ethe, Ethen, Ethian*

Étienne (French) a form of
Stephen.
Etian, Etien, Étienn, Ettien

Ettore (Italian) steadfast.
Etor, Etore

Etu (Native American) sunny.

Euclid (Greek) intelligent.
History: the founder of
Euclidean geometry.

Eugen (German) a form of
Eugene.

Eugene (Greek) born to
nobility. See also Ewan,
Gene, Gino, Iukini, Jenö,
Yevgenyi, Zenda.
*Eoghan, Eugen, Eugéne,
Eugeni, Eugenio, Eugenius,
Evgeny, Ezven*

Eugenio (Spanish) a form of Eugene.

Eulises (Latin) a form of Ulysses.

Eustace (Greek) productive. (Latin) stable, calm. See also Stacey.
Eustache, Eustachius, Eustachy, Eustashe, Eustasius, Eustatius, Eustazio, Eustis, Eustiss

Evan (Irish) young warrior. (English) a form of John. See also Bevan, Owen.
Eavan, Eoin, Ev, Evaine, Evann, Evans, Even, Evens, Evin, Evon, Evyn, Ewan, Ewen

Evangelos (Greek) a form of Andrew.
Evagelos, Evaggelos, Evangelo

Evelyn (English) hazelnut.
Evelin

Everardo (German) strong as a boar.
Everado

Everett (English) a form of Eberhard.
Ev, Evered, Everet, Everette, Everhett, Everit, Everitt, Everrett, Evert, Evrett

Everley (English) boar meadow.
Everlea, Everlee

Everton (English) boar town.

Evgeny (Russian) a form of Eugene. See also Zhek.
Evgeni, Evgenij, Evgenyi

Evin (Irish) a form of Evan.
Evian, Evinn, Evins

Ewald (German) always powerful. (English) powerful lawman.

Ewan (Scottish) a form of Eugene, Evan. See also Keon.
Euan, Euann, Euen, Ewen, Ewhen

Ewert (English) ewe herder, shepherd.
Ewart

Ewing (English) friend of the law.
Ewin, Ewynn

Exavier (Basque) a form of Xavier.
Exaviar, Exavior, Ezavier

Eyota (Native American) great.

Ezekiel (Hebrew) strength of God. Bible: a Hebrew prophet. See also Haskel, Zeke.
Esequiel, Ezakeil, Ezéchiel, Ezeck, Ezeckiel, Ezeeckel, Ezekeial, Ezekeil, Ezekeyial, Ezekial, Ezekielle, Ezell, Ezequiel, Eziakah, Eziechiele

Ezequiel (Hebrew) a form of Ezekiel.
Esequiel, Eziequel

Ezer (Hebrew) a form of Ezra.

Ezra (Hebrew) helper; strong.
Bible: a Jewish priest who
led the Jews back to
Jerusalem.
*Esdras, Esra, Ezer, Ezera,
Ezrah, Ezri, Ezry*

Ezven (Czech) a form of
Eugene.
Esven, Esvin, Ezavin, Ezavine

F

Faber (German) a form of
Fabian.

Fabian (Latin) bean grower.
*Fabain, Fabayan, Fabe, Fabein,
Fabek, Fabeon, Faber, Fabert,
Fabi, Fabiano, Fabien, Fabin,
Fabio, Fabion, Fabius, Fabiyan,
Fabiyus, Fabyan, Fabyen,
Faybian, Faybien*

Fabiano (Italian) a form of
Fabian.
Fabianno, Fabio

Fabio (Latin) a form of
Fabian. (Italian) a short form
of Fabiano.
Fabbio

Fabrizio (Italian) craftsman.
Fabrice, Fabricio, Fabrizius

Fabron (French) little black–
smith; apprentice.
Fabre, Fabroni

Fadey (Ukrainian) a form of
Thaddeus.
*Faday, Faddei, Faddey, Faddy,
Fade, Fadeyka, Fadie, Fady*

Fadi (Arabic) redeemer.
Fadhi

Fadil (Arabic) generous.
Fadeel, Fadel

Fagan (Irish) little fiery one.
Fagin

Fahd (Arabic) lynx.
Fahaad, Fahad

Fai (Chinese) beginning.

Fairfax (English) blond.
Fair, Fax

Faisal (Arabic) decisive.
*Faisel, Faisil, Faisl, Faiyaz,
Faiz, Faizal, Faize, Faizel,
Faizi, Fasel, Fasil, Faysal,
Fayzal, Fayzel*

Fakhir (Arabic) excellent.
Fahkry, Fakher

Fakih (Arabic) thinker; reader
of the Koran.

Falco (Latin) falconer.
Falcon, Falk, Falke, Falken

Falito (Italian) a familiar form
of Rafael, Raphael.

Falkner (English) trainer of
falcons. See also Falco.
*Falconer, Falconner, Faulconer,
Faulconner, Faulkner*

Fane (English) joyful, glad.
Fanes, Faniel

Faraji (Swahili) consolation.

Farid (Arabic) unique.

Faris (Arabic) horseman.
*Faraz, Fares, Farhaz, Farice,
Fariez, Farris*

Farley (English) bull meadow;
sheep meadow. See also Lee.
*Fairlay, Fairlee, Fairleigh,
Fairley, Fairlie, Far, Farlay,
Farlee, Farleigh, Farlie, Farly,
Farrleigh, Farrley*

Farnell (English) fern-covered
hill.
*Farnall, Fernald, Fernall,
Furnald*

Farnham (English) field of
ferns.
Farnam, Farnum, Fernham

Farnley (English) fern
meadow.
*Farnlea, Farnlee, Farnleigh,
Farnly, Fernlea, Fernlee,
Fernleigh, Fernley*

Faroh (Latin) a form of
Pharaoh.

Farold (English) mighty traveler.

Farquhar (Scottish) dear.
*Fark, Farq, Farquar, Farquarson,
Farque, Farquharson, Farquy,
Farqy*

Farr (English) traveler.
*Faer, Farran, Farren, Farrin,
Farrington, Farron*

Farrell (Irish) heroic; courageous.
Farrel, Farrill, Farryll, Ferrell

Farrow (English) piglet.

Farruco (Spanish) a form of
Francis, Francisco.
Frascuelo

Faruq (Arabic) honest.
*Farook, Farooq, Faroque,
Farouk, Faruqh*

Faste (Norwegian) firm.

Fath (Arabic) victor.

Fatin (Arabic) clever.

Faust (Latin) lucky, fortunate.
History: the sixteenth-cen-
tury German necromancer
who inspired many legends.
*Faustino, Faustis, Fausto,
Faustus*

Faustino (Italian) a form of
Faust.

Fausto (Italian) a form of
Faust.

Favian (Latin) understanding.
Favain, Favio, Favyen

Faxon (German) long-haired.

Federico (Italian, Spanish) a
form of Frederick.
Federic, Federigo, Federoquito

Feivel (Yiddish) God aids.

Feliks (Russian) a form of Felix.

Felipe (Spanish) a form of Philip.
Feeleep, Felipino, Felo, Filip, Filippo, Filips, Fillip, Flip

Felippo (Italian) a form of Philip.
Felip, Filippo, Lipp, Lippo, Pip, Pippo

Felix (Latin) fortunate; happy. See also Pitin.
Fee, Felic, Félice, Feliciano, Felicio, Felike, Feliks, Felo, Félix, Felizio, Phelix

Felton (English) field town.
Felten, Feltin

Fenton (English) marshland farm.
Fen, Fennie, Fenny, Fintan, Finton

Feodor (Slavic) a form of Theodore.
Dorek, Fedar, Fedinka, Fedor, Fedya, Fyodor

Feoras (Greek) smooth rock.

Ferdinand (German) daring, adventurous. See also Hernando.
Feranado, Ferd, Ferda, Ferdie, Ferdinánd, Ferdy, Ferdynand, Fernando, Nando

Ferenc (Hungarian) a form of Francis.
Feri, Ferke, Ferko

Fergus (Irish) strong; manly.
Fearghas, Fearghus, Feargus, Ferghus, Fergie, Ferguson, Fergusson

Fermin (French, Spanish) firm, strong.
Ferman, Firmin, Furman

Fernando (Spanish) a form of Ferdinand.
Ferando, Ferdinando, Ferdnando, Ferdo, Fernand, Fernandez, Fernendo

Feroz (Persian) fortunate.

Ferran (Arabic) baker.
Feran, Feron, Ferrin, Ferron

Ferrand (French) iron gray hair.
Farand, Farrand, Farrant, Ferrant

Ferrell (Irish) a form of Farrell.
Ferrel, Ferrill, Ferryl

Ferris (Irish) a form of Peter.
Fares, Faris, Fariz, Farris, Farrish, Feris, Ferriss

Fico (Spanish) a familiar form of Frederick.

Fidel (Latin) faithful. History: Fidel Castro was the Cuban revolutionary who overthrew a dictatorship in 1959 and established a communist regime in Cuba.
Fidele, Fidèle, Fidelio, Fidelis, Fidell, Fido

Field (English) a short form of
Fielding.
Fields

Fielding (English) field; field
worker.
Field

Fife (Scottish) from Fife,
Scotland.
Fyfe

Fifi (Fante) born on Friday.

Fil (Polish) a form of Phil.
Filipek

Filbert (English) brilliant. See
also Bert.
*Filberte, Filberto, Filiberto,
Philbert*

Filiberto (Spanish) a form of
Filbert.

Filip (Greek) a form of Philip.
Filip, Filippo

Fillipp (Russian) a form of
Philip.
*Filip, Filipe, Filipek, Filips, Fill,
Fillip, Filya*

Filmore (English) famous.
*Fillmore, Filmer, Fyllmer,
Fylmer, Philmore*

Filya (Russian) a form of Philip.

Fineas (Irish) a form of Phineas.
Finneas

Finian (Irish) light skinned;
white.
*Finnen, Finnian, Fionan,
Fionn, Phinean*

Finlay (Irish) blond-haired
soldier.
*Findlay, Findley, Finlea, Finlee,
Finley, Finn, Finnlea, Finnley*

Finn (German) from Finland.
(Irish) blond haired; light
skinned. A short form of
Finlay. (Norwegian) from
the Lapland.
Fin, Finnie, Finnis, Finny

Finnegan (Irish) light skinned;
white.
Finegan

Fiorello (Italian) little flower.
Fiore

Firas (Arabic) persistent.

Firman (French) firm; strong.
Ferman, Firmin

Firth (English) woodland.

Fischel (Yiddish) a form of
Phillip.

Fiske (English) fisherman.
Fisk

Fitch (English) weasel, ermine.
Fitche

Fitz (English) son.
Filz

Fitzgerald (English) son of
Gerald.

Fitzhugh (English) son of
Hugh.
Hugh

Fitzpatrick (English) son of Patrick.

Fitzroy (Irish) son of Roy.

Flaminio (Spanish) Religion: Marcantonio Flaminio coauthored one of the most important texts of the Italian Reformation.

Flann (Irish) redhead.
Flainn, Flannan, Flannery

Flavian (Latin) blond, yellow haired.
Flavel, Flavelle, Flavien, Flavio, Flawiusz

Flavio (Italian) a form of Flavian.
Flabio, Flavious, Flavius

Fleming (English) from Denmark; from Flanders.
Flemming, Flemmyng, Flemyng

Fletcher (English) arrow featherer, arrow maker.
Flecher, Fletch

Flint (English) stream; flint stone.
Flynt

Flip (Spanish) a short form of Felipe. (American) a short form of Philip.

Florencio (Italian) a form of Florent.

Florent (French) flowering.
Florenci, Florencio, Florentin, Florentino, Florentyn, Florentz, Florinio, Florino

Florian (Latin) flowering, blooming.
Florien, Florrian, Flory, Floryan

Floyd (English) a form of Lloyd.

Flurry (English) flourishing, blooming.

Flynn (Irish) son of the red-haired man.
Flin, Flinn, Flyn

Folke (German) a form of Volker.
Folker

Foluke (Yoruba) given to God.

Foma (Bulgarian, Russian) a form of Thomas.
Fomka

Fonso (German, Italian) a short form of Alphonso.
Fonzo

Fontaine (French) fountain.

Fonzie (German) a familiar form of Alphonse.
Fons, Fonsie, Fonsy, Fonz

Forbes (Irish) prosperous.
Forbe

Ford (English) a short form of names ending in "ford."

Fordel (Gypsy) forgiving.

Forest (French) a form of
Forrest.
Forestt, Foryst

Forester (English) forest
guardian.
*Forrester, Forrie, Forry, Forster,
Foss, Foster*

Forrest (French) forest;
woodsman.
*Forest, Forester, Forrestar,
Forrester, Forrestt, Forrie*

Fortino (Italian) fortunate,
lucky.

Fortune (French) fortunate,
lucky.
*Fortun, Fortunato, Fortuné,
Fortunio*

Foster (Latin) a short form of
Forester.

Fowler (English) trapper of
wildfowl.

Fran (Latin) a short form of
Francis.
Franh

Francesco (Italian) a form of
Francis.

Franchot (French) a form of
Francis.

Francis (Latin) free; from
France. Religion: Saint
Francis of Assisi was the
founder of the Franciscan
order. See also Farruco,
Ferenc.
Fran, France, Frances, Francesco,

*Franchot, Francisco, Franciskus,
Franco, François, Frang, Frank,
Frannie, Franny, Frans, Franscis,
Fransis, Franta, Frantisek,
Frants, Franus, Frantisek,
Franz, Frencis*

Francisco (Portuguese,
Spanish) a form of Francis.
See also Chilo, Cisco,
Farruco, Paco, Pancho.
*Franco, Fransisco, Fransysco,
Frasco, Frisco*

Franco (Latin) a short form of
Francis.
Franko

François (French) a form of
Francis.
Francoise

Frank (English) a short form
of Francis, Franklin. See also
Palani, Pancho.
*Franc, Franck, Franek, Frang,
Franio, Franke, Frankie, Franko*

Frankie (English) a familiar
form of Frank.
*Francky, Franke, Frankey,
Franki, Franky, Franqui*

Franklin (English) free
landowner.
*Fran, Francklen, Francklin,
Francklyn, Francylen, Frank,
Frankin, Franklen, Franklinn,
Franklyn, Franquelin*

Franklyn (English) a form of
Franklin.
Franklynn

Frans (Swedish) a form of
Francis.
Frants

Frantisek (Czech) a form of
Francis.
Franta

Franz (German) a form of
Francis.
*Fransz, Frantz, Franzen,
Franzie, Franzin, Franzl,
Franzy*

Fraser (French) strawberry.
(English) curly haired.
*Fraizer, Frasier, Fraze, Frazer,
Frazier*

Frayne (French) dweller at the
ash tree. (English) stranger.
*Fraine, Frayn, Frean, Freen,
Freyne*

Fred (German) a short form
of Alfred, Frederick,
Manfred.
Fredd, Fredde, Fredo, Fredson

Freddie (German) a familiar
form of Frederick.
Freddi, Freddy, Fredi, Fredy

Freddy, Fredy (German)
familiar forms of Frederick.

Frederic (German) a form of
Frederick.
*Frédéric, Frederich, Frederric,
Fredric, Fredrich*

Frederick (German) peaceful
ruler. See also Dick, Eric,
Fico, Peleke, Rick.
*Federico, Fico, Fred, Fredderick,
Freddie, Freddrick, Freddy,
Fredek, Frederic, Fréderick,
Frédérick, Frederik, Frederique,
Frederrick, Fredo, Fredrick,
Fredwick, Fredwyck, Fredy,
Friedrich, Fritz*

Frederico (Spanish) a form of
Frederick.
Fredrico, Frederigo

Frederik (German) a form of
Frederick.
Frédérik, Frederrik, Fredrik

Frederique (French) a form of
Frederick.

Fredo (Spanish) a form of
Fred.

Fredrick (German) a form of
Frederick.
Fredric, Fredricka, Fredricks

Freeborn (English) child of
freedom.
Free

Freeman (English) free.
*Free, Freedman, Freemin,
Freemon, Friedman, Friedmann*

Fremont (German) free; noble
protector.

Frewin (English) free; noble
friend.
Frewen

Frey (English) lord.
(Scandinavian) Mythology:
the Norse god who dispenses
peace and prosperity.

Frick (English) bold.

Fridolf (English) peaceful
wolf.
Freydolf, Freydulf, Fridulf

Friedrich (German) a form of
Frederick.
*Friedel, Friedrick, Fridrich,
Fridrick, Friedrike, Friedryk,
Fryderyk*

Frisco (Spanish) a short form
of Francisco.

Fritz (German) a familiar form
of Frederick.
Fritson, Fritts, Fritzchen, Fritzl

Frode (Norwegian) wise.

Fulbright (German) very
bright.
Fulbert

Fuller (English) cloth thickener.

Fulton (English) field near
town.

Funsoni (Nguni) requested.

Fyfe (Scottish) a form of Fife.
Fyffe

Fynn (Ghanaian) Geography:
another name for the Offin
River in Ghana.

Fyodor (Russian) a form of
Theodore.

G

Gabby (American) a familiar
form of Gabriel.
*Gabbi, Gabbie, Gabi, Gabie,
Gaby*

Gabe (Hebrew) a short form
of Gabriel.

Gabino (American) a form of
Gabriel.
Gabin, Gabrino

Gábor (Hungarian) God is my
strength.
Gabbo, Gabko, Gabo

Gabrial (Hebrew) a form of
Gabriel.
*Gaberial, Gabrael, Gabraiel,
Gabrail, Gabreal, Gabriael,
Gabrieal, Gabryalle*

Gabriel (Hebrew) devoted to
God. Bible: the angel of the
Annunciation.
*Gab, Gabe, Gabby, Gabino,
Gabis, Gábor, Gabreil, Gabrel,
Gabrell, Gabrial, Gabriël,
Gabriele, Gabriell, Gabrielle,
Gabrielli, Gabrile, Gabris,
Gabryel, Gabys, Gavril,
Gebereal, Ghabriel, Riel*

Gabrielli (Italian) a form of
Gabriel.
Gabriello

Gadi (Arabic) God is my fortune.
Gad, Gaddy, Gadiel

Gaetan (Italian) from Gaeta, a region in southern Italy.
Gaetano, Gaetono

Gage (French) pledge.
Gager, Gaige, Gaje

Gaige (French) a form of Gage.

Gair (Irish) small.
Gaer, Gearr, Geir

Gaius (Latin) rejoicer. See also Cai.

Galbraith (Irish) Scotsman in Ireland.
Galbrait, Galbreath

Gale (Greek) a short form of Galen.
Gael, Gail, Gaile, Gayle

Galen (Greek) healer; calm. (Irish) little and lively.
Gaelan, Gaelen, Gaelin, Gaelyn, Gailen, Galan, Gale, Galeno, Galin, Galyn, Gaylen

Galeno (Spanish) illuminated child. (Greek, Irish) a form of Galen.

Gallagher (Irish) eager helper.

Galloway (Irish) Scotsman in Ireland.
Gallway, Galway

Galt (Norwegian) high ground.

Galton (English) owner of a rented estate.
Gallton

Galvin (Irish) sparrow.
Gal, Gall, Gallven, Gallvin, Galvan, Galven

Gamal (Arabic) camel. See also Jamal.
Gamall, Gamel, Gamil

Gamble (Scandinavian) old.

Gan (Chinese) daring, adventurous. (Vietnamese) near.

Gannon (Irish) light skinned, white.
Gannan, Gannen, Gannie, Ganny

Ganya (Zulu) clever.

Gar (English) a short form of Gareth, Garnett, Garrett, Garvin.
Garr

Garcia (Spanish) mighty with a spear.

Gardner (English) gardener.
Gard, Gardener, Gardie, Gardiner, Gardy

Garek (Polish) a form of Edgar.

Garen (English) a form of Garry.
Garan, Garen, Garin, Garion, Garon, Garyn, Garyon

Gareth (Welsh) gentle.
*Gar, Garith, Garreth, Garrith,
Garth, Garyth*

Garett (Irish) a form of
Garrett.
*Gared, Garet, Garette, Garhett,
Garit, Garitt, Garritt*

Garfield (English) field of
spears; battlefield.

Garland (French) wreath of
flowers; prize. (English) land
of spears; battleground.
*Garlan, Garlen, Garllan,
Garlund, Garlyn*

Garman (English) spearman.
Garmann, Garrman

Garner (French) army guard,
sentry.
Garnier

Garnett (Latin) pomegranate
seed; garnet stone. (English)
armed with a spear.
Gar, Garnet, Garnie, Garrnett

Garnock (Welsh) dweller by
the alder river.

Garrad (English) a form of
Garrett.
*Gared, Garrard, Garred,
Garrod, Gerred, Gerrid, Gerrod,
Garrode, Jared*

Garret (Irish) a form of
Garrett.
*Garrit, Garyt, Gerret, Garrid,
Gerrit, Gerrot*

Garrett (Irish) brave
spearman. See also Jarrett.
*Gar, Gareth, Garett, Garrad,
Garret, Garrette, Gerrett,
Gerritt, Gerrott*

Garrick (English) oak spear.
*Gaerick, Garek, Garick, Garik,
Garreck, Garrek, Garric,
Garrik, Garryck, Garryk,
Gerreck, Gerrick*

Garren, Garrin (English)
forms of Garry.
*Garran, Garrion, Garron,
Garyn, Gerren, Gerron, Gerryn*

Garrison (French) troops sta-
tioned at a fort; garrison.
Garison, Garisson, Garris

Garroway (English) spear
fighter.
Garraway

Garry (English) a form of
Gary.
*Garen, Garrey, Garri, Garrie,
Garren, Garrin*

Garson (English) son of Gar.

Garth (Scandinavian) garden,
gardener. (Welsh) a short
form of Gareth.

Garvey (Irish) rough peace.
*Garbhán, Garrvey, Garrvie,
Garv, Garvan, Garvie, Garvy*

Garvin (English) comrade in
battle.
Gar, Garvan, Garven, Garvyn,

Garwen, Garwin, Garwyn, Garwynn

Garwood (English) evergreen forest. See also Wood, Woody.
Garrwood

Gary (German) mighty spearman. (English) a familiar form of Gerald. See also Kali.
Gare, Garey, Gari, Garry

Gaspar (French) a form of Casper.
Gáspár, Gaspard, Gaspare, Gaspari, Gasparo, Gasper, Gazsi

Gaston (French) from Gascony, France.
Gascon, Gastaun

Gaute (Norwegian) great.

Gautier (French) a form of Walter.
Galtero, Gaulterio, Gaultier, Gaultiero, Gauthier

Gavin (Welsh) white hawk.
Gav, Gavan, Gaven, Gavinn, Gavino, Gavn, Gavohn, Gavon, Gavyn, Gavynn, Gawain

Gavriel (Hebrew) man of God.
Gav, Gavi, Gavrel, Gavril, Gavy

Gavril (Russian) a form of Gavriel.
Ganya, Gavrilo, Gavrilushka

Gawain (Welsh) a form of Gavin.
Gawaine, Gawayn, Gawayne, Gawen, Gwayne

Gaylen (Greek) a form of Galen.
Gaylin, Gaylinn, Gaylon, Gaylyn

Gaylord (French) merry lord; jailer.
Gaillard, Gallard, Gay, Gayelord, Gayler, Gaylor

Gaynor (Irish) son of the fair-skinned man.
Gainer, Gainor, Gay, Gayner, Gaynnor

Geary (English) variable, changeable.
Gearey, Gery

Gedeon (Bulgarian, French) a form of Gideon.

Geffrey (English) a form of Geoffrey. See also Jeffrey.
Gefery, Geff, Geffery, Geffrard

Gellert (Hungarian) a form of Gerald.

Gena (Russian) a short form of Yevgenyi.
Genka, Genya, Gine

Genaro (Latin) consecrated to God.
Genereo, Genero, Gennaro

Gene (Greek) a short form of Eugene.
Genek

Genek (Polish) a form of
Gene.

Geno (Italian) a form of John.
A short form of Genovese.
Genio, Jeno

Genovese (Italian) from
Genoa, Italy.
Geno, Genovis

Gent (English) gentleman.
Gentle, Gentry

Genty (Irish, English) snow.

Geoff (English) a short form
of Geoffrey.

Geoffery (English) a form of
Geoffrey.
Geofery

Geoffrey (English) a form of
Jeffrey. See also Giotto,
Godfrey, Gottfried, Jeff.
*Geffrey, Geoff, Geoffery, Geoffre,
Geoffrie, Geoffroi, Geoffroy,
Geoffry, Geofrey, Geofri, Gofery*

Geordan (Scottish) a form of
Gordon.
*Geordann, Geordian, Geordin,
Geordon*

Geordie (Scottish) a form of
George.
Geordi, Geordy

Georg (Scandinavian) a form
of George.

George (Greek) farmer. See
also Durko, Egor, Iorgos,
Jerzy, Jiri, Joji, Jörg, Jorge,
Jorgen, Joris, Jorrín, Jur,
Jurgis, Keoki, Mahiái, Semer,
Yegor, Yorgos, Yoyi, Yrjo, Yuri,
Zhora.
*Geordie, Georg, Georgas,
Georges, Georget, Georgi,
Georgii, Georgio, Georgios,
Georgiy, Georgy, Gevork,
Gheorghe, Giorgio, Giorgos,
Goerge, Goran, Gordios, Gorge,
Gorje, Gorya, Grzegorz,
Gyorgy*

Georges (French) a form of
George.
Geórges

Georgio (Italian) a form of
George.

Georgios (Greek) a form of
George.
Georgious, Georgius

Georgy (Greek) a familiar
form of George.
Georgie

Geovanni, Geovanny (Italian)
forms of Giovanni.
*Geovan, Geovani, Geovanne,
Geovannee, Geovannhi,
Geovany*

Geraint (English) old.

Gerald (German) mighty
spearman. See also Fitzgerald,
Jarell, Jarrell, Jerald, Jerry,
Kharald.
*Garald, Garold, Garolds, Gary,
Gearalt, Gellert, Gérald,
Geralde, Geraldo, Gerale,*

*Geraud, Gerek, Gerick, Gerik,
Gerold, Gerrald, Gerrell,
Gérrick, Gerrild, Gerrin, Gerrit,
Gerrold, Gerry, Geryld, Giraldo,
Giraud, Girauld*

Geraldo (Italian, Spanish) a
form of Gerald.

Gerard (English) brave spear-
man. See also Jerard, Jerry.
*Garrard, Garrat, Garratt,
Gearard, Gerad, Gerar, Gérard,
Gerardo, Geraro, Géraud, Gerd,
Gerek, Gerhard, Gerrard,
Gerrit, Gerry, Girard*

Gerardo (Spanish) a form of
Gerard.
Gherardo

Géraud (French) a form of
Gerard.
Gerrad, Gerraud

Gerek (Polish) a form of
Gerard.

Geremia (Hebrew) exalted by
God. (Italian) a form of
Jeremiah.

Geremiah (Italian) a form of
Jeremiah.
Geremia, Gerimiah, Geromiah

Gerhard (German) a form of
Gerard.
*Garhard, Gerhardi, Gerhardt,
Gerhart, Gerhort*

Gerik (Polish) a form of
Edgar.
Geric, Gerick

Germain (French) from
Germany. (English) sprout,
bud. See also Jermaine.
*Germaine, German, Germane,
Germano, Germayn, Germayne*

Gerome (English) a form of
Jerome.

Geronimo (Greek, Italian) a
form of Jerome. History: a
famous Apache chief.
Geronemo

Gerrit (Dutch) a form of
Gerald.

Gerry (English) a familiar
form of Gerald, Gerard. See
also Jerry.
*Geri, Gerre, Gerri, Gerrie,
Gerryson*

Gershom (Hebrew) exiled.
(Yiddish) stranger in exile.
*Gersham, Gersho, Gershon,
Gerson, Geurson, Gursham,
Gurshan*

Gerson (English) son of Gar.
Gersan, Gershawn

Gert (German, Danish)
fighter.

Gervaise (French) honorable.
See also Jervis.
*Garvais, Garvaise, Garvey,
Gervais, Gervase, Gervasio,
Gervaso, Gervayse, Gervis,
Gerwazy*

Gerwin (Welsh) fair love.

Gethin (Welsh) dusky.
Geth

Ghazi (Arabic) conqueror.

Ghilchrist (Irish) servant of
Christ. See also Gil.
*Gilchrist, Gilcrist, Gilie, Gill,
Gilley, Gilly*

Ghislain (French) pledge.

Gi (Korean) brave.

Gia (Vietnamese) family.

Giacinto (Portuguese, Spanish)
a form of Jacinto.
Giacintho

Giacomo (Italian) a form of
Jacob.
*Gaimo, Giacamo, Giaco,
Giacobbe, Giacobo, Giacopo*

Gian (Italian) a form of
Giovanni, John.
*Gianetto, Giann, Gianne,
Giannes, Gianni, Giannis,
Giannos, Ghian*

Giancarlo (Italian) a combination of John + Charles.
Giancarlos, Gianncarlo

Gianluca (Italian) a combination of John + Lucas.

Gianni (Italian) a form of
Johnny.
Giani, Gionni

Gianpaolo (Italian) a combination of John + Paul.
Gianpaulo

Gib (English) a short form of
Gilbert.
Gibb, Gibbie, Gibby

Gibor (Hebrew) powerful.

Gibson (English) son of Gilbert.
*Gibbon, Gibbons, Gibbs, Gillson,
Gilson*

Gideon (Hebrew) tree cutter.
Bible: the judge who
defeated the Midianites.
*Gedeon, Gideone, Gidon,
Hedeon*

Gidon (Hebrew) a form of
Gideon.

Gifford (English) bold giver.
*Giff, Giffard, Gifferd, Giffie,
Giffy*

Gig (English) horse-drawn
carriage.

Gil (Greek) shield bearer.
(Hebrew) happy. (English) a
short form of Ghilchrist,
Gilbert.
*Gili, Gill, Gilli, Gillie, Gillis,
Gilly*

Gilad (Arabic) camel hump;
from Giladi, Saudi Arabia.
Giladi, Gilead

Gilamu (Basque) a form of
William.
Gillen

Gilbert (English) brilliant
pledge; trustworthy. See also
Gil, Gillett.
Gib, Gilberto, Gilburt,

*Giselbert, Giselberto,
Giselbertus, Guilbert*

Gilberto (Spanish) a form of
Gilbert.

Gilby (Scandinavian) hostage's
estate. (Irish) blond boy.
Gilbey, Gillbey, Gillbie, Gillby

Gilchrist (Irish) a form of
Ghilchrist.

Gilen (Basque, German) illustrious pledge.

Giles (French) goatskin shield.
Gide, Gilles, Gyles

Gillean (Irish) Bible: Saint
John's servant.
Gillan, Gillen, Gillian

Gillespie (Irish) son of the
bishop's servant.
Gillis

Gillett (French) young Gilbert.
Gelett, Gelette, Gillette

Gilmer (English) famous
hostage.
Gilmar

Gilmore (Irish) devoted to the
Virgin Mary.
Gillmore, Gillmour, Gilmour

Gilon (Hebrew) circle.

Gilroy (Irish) devoted to the
king.
*Gilderoy, Gildray, Gildroy,
Gillroy, Roy*

Gino (Greek) a familiar form
of Eugene. (Italian) a short
form of names ending in
"gene," "gino."
Ghino

Giona (Italian) a form of
Jonah.

Giordano (Italian) a form of
Jordan.
*Giordan, Giordana, Giordin,
Guordan*

Giorgio (Italian) a form of
George.

Giorgos (Greek) a form of
George.
Georgos, Giorgios

Giosia (Italian) a form of
Joshua.

Giotto (Italian) a form of
Geoffrey.

Giovani (Italian) a form of
Giovanni.
*Giavani, Giovan, Giovane,
Giovanie, Giovon*

Giovanni (Italian) a form of
John. See also Jeovanni,
Jiovanni.
*Geovanni, Geovanny, Gian,
Gianni, Giannino, Giovani,
Giovann, Giovannie, Giovanno,
Giovanny, Giovonathon,
Giovonni, Giovonnia,
Giovonnie, Givonni*

Giovanny (Italian) a form of
Giovanni.
Giovany

Gipsy (English) wanderer.
Gipson, Gypsy

Girvin (Irish) small; tough.
Girvan, Girven, Girvon

Gitano (Spanish) gypsy.

Giuliano (Italian) a form of
Julius.
Giulano, Giulino, Giulliano

Giulio (Italian) a form of
Julius.
Guilano

Giuseppe (Italian) a form of
Joseph.
*Giuseppi, Giuseppino,
Giusseppe, Guiseppe, Guiseppi,
Guiseppie, Guisseppe*

Giustino (Italian) a form of
Justin.
Giusto

Givon (Hebrew) hill; heights.
Givan, Givawn, Givyn

Gladwin (English) cheerful.
See also Win.
*Glad, Gladdie, Gladdy,
Gladwinn, Gladwyn,
Gladwynne*

Glanville (English) village
with oak trees.

Glen (Irish) a form of Glenn.
Glyn

Glendon (Scottish) fortress in
the glen.
*Glenden, Glendin, Glenn,
Glennden, Glennton, Glenton*

Glendower (Welsh) from
Glyndwr, Wales.

Glenn (Irish) a short form of
Glendon.
*Gleann, Glen, Glennie,
Glennis, Glennon, Glenny,
Glynn*

Glentworth (English) from
Glenton, England.

Glenville (Irish) village in the
glen.

Glyn (Welsh) a form of Glen.
Glin, Glynn

Goddard (German) divinely
firm.
*Godard, Godart, Goddart,
Godhardt, Godhart, Gothart,
Gotthard, Gotthardt, Gotthart*

Godfrey (Irish) God's peace.
(German) a form of Jeffrey.
See also Geoffrey, Gottfried.
*Giotto, Godefroi, Godfree,
Godfry, Godofredo, Godoired,
Godrey, Goffredo, Gofraidh,
Gofredo, Gorry*

Godwin (English) friend of
God. See also Win.
*Godewyn, Godwinn, Godwyn,
Goodwin, Goodwyn,
Goodwynn, Goodwynne*

Goel (Hebrew) redeemer.

Goldwin (English) golden friend. See also Win.
Golden, Goldewin, Goldewinn, Goldewyn, Goldwyn, Goldwynn

Goliath (Hebrew) exiled. Bible: the giant Philistine whom David slew with a slingshot.
Golliath

Gomda (Kiowa) wind.

Gomer (Hebrew) completed, finished. (English) famous battle.

Gonza (Rutooro) love.

Gonzalo (Spanish) wolf.
Goncalve, Gonsalo, Gonsalve, Gonzales, Gonzelee, Gonzolo

Gordon (English) triangular-shaped hill.
Geordan, Gord, Gordain, Gordan, Gorden, Gordonn, Gordy

Gordy (English) a familiar form of Gordon.
Gordie

Gore (English) triangular-shaped land; wedge-shaped land.

Gorman (Irish) small; blue eyed.

Goro (Japanese) fifth.

Gosheven (Native American) great leaper.

Gottfried (German) a form of Geoffrey, Godfrey.
Gotfrid, Gotfrids, Gottfrid

Gotzon (German) a form of Angel.

Govert (Dutch) heavenly peace.

Gower (Welsh) pure.

Gowon (Tiv) rainmaker.
Gowan

Gozol (Hebrew) soaring bird.
Gozal

Grady (Irish) noble; illustrious.
Gradea, Gradee, Gradey, Gradleigh, Graidey, Graidy

Graeme (Scottish) a form of Graham.
Graem

Graham (English) grand home.
Graeham, Graehame, Graehme, Graeme, Grahamme, Grahm, Grahame, Grahme, Gram, Grame, Gramm, Grayeme, Grayham

Granger (French) farmer.
Grainger, Grange

Grant (English) a short form of Grantland.
Grand, Grantham, Granthem, Grantley

Grantland (English) great plains.
Grant

Granville (French) large village.
Gran, Granvel, Granvil, Granvile, Granvill, Grenville, Greville

Gray (English) gray haired.
Graye, Grey, Greye

Grayden (English) gray haired.
Graden, Graydan, Graydyn, Greyden

Graydon (English) gray hill.
Gradon, Grayton, Greydon

Grayson (English) bailiff's son. See also Sonny.
Graysen, Greyson

Greeley (English) gray meadow.
Greelea, Greeleigh, Greely

Greenwood (English) green forest.
Green, Greener

Greg, Gregg (Latin) short forms of Gregory.
Graig, Greig, Gregson

Greggory (Latin) a form of Gregory.
Greggery

Gregor (Scottish) a form of Gregory.
Gregoor, Grégor, Gregore

Gregorio (Italian, Portuguese) a form of Gregory.
Gregorios

Gregory (Latin) vigilant watchman. See also Jörn, Krikor.
Gergely, Gergo, Greagoir, Greagory, Greer, Greg, Gregary, Greger, Gregery, Greggory, Grégoire, Gregor, Gregorey, Gregori, Grégorie, Gregorio, Gregorius, Gregors, Gregos, Gregrey, Gregroy, Gregry, Greogry, Gries, Grisha, Grzegorz

Gresham (English) village in the pasture.

Greyson (English) a form of Grayson.
Greysen, Greysten, Greyston

Griffin (Latin) hooked nose.
Griff, Griffen, Griffie, Griffon, Griffy, Gryphon

Griffith (Welsh) fierce chief; ruddy.
Grifen, Griff, Griffeth, Griffie, Griffy, Griffyn, Griffynn, Gryphon

Grigori (Bulgarian) a form of Gregory.
Grigoi, Grigor, Grigore, Grigorios, Grigorov, Grigory

Grimshaw (English) dark woods.

Grisha (Russian) a form of Gregory.

Griswold (German, French) gray forest.
Gris, Griz, Grizwald

Grosvener (French) big
hunter.

Grover (English) grove.
Grove

Guadalupe (Arabic) river of
black stones.
Guadalope

Gualberto (Spanish) a form of
Walter.
Gualterio

Gualtiero (Italian) a form of
Walter.
Gualterio

Guglielmo (Italian) a form of
William.

Guido (Italian) a form of Guy.

Guilford (English) ford with
yellow flowers.
Guildford

Guilherme (Portuguese) a
form of William.

Guillaume (French) a form of
William.
*Guillaums, Guilleaume,
Guilem, Guyllaume*

Guillermo (Spanish) a form of
William.
Guillerrmo

Gunnar (Scandinavian) a form
of Gunther.
Guner, Gunner

Gunther (Scandinavian) battle
army; warrior.
Guenter, Guenther, Gun,
Gunnar, Guntar, Gunter,
Guntero, Gunthar, Günther

Guotin (Chinese) polite;
strong leader.

Gurion (Hebrew) young lion.
Gur, Guri, Guriel

Gurpreet (Sikh) devoted to
the guru; devoted to the
Prophet.
Gurjeet, Gurmeet, Guruprit

Gurvir (Sikh) guru's warrior.
Gurveer

Gus (Scandinavian) a short
form of Angus, Augustine,
Gustave.
Guss, Gussie, Gussy, Gusti,
Gustry, Gusty

Gustaf (Swedish) a form of
Gustave.
Gustaaf, Gustaff

Gustave (Scandinavian) staff of
the Goths. History: Gustavus
Adolphus was a king of
Sweden. See also Kosti, Tabo,
Tavo.
Gus, Gustaf, Gustaff, Gustaof,
Gustav, Gustáv, Gustava,
Gustaves, Gustavo, Gustavs,
Gustavus, Gustik, Gustus,
Gusztav

Gustavo (Italian, Spanish) a
form of Gustave.
Gustabo

Guthrie (German) war hero.
(Irish) windy place.
Guthrey, Guthry

Gutierre (Spanish) a form of
Walter.

Guy (Hebrew) valley.
(German) warrior. (French)
guide. See also Guido.
Guyon

Guyapi (Native American)
candid.

Gwayne (Welsh) a form of
Gawain.
Gwaine, Gwayn

Gwidon (Polish) life.

Gwilym (Welsh) a form of
William.
Gwillym

Gwyn (Welsh) fair; blessed.
Gwynn, Gwynne

Gyasi (Akan) marvelous baby.

Gyorgy (Russian) a form of
George.
Gyoergy, György, Gyuri,
Gyurka

Gyula (Hungarian) youth.
Gyala, Gyuszi

H

Habib (Arabic) beloved.

Hackett (German, French)
little wood cutter.
Hacket, Hackit, Hackitt

Hackman (German, French)
wood cutter.

Hadar (Hebrew) glory.

Haddad (Arabic) blacksmith.

Hadden (English) heather-
covered hill.
Haddan, Haddon, Haden

Haden (English) a form of
Hadden.
Hadin, Hadon, Hadyn, Haeden

Hadi (Arabic) guiding to the
right.
Hadee, Hady

Hadley (English) heather-cov-
ered meadow.
Had, Hadlea, Hadlee, Hadleigh,
Hadly, Lee, Leigh

Hadrian (Latin, Swedish) dark.
Adrian, Hadrien

Hadwin (English) friend in a
time of war.
Hadwinn, Hadwyn, Hadwynn,
Hadwynne

Hagan (German) strong
defense.
Haggan

Hagen (Irish) young, youthful.

Hagley (English) enclosed
meadow.

Hagos (Ethiopian) happy.

Hahnee (Native American) beggar.

Hai (Vietnamese) sea.

Haidar (Arabic) lion.
Haider

Haiden (English) a form of Hayden.
Haidyn

Haig (English) enclosed with hedges.

Hailey (Irish) a form of Haley.
Haile, Haille, Haily, Halee

Haji (Swahili) born during the pilgrimage to Mecca.

Hakan (Native American) fiery.

Hakeem (Arabic) a form of Hakim.
Hakam, Hakem

Hakim (Arabic) wise. (Ethiopian) doctor.
Hakeem, Hakiem

Hakon (Scandinavian) of Nordic ancestry.
Haaken, Haakin, Haakon, Haeo, Hak, Hakan, Hako

Hal (English) a short form of Halden, Hall, Harold.

Halbert (English) shining hero.
Bert, Halburt

Halden (Scandinavian) half-Danish. See also Dane.
Hal, Haldan, Haldane, Halfdan, Halvdan

Hale (English) a short form of Haley. (Hawaiian) a form of Harry.
Hayle, Heall

Halen (Swedish) hall.
Hale, Hallen, Haylan, Haylen

Haley (Irish) ingenious.
Hailey, Hale, Haleigh, Halley, Hayleigh, Hayley, Hayli

Halford (English) valley ford.

Hali (Greek) sea.

Halian (Zuni) young.

Halil (Turkish) dear friend.
Halill

Halim (Arabic) mild, gentle.
Haleem

Hall (English) manor, hall.
Hal, Halstead, Halsted

Hallam (English) valley.

Hallan (English) dweller at the hall; dweller at the manor.
Halin, Hallene, Hallin

Halley (English) meadow near the hall; holy.
Hallie

Halliwell (English) holy well.
Hallewell, Hellewell, Helliwell

Hallward (English) hall guard.

Halsey (English) Hal's island.

Halstead (English) manor grounds.
Halsted

Halton (English) estate on the hill.

Halvor (Norwegian) rock; protector.
Halvard

Ham (Hebrew) hot. Bible: one of Noah's sons.

Hamal (Arabic) lamb. Astronomy: a bright star in the constellation of Aries.

Hamar (Scandinavian) hammer.

Hamid (Arabic) praised. See also Muhammad.
Haamid, Hamaad, Hamadi, Hamd, Hamdrem, Hamed, Hamedo, Hameed, Hamidi, Hammad, Hammed, Humayd

Hamill (English) scarred.
Hamel, Hamell, Hammill

Hamilton (English) proud estate.
Hamel, Hamelton, Hamil, Hamill, Tony

Hamish (Scottish) a form of Jacob, James.

Hamisi (Swahili) born on Thursday.

Hamlet (German, French) little village; home. Literature: one of Shakespeare's tragic heroes.

Hamlin (German, French) loves his home.
Hamblin, Hamelen, Hamelin, Hamlen, Hamlyn, Lin

Hammet (English, Scandinavian) village.
Hammett, Hamnet, Hamnett

Hammond (English) village.
Hamond

Hampton (English) Geography: a town in England.
Hamp

Hamza (Arabic) powerful.
Hamzah, Hamze, Hamzeh, Hamzia

Hanale (Hawaiian) a form of Henry.
Haneke

Hanan (Hebrew) grace.
Hananel, Hananiah, Johanan

Hanbal (Arabic) pure. History: Ahmad Ibn Hanbal founded an Islamic school of thought.

Handel (German, English) a form of John. Music: George Frideric Handel was a German composer whose works include *Messiah* and *Water Music*.

Hanford (English) high ford.

Hanif (Arabic) true believer.
Haneef, Hanef

Hank (American) a familiar form of Henry.

Hanley (English) high meadow.
Handlea, Handleigh, Handley,

Hanlea, Hanlee, Hanleigh, Hanly, Henlea, Henlee, Henleigh, Henley

Hannes (Finnish) a form of John.

Hannibal (Phoenician) grace of God. History: a famous Carthaginian general who fought the Romans.
Anibal

Hanno (German) a short form of Johan.
Hanna, Hannah, Hannon, Hannu, Hanon

Hans (Scandinavian) a form of John.
Hanschen, Hansel, Hants, Hanz

Hansel (Scandinavian) a form of Hans.
Haensel, Hansell, Hansl, Hanzel

Hansen (Scandinavian) son of Hans.
Hanson

Hansh (Hindi) god; godlike.

Hanson (Scandinavian) a form of Hansen.
Hansen, Hanssen, Hansson

Hanus (Czech) a form of John.

Haoa (Hawaiian) a form of Howard.

Hara (Hindi) seizer. Religion: another name for the Hindu god Shiva.

Harald (Scandinavian) a form of Harold.
Haraldo, Haralds, Haralpos

Harb (Arabic) warrior.

Harbin (German, French) little bright warrior.
Harben, Harbyn

Harcourt (French) fortified dwelling.
Court, Harcort

Hardeep (Punjabi) a form of Harpreet.

Harden (English) valley of the hares.
Hardian, Hardin

Harding (English) brave; hardy.
Hardin

Hardwin (English) brave friend.

Hardy (German) bold, daring.
Hardie

Harel (Hebrew) mountain of God.
Harell, Hariel, Harrell

Harford (English) ford of the hares.

Hargrove (English) grove of the hares.
Hargreave, Hargreaves

Hari (Hindi) tawny.
Hariel, Harin

Harith (Arabic) cultivator.

Harjot (Sikh) light of God.
Harjeet, Harjit, Harjodh

Harkin (Irish) dark red.
Harkan, Harken

Harlan (English) hare's land;
army land.
*Harland, Harlen, Harlenn,
Harlin, Harlon, Harlyn,
Harlynn*

Harland (English) a form of
Harlan.
Harlend

Harley (English) hare's
meadow; army meadow.
*Arley, Harlea, Harlee, Harleigh,
Harly*

Harlow (English) hare's hill;
army hill. See also Arlo.

Harman, Harmon (English)
forms of Herman.
*Harm, Harmen, Harmond,
Harms*

Harold (Scandinavian) army
ruler. See also Jindra.
*Araldo, Garald, Garold, Hal,
Harald, Haraldas, Haraldo,
Haralds, Harry, Heraldo, Herold,
Heronim, Herrick, Herryck*

Haroun (Arabic) lofty; exalted.
*Haarun, Harin, Haron, Haroon,
Harron, Harun*

Harper (English) harp player.
Harp, Harpo

Harpreet (Punjabi) loves God,
devoted to God.
Hardeep

Harris (English) a short form
of Harrison.
Haris, Hariss

Harrison (English) son of
Harry.
*Harison, Harreson, Harris,
Harrisen, Harrisson*

Harrod (Hebrew) hero; conqueror.

Harry (English) a familiar
form of Harold. See also
Arrigo, Hale, Parry.
*Harm, Harray, Harrey, Harri,
Harrie*

Hart (English) a short form of
Hartley.

Hartley (English) deer
meadow.
*Hart, Hartlea, Hartlee,
Hartleigh, Hartly*

Hartman (German) hard;
strong.

Hartwell (English) deer well.
Harwell, Harwill

Hartwig (German) strong
advisor.

Hartwood (English) deer forest.
Harwood

Harvey (German) army warrior.
Harv, Hervé, Hervey, Hervie, Hervy

Harvir (Sikh) God's warrior.
Harvier

Hasad (Turkish) reaper, harvester.

Hasan (Arabic) a form of Hassan.
Hasaan, Hasain, Hasaun, Hashaan, Hason

Hasani (Swahili) handsome.
Hasan, Hasanni, Hassani, Heseny, Hassen, Hassian, Husani

Hashim (Arabic) destroyer of evil.
Haashim, Hasham, Hasheem, Hashem

Hasin (Hindi) laughing.
Haseen, Hasen, Hassin, Hazen, Hesen

Haskel (Hebrew) a form of Ezekiel.
Haskell

Haslett (English) hazel-tree land.
Haze, Hazel, Hazlett, Hazlitt

Hassan (Arabic) handsome.
Hasan, Hassen, Hasson

Hassel (German, English) witches' corner.
Hassal, Hassall, Hassell, Hazael, Hazell

Hastin (Hindi) elephant.

Hastings (Latin) spear. (English) house council.
Hastie, Hasty

Hatim (Arabic) judge.
Hateem, Hatem

Hauk (Norwegian) hawk.
Haukeye

Havelock (Norwegian) sea battler.

Haven (Dutch, English) harbor, port; safe place.
Haeven, Havin, Hevin, Hevon, Hovan

Havika (Hawaiian) a form of David.

Hawk (English) hawk.
Hawke, Hawkin, Hawkins

Hawley (English) hedged meadow.
Hawleigh, Hawly

Hawthorne (English) hawthorn tree.

Hayden (English) hedged valley.
Haiden, Haydan, Haydenn, Haydn, Haydon

Hayes (English) hedged valley.
Hayse

Hayward (English) guardian of the hedged area.
Haward, Heyvard, Heyward

Haywood (English) hedged forest.
Heywood, Woody

Hearn (Scottish, English) a short form of Ahearn.
Hearne, Herin, Hern

Heath (English) heath.
Heathe, Heith

Heathcliff (English) cliff near the heath. Literature: the hero of Emily Brontë's novel *Wuthering Heights.*

Heaton (English) high place.

Heber (Hebrew) ally, partner.

Hector (Greek) steadfast. Mythology: the greatest hero of the Trojan War in Homer's epic poem *Iliad.*

Hedley (English) heather-filled meadow.
Headley, Headly, Hedly

Heinrich (German) a form of Henry.
Heindrick, Heiner, Heinreich, Heinrick, Heinrik, Hinrich

Heinz (German) a familiar form of Henry.

Helaku (Native American) sunny day.

Helge (Russian) holy.

Helki (Moquelumnan) touching.

Helmer (German) warrior's wrath.

Helmut (German) courageous.
Helmuth

Heman (Hebrew) faithful.

Henderson (Scottish, English) son of Henry.
Hendrie, Hendries, Hendron, Henryson

Hendrick (Dutch) a form of Henry.
Hendricks, Hendrickson, Hendrik, Hendriks, Hendrikus, Hendrix, Henning

Heniek (Polish) a form of Henry.
Henier

Henley (English) high meadow.

Henning (German) a form of Hendrick, Henry.

Henoch (Yiddish) initiator.
Enoch, Henock, Henok

Henri (French) a form of Henry.
Henrico, Henrri

Henrick (Dutch) a form of Henry.
Heinrick, Henerik, Henrich, Henrik, Henryk

Henrique (Portuguese) a form of Henry.

Henry (German) ruler of the household. See also Arrigo,

Enric, Enrick, Enrico,
Enrikos, Enrique, Hanale,
Honok, Kiki.
Hagan, Hank, Harro, Harry,
Heike, Heinrich, Heinz,
Hendrick, Henery, Heniek,
Henning, Henraoi, Henri,
Henrick, Henrim, Henrique,
Henrry, Heromin, Hersz

Heraldo (Spanish) a form of
Harold.
Herald, Hiraldo

Herb (German) a short form
of Herbert.
Herbie, Herby

Herbert (German) glorious
soldier.
Bert, Erbert, Eriberto, Harbert,
Hebert, Hébert, Heberto, Herb,
Heriberto, Hurbert

Hercules (Latin) glorious gift.
Mythology: a Greek hero of
fabulous strength, renowned
for his twelve labors.
Herakles, Herc, Hercule, Herculie

Heriberto (Spanish) a form of
Herbert.
Heribert

Herman (Latin) noble.
(German) soldier. See also
Armand, Ermanno, Ermano,
Mandek.
Harmon, Hermaan, Hermann,
Hermie, Herminio, Hermino,
Hermon, Hermy, Heromin

Hermes (Greek) messenger.
Mythology: the divine herald
of Greek mythology.

Hernan (German)
peacemaker.

Hernando (Spanish) a form of
Ferdinand.
Hernandes, Hernandez

Herrick (German) war ruler.
Herrik, Herryck

Herschel (Hebrew) a form of
Hershel.
Herchel, Hersch, Herschel,
Herschell

Hersh (Hebrew) a short form
of Hershel.
Hersch, Hirsch

Hershel (Hebrew) deer.
Herschel, Hersh, Hershal,
Hershall, Hershell, Herzl,
Hirschel, Hirshel

Hertz (Yiddish) my strife.
Herzel

Hervé (French) a form of
Harvey.

Hesperos (Greek) evening
star.
Hespero

Hesutu (Moquelumnan) pick-
ing up a yellow jacket's nest.

Hew (Welsh) a form of Hugh.
Hewe, Huw

Hewitt (German, French) little smart one.
Hewe, Hewet, Hewett, Hewie, Hewit, Hewlett, Hewlitt, Hugh

Hewson (English) son of Hugh.

Hezekiah (Hebrew) God gives strength.
Hezekyah, Hazikiah, Hezikyah

Hiamovi (Cheyenne) high chief.

Hibah (Arabic) gift.

Hideaki (Japanese) smart, clever.
Hideo

Hieremias (Greek) God will uplift.

Hieronymos (Greek) a form of Jerome. Art: Hieronymus Bosch was a fifteenth-century Dutch painter.
Hierome, Hieronim, Hieronimo, Hieronimos, Hieronymo, Hieronymus

Hieu (Vietnamese) respectful.

Hilario (Spanish) a form of Hilary.

Hilary (Latin) cheerful. See also Ilari.
Hi, Hilair, Hilaire, Hilarie, Hilario, Hilarion, Hilarius, Hil, Hill, Hillary, Hillery, Hilliary, Hillie, Hilly

Hildebrand (German) battle sword.
Hildebrando, Hildo

Hilel (Arabic) new moon.

Hillel (Hebrew) greatly praised. Religion: Rabbi Hillel originated the Talmud.

Hilliard (German) brave warrior.
Hillard, Hiller, Hillier, Hillierd, Hillyard, Hillyer, Hillyerd

Hilmar (Swedish) famous noble.

Hilton (English) town on a hill.
Hylton

Hinto (Dakota) blue.

Hinun (Native American) spirit of the storm.

Hippolyte (Greek) horseman.
Hipolito, Hippolit, Hippolitos, Hippolytus, Ippolito

Hiram (Hebrew) noblest; exalted.
Hi, Hirom, Huram, Hyrum

Hiromasa (Japanese) fair, just.

Hiroshi (Japanese) generous.

Hisoka (Japanese) secretive, reserved.

Hiu (Hawaiian) a form of Hugh.

Ho (Chinese) good.

Hoang (Vietnamese) finished.

Hobart (German) Bart's hill.
Hobard, Hobbie, Hobby, Hobie,
Hoebart

Hobert (German) Bert's hill.
Hobey

Hobson (English) son of
Robert.
Hobbs, Hobs

Hoc (Vietnamese) studious.

Hod (Hebrew) a short form of
Hodgson.

Hodgson (English) son of
Roger.
Hod

Hogan (Irish) youth.
Hogin

Holbrook (English) brook in
the hollow.
Brook, Holbrooke

Holden (English) hollow in
the valley.
Holdan, Holdin, Holdon,
Holdun, Holdyn

Holic (Czech) barber.

Holland (French) Geography:
a former province of the
Netherlands.

Holleb (Polish) dove.
Hollub, Holub

Hollis (English) grove of holly
trees.
Hollie, Holly

Holmes (English) river islands.

Holt (English) forest.
Holten, Holton

Homer (Greek) hostage;
pledge; security. Literature: a
renowned Greek epic poet.
Homar, Homere, Homère,
Homero, Homeros, Homerus

Hondo (Shona) warrior.

Honesto (Filipino) honest.

Honi (Hebrew) gracious.
Choni

Honok (Polish) a form of
Henry.

Honon (Moquelumnan) bear.

Honorato (Spanish) honorable.

Honoré (Latin) honored.
Honor, Honoratus, Honoray,
Honorio, Honorius

Honovi (Native American)
strong.

Honza (Czech) a form of
John.

Hop (Chinese) agreeable.

Horace (Latin) keeper of the
hours. Literature: a famous
Roman lyric poet and
satirist.
Horacio, Horaz

Horacio (Latin) a form of
Horace.

Horatio (Latin) clan name. See also Orris.
Horatius, Oratio

Horst (German) dense grove; thicket.
Hurst

Horton (English) garden estate.
Hort, Horten, Orton

Hosa (Arapaho) young crow.

Hosea (Hebrew) salvation. Bible: a Hebrew prophet.
Hose, Hoseia, Hoshea, Hosheah

Hotah (Lakota) white.

Hototo (Native American) whistler.

Houghton (English) settlement on the headland.

Houston (English) hill town. Geography: a city in Texas.
Housten, Houstin, Hustin, Huston

Howard (English) watchman. See also Haoa.
Howie, Ward

Howe (German) high.
Howey, Howie

Howell (Welsh) remarkable.
Howel

Howi (Moquelumnan) turtledove.

Howie (English) a familiar form of Howard, Howland.
Howey

Howin (Chinese) loyal swallow.

Howland (English) hilly land.
Howie, Howlan, Howlen

Hoyt (Irish) mind; spirit.

Hu (Chinese) tiger.

Hubbard (German) a form of Hubert.

Hubert (German) bright mind; bright spirit. See also Beredei, Uberto.
Bert, Hobart, Hubbard, Hubbert, Huber, Hubertek, Huberto, Hubertson, Hubie, Huey, Hugh, Hugibert, Huibert, Humberto

Huberto (Spanish) a form of Hubert.
Humberto

Hubie (English) a familiar form of Hubert.
Hube, Hubi

Hud (Arabic) Religion: a Muslim prophet.

Hudson (English) son of Hud.

Huey (English) a familiar form of Hugh.
Hughey, Hughie, Hughy, Hui

Hugh (English) a short form of Hubert. See also Ea, Hewitt, Huxley, Maccoy, Ugo.
Fitzhugh, Hew, Hiu, Hue, Huey, Hughes, Hugo, Hugues

Hugo (Latin) a form of Hugh.
Ugo

Hulbert (German) brilliant
grace.
*Bert, Hulbard, Hulburd,
Hulburt, Hull*

Humbert (German) brilliant
strength. See also Umberto.
Hum, Humberto

Humberto (Portuguese) a
form of Humbert.

Humphrey (German) peaceful
strength. See also Onofrio,
Onufry.
*Hum, Humfredo, Humfrey,
Humfrid, Humfried, Humfry,
Hump, Humph, Humphery,
Humphry, Humphrys, Hunfredo*

Hung (Vietnamese) brave.

Hunt (English) a short form of
names beginning with
"Hunt."

Hunter (English) hunter.
Hunt, Huntur

Huntington (English) hunting
estate.
Hunt, Huntingdon

Huntley (English) hunter's
meadow.
*Hunt, Huntlea, Huntlee,
Huntleigh, Huntly*

Hurley (Irish) sea tide.
Hurlee, Hurleigh

Hurst (English) a form of
Horst.
Hearst, Hirst

Husam (Arabic) sword.

Husamettin (Turkish) sharp
sword.

Huslu (Native American) hairy
bear.

Hussain (Arabic) a form of
Hussein.
*Hossain, Husain, Husani,
Husayn, Hussan, Hussayn*

Hussein (Arabic) little; hand-
some.
*Hossein, Houssein, Houssin,
Huissien, Huossein, Husein,
Husien, Hussain, Hussien*

Hussien (Arabic) a form of
Hussein.
Husian, Hussin

Hutchinson (English) son of
the hutch dweller.
Hutcheson

Hute (Native American) star.

Hutton (English) house on the
jutting ledge.
Hut, Hutt, Huttan

Huxley (English) Hugh's
meadow.
*Hux, Huxlea, Huxlee,
Huxleigh, Lee*

Huy (Vietnamese) glorious.

Hy (Vietnamese) hopeful. (English) a short form of Hyman.

Hyacinthe (French) hyacinth.

Hyatt (English) high gate.
Hyat

Hyde (English) cache; measure of land equal to 120 acres; animal hide.

Hyder (English) tanner, preparer of animal hides for tanning.

Hyman (English) a form of Chaim.
Haim, Hayim, Hayvim, Hayyim, Hy, Hyam, Hymie

Hyun-Ki (Korean) wise.

Hyun-Shik (Korean) clever.

I

Iago (Spanish, Welsh) a form of Jacob, James. Literature: the villain in Shakespeare's *Othello*.
Jago

Iain (Scottish) a form of Ian.

Iakobos (Greek) a form of Jacob.
Iakov, Iakovos, Iakovs

Ian (Scottish) a form of John. See also Ean, Eion.
Iain, Iane, Iann

Ianos (Czech) a form of John.
Iannis

Ib (Phoenician, Danish) oath of Baal.

Iban (Basque) a form of John.

Ibon (Basque) a form of Ivor.

Ibrahim (Hausa) my father is exalted.
Ibrahaim, Ibraham, Ibraheem, Ibrahem, Ibrahiem, Ibrahiim, Ibrahmim

Ichabod (Hebrew) glory is gone. Literature: Ichabod Crane is the main character of Washington Irving's story "The Legend of Sleepy Hollow."

Idi (Swahili) born during the Idd festival.

Idris (Welsh) eager lord. (Arabic) Religion: a Muslim prophet.
Idrease, Idrees, Idres, Idress, Idreus, Idriece, Idriss, Idrissa, Idriys

Iestyn (Welsh) a form of Justin.

Igashu (Native American) wanderer; seeker.
Igasho

Iggy (Latin) a familiar form of Ignatius.

Ignacio (Italian) a form of Ignatius.
Ignazio

Ignatius (Latin) fiery, ardent. Religion: Saint Ignatius of Loyola founded the Jesuit order. See also Inigo, Neci.
Iggie, Iggy, Ignac, Ignác, Ignace, Ignacio, Ignacius, Ignatios, Ignatious, Ignatz, Ignaz, Ignazio

Igor (Russian) a form of Inger, Ingvar. See also Egor, Yegor.
Igoryok

Ihsan (Turkish) compassionate.

Ike (Hebrew) a familiar form of Isaac. History: the nickname of the thirty-fourth U.S. president Dwight D. Eisenhower.
Ikee, Ikey

Iker (Basque) visitation.

Ilan (Hebrew) tree. (Basque) youth.

Ilari (Basque) a form of Hilary.
Ilario

Ilias (Greek) a form of Elijah.
Illias, Illyas, Ilyas, Ilyes

Illan (Basque, Latin) youth.

Ilom (Ibo) my enemies are many.

Ilya (Russian) a form of Elijah.
Ilia, Ilie, Ilija, Iliya, Ilja, Illia, Illya

Imad (Arabic) supportive; mainstay.

Iman (Hebrew) a short form of Immanuel.
Imani, Imanni

Immanuel (Hebrew) a form of Emmanuel.
Iman, Imanol, Imanuel, Immanual, Immanuele, Immuneal

Imran (Arabic) host.
Imraan

Imre (Hungarian) a form of Emery.
Imri

Imrich (Czech) a form of Emery.
Imrus

Inay (Hindi) god; godlike.

Ince (Hungarian) innocent.

Inder (Hindi) god; godlike.
Inderbir, Inderdeep, Inderjeet, Inderjit, Inderpal, Inderpreet, Inderveer, Indervir, Indra, Indrajit

Indiana (Hindi) from India.
Indi, Indy

Inek (Welsh) a form of Irvin.

Ing (Scandinavian) a short form of Ingmar.
Inge

Ingelbert (German) a form of Engelbert.
Inglebert

Inger (Scandinavian) son's army.
Igor, Ingemar, Ingmar

Ingmar (Scandinavian) famous son.
Ing, Ingamar, Ingamur, Ingemar

Ingram (English) angel.
Inglis, Ingra, Ingraham, Ingrim

Ingvar (Scandinavian) Ing's soldier.
Igor, Ingevar

Inigo (Basque) a form of Ignatius.
Iñaki, Iniego, Iñigo

Iniko (Ibo) born during bad times.

Innis (Irish) island.
Innes, Inness, Inniss

Innocenzio (Italian) innocent.
Innocenty, Inocenci, Inocencio, Inocente, Inosente

Inteus (Native American) proud; unashamed.

Ioakim (Russian) a form of Joachim.
Ioachime, Ioakimo, Iov

Ioan (Greek, Bulgarian, Romanian) a form of John.
Ioane, Ioann, Ioannes, Ioannikios, Ioannis, Ionel

Iokepa (Hawaiian) a form of Joseph.
Keo

Iolo (Welsh) the Lord is worthy.
Iorwerth

Ionakana (Hawaiian) a form of Jonathan.

Iorgos (Greek) a form of George.

Iosif (Greek, Russian) a form of Joseph.

Iosua (Romanian) a form of Joshua.

Ipyana (Nyakyusa) graceful.

Ira (Hebrew) watchful.

Iram (English) bright.

Irumba (Rutooro) born after twins.

Irv (Irish, Welsh, English) a short form of Irvin, Irving.

Irvin (Irish, Welsh, English) a short form of Irving. See also Ervine.
Inek, Irv, Irven, Irvine, Irvinn, Irvon

Irving (Irish) handsome. (Welsh) white river. (English) sea friend. See also Ervin, Ervine.
Irv, Irvin, Irvington, Irwin, Irwing

Irwin (English) a form of
Irving. See also Ervin.
Irwinn, Irwyn

Isa (Arabic) a form of Jesus.
Isaah

Isaac (Hebrew) he will laugh.
Bible: the son of Abraham
and Sarah. See also Itzak,
Izak, Yitzchak.
*Aizik, Icek, Ike, Ikey, Ikie,
Isaak, Isaakios, Isac, Isacc, Isacco,
Isack, Isaic, Ishaq, Isiac, Isiacc,
Issac, Issca, Itzak, Izak, Izzy*

Isaak (Hebrew) a form of
Isaac.
Isack, Isak, Isik, Issak

Isaiah (Hebrew) God is my
salvation. Bible: a Hebrew
prophet.
*Isa, Isai, Isaia, Isaias, Isaid,
Isaih, Isaish, Ishaq, Isia, Isiah,
Isiash, Issia, Issiah, Izaiah,
Izaiha, Izaya, Izayah, Izayaih,
Izayiah, Izeyah, Izeyha*

Isaias (Hebrew) a form of
Isaiah.
Isaiahs, Isais, Izayus

Isam (Arabic) safeguard.

Isas (Japanese) meritorious.

Isekemu (Native American)
slow-moving creek.

Isham (English) home of the
iron one.

Ishan (Hindi) direction.
Ishaan, Ishaun

Ishaq (Arabic) a form of Isaac.
Ishaac, Ishak

Ishmael (Hebrew) God will
hear. Literature: the narrator
of Herman Melville's novel
Moby-Dick.
*Isamael, Isamail, Ishma,
Ishmail, Ishmale, Ishmeal,
Ishmeil, Ishmel, Ishmil, Ismael,
Ismail*

Isidore (Greek) gift of Isis. See
also Dorian, Ysidro.
*Isador, Isadore, Isadorios, Isidor,
Isidro, Issy, Ixidor, Izadore,
Izidor, Izidore, Izydor, Izzy*

Isidro (Greek) a form of
Isidore.
Isidoro, Isidoros

Iskander (Afghan) a form of
Alexander.

Ismael (Arabic) a form of
Ishmael.

Ismail (Arabic) a form of
Ishmael.
Ismeil, Ismiel

Israel (Hebrew) prince of
God; wrestled with God.
History: the nation of Israel
took its name from the name
given Jacob after he wrestled
with the angel of the Lord.
See also Yisrael.
*Iser, Isreal, Israhel, Isrell, Isrrael,
Isser, Izrael, Izzy, Yisrael*

Isreal (Hebrew) a form of
Israel.
Isrieal

Issa (Swahili) God is our salvation.

Issac (Hebrew) a form of Isaac.
Issacc, Issaic, Issiac

Issiah (Hebrew) a form of
Isaiah.
Issaiah, Issia

Istu (Native American) sugar
pine.

István (Hungarian) a form of
Stephen.
Isti, Istvan, Pista

Ithel (Welsh) generous lord.

Ittamar (Hebrew) island of
palms.
Itamar

Itzak (Hebrew) a form of
Isaac, Yitzchak.
Itzik

Iukini (Hawaiian) a form of
Eugene.
Kini

Iustin (Bulgarian, Russian) a
form of Justin.

Ivan (Russian) a form of John.
*Iván, Ivanchik, Ivanichek, Ivann,
Ivano, Ivas, Iven, Ivin, Ivon,
Ivyn, Vanya*

Ivar (Scandinavian) a form of
Ivor. See also Yves, Yvon.
Iv, Iva

Ives (English) young archer.
Ive, Iven, Ivey, Yves

Ivo (German) yew wood; bow
wood.
*Ibon, Ivar, Ives, Ivon, Ivonnie,
Ivor, Yvo*

Ivor (Scandinavian) a form of
Ivo.
Ibon, Ifor, Ivar, Iver, Ivory, Ivry

Iwan (Polish) a form of John.

Iyapo (Yoruba) many trials;
many obstacles.

Iye (Native American) smoke.

Izak (Czech) a form of Isaac.
*Itzhak, Ixaka, Izaac, Izaak,
Izac, Izaic, Izak, Izec, Izeke,
Izick, Izik, Izsak, Izsák, Izzak*

Izzy (Hebrew) a familiar form
of Isaac, Isidore, Israel.
Issy

J

J (American) an initial used as
a first name.
J.

Ja (Korean) attractive,
magnetic.

Jaali (Swahili) powerful.

Jaan (Estonian) a form of
Christian.

Jaap (Dutch) a form of Jim.

Jabari (Swahili) fearless, brave.
Jabaar, Jabahri, Jabar, Jabarae, Jabare, Jabaree, Jabarei, Jabarie, Jabarri, Jabarrie, Jabary, Jabbar, Jabbaree, Jabbari, Jaber, Jabiari, Jabier, Jabori, Jaborie

Jabez (Hebrew) born in pain.
Jabe, Jabes, Jabesh

Jabin (Hebrew) God has created.
Jabain, Jabien, Jabon

Jabir (Arabic) consoler, comforter.
Jabiri, Jabori

Jabril (Arabic) a form of Jibril.
Jabrail, Jabree, Jabreel, Jabrel, Jabrell, Jabrelle, Jabri, Jabrial, Jabrie, Jabriel, Jabrielle, Jabrille

Jabulani (Shona) happy.

Jacan (Hebrew) trouble.
Jachin

Jacari (American) a form of Jacorey.
Jacarey, Jacaris, Jacarius, Jacarre, Jacarri, Jacarrus, Jacarus, Jacary, Jacaure, Jacauri, Jaccar, Jaccari

Jace (American) a combination of the initials J. + C.
JC, J.C., Jacee, Jacek, Jacey, Jacie, Jaice, Jaicee

Jacen (Greek) a form of Jason.
Jaceon

Jacinto (Portuguese, Spanish) hyacinth. See also Giacinto.
Jacindo, Jacint, Jacinta

Jack (American) a familiar form of Jacob, John. See also Keaka.
Jackie, Jacko, Jackub, Jak, Jax, Jock, Jocko

Jackie, Jacky (American) familiar forms of Jack.
Jackey

Jackson (English) son of Jack.
Jacksen, Jacksin, Jacson, Jakson, Jaxon

Jaco (Portuguese) a form of Jacob.

Jacob (Hebrew) supplanter, substitute. Bible: son of Isaac, brother of Esau. See also Akiva, Chago, Checha, Coby, Diego, Giacomo, Hamish, Iago, Iakobos, James, Kiva, Koby, Kuba, Tiago, Yakov, Yasha, Yoakim.
Jaap, Jachob, Jack, Jackob, Jackub, Jaco, Jacobb, Jacobe, Jacobi, Jacobo, Jacoby, Jacolbi, Jacolby, Jacque, Jacques, Jacub, Jaecob, Jago, Jaicob, Jaime, Jake, Jakob, Jalu, Jasha, Jaycob, Jecis, Jeks, Jeska, Jim, Jocek, Jock, Jocob, Jocobb, Jocoby, Jocolby, Jokubas

Jacobi, Jacoby (Hebrew) forms of Jacob.
Jachobi, Jacobbe, Jacobee, Jacobey, Jacobie, Jacobii, Jacobis

Jacobo (Hebrew) a form of Jacob.

Jacobson (English) son of Jacob.
Jacobs, Jacobsen, Jacobsin, Jacobus

Jacorey (American) a combination of Jacob + Corey.
Jacari, Jacori, Jacoria, Jacorie, Jacoris, Jacorius, Jacorrey, Jacorrien, Jacorry, Jacory, Jacouri, Jacourie, Jakari

Jacque (French) a form of Jacob.
Jacquay, Jacqui, Jocque, Jocqui

Jacques (French) a form of Jacob, James. See also Coco.
Jackque, Jackques, Jackquise, Jacot, Jacquan, Jacquees, Jacquese, Jacquess, Jacquet, Jacquett, Jacquez, Jacquis, Jacquise, Jaquez, Jarques, Jarquis

Jacquez, Jaquez (French) forms of Jacques.
Jaques, Jaquese, Jaqueus, Jaqueze, Jaquis, Jaquise, Jaquze, Jocquez

Jacy (Tupi-Guarani) moon.
Jaicy, Jaycee

Jade (Spanish) jade, precious stone.
Jaeid, Jaid, Jaide

Jaden (Hebrew) a form of Jadon.
Jadee, Jadeen, Jadenn, Jadeon, Jadin, Jaeden

Jadon (Hebrew) God has heard.
Jaden, Jadyn, Jaedon, Jaiden, Jaydon

Jadrien (American) a combination of Jay + Adrien.
Jad, Jada, Jadd, Jader, Jadrian

Jadyn (Hebrew) a form of Jadon.
Jadyne, Jaedyn

Jaegar (German) hunter.
Jaager, Jaeger, Jagur

Jae-Hwa (Korean) rich, prosperous.

Jael (Hebrew) mountain goat.
Yael

Jaelen (American) a form of Jalen.
Jaelan, Jaelaun, Jaelin, Jaelon, Jaelyn

Ja'far (Sanskrit) little stream.
Jafar, Jafari, Jaffar, Jaffer, Jafur

Jagger (English) carter.
Jagar, Jager, Jaggar

Jago (English) a form of James.

Jaguar (Spanish) jaguar.
Jagguar

Jahi (Swahili) dignified.

Jahlil (Hindi) a form of Jalil.
Jahlal, Jahlee, Jahleel, Jahliel

Jahmar (American) a form of Jamar.
Jahmare, Jahmari, Jahmarr, Jahmer

Jahvon (Hebrew) a form of
Javan.
*Jahvan, Jahvine, Jahwaan,
Jahwon*

Jai (Tai) heart.
Jaie, Jaii

Jaiden (Hebrew) a form of
Jadon.
Jaidan, Jaidon, Jaidyn

Jailen (American) a form of
Jalen.
*Jailan, Jailani, Jaileen, Jailen,
Jailon, Jailyn, Jailynn*

Jaime (Spanish) a form of
Jacob, James.
*Jaimee, Jaimey, Jaimie, Jaimito,
Jaimy, Jayme, Jaymie*

Jairo (Spanish) God enlight-
ens.
Jair, Jairay, Jaire, Jairus, Jarius

Jaison (Greek) a form of
Jason.
Jaisan, Jaisen, Jaishon, Jaishun

Jaivon (Hebrew) a form of
Javan.
Jaiven, Jaivion, Jaiwon

Jaja (Ibo) honored.

Jajuan (American) a combina-
tion of the prefix Ja + Juan.
*Ja Juan, Jauan, Jawaun, Jejuan,
Jujuan, Juwan*

Jakari (American) a form
of Jacorey.
Jakaire, Jakar, Jakaray, Jakarie,

*Jakarious, Jakarius, Jakarre,
Jakarri, Jakarus*

Jake (Hebrew) a short form of
Jacob.
Jakie, Jayk, Jayke

Jakeem (Arabic) uplifted.

Jakob (Hebrew) a form of
Jacob.
*Jaekob, Jaikab, Jaikob, Jakab,
Jakeb, Jakeob, Jakeub, Jakib,
Jakiv, Jakobe, Jakobi, Jakobus,
Jakoby, Jakov, Jakovian, Jakub,
Jakubek, Jekebs*

Jakome (Basque) a form of
James.
Xanti

Jal (Gypsy) wanderer.

Jalan (American) a form of
Jalen.
*Jalaan, Jalaen, Jalain, Jaland,
Jalane, Jalani, Jalanie, Jalann,
Jalaun, Jalean, Jallan*

Jaleel (Hindi) a form of Jalil.
Jaleell, Jaleil, Jalel

Jalen (American) a combina-
tion of the prefix Ja + Len.
*Jaelen, Jailen, Jalan, Jaleen,
Jalend, Jalene, Jalin, Jallen,
Jalon, Jalyn*

Jalil (Hindi) revered.
Jahlil, Jalaal, Jalal

Jalin, Jalyn (American) forms
of Jalen.
Jalian, Jaline, Jalynn, Jalynne

Jalon (American) a form of
Jalen.
Jalone, Jaloni, Jalun

Jam (American) a short form
of Jamal, Jamar.
Jama

Jamaal (Arabic) a form of
Jamal.

Jamaine (Arabic) a form of
Germain.

Jamal (Arabic) handsome. See
also Gamal.
*Jahmal, Jahmall, Jahmalle,
Jahmeal, Jahmeel, Jahmeil,
Jahmel, Jahmelle, Jahmil,
Jahmile, Jaimal, Jam, Jamaal,
Jamael, Jamahl, Jamail, Jamaile,
Jamala, Jamale, Jamall, Jamalle,
Jamar, Jamaul, Jamel, Jamil,
Jammal, Jamor, Jamual, Jarmal,
Jaumal, Jemal, Jermal, Jomal,
Jomall*

Jamar (American) a form of
Jamal.
*Jam, Jamaar, Jamaari, Jamahrae,
Jamair, Jamara, Jamaras,
Jamaraus, Jamarl, Jamarr,
Jamarre, Jamarrea, Jamarree,
Jamarri, Jamarvis, Jamaur, Jamir,
Jamire, Jamiree, Jammar, Jarmar,
Jarmarr, Jaumar, Jemaar, Jemar,
Jimar, Jomar*

Jamarcus (American) a com-
bination of the prefix Ja +
Marcus.
*Jamarco, Jamarkus, Jemarcus,
Jimarcus*

Jamari (American) a form of
Jamario.
*Jamare, Jamarea, Jamaree,
Jamareh, Jamaria, Jamarie,
Jamaul*

Jamario (American) a combi-
nation of the prefix Ja +
Mario.
*Jamareo, Jamari, Jamariel,
Jamarious, Jamaris, Jamarius,
Jamariya, Jemario, Jemarus*

Jamarquis (American) a com-
bination of the prefix Ja +
Marquis.
*Jamarkees, Jamarkeus, Jamarkis,
Jamarqese, Jamarqueis,
Jamarques, Jamarquez,
Jamarquios, Jamarqus*

Jamel (Arabic) a form of
Jamal.
*Jameel, Jamele, Jamell, Jamelle,
Jammel, Jamuel, Jamul, Jarmel,
Jaumal, Jaumell, Je-Mell, Jimell*

James (Hebrew) supplanter,
substitute. (English) a form of
Jacob. Bible: James the Great
and James the Less were two
of the Twelve Apostles. See
also Diego, Hamish, Iago,
Kimo, Santiago, Seamus,
Seumas, Yago, Yasha.
*Jacques, Jago, Jaime, Jaimes,
Jakome, Jamesie, Jamesy, Jamez,
Jameze, Jamie, Jamies, Jamse,
Jamyes, Jamze, Jas, Jasha, Jay,
Jaymes, Jem, Jemes, Jim*

Jameson (English) son of
James.
Jamerson, Jamesian, Jamison,
Jaymeson

Jamie (English) a familiar form
of James.
Jaime, Jaimey, Jaimie, Jame,
Jamee, Jamey, Jameyel, Jami,
Jamia, Jamiah, Jamian, Jamme,
Jammie, Jamiee, Jammy, Jamy,
Jamye, Jayme, Jaymee, Jaymie

Jamil (Arabic) a form of Jamal.
Jamiel, Jamiell, Jamielle, Jamile,
Jamill, Jamille, Jamyl, Jarmil

Jamin (Hebrew) favored.
Jamen, Jamian, Jamien, Jamion,
Jamionn, Jamon, Jamun, Jamyn,
Jarmin, Jarmon, Jaymin

Jamison (English) son of
James.
Jamiesen, Jamieson, Jamis,
Jamisen, Jamyson, Jaymison

Jamon (Hebrew) a form of
Jamin.
Jamohn, Jamone, Jamoni

Jamond (American) a combi-
nation of James + Raymond.
Jamod, Jamont, Jamonta,
Jamontae, Jamontay, Jamonte,
Jarmond

Jamor (American) a form of
Jamal.
Jamoree, Jamori, Jamorie,
Jamorius, Jamorrio, Jamorris,
Jamory, Jamour

Jamsheed (Persian) from
Persia.
Jamshaid, Jamshed

Jan (Dutch, Slavic) a form of
John.
Jaan, Jana, Janae, Jann, Janne,
Jano, Janson, Jenda, Yan

Janco (Czech) a form of John.
Jancsi, Janke, Janko

Jando (Spanish) a form of
Alexander.
Jandino

Janeil (American) a combina-
tion of the prefix Ja + Neil.
Janal, Janel, Janell, Janelle,
Janiel, Janielle, Janile, Janille,
Jarnail, Jarneil, Jarnell

Janek (Polish) a form of John.
Janak, Janik, Janika, Janka,
Jankiel, Janko

Janis (Latvian) a form of John.
Ansis, Jancis, Zanis

Janne (Finnish) a form of
John.
Jann, Jannes

János (Hungarian) a form of
John.
Jancsi, Jani, Jankia, Jano

Janson (Scandinavian) son of
Jan.
Janse, Jansen, Jansin, Janssen,
Jansun, Jantzen, Janzen, Jensen,
Jenson

Jantzen (Scandinavian) a form of Janson.
Janten, Jantsen, Jantson

Janus (Latin) gate, passageway; born in January. Mythology: the Roman god of beginnings and endings.
Jannese, Jannus, Januario, Janusz

Japheth (Hebrew) handsome. (Arabic) abundant. Bible: a son of Noah. See also Yaphet.
Japeth, Japhet

Jaquan (American) a combination of the prefix Ja + Quan.
Jaequan, Jaiqaun, Jaiquan, Jaqaun, Jaqawan, Jaquaan, Jaquain, Ja'quan, Jaquane, Jaquann, Jaquanne, Jaquavius, Jaquawn, Jaquin, Jaquon, Jaqwan

Jaquarius (American) a combination of Jaquan + Darius.
Jaquari, Jaquarious, Jaquaris

Jaquavius (American) a form of Jaquan.
Jaquavas, Jaquaveis, Jaquaveius, Jaquaveon, Jaquaveous, Jaquavias, Jaquavious, Jaquavis, Jaquavus

Jaquon (American) a form of Jaquan.
Jaequon, Jaqoun, Jaquinn, Jaqune, Jaquoin, Jaquone, Jaqwon

Jarad (Hebrew) a form of Jared.
Jaraad, Jaraed

Jarah (Hebrew) sweet as honey.
Jerah

Jardan (Hebrew) a form of Jordan.
Jarden, Jardin, Jardon

Jareb (Hebrew) contending.
Jarib

Jared (Hebrew) a form of Jordan.
Jahred, Jaired, Jarad, Jaredd, Jareid, Jarid, Jarod, Jarred, Jarrett, Jarrod, Jarryd, Jerad, Jered, Jerod, Jerrad, Jerred, Jerrod, Jerryd, Jordan

Jarek (Slavic) born in January.
Janiuszck, Januarius, Januisz, Jarec, Jarrek, Jarric, Jarrick

Jarell (Scandinavian) a form of Gerald.
Jairell, Jarael, Jareil, Jarel, Jarelle, Jariel, Jarrell, Jarryl, Jayryl, Jerel, Jerell, Jerrell, Jharell

Jaren (Hebrew) a form of Jaron.
Jarian, Jarien, Jarin, Jarion

Jareth (American) a combination of Jared + Gareth.
Jarreth, Jereth, Jarreth

Jarett (English) a form of Jarrett.
Jaret, Jarette

Jarl (Scandinavian) earl, noble-man.

Jarlath (Latin) in control.
Jarl, Jarlen

Jarman (German) from Germany.
Jerman

Jarod (Hebrew) a form of Jared.
Jarodd, Jaroid

Jaron (Hebrew) he will sing; he will cry out.
Jaaron, Jairon, Jaren, Jarone, Jarren, Jarron, Jaryn, Jayron, Jayronn, Je Ronn, J'ron

Jaroslav (Czech) glory of spring.
Jarda

Jarred (Hebrew) a form of Jared.
Ja'red, Jarrad, Jarrayd, Jarrid, Jarrod, Jarryd, Jerrid

Jarrell (English) a form of Gerald.
Jarel, Jarell, Jarrel, Jerall, Jerel, Jerell

Jarren (Hebrew) a form of Jaron.
Jarrain, Jarran, Jarrian, Jarrin

Jarrett (English) a form of Garrett, Jared.
Jairett, Jareth, Jarett, Jaretté, Jarhett, Jarratt, Jarret, Jarrette, Jarrot, Jarrott, Jerrett

Jarrod (Hebrew) a form of Jared.
Jarod, Jerod, Jerrod

Jarryd (Hebrew) a form of Jared.
Jarrayd, Jaryd

Jarvis (German) skilled with a spear.
Jaravis, Jarv, Jarvaris, Jarvas, Jarvaska, Jarvey, Jarvez, Jarvie, Jarvios, Jarvious, Jarvius, Jarvorice, Jarvoris, Jarvous, Jarvus, Javaris, Jervey, Jervis

Jaryn (Hebrew) a form of Jaron.
Jarryn, Jarynn, Jaryon

Jas (Polish) a form of John. (English) a familiar form of James.
Jasio

Jasha (Russian) a familiar form of Jacob, James.
Jascha

Jashawn (American) a combination of the prefix Ja + Shawn.
Jasean, Jashan, Jashaun, Jashion, Jashon

Jaskaran (Sikh) sings praises to the Lord.
Jaskaren, Jaskarn, Jaskiran

Jasmin (Persian) jasmine flower.
Jasman, Jasmanie, Jasmine, Jasmon, Jasmond

Jason (Greek) healer.
Mythology: the hero who
led the Argonauts in search
of the Golden Fleece.
*Jacen, Jaeson, Jahson, Jaison,
Jasan, Jasaun, Jase, Jasen, Jasin,
Jasson, Jasten, Jasun, Jasyn,
Jathan, Jathon, Jay, Jayson*

Jaspal (Punjabi) living a virtuous lifestyle.

Jasper (French) brown, red, or
yellow ornamental stone.
(English) a form of Casper.
See also Kasper.
Jaspar, Jazper, Jespar, Jesper

Jasson (Greek) a form of
Jason.
Jassen, Jassin

Jatinra (Hindi) great Brahmin
sage.

Javan (Hebrew) Bible: son of
Japheth.
*Jaewan, Jahvaughan, Jahvon,
Jaivon, Javante, Javaon,
JaVaughn, Javen, Javian, Javien,
Javin, Javine, Javoanta, Javon,
Javona, Javone, Javonte, Jayvin,
Jayvion, Jayvon, Jevan, Jevon*

Javante (American) a form of
Javan.
*Javantae, Javantai, Javantée,
Javanti*

Javaris (English) a form of
Jarvis.
*Javaor, Javar, Javaras, Javare,
Javares, Javari, Javarias, Javaries,*

*Javario, Javarius, Javaro, Javaron,
Javarous, Javarre, Javarreis,
Javarri, Javarrious, Javarris,
Javarro, Javarous, Javarte, Javarus,
Javorious, Javoris, Javorius,
Javouris*

Javas (Sanskrit) quick, swift.
Jayvas, Jayvis

Javier (Spanish) owner of a
new house. See also Xavier.
Jabier, Javer, Javere, Javiar

Javon (Hebrew) a form of
Javan.
*Jaavon, Jaevin, Jaevon, Jaewon,
Javeon, Javion, Javionne, Javohn,
Javona, Javone, Javoney, Javoni,
Javonn, Javonne, Javonni,
Javonnie, Javonnte, Javoun,
Jayvon*

Javonte (American) a form of
Javan.
*Javona, Javontae, Javontai,
Javontay, Javontaye, Javonté,
Javontee, Javonteh, Javontey*

Jawaun (American) a form of
Jajuan.
*Jawaan, Jawan, Jawann, Jawn,
Jawon, Jawuan*

Jawhar (Arabic) jewel; essence.

Jaxon (English) a form of
Jackson.
*Jaxen, Jaxsen, Jaxson, Jaxsun,
Jaxun*

Jay (French) blue jay. (English)
a short form of James, Jason.
Jae, Jai, Jave, Jaye, Jeays, Jeyes

Jayce (American) a combination of the initials J. + C.
JC, J.C., Jayc, Jaycee, Jay Cee, Jaycey, Jecie

Jaycob (Hebrew) a form of Jacob.
Jaycub, Jaykob

Jayde (American) a combination of the initials J. + D.
JD, J.D., Jayd, Jaydee, Jayden

Jayden (American) a form of Jayde.
Jaydan, Jaydin, Jaydn, Jaydon

Jaylee (American) a combination of Jay + Lee.
Jayla, Jayle, Jaylen

Jaylen (American) a combination of Jay + Len.
Jaylaan, Jaylan, Jayland, Jayleen, Jaylend, Jaylin, Jayln, Jaylon, Jaylun, Jaylund, Jaylyn

Jaylin (American) a form of Jaylen.
Jaylian, Jayline

Jaylon (American) a form of Jaylen.
Jayleon

Jaylyn (American) a form of Jaylen.
Jaylynd, Jaylynn, Jaylynne

Jayme (English) a form of Jamie.
Jaymie

Jaymes (English) a form of James.
Jaymis, Jayms, Jaymz

Jayquan (American) a combination of Jay + Quan.
Jaykwan, Jaykwon, Jayqon, Jayquawn, Jayqunn

Jayson (Greek) a form of Jason.
Jaycent, Jaysean, Jaysen, Jayshaun, Jayshawn, Jayshon, Jayshun, Jaysin, Jaysn, Jayssen, Jaysson, Jaysun

Jayvon (American) a form of Javon.
Jayvion, Jayvohn, Jayvone, Jayvonn, Jayvontay, Jayvonte, Jaywan, Jaywaun, Jaywin

Jazz (American) jazz.
Jaz, Jazze, Jazzlee, Jazzman, Jazzmen, Jazzmin, Jazzmon, Jazztin, Jazzton, Jazzy

Jean (French) a form of John.
Jéan, Jeane, Jeannah, Jeannie, Jeannot, Jeano, Jeanot, Jeanty, Jene

Jeb (Hebrew) a short form of Jebediah.
Jebb, Jebi, Jeby

Jebediah (Hebrew) a form of Jedidiah.
Jeb, Jebadia, Jebadiah, Jebadieh, Jebidiah

Jed (Hebrew) a short form of Jedidiah. (Arabic) hand.
Jedd, Jeddy, Jedi

Jediah (Hebrew) hand of
God.
*Jedaia, Jedaiah, Jedeiah, Jedi,
Yedaya*

Jedidiah (Hebrew) friend of
God, beloved of God. See
also Didi.
*Jebediah, Jed, Jedadiah,
Jeddediah, Jedediah, Jedediha,
Jedidia, Jedidiah, Jedidiyah,
Yedidya*

Jedrek (Polish) strong; manly.
Jedric, Jedrik, Jedrus

Jeff (English) a short form of
Jefferson, Jeffrey. A familiar
form of Geoffrey.
*Jef, Jefe, Jeffe, Jeffey, Jeffie, Jeffy,
Jhef*

Jefferson (English) son of Jeff.
History: Thomas Jefferson
was the third U.S. president.
Jeferson, Jeff, Jeffers

Jeffery (English) a form of
Jeffrey.
*Jefery, Jeffari, Jeffary, Jeffeory,
Jefferay, Jeffereoy, Jefferey, Jefferie,
Jeffory*

Jefford (English) Jeff's ford.

Jeffrey (English) divinely
peaceful. See also Geffrey,
Geoffrey, Godfrey.
*Jeff, Jefferies, Jeffery, Jeffre, Jeffree,
Jeffrie, Jeffrery, Jeffrie, Jeffries,
Jeffry, Jefre, Jefri, Jefry, Jeoffroi,
Joffre, Joffrey*

Jeffry (English) a form of
Jeffrey.

Jehan (French) a form of
John.
Jehann

Jehu (Hebrew) God lives.
Bible: a military commander
and king of Israel.
Yehu

Jelani (Swahili) mighty.
Jel, Jelan, Jelanie, Jelaun

Jem (English) a short form of
James, Jeremiah.
Jemmie, Jemmy

Jemal (Arabic) a form of
Jamal.
Jemaal, Jemael, Jemale, Jemel

Jemel (Arabic) a form of
Jemal.
*Jemeal, Jemehl, Jemehyl, Jemell,
Jemelle, Jemello, Jemeyle, Jemile,
Jemmy*

Jemond (French) worldly.
Jemon, Jémond, Jemonde, Jemone

Jenkin (Flemish) little John.
*Jenkins, Jenkyn, Jenkyns,
Jennings*

Jenö (Hungarian) a form of
Eugene.
Jenci, Jency, Jenoe, Jensi, Jensy

Jens (Danish) a form of John.
*Jense, Jensen, Jenson, Jenssen,
Jensy, Jentz*

Jeovanni (Italian) a form of Giovanni.
Jeovahny, Jeovan, Jeovani, Jeovany

Jequan (American) a combination of the prefix Je + Quan.
Jeqaun, Jequann, Jequon

Jerad, Jerrad (Hebrew) forms of Jared.
Jeread, Jeredd

Jerahmy (Hebrew) a form of Jeremy.
Jerahmeel, Jerahmeil, Jerahmey

Jerald (English) a form of Gerald.
Jeraldo, Jerold, Jerral, Jerrald, Jerrold, Jerry

Jerall (English) a form of Jarrell.
Jerael, Jerai, Jerail, Jeraile, Jeral, Jerale, Jerall, Jerrail, Jerral, Jerrel, Jerrell, Jerrelle

Jeramie, Jeramy (Hebrew) forms of Jeremy.
Jerame, Jeramee, Jeramey, Jerami, Jerammie

Jerard (French) a form of Gerard.
Jarard, Jarrard, Jerardo, Jeraude, Jerrard

Jere (Hebrew) a short form of Jeremiah, Jeremy.
Jeré, Jeree

Jered, Jerred (Hebrew) forms of Jared.
Jereed, Jerid, Jerryd, Jeryd

Jerel, Jerell, Jerrell (English) forms of Jarell.
Jerelle, Jeriel, Jeril, Jerrail, Jerral, Jerrall, Jerrel, Jerrill, Jerrol, Jerroll, Jerryl, Jerryll, Jeryl, Jeryle

Jereme, Jeremey (Hebrew) forms of Jeremy.
Jarame

Jeremiah (Hebrew) God will uplift. Bible: a Hebrew prophet. See also Dermot, Yeremey, Yirmaya.
Geremiah, Jaramia, Jem, Jemeriah, Jemiah, Jeramiah, Jeramiha, Jere, Jereias, Jeremaya, Jeremi, Jeremia, Jeremial, Jeremias, Jeremija, Jeremy, Jerimiah, Jerimiha, Jerimya, Jermiah, Jermija, Jerry

Jeremie, Jérémie (Hebrew) forms of Jeremy.
Jeremi, Jérémie, Jeremii

Jeremy (English) a form of Jeremiah.
Jaremay, Jaremi, Jaremy, Jem, Jemmy, Jerahmy, Jeramie, Jeramy, Jere, Jereamy, Jereme, Jeremee, Jeremey, Jeremie, Jérémie, Jeremry, Jérémy, Jeremye, Jereomy, Jeriemy, Jerime, Jerimy, Jermey, Jeromy, Jerremy

Jeriah (Hebrew) Jehovah has seen.

Jericho (Arabic) city of the moon. Bible: a city conquered by Joshua.
Jeric, Jerick, Jerico, Jerik, Jerric, Jerrick, Jerrico, Jerricoh, Jerryco

Jermaine (French) a form of Germain. (English) sprout, bud.
Jarman, Jeremaine, Jeremane, Jerimane, Jermain, Jerman, Jermane, Jermanie, Jermanne, Jermany, Jermayn, Jermayne, Jermiane, Jermine, Jer-Mon, Jermone, Jermoney, Jhirmaine

Jermal (Arabic) a form of Jamal.
Jermael, Jermail, Jermall, Jermaul, Jermel, Jermell, Jermil, Jermol, Jermyll

Jermey (English) a form of Jeremy.
Jerme, Jermee, Jermere, Jermery, Jermie, Jermy, Jhermie

Jermiah (Hebrew) a form of Jeremiah.
Jermiha, Jermiya

Jerney (Slavic) a form of Bartholomew.

Jerod, Jerrod (Hebrew) forms of Jarrod.
Jerode, Jeroid

Jerolin (Basque, Latin) holy.

Jerome (Latin) holy. See also Geronimo, Hieronymos.
Gerome, Jere, Jeroen, Jerom, Jérome, Jérôme, Jeromo, Jeromy, Jeron, Jerónimo, Jerrome, Jerromy

Jeromy (Latin) a form of Jerome.
Jeromee, Jeromey, Jeromie

Jeron (English) a form of Jerome.
Jéron, Jerone, Jeronimo, Jerrin, Jerrion, Jerron, Jerrone, J'ron

Jerrett (Hebrew) a form of Jarrett.
Jeret, Jerett, Jeritt, Jerret, Jerrette, Jerriot, Jerritt, Jerrot, Jerrott

Jerrick (American) a combination of Jerry + Derrick.
Jaric, Jarrick, Jerick, Jerrik

Jerry (German) mighty spearman. (English) a familiar form of Gerald, Gerard. See also Gerry, Kele.
Jehri, Jere, Jeree, Jeris, Jerison, Jerri, Jerrie, Jery

Jervis (English) a form of Gervaise, Jarvis.

Jerzy (Polish) a form of George.
Jersey, Jerzey, Jurek

Jeshua (Hebrew) a form of Joshua.
Jeshuah

Jess (Hebrew) a short form of Jesse.

Jesse (Hebrew) wealthy. Bible: the father of David. See also Yishai.
Jese, Jesee, Jesi, Jess, Jessé, Jessee, Jessie, Jessy

Jessie (Hebrew) a form of Jesse.
Jesie, Jessi, Jessi

Jessy (Hebrew) a form of Jesse.
Jescey, Jessey, Jessye, Jessyie, Jesy

Jestin (Welsh) a form of Justin.
Jessten, Jesten, Jeston, Jesstin, Jesston

Jesus (Hebrew) a form of Joshua. Bible: son of Mary and Joseph, believed by Christians to be the Son of God. See also Chucho, Isa, Yosu.
Jecho, Jessus, Jesu, Jesús, Josu

Jesús (Hispanic) a form of Jesus.

Jethro (Hebrew) abundant. Bible: the father-in-law of Moses. See also Yitro.
Jeth, Jethroe, Jetro, Jett

Jett (English) hard, black mineral. (Hebrew) a short form of Jethro.
Jet, Jetson, Jetter, Jetty

Jevan (Hebrew) a form of Javan.
Jevaun, Jeven, Jevin

Jevon (Hebrew) a form of Javan.
Jevion, Jevohn, Jevone, Jevonn, Jevonne, Jevonnie

Jevonte (American) a form of Jevon.
Jevonta, Jevontae, Jevontaye, Jevonté

Jibade (Yoruba) born close to royalty.

Jibben (Gypsy) life.
Jibin

Jibril (Arabic) archangel of Allah.
Jabril, Jibreel, Jibriel

Jilt (Dutch) money.

Jim (Hebrew, English) a short form of James. See also Jaap.
Jimbo, Jimm, Jimmy

Jimbo (American) a familiar form of Jim.
Jimboo

Jimell (Arabic) a form of Jamel.
Jimel, Jimelle, Jimill, Jimmell, Jimmelle, Jimmiel, Jimmil

Jimiyu (Abaluhya) born in the dry season.

Jimmie (English) a form of Jimmy.
Jimi, Jimie, Jimmee, Jimmi

Jimmy (English) a familiar form of Jim.
Jimmey, Jimmie, Jimmye, Jimmyjo, Jimy

Jimoh (Swahili) born on Friday.

Jin (Chinese) gold.
Jinn

Jindra (Czech) a form of
Harold.

Jing-Quo (Chinese) ruler of
the country.

Jiovanni (Italian) a form of
Giovanni.
Jio, Jiovani, Jiovanie, Jiovann,
Jiovannie, Jiovanny, Jiovany,
Jiovoni, Jivan

Jirair (Armenian) strong; hard
working.

Jiri (Czech) a form of George.
Jirka

Jiro (Japanese) second son.

Jivin (Hindi) life giver.
Jivanta

Jo (Hebrew, Japanese) a form
of Joe.

Joab (Hebrew) God is father.
See also Yoav.
Joabe, Joaby

Joachim (Hebrew) God will
establish. See also Akeem,
Ioakim, Yehoyakem.
Joacheim, Joakim, Joaquim,
Joaquín, Jokin, Jov

João (Portuguese) a form of
John.

Joaquim (Portuguese) a form
of Joachim.

Joaquín (Spanish) a form of
Joachim, Yehoyakem.
Jehoichin, Joaquin, Jocquin,
Jocquinn, Joquin, Juaquin

Job (Hebrew) afflicted. Bible: a
righteous man whose faith in
God survived the test of
many afflictions.
Jobe, Jobert, Jobey, Jobie, Joby

Joben (Japanese) enjoys clean-
liness.
Joban, Jobin

Jobo (Spanish) a familiar form
of Joseph.

Joby (Hebrew) a familiar form
of Job.
Jobie

Jock (American) a familiar
form of Jacob.
Jocko, Joco, Jocoby, Jocolby

Jocquez (French) a form of
Jacquez.
Jocques, Jocquis, Jocquise

Jodan (Hebrew) a combina-
tion of Jo + Dan.
Jodahn, Joden, Jodhan, Jodian,
Jodin, Jodon, Jodonnis

Jody (Hebrew) a familiar form
of Joseph.
Jodey, Jodi, Jodie, Jodiha, Joedy

Joe (Hebrew) a short form of
Joseph.
Jo, Joely, Joey

Joel (Hebrew) God is willing.
Bible: an Old Testament
Hebrew prophet.
*Jôel, Joël, Joell, Joelle, Joely, Jole,
Yoel*

Joeseph (Hebrew) a form of
Joseph.
Joesph

Joey (Hebrew) a familiar form
of Joe, Joseph.

Johan, Johann (German)
forms of John. See also
Anno, Hanno, Yoan, Yohan.
*Joahan, Joan, Joannes, Johahn,
Johan, Johanan, Johane,
Johannan, Johannes, Johanthan,
Johatan, Johathan, Johathon,
Johaun, Johon*

Johannes (German) a form of
Johan, Johann.
*Johanes, Johannas, Johannus,
Johansen, Johanson, Johonson*

John (Hebrew) God is
gracious. Bible: the name
honoring John the Baptist
and John the Evangelist. See
also Elchanan, Evan, Geno,
Gian, Giovanni, Handel,
Hannes, Hans, Hanus,
Honza, Ian, Ianos, Iban, Ioan,
Ivan, Iwan, Keoni, Kwam,
Ohannes, Sean, Ugutz, Yan,
Yanka, Yanni, Yochanan,
Yohance, Zane.
*Jack, Jacsi, Jaenda, Jahn, Jan,
Janak, Janco, Janek, Janis, Janne,
János, Jansen, Jantje, Jantzen,*
*Jas, Jean, Jehan, Jen, Jenkin,
Jenkyn, Jens, Jhan, Jhanick,
Jhon, Jian, Joáo, João, Jock, Joen,
Johan, Johann, Johne, Johnl,
Johnlee, Johnnie, Johnny,
Johnson, Jon, Jonam, Jonas, Jone,
Jones, Jonny, Jonté, Jovan, Juan,
Juhana*

Johnathan (Hebrew) a form
of Jonathan.
*Jhonathan, Johathe, Johnatan,
Johnathann, Johnathaon,
Johnathen, Johnathyne,
Johnatten, Johniathin,
Johnothan, Johnthan*

Johnathon (Hebrew) a form
of Jonathon. See also Yanton.
Johnaton

Johnnie (Hebrew) a familiar
form of John.
*Johnie, Johnier, Johnni, Johnsie,
Jonni, Jonnie*

Johnny (Hebrew) a familiar
form of John. See also
Gianni.
*Jantje, Jhonny, Johney, Johnney,
Johny, Jonny*

Johnson (English) son of
John.
Johnston, Jonson

Joji (Japanese) a form of
George.

Jojo (Fante) born on Monday.

Jokim (Basque) a form of
Joachim.

Jolon (Native American) valley of the dead oaks.
Jolyon

Jomar (American) a form of Jamar.
Jomari, Jomarie, Jomarri

Jomei (Japanese) spreads light.

Jon (Hebrew) a form of John. A short form of Jonathan.
J'on, Joni, Jonn, Jonnie, Jonny, Jony

Jonah (Hebrew) dove. Bible: an Old Testament prophet who was swallowed by a large fish.
Giona, Jona, Yonah, Yunus

Jonas (Hebrew) he accomplishes. (Lithuanian) a form of John.
Jonahs, Jonass, Jonaus, Jonelis, Jonukas, Jonus, Jonutis, Joonas

Jonatan (Hebrew) a form of Jonathan.
Jonatane, Jonate, Jonattan, Jonnattan

Jonathan (Hebrew) gift of God. Bible: the son of King Saul who became a loyal friend of David. See also Ionakana, Yanton, Yonatan.
Janathan, Johnathan, Johnathon, Jon, Jonatan, Jonatha, Jonathen, Jonathin, Jonathon, Jonathun, Jonathyn, Jonethen, Jonnatha, Jonnathan, Jonnathun, Jonothan, Jonthan

Jonathon (Hebrew) a form of Jonathan.
Joanathon, Johnathon, Jonnathon, Jonothon, Jonthon, Jounathon, Yanaton

Jones (Welsh) son of John.
Joenns, Joness, Jonesy

Jonny (Hebrew) a familiar form of John.
Jonhy, Joni, Jonnee, Jony

Jontae (French) a combination of Jon + the suffix Tae.
Johntae, Jontay, Jontea, Jonteau, Jontez

Jontay (American) a form of Jontae.
Johntay, Johnte, Johntez, Jontai, Jonte, Jonté, Jontez

Joop (Dutch) a familiar form of Joseph.
Jopie

Joost (Dutch) just.

Joquin (Spanish) a form of Joaquin.
Joquan, Joquawn, Joqunn, Joquon

Jora (Hebrew) teacher.
Yora, Jorah

Joram (Hebrew) Jehovah is exalted.
Joran, Jorim

Jordan (Hebrew) descending. See also Giordano, Yarden.
Jardan, Jared, Jordaan, Jordae, Jordain, Jordaine, Jordane,

Jordani, Jordanio, Jordann,
Jordanny, Jordano, Jordany,
Jordáo, Jordayne, Jorden, Jordian,
Jordin, Jordon, Jordun, Jordy,
Jordyn, Jorrdan, Jory, Jourdan

Jorden (Hebrew) a form of
Jordan.
Jordenn

Jordon (Hebrew) a form of
Jordan.
Jeordon, Johordan

Jordy (Hebrew) a familiar
form of Jordan.
Jordi, Jordie

Jordyn (Hebrew) a form of
Jordan.

Jorell (American) he saves.
Literature: a name inspired
by the fictional character Jor-
El, Superman's father.
Jorel, Jor-El, Jorelle, Jorl, Jorrel,
Jorrell

Jörg (German) a form of
George.
Jeorg, Juergen, Jungen, Jürgen

Jorge (Spanish) a form of
George.
Jorrín

Jorgen (Danish) a form of
George.
Joergen, Jorgan, Jörgen

Joris (Dutch) a form of
George.

Jörn (German) a familiar form
of Gregory.

Jorrín (Spanish) a form of
George.
Jorian, Jorje

Jory (Hebrew) a familiar form
of Jordan.
Joar, Joary, Jorey, Jori, Jorie, Jorrie

José (Spanish) a form of
Joseph. See also Ché, Pepe.
Josean, Josecito, Josee, Joseito,
Joselito, Josey

Josef (German, Portuguese,
Czech, Scandinavian) a form
of Joseph.
Joosef, Joseff, Josif, Jozef, József,
Juzef

Joseluis (Spanish) a combination of Jose + Luis.

Joseph (Hebrew) God will
add, God will increase. Bible:
in the Old Testament, the son
of Jacob who came to rule
Egypt; in the New
Testament, the husband of
Mary. See also Beppe,
Cheche, Chepe, Giuseppe,
Iokepa, Iosif, Osip, Pepa,
Peppe, Pino, Sepp, Yeska,
Yosef, Yousef, Youssel, Yusif,
Yusuf, Zeusef.
Jazeps, Jo, Jobo, Jody, Joe,
Joeseph, Joey, Jojo, Joop, Joos,
Jooseppi, Jopie, José, Joseba, Josef,
Josep, Josephat, Josephe, Josephie,
Josephus, Josheph, Josip, Jóska,
Joza, Joze, Jozef, Jozeph, Jozhe,
Jozio, Jozka, Jozsi, Jozzepi,
Jupp, Juziu

Josh (Hebrew) a short form of
Joshua.
Joshe

Josha (Hindi) satisfied.

Joshi (Swahili) galloping.

Joshua (Hebrew) God is my
salvation. Bible: led the
Israelites into the Promised
Land. See also Giosia, Iosua,
Jesus, Yehoshua.
*Jeshua, Johsua, Johusa, Josh,
Joshau, Joshaua, Joshauh,
Joshawa, Joshawah, Joshia,
Joshu, Joshuaa, Joshuah,
Joshuea, Joshuia, Joshula, Joshus,
Joshusa, Joshuwa, Joshwa, Josue,
Jousha, Jozshua, Jozsua, Jozua,
Jushua*

Josiah (Hebrew) fire of the
Lord. See also Yoshiyahu.
*Joshiah, Josia, Josiahs, Josian,
Josias, Josie*

Joss (Chinese) luck; fate.
Josse, Jossy

Josue (Hebrew) a form of
Joshua.
*Joshue, Jossue, Josu, Josua,
Josuha, Jozus*

Jotham (Hebrew) may God
complete. Bible: a king of
Judah.

Jourdan (Hebrew) a form of
Jordan.
*Jourdain, Jourden, Jourdin,
Jourdon, Jourdyn*

Jovan (Latin) Jove-like, majes-
tic. (Slavic) a form of John.
Mythology: Jove, also known
as Jupiter, was the supreme
Roman deity.
*Johvan, Johvon, Jovaan, Jovane,
Jovani, Jovanic, Jovann, Jovanni,
Jovannis, Jovanny, Jovany,
Jovaughn, Jovaun, Joven,
Jovenal, Jovenel, Jovi, Jovian,
Jovin, Jovito, Jovoan, Jovon,
Jovone, Jovonn, Jovonne, Jowan,
Jowaun, Yovan, Yovani*

Jovani, Jovanni (Latin) forms
of Jovan.
*Jovanie, Jovannie, Jovoni,
Jovonie, Jovonni*

Jovanny, Jovany (Latin) forms
of Jovan.
Jovony

Jr (Latin) a short form of
Junior.
Jr.

Juan (Spanish) a form of John.
See also Chan.
*Juanch, Juanchito, Juane, Juanito,
Juann, Juaun*

Juancarlos (Spanish) a combination of Juan + Carlos.

Juaquin (Spanish) a form of
Joaquín.
*Juaqin, Juaqine, Juquan,
Juaquine*

Jubal (Hebrew) ram's horn.
Bible: a musician and a
descendant of Cain.

Judah (Hebrew) praised. Bible: the fourth of Jacob's sons. See also Yehudi.
Juda, Judas, Judd, Jude

Judas (Latin) a form of Judah. Bible: Judas Iscariot was the disciple who betrayed Jesus.
Jude

Judd (Hebrew) a short form of Judah.
Jud, Judson

Jude (Latin) a short form of Judah, Judas. Bible: one of the Twelve Apostles, author of "The Epistle of Jude."

Judson (English) son of Judd.

Juhana (Finnish) a form of John.
Juha, Juho

Juku (Estonian) a form of Richard.
Jukka

Jules (French) a form of Julius.
Joles, Jule

Julian (Greek, Latin) a form of Julius.
Jolyon, Julean, Juliaan, Julianne, Juliano, Julien, Jullian, Julyan

Julien (Latin) a form of Julian.
Juliene, Julienn, Julienne, Jullien, Jullin

Julio (Hispanic) a form of Julius.

Julius (Greek, Latin) youthful, downy bearded. History: Julius Caesar was a great Roman dictator. See also Giuliano.
Jolyon, Julas, Jule, Jules, Julen, Jules, Julian, Julias, Julie, Julio, Juliusz, Jullius, Juluis

Jumaane (Swahili) born on Tuesday.

Jumah (Arabic, Swahili) born on Friday, a holy day in the Islamic religion.
Jimoh, Juma

Jumoke (Yoruba) loved by everyone.

Jun (Chinese) truthful. (Japanese) obedient; pure.
Junnie

Junior (Latin) young.
Jr, Junious, Junius, Junor

Jupp (German) a form of Joseph.

Jur (Czech) a form of George.
Juraz, Jurek, Jurik, Jurko, Juro

Jurgis (Lithuanian) a form of George.
Jurgi, Juri

Juro (Japanese) best wishes; long life.

Jurrien (Dutch) God will uplift.
Jore, Jurian, Jurre

Justen (Latin) a form of Justin.
Jasten

Justice (Latin) a form of Justis.
Justic, Justiz, Justyc, Justyce

Justin (Latin) just, righteous.
See also Giustino, Iestyn,
Iustin, Tutu, Ustin, Yustyn.
*Jastin, Jaston, Jestin, Jobst, Joost,
Jost, Jusa, Just, Justain, Justan,
Justas, Justek, Justen, Justian,
Justinas, Justine, Justinian,
Justinius, Justinn, Justino,
Justins, Justinus, Justo, Juston,
Justton, Justukas, Justun, Justyn*

Justis (French) just.
Justice, Justs, Justus, Justyse

Justyn (Latin) a form of Justin.
Justn, Justyne, Justynn

Juvenal (Latin) young.
Literature: a Roman satirist.
Juvon, Juvone

Juwan (American) a form of
Jajuan.
*Juvon, Juvone, Juvaun, Juwaan,
Juwain, Juwane, Juwann,
Juwaun, Juwon, Juwonn,
Juwuan, Juwuane, Juwvan,
Jwan, Jwon*

K

Kabiito (Rutooro) born while
foreigners are visiting.

Kabil (Turkish) a form of
Cain.
Kabel

Kabir (Hindi) History: an
Indian mystic poet.
Kabar, Kabeer, Kabier

Kabonero (Runyankore) sign.

Kabonesa (Rutooro) difficult
birth.

Kacey (Irish) a form of Casey.
(American) a combination of
the initials K. + C. See also
KC.
*Kace, Kacee, Kaci, Kacy, Kaesy,
Kase, Kasey, Kasie, Kasy,
Kaycee*

Kadar (Arabic) powerful.
Kader

Kadarius (American) a com-
bination of Kade + Darius.
*Kadairious, Kadarious, Kadaris,
Kadarrius, Kadarus, Kaddarrius,
Kaderious, Kaderius*

Kade (Scottish) wetlands.
(American) a combination of
the initials K. + D.
*Kadee, Kady, Kaid, Kaide,
Kaydee*

Kadeem (Arabic) servant.
Kadim, Khadeem

Kaden (Arabic) a form of
Kadin.
*Kadeen, Kadein, Kaidan,
Kaiden*

Kadin (Arabic) friend, companion.
Caden, Kaden, Kadyn, Kaeden, Kayden

Kadir (Arabic) spring greening.
Kadeer

Kado (Japanese) gateway.

Kaeden (Arabic) a form of Kadin.
Kaedin, Kaedon, Kaedyn

Kaelan, Kaelin (Irish) forms of Kellen.
Kael, Kaelen, Kaelon, Kaelyn

Kaeleb (Hebrew) a form of Kaleb.
Kaelib, Kaelob, Kaelyb, Kailab, Kaileb

Kaemon (Japanese) joyful; right-handed.
Kaeman, Kaemen, Kaemin

Kaenan (Irish) a form of Keenan.
Kaenen, Kaenin, Kaenyn

Ka'eo (Hawaiian) victorious.

Kafele (Nguni) worth dying for.

Kaga (Native American) writer.

Kagan (Irish) a form of Keegan.
Kage, Kagen, Kaghen, Kaigan

Kahale (Hawaiian) home.

Kahil (Turkish) young; inexperienced; naive.
Cahil, Kaheel, Kale, Kayle

Kahlil (Arabic) a form of Khalíl.
Kahleal, Kahlee, Kahleel, Kahleil, Kahli, Kahliel, Kahlill, Kalel, Kalil

Kaholo (Hawaiian) runner.

Kahraman (Turkish) hero.

Kai (Welsh) keeper of the keys. (German) a form of Kay. (Hawaiian) sea.
Kae, Kaie, Kaii

Kaikara (Runyoro) Religion: a Banyoro deity.

Kailen (Irish) a form of Kellen.
Kail, Kailan, Kailey, Kailin, Kailon, Kailyn

Kaili (Hawaiian) Religion: a Hawaiian god.
Kailli

Kain (Welsh, Irish) a form of Kane.
Kainan, Kaine, Kainen, Kainin, Kainon

Kainoa (Hawaiian) name.

Kaipo (Hawaiian) sweetheart.

Kairo (Arabic) a form of Cairo.
Kaire, Kairee, Kairi

Kaiser (German) a form of
Caesar.
Kaesar, Kaisar, Kaizer

Kaiven (American) a form of
Kevin.
*Kaivan, Kaiven, Kaivon,
Kaiwan*

Kaj (Danish) earth.
Kai, Kaje

Kakar (Hindi) grass.

Kala (Hindi) black; phase.
(Hawaiian) sun.

Kalama (Hawaiian) torch.
Kalam

Kalan (Irish) a form of Kalen.
Kalane, Kallan

Kalani (Hawaiian) sky; chief.
Kalan

Kale (Arabic) a short form of
Kahlil. (Hawaiian) a familiar
form of Carl.
*Kalee, Kalen, Kaleu, Kaley,
Kali, Kalin, Kalle, Kayle*

Kaleb (Hebrew) a form of
Caleb.
*Kaeleb, Kal, Kalab, Kalabe,
Kalb, Kale, Kaleob, Kalev,
Kalib, Kalieb, Kallb, Kalleb,
Kalob, Kaloeb, Kalub, Kalyb,
Kilab*

Kalen, Kalin (Arabic,
Hawaiian) forms of Kale.
(Irish) forms of Kellen.
Kalan

Kalevi (Finnish) hero.

Kali (Arabic) a short form of
Kalil. (Hawaiian) a form of
Gary.

Kalil (Arabic) a form of Khalíl.
*Kaleel, Kalell, Kali, Kaliel,
Kaliil*

Kaliq (Arabic) a form of
Khaliq.
Kalic, Kalique

Kalkin (Hindi) tenth.
Religion: Kalki is the final
incarnation of the Hindu
god Vishnu.
Kalki

Kalle (Scandinavian) a form of
Carl. (Arabic, Hawaiian) a
form of Kale.

Kallen (Irish) a form of
Kellen.
*Kallan, Kallin, Kallion, Kallon,
Kallun, Kalun*

Kalon, Kalyn (Irish) forms of
Kellen.
*Kalone, Kalonn, Kalyen,
Kalyne, Kalynn*

Kaloosh (Armenian) blessed
event.

Kalvin (Latin) a form of
Calvin.
*Kal, Kalv, Kalvan, Kalven,
Kalvon, Kalvyn, Vinny*

Kamaka (Hawaiian) face.

Kamakani (Hawaiian) wind.

Kamal (Hindi) lotus. (Arabic) perfect, perfection.
Kamaal, Kamel, Kamil

Kamau (Kikuyu) quiet warrior.

Kamden (Scottish) a form of Camden.
Kamdon

Kameron (Scottish) a form of Cameron.
Kam, Kamaren, Kamaron, Kameran, Kameren, Kamerin, Kamerion, Kamerron, Kamerun, Kameryn, Kamey, Kammeren, Kammeron, Kammy, Kamoryn, Kamran, Kamron

Kami (Hindi) loving.

Kamil (Arabic) a form of Kamal.
Kameel

Kamran, Kamron (Scottish) forms of Kameron.
Kammron, Kamrein, Kamren, Kamrin, Kamrun, Kamryn

Kamuela (Hawaiian) a form of Samuel.

Kamuhanda (Runyankore) born on the way to the hospital.

Kamukama (Runyankore) protected by God.

Kamuzu (Nguni) medicine.

Kamya (Luganda) born after twin brothers.

Kana (Japanese) powerful; capable. (Hawaiian) Mythology: a demigod.

Kanaiela (Hawaiian) a form of Daniel.
Kana, Kaneii

Kane (Welsh) beautiful. (Irish) tribute. (Japanese) golden. (Hawaiian) eastern sky. (English) a form of Keene. See Kahan, Kain, Kaney, Kayne.

Kange (Lakota) raven.
Kang, Kanga

Kaniel (Hebrew) stalk, reed.
Kan, Kani, Kannie, Kanny

Kannan (Hindi) Religion: another name for the Hindu god Krishna.
Kanaan, Kanan, Kanen, Kanin, Kanine, Kannen

Kannon (Polynesian) free. (French) A form of Cannon.
Kanon

Kanoa (Hawaiian) free.

Kantu (Hindi) happy.

Kanu (Swahili) wildcat.

Kaori (Japanese) strong.

Kapila (Hindi) ancient prophet.
Kapil

Kapono (Hawaiian) righteous.
Kapena

Kardal (Arabic) mustard seed.
Karandal, Kardell

Kare (Norwegian) enormous.
Karee

Kareem (Arabic) noble; distinguished.
Karee, Karem, Kareme, Karim, Karriem

Karel (Czech) a form of Carl.
Karell, Karil, Karrell

Karey (Greek) a form of Carey.
Karee, Kari, Karry, Kary

Karif (Arabic) born in autumn.
Kareef

Kariisa (Runyankore) herdsman.

Karim (Arabic) a form of Kareem.

Karl (German) a form of Carl.
Kaarle, Kaarlo, Kale, Kalle, Kalman, Kálmán, Karcsi, Karel, Kari, Karlen, Karlitis, Karlo, Karlos, Karlton, Karlus, Karol, Kjell

Karlen (Latvian, Russian) a form of Carl.
Karlan, Karlens, Karlik, Karlin, Karlis, Karlon

Karmel (Hebrew) a form of Carmel.

Karney (Irish) a form of Carney.

Karol (Czech, Polish) a form of Carl.
Karal, Karolek, Karolis, Karalos, Károly, Karrel, Karrol

Karr (Scandinavian) a form of Carr.

Karson (English) a form of Carson.
Karrson, Karsen

Karsten (Greek) anointed.
Carsten, Karstan, Karston

Karu (Hindi) cousin.
Karun

Karutunda (Runyankore) little.

Karwana (Rutooro) born during wartime.

Kaseem (Arabic) divided.
Kasceem, Kaseam, Kaseym, Kasim, Kasseem, Kassem, Kazeem

Kaseko (Rhodesian) mocked, ridiculed.

Kasem (Tai) happiness.

Kasen (Basque) protected with a helmet.
Kasean, Kasene, Kaseon, Kasin, Kason, Kassen

Kasey (Irish) a form of Casey.
Kaese, Kaesy, Kasay, Kassey

Kashawn (American) a combination of the prefix Ka + Shawn.
Kashain, Kashan, Kashaun, Kashen, Kashon

Kasib (Arabic) fertile.

Kasim (Arabic) a form of Kaseem.
Kassim

Kasimir (Arabic) peace. (Slavic) a form of Casimir.
Kasim, Kazimierz, Kazimir, Kazio, Kazmer, Kazmér, Kázmér

Kasiya (Nguni) separate.

Kasper (Persian) treasurer. (German) a form of Casper.
Jasper, Kaspar, Kaspero

Kass (German) blackbird.
Kaese, Kasch, Kase

Kassidy (Irish) a form of Cassidy.
Kassady, Kassie, Kassy

Kateb (Arabic) writer.

Kato (Runyankore) second of twins.

Katungi (Runyankore) rich.

Kavan (Irish) handsome.
Cavan, Kavanagh, Kavaugn, Kaven, Kavenaugh, Kavin, Kavon, Kayvan

Kaveh (Persian) ancient hero.

Kavi (Hindi) poet.

Kavin, Kavon (Irish) forms of Kavan.
Kaveon, Kavion, Kavone, Kayvon, Kaywon

Kawika (Hawaiian) a form of David.

Kay (Greek) rejoicing. (German) fortified place. Literature: one of King Arthur's knights of the Round Table.
Kai, Kaycee, Kaye, Kayson

Kayden (Arabic) a form of Kadin.
Kayde, Kaydee, Kaydin, Kaydn, Kaydon

Kayin (Nigerian) celebrated. (Yoruba) long-hoped-for child.

Kayle (Hebrew) faithful dog. (Arabic) a short form of Kahlil.
Kayl, Kayla, Kaylee

Kayleb (Hebrew) a form of Caleb.
Kaylib, Kaylob, Kaylub

Kaylen (Irish) a form of Kellen.
Kaylan, Kaylin, Kaylon, Kaylyn, Kaylynn

Kayne (Hebrew) a form of Cain.
Kaynan, Kaynen, Kaynon

Kayode (Yoruba) he brought joy.

Kayonga (Runyankore) ash.

Kazio (Polish) a form of Casimir, Kasimir. See also Cassidy.

Kazuo (Japanese) man of peace.

KC (American) a combination of the initials K. + C. See also Kacey.
Kc, K.C., Kcee, Kcey

Keagan (Irish) a form of Keegan.
Keagean, Keagen, Keaghan, Keagyn

Keahi (Hawaiian) flames.

Keaka (Hawaiian) a form of Jack.

Kealoha (Hawaiian) fragrant.
Ke'ala

Keanan (Irish) a form of Keenan.
Keanen, Keanna, Keannan, Keanon

Keandre (American) a combination of the prefix Ke + Andre.
Keandra, Keandray, Keandré, Keandree, Keandrell, Keondre

Keane (German) bold; sharp. (Irish) handsome. (English) a form of Keene.
Kean

Keanu (Irish) a form of Keenan.
Keaneu, Keani, Keanno, Keano, Keanue, Keeno, Keenu, Kianu

Kearn (Irish) a short form of Kearney.
Kearne

Kearney (Irish) a form of Carney.
Kar, Karney, Karny, Kearn, Kearny

Keary (Irish) a form of Kerry.
Kearie

Keaton (English) where hawks fly.
Keatan, Keaten, Keatin, Keatton, Keatyn, Keeton, Keetun

Keaven (Irish) a form of Kevin.
Keavan, Keavon

Keawe (Hawaiian) strand.

Keb (Egyptian) earth. Mythology: an ancient earth god, also known as Geb.

Kedar (Hindi) mountain lord. (Arabic) powerful. Religion: another name for the Hindu god Shiva.
Kadar, Kedaar, Keder

Keddy (Scottish) a form of Adam.
Keddie

Kedem (Hebrew) ancient.

Kedrick (English) a form of Cedric.
Keddrick, Kederick, Kedrek, Kedric, Kiedric, Kiedrick

Keefe (Irish) handsome; loved.

Keegan (Irish) little; fiery.
Kaegan, Kagan, Keagan,

Keagen, Keeghan, Keegon, Keegun, Kegan, Keigan

Keelan (Irish) little; slender.
Keelen, Keelin, Keelyn, Keilan, Kelan

Keeley (Irish) handsome.
Kealey, Kealy, Keeli, Keelian, Keelie, Keely

Keenan (Irish) little Keene.
Kaenan, Keanan, Keanu, Keenen, Keennan, Keenon, Kenan, Keynan, Kienan, Kienon

Keene (German) bold; sharp. (English) smart. See also Kane.
Kaene, Keane, Keen, Keenan

Keenen (Irish) a form of Keenan.
Keenin, Kienen

Kees (Dutch) a form of Kornelius.
Keese, Keesee, Keyes

Keevon (Irish) a form of Kevin.
Keevan, Keeven, Keevin, Keewan, Keewin

Kegan (Irish) a form of Keegan.
Kegen, Keghan, Kegon, Kegun

Kehind (Yoruba) second-born twin.
Kehinde

Keiffer (German) a form of Cooper.
Keefer, Keifer, Kiefer

Keigan (Irish) a form of Keegan.
Keighan, Keighen

Keiji (Japanese) cautious ruler.

Keilan (Irish) a form of Keelan.
Keilen, Keilin, Keillene, Keillyn, Keilon, Keilynn

Keir (Irish) a short form of Kieran.

Keitaro (Japanese) blessed.
Keita

Keith (Welsh) forest. (Scottish) battle place. See also Kika.
Keath, Keeth, Keithen

Keithen (Welsh, Scottish) a form of Keith.
Keithan, Keitheon, Keithon

Keivan (Irish) a form of Kevin.
Keiven, Keivn, Keivon, Keivone

Kekapa (Hawaiian) tapa cloth.

Kekipi (Hawaiian) rebel.

Kekoa (Hawaiian) bold, courageous.

Kelby (German) farm by the spring.
Keelby, Kelbee, Kelbey, Kelbi, Kellby

Kele (Hopi) sparrow hawk.
(Hawaiian) a form of Jerry.
Kelle

Kelemen (Hungarian) gentle;
kind.
Kellman

Kelevi (Finnish) hero.

Keli (Hawaiian) a form of
Terry.

Keli'i (Hawaiian) chief.

Kelile (Ethiopian) protected.

Kell (Scandinavian) spring.

Kellan (Irish) a form of
Kellen.
Keillan

Kellen (Irish) mighty warrior.
*Kaelan, Kailen, Kalan, Kalen,
Kalin, Kallen, Kalon, Kalyn,
Kaylen, Keelan, Kelden, Kelin,
Kellan, Kelle, Kellin, Kellyn,
Kelyn, Kelynn*

Keller (Irish) little companion.

Kelly (Irish) warrior.
*Kelle, Kellen, Kelley, Kelli,
Kellie, Kely*

Kelmen (Basque) merciful.
Kelmin

Kelsey (Scandinavian) island
of ships.
*Kelcy, Kelse, Kelsea, Kelsi,
Kelsie, Kelso, Kelsy, Kesley,
Kesly*

Kelton (English) keel town;
port.
*Kelden, Keldon, Kelson,
Kelston, Kelten, Keltin,
Keltonn, Keltyn*

Kelvin (Irish, English) narrow
river. Geography: a river in
Scotland.
*Kelvan, Kelven, Kelvon,
Kelvyn, Kelwin, Kelwyn*

Kemal (Turkish) highest
honor.

Kemen (Basque) strong.

Kemp (English) fighter; champion.

Kempton (English) military
town.

Ken (Japanese) one's own
kind. (Scottish) a short form
of Kendall, Kendrick,
Kenneth.
Kena, Kenn, Keno

Kenan (Irish) a form of
Keenan.

Kenaz (Hebrew) bright.

Kendal (English) a form of
Kendall.
*Kendale, Kendali, Kendel,
Kendul, Kendyl*

Kendall (English) valley of the
river Kent.
*Ken, Kendal, Kendell, Kendrall,
Kendryll, Kendyll, Kyndall*

Kendarius (American) a combination of Ken + Darius.
Kendarious, Kendarrious, Kendarrius, Kenderious, Kenderius, Kenderyious

Kendell (English) a form of Kendall.
Kendelle, Kendrel, Kendrell

Kendrew (Scottish) a form of Andrew.

Kendrick (Irish) son of Henry. (Scottish) royal chieftain.
Ken, Kenderrick, Kendric, Kendrich, Kenedrick, Kendricks, Kendrik, Kendrix, Kendryck, Kenndrick, Keondric, Keondrick

Kenley (English) royal meadow.
Kenlea, Kenlee, Kenleigh, Kenlie, Kenly

Kenn (Scottish) a form of Ken.

Kennan (Scottish) little Ken.
Kenna, Kenan, Kenen, Kennen, Kennon

Kennard (Irish) brave chieftain.
Kenner

Kennedy (Irish) helmeted chief. History: John F. Kennedy was the thirty-fifth U.S. president.
Kenedy, Kenidy, Kennady, Kennedey

Kenneth (Irish) handsome. (English) royal oath.
Ken, Keneth, Kenneith, Kennet, Kennethen, Kennett, Kennieth, Kennith, Kennth, Kenny, Kennyth, Kenya

Kenny (Scottish) a familiar form of Kenneth.
Keni, Kenney, Kenni, Kennie, Kinnie

Kenrick (English) bold ruler; royal ruler.
Kenric, Kenricks, Kenrik

Kent (Welsh) white; bright. (English) a short form of Kenton. Geography: a region in England.

Kentaro (Japanese) big boy.

Kenton (English) from Kent, England.
Kent, Kenten, Kentin, Kentonn

Kentrell (English) king's estate.
Kenreal, Kentrel, Kentrelle

Kenward (English) brave; royal guardian.

Kenya (Hebrew) animal horn. (Russian) a form of Kenneth. Geography: a country in east-central Africa.
Kenyatta

Kenyatta (American) a form of Kenya.
Kenyata, Kenyatae, Kenyatee, Kenyatter, Kenyatti, Kenyotta

Kenyon (Irish) white haired,
blond.
Kenyan, Kenynn, Keonyon

Kenzie (Scottish) wise leader.
See also Mackenzie.
Kensie

Keoki (Hawaiian) a form of
George.

Keola (Hawaiian) life.

Keon (Irish) a form of Ewan.
*Keeon, Keion, Keionne,
Keondre, Keone, Keonne,
Keonte, Keony, Keyon, Kian,
Kion*

Keoni (Hawaiian) a form of
John.

Keonte (American) a form of
Keon.
*Keonntay, Keonta, Keontae,
Keontay, Keontaye, Keontez,
Keontia, Keontis, Keontrae,
Keontre, Keontrey, Keontrye*

Kerbasi (Basque) warrior.

Kerel (Afrikaans) young.
Kerell

Kerem (Turkish) noble; kind.
Kereem

Kerey (Gypsy) homeward
bound.
Ker

Kerman (Basque) from
Germany.

Kermit (Irish) a form of
Dermot.
*Kermey, Kermie, Kermitt,
Kermy*

Kern (Irish) a short form of
Kieran.
Kearn, Kerne

Kerr (Scandinavian) a form of
Carr.
Karr

Kerrick (English) king's rule.

Kerry (Irish) dark; dark haired.
*Keary, Keri, Kerrey, Kerri,
Kerrie*

Kers (Todas) Botany: an
Indian plant.

Kersen (Indonesian) cherry.

Kerstan (Dutch) a form of
Christian.

Kerwin (Irish) little; dark.
(English) friend of the
marshlands.
*Kervin, Kervyn, Kerwinn,
Kerwyn, Kerwynn, Kirwin,
Kirwyn*

Kesar (Russian) a form of
Caesar.
Kesare

Keshawn (American) a com-
bination of the prefix Ke +
Shawn.
*Keeshaun, Keeshawn, Keeshon,
Kesean, Keshan, Keshane,
Keshaun, Keshayne, Keshion,*

*Keshon, Keshone, Keshun,
Kishan*

Kesin (Hindi) long-haired
beggar.

Kesse (Ashanti, Fante) chubby
baby.
Kessie

Kester (English) a form of
Christopher.

Kestrel (English) falcon.
Kes

Keung (Chinese) universe.

Kevan (Irish) a form of Kevin.
*Kavan, Kewan, Kewane,
Kewaun, Keyvan, Kiwan,
Kiwane*

Keven (Irish) a form of Kevin.
Keve, Keveen, Kiven

Kevin (Irish) handsome. See
also Cavan.
*Kaiven, Keaven, Keevon,
Keivan, Kev, Kevan, Keven,
Keverne, Kevian, Kevien,
Kévin, Kevinn, Kevins, Kevis,
Kevn, Kevon, Kevvy, Kevyn,
Kyven*

Kevon (Irish) a form of Kevin.
*Keveon, Kevion, Kevone,
Kevonne, Kevontae, Kevonte,
Kevoyn, Kevron, Kewon,
Kewone, Keyvon, Kivon*

Kevyn (Irish) a form of Kevin.
Kevyon

Key (English) key; protected.

Keyon (Irish) a form of Keon.
Keyan, Keyen, Keyin, Keyion

Keyshawn (American) a com-
bination of Key + Shawn.
*Keyshan, Keyshaun, Keyshon,
Keyshun*

Khachig (Armenian) small
cross.
Khachik

Khaim (Russian) a form of
Chaim.

Khaldun (Arabic) forever.
Khaldoon, Khaldoun

Khalfani (Swahili) born to
lead.
Khalfan

Khälid (Arabic) eternal.
Khaled, Khallid, Khalyd

Khalîl (Arabic) friend.
*Kahlil, Kaleel, Kalil, Khahlil,
Khailil, Khailyl, Khalee,
Khaleel, Khaleil, Khali,
Khalial, Khaliel, Khalihl,
Khalill, Khaliyl*

Khaliq (Arabic) creative.
Kaliq, Khalique

Khamisi (Swahili) born on
Thursday.
Kham

Khan (Turkish) prince.
Khanh

Kharald (Russian) a form of
Gerald.

Khayru (Arabic) benevolent.
Khiri, Khiry, Kiry

Khoury (Arabic) priest.
Khory

Khristian (Greek) a form of
Christian, Kristian.
*Khris, Khristan, Khristin,
Khriston, Khrystian*

Khristopher (Greek) a form
of Kristopher.
*Khristofer, Khristophar,
Khrystopher*

Khristos (Greek) a form of
Christos.
*Khris, Khristophe, Kristo,
Kristos*

Kibo (Uset) worldly; wise.

Kibuuka (Luganda) brave warrior. History: a Ganda warrior deity.

Kidd (English) child; young
goat.

Kiefer (German) a form of
Keifer.
*Kief, Kieffer, Kiefor, Kiffer,
Kiiefer*

Kiel (Irish) a form of Kyle.
Kiell

Kiele (Hawaiian) gardenia.

Kieran (Irish) little and dark;
little Keir.
*Keiran, Keiren, Keiron, Kiaron,
Kiarron, Kier, Kieren, Kierian,
Kierien, Kierin, Kiernan,*

**Kieron, Kierr, Kierre, Kierron,
Kyran**

Kiernan (Irish) a form of
Kieran.
Kern, Kernan, Kiernen

Kiet (Tai) honor.

Kifeda (Luo) only boy among
girls.

Kiho (Rutooro) born on a
foggy day.

Kijika (Native American)
quiet walker.

Kika (Hawaiian) a form of
Keith.

Kiki (Spanish) a form of
Henry.

Kile (Irish) a form of Kyle.
Kilee, Kilen, Kiley, Kiyl, Kiyle

Killian (Irish) little Kelly.
*Kilean, Kilian, Kilien, Killie,
Killien, Killiean, Killion, Killy*

Kim (English) a short form of
Kimball.
Kimie, Kimmy

Kimball (Greek) hollow ves-
sel. (English) warrior chief.
*Kim, Kimbal, Kimbel, Kimbell,
Kimble*

Kimo (Hawaiian) a form of
James.

Kimokeo (Hawaiian) a form
of Timothy.

Kin (Japanese) golden.

Kincaid (Scottish) battle chief.
Kincade, Kinkaid

Kindin (Basque) fifth.

King (English) king. A short form of names beginning with "King."

Kingsley (English) king's meadow.
King, Kings, Kingslea, Kingslie, Kingsly, Kingzlee, Kinslea, Kinslee, Kinsley, Kinslie, Kinsly

Kingston (English) king's estate.
King, Kinston

Kingswell (English) king's well.
King

Kini (Hawaiian) a short form of Iukini.

Kinnard (Irish) tall slope.

Kinsey (English) victorious royalty.
Kinze, Kinzie

Kinton (Hindi) crowned.

Kion (Irish) a form of Keon.
Kione, Kionie, Kionne

Kioshi (Japanese) quiet.

Kipp (English) pointed hill.
Kip, Kippar, Kipper, Kippie, Kippy

Kir (Bulgarian) a familiar form of Cyrus.

Kiral (Turkish) king; supreme leader.

Kiran (Sanskrit) beam of light.
Kyran

Kirby (Scandinavian) church village. (English) cottage by the water.
Kerbey, Kerbie, Kerby, Kirbey, Kirbie, Kirkby

Kiri (Cambodian) mountain.

Kiril (Slavic) a form of Cyril.
Kirill, Kiryl, Kyrillos

Kiritan (Hindi) wearing a crown.

Kirk (Scandinavian) church.
Kerk

Kirkland (English) church land.
Kirklin, Kirklind, Kirklynd

Kirkley (English) church meadow.

Kirklin (English) a form of Kirkland.
Kirklan, Kirklen, Kirkline, Kirkloun, Kirklun, Kirklyn, Kirklynn

Kirkwell (English) church well; church spring.

Kirkwood (English) church forest.

Kirton (English) church town.

Kishan (American) a form of Keshawn.
Kishaun, Kishawn, Kishen, Kishon, Kyshon, Kyshun

Kistna (Hindi) sacred, holy. Geography: a sacred river in India.

Kistur (Gypsy) skillful rider.

Kit (Greek) a familiar form of Christian, Christopher, Kristopher.
Kitt, Kitts

Kito (Swahili) jewel; precious child.

Kitwana (Swahili) pledged to live.

Kiva (Hebrew) a short form of Akiva, Jacob.
Kiba, Kivi, Kiwa

Kiyoshi (Japanese) quiet; peaceful.

Kizza (Luganda) born after twins.
Kizzy

Kjell (Swedish) a form of Karl.
Kjel

Klaus (German) a short form of Nicholas. A form of Claus.
Klaas, Klaes, Klas, Klause

Klay (English) a form of Clay.

Klayton (English) a form of Clayton.

Kleef (Dutch) cliff.

Klement (Czech) a form of Clement.
Klema, Klemenis, Klemens, Klemet, Klemo, Klim, Klimek, Kliment, Klimka

Kleng (Norwegian) claw.

Knight (English) armored knight.
Knightly

Knoton (Native American) a form of Nodin.

Knowles (English) grassy slope.
Knolls, Nowles

Knox (English) hill.

Knute (Scandinavian) a form of Canute.
Knud, Knut

Koby (Polish) a familiar form of Jacob.
Kobby, Kobe, Kobey, Kobi, Kobia, Kobie

Kodi (English) a form of Kody.
Kode, Kodee, Kodie

Kody (English) a form of Cody.
Kodey, Kodi, Kodye, Koty

Kofi (Twi) born on Friday.

Kohana (Lakota) swift.

Koi (Choctaw) panther. (Hawaiian) a form of Troy.

Kojo (Akan) born on Monday.

Koka (Hawaiian) Scotsman.

Kokayi (Shona) gathered together.

Kolby (English) a form of Colby.
Kelby, Koalby, Koelby, Kohlbe, Kohlby, Kolbe, Kolbey, Kolbi, Kolbie, Kolebe, Koleby, Kollby

Kole (English) a form of Cole.
Kohl, Kohle

Koleman (English) a form of Coleman.
Kolemann, Kolemen

Kolin (English) a form of Colin.
Kolen, Kollen, Kollin, Kollyn, Kolyn

Kolton (English) a form of Colton.
Kolt, Koltan, Kolte, Kolten, Koltin, Koltn, Koltyn

Kolya (Russian) a familiar form of Nikolai, Nikolos.
Kola, Kolenka, Kolia, Kolja

Kona (Hawaiian) a form of Don.
Konala

Konane (Hawaiian) bright moonlight.

Kondo (Swahili) war.

Kong (Chinese) glorious; sky.

Konner (Irish) a form of Conner, Connor.
Konar, Koner

Konnor (Irish) a form of Connor.
Kohner, Kohnor, Konor

Kono (Moquelumnan) squirrel eating a pine nut.

Konrad (German) a form of Conrad.
Khonrad, Koen, Koenraad, Kon, Konn, Konney, Konni, Konnie, Konny, Konrád, Konrade, Konrado, Kord, Kort, Kunz

Konstantin (German, Russian) a form of Constantine. See also Dinos.
Konstancji, Konstadine, Konstadino, Konstandinos, Konstantinas, Konstantine, Konstantinos, Konstantio, Konstanty, Konstantyn, Konstanz, Konstatino, Kostadino, Kostadinos, Kostandino, Kostandinos, Kostantin, Kostantino, Kostas, Kostenka, Kostya, Kotsos

Kontar (Akan) only child.

Korb (German) basket.

Korbin (English) a form of Corbin.
Korban, Korben, Korbyn

Kordell (English) a form of Cordell.
Kordel

Korey (Irish) a form of Corey, Kory.
Kore, Koree, Korei, Korio, Korre, Korria, Korrye

Kornel (Latin) a form of Cornelius, Kornelius.
Kees, Korneil, Kornél, Korneli, Kornelisz, Kornell, Krelis, Soma

Kornelius (Latin) a form of Cornelius. See also Kees, Kornel.
Karnelius, Korneilius, Korneliaus, Kornelious, Kornellius

Korrigan (Irish) a form of Corrigan.
Korigan, Korigan, Korrigon, Korrigun

Kort (German, Dutch) a form of Cort, Kurt.
Kourt

Kortney (English) a form of Courtney.
Kortni, Kourtney

Korudon (Greek) helmeted one.

Kory (Irish) a form of Corey.
Korey, Kori, Korie, Korrey, Korri, Korrie, Korry

Kosey (African) lion.
Kosse

Kosmo (Greek) a form of Cosmo.
Kosmy, Kozmo

Kostas (Greek) a short form of Konstantin.

Kosti (Finnish) a form of Gustave.

Kosumi (Moquelumnan) spear fisher.

Koukalaka (Hawaiian) a form of Douglas.

Kourtland (English) a form of Courtland.
Kortlan, Kortland, Kortlend, Kortlon, Kourtlin

Kovit (Tai) expert.

Kraig (Irish, Scottish) a form of Craig.
Kraggie, Kraggy, Krayg, Kreg, Kreig, Kreigh

Krikor (Armenian) a form of Gregory.

Kris (Greek) a form of Chris. A short form of Kristian, Kristofer, Kristopher.
Kriss, Krys

Krischan (German) a form of Christian.
Krishan, Krishaun, Krishawn, Krishon, Krishun

Krishna (Hindi) delightful, pleasurable. Religion: the eighth and principal avatar of the Hindu god Vishnu.
Kistna, Kistnah, Krisha, Krishnah

Krispin (Latin) a form of Crispin.
Krispian, Krispino, Krispo

Krister (Swedish) a form of Christian.
Krist, Kristar

Kristian (Greek) a form of Christian, Khristian.
Kerstan, Khristos, Kit, Kris, Krischan, Krist, Kristan, Kristar, Kristek, Kristen, Krister, Kristien, Kristin, Kristine, Kristinn, Kristion, Kristjan, Kristo, Kristos, Krists, Krystek, Krystian, Khrystiyan

Kristo (Greek) a short form of Khristos.

Kristofer (Swedish) a form of Kristopher.
Kris, Kristafer, Kristef, Kristifer, Kristoff, Kristoffer, Kristofo, Kristofor, Kristofyr, Kristufer, Kristus, Krystofer

Kristoff (Greek) a short form of Kristofer, Kristopher.
Kristof, Kristóf

Kristophe (French) a form of Kristopher.

Kristopher (Greek) a form of Christopher. See also Topher.
Khristopher, Kit, Kris, Krisstopher, Kristapher, Kristepher, Kristfer, Kristfor, Kristo, Kristofer, Kristoff, Kristoforo, Kristoph, Kristophe, Kristophor, Kristos, Krists,

Krisus, Krystopher, Krystupas, Krzysztof

Kruz (Spanish) a form of Cruz.
Kruise, Kruize, Kruse, Kruze

Krystian (Polish) a form of Christian.
Krys, Krystek, Krystien, Krystin

Kuba (Czech) a form of Jacob.
Kubo, Kubus

Kueng (Chinese) universe.

Kugonza (Rutooro) love.

Kuiril (Basque) lord.

Kumar (Sanskrit) prince.

Kunle (Yoruba) home filled with honors.

Kuper (Yiddish) copper.

Kurt (Latin, German, French) a short form of Kurtis. A form of Curt.
Kirt, Kort, Kuno, Kurtt

Kurtis (Latin, French) a form of Curtis.
Kirtis, Kirtus, Kurt, Kurtes, Kurtez, Kurtice, Kurties, Kurtiss, Kurtus, Kurtys

Kuruk (Pawnee) bear.

Kuzih (Carrier) good speaker.

Kwabena (Akan) born on Tuesday.

Kwacha (Nguni) morning.

Kwako (Akan) born on
Wednesday.
Kwaka, Kwaku

Kwam (Zuni) a form of John.

Kwame (Akan) born on
Saturday.
Kwamen, Kwami, Kwamin

Kwan (Korean) strong.
Kwane

Kwasi (Akan) born on Sunday.
(Swahili) wealthy.
Kwasie, Kwazzi, Kwesi

Kwayera (Nguni) dawn.

Kwende (Nguni) let's go.

Kyele (Irish) a form of Kyle.

Kylan (Irish) a form of Kyle.
*Kyelen, Kyleen, Kylen, Kylin,
Kyline, Kylon, Kylun*

Kyle (Irish) narrow piece of
land; place where cattle
graze. (Yiddish) crowned
with laurels.
*Cyle, Kiel, Kilan, Kile, Kilen,
Kiley, Ky, Kye, Kyel, Kyele,
Kylan, Kylee, Kyler, Kyley,
Kylie, Kyll, Kylle, Kyrell*

Kyler (English) a form of
Kyle.
Kylar, Kylor

Kynan (Welsh) chief.

Kyndall (English) a form of
Kendall.
*Kyndal, Kyndel, Kyndell,
Kyndle*

Kyne (English) royal.

Kyran (Sanskrit) a form of
Kiran.
Kyren, Kyron, Kyrone

Kyros (Greek) master.

Kyven (American) a form of
Kevin.
*Kyvan, Kyvaun, Kyvon,
Kywon, Kywynn*

L

Laban (Hawaiian) white.
Labon, Lebaan, Leban, Liban

Labaron (American) a combi-
nation of the prefix La +
Baron.
*Labaren, Labarren, Labarron,
Labearon, Labron*

Labib (Arabic) sensible; intelligent.

Labrentsis (Russian) a form
of Lawrence.
Labhras, Labhruinn, Labrencis

Lachlan (Scottish) land of
lakes.
*Lache, Lachlann, Lachunn,
Lakelan, Lakeland*

Ladarian (American) a com-
bination of the prefix La +
Darian.
*Ladarien, Ladarin, Ladarion,
Ladarren, Ladarrian, Ladarrien,*

Ladarrin, Ladarrion, Laderion, Laderrian, Laderrion

Ladarius (American) a combination of the prefix La + Darius.
Ladarious, Ladaris, Ladarrius, Ladauris, Laderius, Ladirus

Ladarrius (American) a form of Ladarius.
Ladarrias, Ladarries, Ladarrious, Laderrious, Laderris

Ladd (English) attendant.
Lad, Laddey, Laddie, Laddy

Laderrick (American) a combination of the prefix La + Derrick.
Ladarrick, Ladereck, Laderic, Laderricks

Ladislav (Czech) a form of Walter.
Laco, Lada, Ladislaus

Lado (Fante) second-born son.

Lafayette (French) History: Marquis de Lafayette was a French soldier and politician who aided the American Revolution.
Lafaiete, Lafayett, Lafette, Laffyette

Laine (English) a form of Lane.
Lain

Laird (Scottish) wealthy landowner.

Lais (Arabic) lion.

Lajos (Hungarian) famous; holy.
Lajcsi, Laji, Lali

Lake (English) lake.
Lakan, Lakane, Lakee, Laken, Lakin

Lakota (Dakota) a tribal name.
Lakoda

Lal (Hindi) beloved.

Lamar (German) famous throughout the land. (French) sea, ocean.
Lamair, Lamario, Lamaris, Lamarr, Lamarre, Larmar, Lemar

Lambert (German) bright land.
Bert, Lambard, Lamberto, Lambirt, Lampard, Landbert

Lamond (French) world.
Lammond, Lamon, Lamonde, Lamondo, Lamondre, Lamund, Lemond

Lamont (Scandinavian) lawyer.
Lamaunt, Lamonta, Lamonte, Lamontie, Lamonto, Lamount, Lemont

Lance (German) a short form of Lancelot.
Lancy, Lantz, Lanz, Launce

Lancelot (French) attendant. Literature: the knight who loved King Arthur's wife, Queen Guinevere.
Lance, Lancelott, Launcelet, Launcelot

Landen (English) a form of
Landon.
Landenn

Lander (Basque) lion man.
(English) landowner.
Landers, Landor

Lando (Portuguese, Spanish) a
short form of Orlando,
Rolando.

Landon (English) open, grassy
meadow.
*Landan, Landen, Landin,
Landyn*

Landry (French, English)
ruler.
Landre, Landré, Landrue

Lane (English) narrow road.
Laine, Laney, Lanie, Layne

Lang (Scandinavian) tall man.
Lange

Langdon (English) long hill.
Landon, Langsdon, Langston

Langford (English) long ford.
Lanford, Lankford

Langley (English) long
meadow.
*Langlea, Langlee, Langleigh,
Langly*

Langston (English) long, narrow town.
Langsden, Langsdon

Langundo (Native American)
peaceful.

Lani (Hawaiian) heaven.

Lanny (American) a familiar
form of Lawrence, Laurence.
Lanney, Lannie, Lennie

Lanu (Moquelumnan) running
around the pole.

Lanz (Italian) a form of Lance.
Lanzo, Lonzo

Lao (Spanish) a short form of
Stanislaus.

Lap (Vietnamese) independent.

Lapidos (Hebrew) torches.
Lapidoth

Laquan (American) a combi-
nation of the prefix La +
Quan.
*Laquain, Laquann, Laquanta,
Laquantae, Laquante, Laquawn,
Laquawne, Laquin, Laquinn,
Laqun, Laquon, Laquone,
Laqwan, Laqwon*

Laquintin (American) a com-
bination of the prefix La +
Quintin.
*Laquentin, Laquenton,
Laquintas, Laquinten,
Laquintiss, Laquinton*

Laramie (French) tears of love.
Geography: a town in
Wyoming on the Overland
Trail.
Larami, Laramy, Laremy

Larenzo (Italian, Spanish) a
form of Lorenzo.
*Larenz, Larenza, Larinzo,
Laurenzo*

Larkin (Irish) rough; fierce.
Larklin

Larnell (American) a combination of Larry + Darnell.

Laron (French) thief.
Laran, La'ron, La Ron, Larone, Laronn, Larron, La Ruan

Larrimore (French) armorer.
Larimore, Larmer, Larmor

Larry (Latin) a familiar form of Lawrence.
Larrie, Lary

Lars (Scandinavian) a form of Lawrence.
Laris, Larris, Larse, Larsen, Larson, Larsson, Larz, Lasse, Laurans, Laurits, Lavrans, Lorens

LaSalle (French) hall.
Lasal, Lasalle, Lascell, Lascelles

Lash (Gypsy) a form of Louis.
Lashi, Lasho

Lashawn (American) a combination of the prefix La + Shawn.
Lasaun, Lasean, Lashajaun, Lashan, Lashane, Lashaun, Lashon, Lashun

Lashon (American) a form of Lashawn.
Lashone, Lashonne

Lasse (Finnish) a form of Nicholas.

László (Hungarian) famous ruler.
Laci, Lacko, Laslo, Lazlo

Lateef (Arabic) gentle; pleasant.
Latif, Letif

Latham (Scandinavian) barn. (English) district.
Laith, Lathe, Lay

Lathan (American) a combination of the prefix La + Nathan.
Lathaniel, Lathen, Lathyn, Leathan

Lathrop (English) barn, farmstead.
Lathe, Lathrope, Lay

Latimer (English) interpreter.
Lat, Latimor, Lattie, Latty, Latymer

Latravis (American) a combination of the prefix La + Travis.
Latavious, Latavius, Latraveus, Latraviaus, Latravious, Latravius, Latrayvious, Latrayvous, Latrivis

Latrell (American) a combination of the prefix La + Kentrell.
Latreal, Latreil, Latrel, Latrelle, Letreal, Letrel, Letrell, Letrelle

Laudalino (Portuguese) praised.
Lino

Laughlin (Irish) servant of
Saint Secundinus.
Lanty, Lauchlin, Leachlainn

Laurence (Latin) crowned
with laurel. A form of
Lawrence. See also Rance,
Raulas, Raulo, Renzo.
*Lanny, Lauran, Laurance,
Laureano, Lauren, Laurencho,
Laurencio, Laurens, Laurent,
Laurentij, Laurentios, Laurentiu,
Laurentius, Laurentz,
Laurentzi, Laurie, Laurin,
Lauris, Laurits, Lauritz,
Laurnet, Lauro, Laurus,
Lavrenti, Lurance*

Laurencio (Spanish) a form of
Laurence.

Laurens (Dutch) a form of
Laurence.
Laurenz

Laurent (French) a form of
Laurence.
Laurente

Laurie (English) a familiar
form of Laurence.
Lauri, Laury, Lorry

Lauris (Swedish) a form of
Laurence.

Lauro (Filipino) a form of
Laurence.

LaValle (French) valley.
*Lavail, Laval, Lavalei, Lavalle,
Lavell*

Lavan (Hebrew) white.
*Lavane, Lavaughan, Laven,
Lavon, Levan*

Lavaughan (American) a form
of Lavan.
*Lavaughn, Levaughan,
Levaughn*

Lave (Italian) lava. (English)
lord.

Lavell (French) a form of
LaValle.
*Lavel, Lavele, Lavelle, Levele,
Levell, Levelle*

Lavi (Hebrew) lion.

Lavon (American) a form of
Lavan.
*Lavion, Lavone, Lavonn,
Lavonne, Lavont, Lavonte*

Lavrenti (Russian) a form of
Lawrence.
*Larenti, Lavrentij, Lavrusha,
Lavrik, Lavro*

Lawerence (Latin) a form of
Lawrence.
Lawerance

Lawford (English) ford on the
hill.
Ford, Law

Lawler (Irish) soft-spoken.
Lawlor, Lollar, Loller

Lawrence (Latin) crowned
with laurel. See also Brencis,
Chencho.
*Labrentsis, Laiurenty, Lanny,
Lanty, Larance, Laren, Larian,*

Larien, Laris, Larka, Larrance,
Larrence, Larry, Lars, Larya,
Laurence, Lavrenti, Law,
Lawerence, Lawrance, Lawren,
Lawrey, Lawrie, Lawron, Lawry,
Lencho, Lon, Lóránt, Loreca,
Loren, Loretto, Lorenzo, Lorne,
Lourenco, Lowrance

Lawson (English) son of
Lawrence.
Lawsen, Layson

Lawton (English) town on the
hill.
Laughton, Law

Layne (English) a form of
Lane.
Layn, Laynee

Layton (English) a form of
Leighton.
Laydon, Layten, Layth,
Laythan, Laython

Lazaro (Italian) a form of
Lazarus.
Lazarillo, Lazarito, Lazzaro

Lazarus (Greek) a form of
Eleazar. Bible: Lazarus was
raised from the dead by
Jesus.
Lazar, Lázár, Lazare, Lazarius,
Lazaro, Lazaros, Lazorus

Leander (Greek) lion-man;
brave as a lion.
Ander, Leandro

Leandro (Spanish) a form of
Leander.
Leandra, Léandre, Leandrew,
Leandros

Leben (Yiddish) life.
Laben, Lebon

Lebna (Ethiopian) spirit; heart.

Ledarius (American) a combi-
nation of the prefix Le +
Darius.
Ledarrious, Ledarrius, Lederious,
Lederris

Lee (English) a short form of
Farley, Leonard, and names
containing "lee."
Leigh

Leggett (French) one who is
sent; delegate.
Legate, Legette, Leggitt, Liggett

Lei (Chinese) thunder.
(Hawaiian) a form of Ray.

Leib (Yiddish) roaring lion.
Leibel

Leif (Scandinavian) beloved.
Laif, Leife, Lief

Leigh (English) a form of Lee.

Leighton (English) meadow
farm.
Lay, Layton, Leigh, Leyton

Leith (Scottish) broad river.

Lek (Tai) small.

Lekeke (Hawaiian) powerful
ruler.

Leks (Estonian) a familiar form of Alexander.
Leksik, Lekso

Lel (Gypsy) taker.

Leland (English) meadowland; protected land.
Lealand, Lee, Leeland, Leigh, Leighland, Lelan, Lelann, Lelend, Lelund, Leyland

Lemar (French) a form of Lamar.
Lemario, Lemarr

Lemuel (Hebrew) devoted to God.
Lem, Lemmie, Lemmy

Len (Hopi) flute. (German) a short form of Leonard.

Lenard (German) a form of Leonard.
Lennard

Lencho (Spanish) a form of Lawrence.
Lenci, Lenzy

Lennart (Swedish) a form of Leonard.
Lennerd

Lenno (Native American) man.

Lennon (Irish) small cloak; cape.
Lenon

Lennor (Gypsy) spring; summer.

Lennox (Scottish) with many elms.
Lennix, Lenox

Lenny (German) a familiar form of Leonard.
Leni, Lennie, Leny

Leo (Latin) lion. (German) a short form of Leon, Leopold.
Lavi, Leão, Lee, Leib, Leibel, Leos, Leosko, Léo, Léocadie, Leos, Leosoko, Lev, Lio, Lion, Liutas, Lyon, Nardek

Leobardo (Italian) a form of Leonard.

Leon (Greek, German) a short form of Leonard, Napoleon.
Leo, Léon, Leonas, Léonce, Leoncio, Leondris, Leone, Leonek, Leonetti, Leoni, Leonid, Leonidas, Leonirez, Leonizio, Leonon, Leons, Leontes, Leontios, Leontrae, Liutas

Leonard (German) brave as a lion.
Leanard, Lee, Len, Lena, Lenard, Lennart, Lenny, Leno, Leobardo, Leon, Léonard, Leonardis, Leonardo, Leonart, Leonerd, Leonhard, Leonidas, Leonnard, Leontes, Lernard, Lienard, Linek, Lnard, Lon, Londard, Lonnard, Lonya, Lynnard

Leonardo (Italian) a form of Leonard.
Leonaldo, Lionardo

Leonel (English) little lion. See also Lionel.
Leonell

Leonhard (German) a form of Leonard.
Leonhards

Leonid (Russian) a form of Leonard.
Leonide, Lyonechka, Lyonya

Leonidas (Greek) a form of Leonard.
Leonida, Leonides

Leopold (German) brave people.
Leo, Leopoldo, Leorad, Lipót, Lopolda, Luepold, Luitpold, Poldi

Leopoldo (Italian) a form of Leopold.

Leor (Hebrew) my light.
Leory, Lior

Lequinton (American) a combination of the prefix Le + Quinton.
Lequentin, Lequenton, Lequinn

Leron (French) round, circle. (American) a combination of the prefix Le + Ron.
Leeron, Le Ron, Lerone, Liron, Lyron

Leroy (French) king. See also Delroy, Elroy.
Lee, Leeroy, LeeRoy, Leigh, Lerai, Leroi, LeRoi, LeRoy, Roy

Les (Scottish, English) a short form of Leslie, Lester.
Lessie

Lesharo (Pawnee) chief.

Leshawn (American) a combination of the prefix Le + Shawn.
Lashan, Lesean, Leshaun, Leshon, Leshun

Leslie (Scottish) gray fortress.
Lee, Leigh, Les, Leslea, Leslee, Lesley, Lesli, Lesly, Lezlie, Lezly

Lester (Latin) chosen camp. (English) from Leicester, England.
Leicester, Les

Lev (Hebrew) heart. (Russian) a form of Leo. A short form of Leverett, Levi.
Leb, Leva, Levka, Levko, Levushka

Leverett (French) young hare.
Lev, Leveret, Leverit, Leveritt

Levi (Hebrew) joined in harmony. Bible: the third son of Jacob; Levites are the priestly tribe of the Israelites.
Leavi, Leevi, Leevie, Lev, Levey, Levie, Levin, Levitis, Levy, Lewi, Leyvi

Levin (Hebrew) a form of Levi.
Levine, Levion

Levon (American) a form of
Lavon.
Leevon, Levone, Levonn,
Levonne, Levonte, Lyvonne

Lew (English) a short form of
Lewis.

Lewin (English) beloved
friend.

Lewis (Welsh) a form of
Llewellyn. (English) a form
of Louis.
Lew, Lewes, Lewie, Lewy

Lex (English) a short form of
Alexander.
Lexi, Lexie, Lexin

Lexus (Greek) a short form of
Alexander.
Lexis, Lexius, Lexxus

Leyati (Moquelumnan) shape
of an abalone shell.

Lí (Chinese) strong.

Liam (Irish) a form of
William.
Liem, Lliam, Lyam

Liang (Chinese) good, excellent.

Liban (Hawaiian) a form of
Laban.
Libaan, Lieban

Liberio (Portuguese) libera-
tion.
Liberaratore, Liborio

Lidio (Greek, Portuguese)
ancient.

Ligongo (Yao) who is this?

Likeke (Hawaiian) a form of
Richard.

Liko (Chinese) protected by
Buddha. (Hawaiian) bud.
Like

Lin (Burmese) bright. (English)
a short form of Lyndon.
Linh, Linn, Linny, Lyn, Lynn

Linc (English) a short form of
Lincoln.
Link

Lincoln (English) settlement
by the pool. History:
Abraham Lincoln was the
sixteenth U.S. president.
Linc, Lincon, Lyncoln

Lindberg (German) mountain
where linden grow.
Lindbergh, Lindburg, Lindy

Lindell (English) valley of the
linden.
Lendall, Lendel, Lendell,
Lindall, Lindel, Lyndale,
Lyndall, Lyndel, Lyndell

Linden (English) a form of
Lyndon.

Lindley (English) linden field.
Lindlea, Lindlee, Lindleigh,
Lindly

Lindon (English) a form of
Lyndon.
Lin, Lindan

Lindsay (English) a form of
Lindsey.
Linsay

Lindsey (English) linden-tree
island.
*Lind, Lindsay, Lindsee, Lindsie,
Lindsy, Lindzy, Linsey, Linzie,
Linzy, Lyndsay, Lyndsey,
Lyndsie, Lynzie*

Linford (English) linden ford.
Lynford

Linfred (German) peaceful,
calm.

Linley (English) flax meadow.
Linlea, Linlee, Linleigh, Linly

Linton (English) flax town.
Lintonn, Lynton, Lyntonn

Linu (Hindi) lily.

Linus (Greek) flaxen haired.
Linas, Linux

Linwood (English) flax wood.

Lio (Hawaiian) a form of Leo.

Lionel (French) lion cub. See
also Leonel.
*Lional, Lionell, Lionello, Lynel,
Lynell, Lyonel*

Liron (Hebrew) my song.
Lyron

Lise (Moquelumnan) salmon's
head coming out of the
water.

Lisimba (Yao) lion.
Simba

Lister (English) dyer.

Litton (English) town on the
hill.
Liton

Liu (African) voice.

Liuz (Polish) light.
Lius

Livingston (English) Leif's
town.
Livingstone

Liwanu (Moquelumnan)
growling bear.

Llewellyn (Welsh) lionlike.
*Lewis, Llewelin, Llewellen,
Llewelleyn, Llewellin, Llewlyn,
Llywellyn, Llywellynn, Llywelyn*

Lloyd (Welsh) gray haired;
holy. See also Floyd.
Loy, Loyd, Loyde, Loydie

Lobo (Spanish) wolf.

Lochlain (Irish, Scottish) land
of lakes.
*Laughlin, Lochlan, Lochlann,
Lochlin, Locklynn*

Locke (English) forest.
Lock, Lockwood

Loe (Hawaiian) a form of
Roy.

Logan (Irish) meadow.
*Llogan, Loagan, Loagen,
Loagon, Logann, Logen,
Loggan, Loghan, Logon, Logn,
Logun, Logunn, Logyn*

Lok (Chinese) happy.

Lokela (Hawaiian) a form of Roger.

Lokni (Moquelumnan) raining through the roof.

Lomán (Irish) bare. (Slavic) sensitive.

Lombard (Latin) long bearded.
Bard, Barr

Lon (Irish) fierce. (Spanish) a short form of Alonso, Alonzo, Leonard, Lonnie.
Lonn

Lonan (Zuni) cloud.

Lonato (Native American) flint stone.

London (English) fortress of the moon. Geography: the capital of the United Kingdom.
Londen, Londyn, Lunden, Lundon

Long (Chinese) dragon. (Vietnamese) hair.

Lonnie (German, Spanish) a familiar form of Alonso, Alonzo.
Lon, Loni, Lonie, Lonnell, Lonney, Lonni, Lonniel, Lonny

Lono (Hawaiian) Mythology: the god of learning and intellect.

Lonzo (German, Spanish) a short form of Alonso, Alonzo.
Lonso

Lootah (Lakota) red.

Lopaka (Hawaiian) a form of Robert.

Loránd (Hungarian) a form of Roland.

Lóránt (Hungarian) a form of Lawrence.
Lorant

Lorcan (Irish) little; fierce.

Lord (English) noble title.

Loren (Latin) a short form of Lawrence.
Lorin, Lorren, Lorrin, Loryn

Lorenzo (Italian, Spanish) a form of Lawrence.
Larenzo, Lerenzo, Lewrenzo, Lorenc, Lorence, Lorenco, Lorencz, Lorens, Lorenso, Lorentz, Lorenz, Lorenza, Loretto, Lorinc, Lörinc, Lorinzo, Loritz, Lorrenzo, Lorrie, Lorry, Lourenza, Lourenzo, Lowrenzo, Renzo, Zo

Loretto (Italian) a form of Lawrence.
Loreto

Lorimer (Latin) harness maker.
Lorrie, Lorrimer, Lorry

Loring (German) son of the famous warrior.
Lorrie, Lorring, Lorry

Loris (Dutch) clown.

Loritz (Latin, Danish) laurel.
Lauritz

Lorne (Latin) a short form of Lawrence.
Lorn, Lornie

Lorry (English) a form of Laurie.
Lori, Lorri, Lory

Lot (Hebrew) hidden, covered. Bible: Lot fled from Sodom, but his wife glanced back upon its destruction and was transformed into a pillar of salt.
Lott

Lothar (German) a form of Luther.
Lotaire, Lotarrio, Lothair, Lothaire, Lothario, Lotharrio

Lou (German) a short form of Louis.

Loudon (German) low valley.
Loudan, Louden, Loudin, Lowden

Louie (German) a familiar form of Louis.

Louis (German) famous warrior. See also Aloisio, Aloysius, Clovis, Luigi.
Lash, Lashi, Lasho, Lewis, Lou, Loudovicus, Louie, Louies,
Louise, Lucho, Lude, Ludek, Ludirk, Ludis, Ludko, Ludwig, Lughaidh, Lui, Luigi, Luis, Luiz, Luki, Lutek

Lourdes (French) from Lourdes, France. Religion: a place where the Virgin Mary was said to have appeared.

Louvain (English) Lou's vanity. Geography: a city in Belgium.
Louvin

Lovell (English) a form of Lowell.
Louvell, Lovel, Lovelle, Lovey

Lowell (French) young wolf. (English) beloved.
Lovell, Lowe, Lowel

Loyal (English) faithful, loyal.
Loy, Loyall, Loye, Lyall, Lyell

Lubomir (Polish) lover of peace.

Luboslaw (Polish) lover of glory.
Lubs, Lubz

Luc (French) a form of Luke.
Luce

Luca (Italian) a form of Lucius.
Lucca, Luka

Lucas (German, Irish, Danish, Dutch) a form of Lucius.
Lucais, Lucassie, Lucaus, Luccas, Luccus, Luckas, Lucus

Lucian (Latin) a form of
Lucius.
Liuz, Lucan, Lucanus, Luciano,
Lucianus, Lucias, Lucjan,
Lukianos, Lukyan

Luciano (Italian) a form of
Lucian.
Luca, Lucca, Lucino, Lucio

Lucien (French) a form of
Lucius.

Lucio (Italian) a form of
Lucius.

Lucius (Latin) light; bringer of
light.
Loukas, Luc, Luca, Lucais,
Lucanus, Lucas, Luce, Lucian,
Lucien, Lucio, Lucious, Lucis,
Luke, Lusio

Lucky (American) fortunate.
Luckee, Luckie, Luckson, Lucson

Ludlow (English) prince's hill.

Ludovic (German) a form of
Ludwig.
Ludovick, Ludovico

Ludwig (German) a form of
Louis. Music: Ludwig van
Beethoven was a famous
nineteenth-century German
composer.
Ludovic, Ludvig, Ludvik,
Ludwik, Lutz

Lui (Hawaiian) a form of
Louis.

Luigi (Italian) a form of Louis.
Lui, Luiggi, Luigino, Luigy

Luis, Luiz (Spanish) forms of
Louis.
Luise

Lukas, Lukus (Greek, Czech,
Swedish) forms of Luke.
Loukas, Lukais, Lukash,
Lukasha, Lukass, Lukasz,
Lukaus, Lukkas

Luke (Latin) a form of Lucius.
Bible: companion of Saint
Paul and author of the third
Gospel of the New
Testament.
Luc, Luchok, Luck, Lucky, Luk,
Luka, Lúkács, Lukas, Luken,
Lukes, Lukus, Lukyan, Lusio

Lukela (Hawaiian) a form of
Russel.

Luken (Basque) bringer of
light.
Lucan, Lucane, Lucano, Luk

Luki (Basque) famous warrior.

Lukman (Arabic) prophet.
Luqman

Lulani (Hawaiian) highest
point in heaven.

Lumo (Ewe) born facedown.

Lundy (Scottish) grove by the
island.

Lunn (Irish) warlike.
Lon, Lonn

Lunt (Swedish) grove.

Lusila (Hindi) leader.

Lusio (Zuni) a form of Lucius.

Lutalo (Luganda) warrior.

Lutfi (Arabic) kind, friendly.

Luther (German) famous warrior. History: Martin Luther was one of the central figures of the Reformation.
Lothar, Lutero, Luthor

Lutherum (Gypsy) slumber.

Luyu (Moquelumnan) head shaker.

Lyall, Lyell (Scottish) loyal.

Lyle (French) island.
Lisle, Ly, Lysle

Lyman (English) meadow.
Leaman, Leeman, Lymon

Lynch (Irish) mariner.
Linch

Lyndal (English) valley of lime trees.
Lyndale, Lyndall, Lyndel, Lyndell

Lyndon (English) linden hill. History: Lyndon B. Johnson was the thirty-sixth U.S. president.
Lin, Linden, Lindon, Lyden, Lydon, Lyn, Lyndan, Lynden, Lynn

Lynn (English) waterfall; brook.
Lyn, Lynell, Lynette, Lynnard, Lynoll

Lyron (Hebrew) a form of Leron, Liron.

Lysander (Greek) liberator.
Lyzander, Sander

M

Maalik (Punjabi) a form of Malik.
Maalek, Maaliek

Mac (Scottish) son.
Macs

Macadam (Scottish) son of Adam.
MacAdam, McAdam

Macallister (Irish) son of Alistair.
Macalaster, Macalister, MacAlister, McAlister, McAllister

Macario (Spanish) a form of Makarios.

Macarthur (Irish) son of Arthur.
MacArthur, McArthur

Macaulay (Scottish) son of righteousness.
Macaulee, Macauley, Macaully, Macauly, Maccauley, Mackauly, Macualay, McCauley

Macbride (Scottish) son of a follower of Saint Brigid.
Macbryde, Mcbride, McBride

Maccoy (Irish) son of Hugh,
Coy.
MacCoy, Mccoy, McCoy

Maccrea (Irish) son of grace.
*MacCrae, MacCray, MacCrea,
Macrae, Macray, Makray,
Mccrea, McCrea*

Macdonald (Scottish) son of
Donald.
*MacDonald, Mcdonald,
McDonald, Mcdonna,
Mcdonnell, McDonnell*

Macdougal (Scottish) son of
Dougal.
*MacDougal, Mcdougal,
McDougal, McDougall, Dougal*

Mace (French) club. (English)
a short form of Macy,
Mason.
*Macean, Maceo, Macer, Macey,
Macie, Macy*

Macgregor (Scottish) son of
Gregor.
Macgreggor

Machas (Polish) a form of
Michael.

Mack (Scottish) a short form
of names beginning with
"Mac" and "Mc."
*Macke, Mackey, Mackie,
Macklin, Macks, Macky*

Mackenzie (Irish) son of
Kenzie.
*Mackensy, Mackenxo,
Mackenze, Mackenzey,
Mackenzi, MacKenzie,
Mackenzly, Mackenzy,
Mackienzie, Mackinsey,
Mackinzie, Makenzie,
McKenzie, Mickenzie*

Mackinnley (Irish) son of the
learned ruler.
*Mackinley, MacKinnley,
Mackinnly, Mckinley*

Macklain (Irish) a form of
Maclean.
Macklaine, Macklane

Maclean (Irish) son of
Leander.
*Machlin, Macklain, MacLain,
MacLean, Maclin, Maclyn,
Makleen, McLaine, McLean*

Macmahon (Irish) son of
Mahon.
MacMahon, McMahon

Macmurray (Irish) son of
Murray.
McMurray

Macnair (Scottish) son of the
heir.
Macknair

Maco (Hungarian) a form of
Emmanuel.

Macon (German, English)
maker.

Macy (French) Matthew's
estate.
Mace, Macey

Maddock (Welsh) generous.
Madoc, Madock, Madog

Maddox (Welsh, English) benefactor's son.
Maddux, Madox

Madhar (Hindi) full of intoxication; relating to spring.

Madison (English) son of Maude; good son.
Maddie, Maddison, Maddy, Madisen, Madisson, Madisyn, Madsen, Son, Sonny

Madongo (Luganda) uncircumcised.

Madu (Ibo) people.

Magar (Armenian) groom's attendant.
Magarious

Magee (Irish) son of Hugh.
MacGee, MacGhee, McGee

Magen (Hebrew) protector.

Magnar (Norwegian) strong; warrior.
Magne

Magnus (Latin) great.
Maghnus, Magnes, Manius, Mayer

Magomu (Luganda) younger of twins.

Maguire (Irish) son of the beige one.
MacGuire, McGuire, McGwire

Mahammed (Arabic) a form of Muhammad.
Mahamad, Mahamed

Mahdi (Arabic) guided to the right path.
Mahde, Mahdee, Mahdy

Mahesa (Hindi) great lord. Religion: another name for the Hindu god Shiva.

Mahi'ai (Hawaiian) a form of George.

Mahir (Arabic, Hebrew) excellent; industrious.
Maher

Mahkah (Lakota) earth.

Mahmoud (Arabic) a form of Muhammad.
Mahamoud, Mahmmoud, Mahmuod

Mahmúd (Arabic) a form of Muhammad.
Mahmed, Mahmood, Mahmut

Mahomet (Arabic) a form of Muhammad.
Mehemet, Mehmet

Mahon (Irish) bear.

Mahpee (Lakota) sky.

Maimun (Arabic) lucky.
Maimon

Mairtin (Irish) a form of Martin.
Martain, Martainn

Maitias (Irish) a form of Mathias.
Maithias

Maitiú (Irish) a form of
Matthew.

Maitland (English) meadowland.

Majid (Arabic) great, glorious.
Majd, Majde, Majdi, Majdy,
Majed, Majeed

Major (Latin) greater; military
rank.
Majar, Maje, Majer, Mayer,
Mayor

Makaio (Hawaiian) a form of
Matthew.

Makalani (Mwera) writer.

Makani (Hawaiian) wind.

Makarios (Greek) happy;
blessed.
Macario, Macarios, Maccario,
Maccarios

Makenzie (Irish) a form of
Mackenzie.
Makensie, Makenzy

Makin (Arabic) strong.
Makeen

Makis (Greek) a form of
Michael.

Makoto (Japanese) sincere.

Maks (Hungarian) a form of
Max.
Makszi

Maksim (Russian) a form of
Maximilian.
Maksimka, Maksym, Maxim

Maksym (Polish) a form of
Maximilian.
Makimus, Maksim,
Maksymilian

Makyah (Hopi) eagle hunter.

Mal (Irish) a short form of
names beginning with "Mal."

Malachi (Hebrew) angel of
God. Bible: the last canonical
Hebrew prophet.
Maeleachlainn, Mal, Malachai,
Malachia, Malachie, Malachy,
Malakai, Malake, Malaki,
Malchija, Malechy, Málik

Malachy (Irish) a form of
Malachi.

Malajitm (Sanskrit) garland of
victory.

Malcolm (Scottish) follower of
Saint Columba who
Christianized North
Scotland. (Arabic) dove.
Mal, Malcalm, Malcohm,
Malcolum, Malcom, Malkolm

Malcom (Scottish) a form of
Malcolm.
Malcome, Malcum, Malkom,
Malkum

Malden (English) meeting
place in a pasture.
Mal, Maldon

Malek (Arabic) a form of
Málik.
Maleak, Maleek, Maleik,
Maleka, Maleke, Mallek

Maleko (Hawaiian) a form of Mark.

Málik (Punjabi) lord, master. (Arabic) a form of Malachi.
Maalik, Mailik, Malak, Malic, Malick, Malicke, Maliek, Maliik, Malik, Malike, Malikh, Maliq, Malique, Mallik, Malyk, Malyq

Malin (English) strong, little warrior.
Mal, Mallin, Mallon

Mallory (German) army counselor. (French) wild duck.
Lory, Mal, Mallery, Mallori, Mallorie, Malory

Maloney (Irish) church going.
Malone, Malony

Malvern (Welsh) bare hill.
Malverne

Malvin (Irish, English) a form of Melvin.
Mal, Malvinn, Malvyn, Malvynn

Mamo (Hawaiian) yellow flower; yellow bird.

Manchu (Chinese) pure.

Manco (Peruvian) supreme leader. History: a sixteenth-century Incan king.

Mandala (Yao) flowers.
Manda, Mandela

Mandeep (Punjabi) mind full of light.
Mandieep

Mandel (German) almond.
Mandell

Mandek (Polish) a form of Armand, Herman.
Mandie

Mander (Gypsy) from me.

Manford (English) small ford.

Manfred (English) man of peace. See also Fred.
Manfret, Manfrid, Manfried, Maniferd, Mannfred, Mannfryd

Manger (French) stable.

Mango (Spanish) a familiar form of Emmanuel, Manuel.

Manheim (German) servant's home.

Manipi (Native American) living marvel.

Manius (Scottish) a form of Magnus.
Manus, Manyus

Manley (English) hero's meadow.
Manlea, Manleigh, Manly

Mann (German) man.
Manin

Manning (English) son of the hero.

Mannix (Irish) monk.
Mainchin

Manny (German, Spanish) a familiar form of Manuel.
Mani, Manni, Mannie, Many

Mano (Hawaiian) shark. (Spanish) a short form of Manuel.
Manno, Manolo

Manoj (Sanskrit) cupid.

Mansa (Swahili) king. History: a fourteenth-century king of Mali.

Mansel (English) manse; house occupied by a clergyman.
Mansell

Mansfield (English) field by the river; hero's field.

Man-Shik (Korean) deeply rooted.

Mansür (Arabic) divinely aided.
Mansoor, Mansour

Manton (English) man's town; hero's town.
Mannton, Manten

Manu (Hindi) lawmaker. History: the reputed writer of the Hindi compendium of sacred laws and customs. (Hawaiian) bird. (Ghanaian) second-born son.

Manuel (Hebrew) a short form of Emmanuel.
Maco, Mango, Mannuel, Manny, Mano, Manolón, Manual, Manuale, Manue,

Manuelli, Manuelo, Manuil, Manyuil, Minel

Manville (French) worker's village. (English) hero's village.
Mandeville, Manvel, Manvil

Man-Young (Korean) ten thousand years of prosperity.

Manzo (Japanese) third son.

Maona (Winnebago) creator, earth maker.

Mapira (Yao) millet.

Marc (French) a form of Mark.

Marcel (French) a form of Marcellus.
Marcell, Marsale, Marsel

Marcelino (Italian) a form of Marcellus.
Marceleno, Marcelin, Marcellin, Marcellino

Marcelo, Marcello (Italian) forms of Marcellus.
Marchello, Marsello, Marselo

Marcellus (Latin) a familiar form of Marcus.
Marceau, Marcel, Marceles, Marcelias, Marcelino, Marcelis, Marcelius, Marcellas, Marcelleous, Marcellis, Marcellous, Marcelluas, Marcelo, Marcelus, Marcely, Marciano, Marcilka, Marcsseau, Marquel, Marsalis

March (English) dweller by a boundary.

Marciano (Italian) a form of Martin.
Marci, Marcio

Marcilka (Hungarian) a form of Marcellus.
Marci, Marcilki

Marcin (Polish) a form of Martin.

Marco (Italian) a form of Marcus. History: Marco Polo was a thirteenth-century Venetian traveler who explored Asia.
Marcko, Marko

Marcos (Spanish) a form of Marcus.
Marckos, Marcous, Markos, Markose

Marcus (Latin) martial, war-like.
Marc, Marcas, Marcellus, Marcio, Marckus, Marco, Marcos, Marcous, Marcuss, Marcuus, Marcux, Marek, Mark, Markov, Markus

Marek (Slavic) a form of Marcus.

Maren (Basque) sea.

Mareo (Japanese) uncommon.

Marian (Polish) a form of Mark.

Mariano (Italian) a form of Mark.

Marid (Arabic) rebellious.

Marin (French) sailor.
Marine, Mariner, Marino, Marius, Marriner

Marino (Italian) a form of Marin.
Marinos, Marinus, Mario, Mariono

Mario (Italian) a form of Marino.
Marios, Marrio

Marion (French) bitter; sea of bitterness.
Mareon, Mariano

Marius (Latin) a form of Marin.
Marious

Mark (Latin) a form of Marcus. Bible: author of the second Gospel in the New Testament. See also Maleko.
Marc, Marek, Marian, Mariano, Marke, Markee, Markel, Markell, Markey, Marko, Markos, Márkus, Markusha, Marque, Martial, Marx

Markanthony (Italian) a combination of Mark + Anthony.

Marke (Polish) a form of Mark.

Markel, Markell (Latin) forms of Mark.
Markelle, Markelo

Markes (Portuguese) a form of Marques.
Markess, Markest

Markese (French) a form of Marquis.
Markease, Markeece, Markees, Markeese, Markei, Markeice, Markeis, Markeise, Markes, Markez, Markeze, Markice

Markham (English) homestead on the boundary.

Markis (French) a form of Marquis.
Markies, Markiese, Markise, Markiss, Markist

Marko (Latin) a form of Marco, Mark.
Markco

Markus (Latin) a form of Marcus.
Markas, Markcus, Markcuss, Markys, Marqus

Marland (English) lake land.

Marley (English) lake meadow.
Marlea, Marleigh, Marly, Marrley

Marlin (English) deep-sea fish.
Marlen, Marlion, Marlyn

Marlon (French) a form of Merlin.

Marlow (English) hill by the lake.
Mar, Marlo, Marlowe

Marmion (French) small.
Marmyon

Marnin (Hebrew) singer; bringer of joy.

Maro (Japanese) myself.

Marquan (American) a combination of Mark + Quan.
Marquane, Marquante

Marquel (American) a form of Marcellus.
Marqueal, Marquelis, Marquell, Marquelle, Marquellis, Marquiel, Marquil, Marquiles, Marquill, Marquille, Marquillus, Marqwel, Marqwell

Marques (Portuguese) nobleman.
Markes, Markqes, Markques, Markquese, Marqese, Marqesse, Marqez, Marqeze, Marquees, Marquese, Marquess, Marquesse, Marquest, Markqueus, Marquez, Marqus

Marquez (Portuguese) a form of Marques.
Marqueze, Marquiez

Marquice (American) a form of Marquis.
Marquaice, Marquece

Marquis, Marquise (French) nobleman.
Marcquis, Marcuis, Markis,

Markquis, Markquise, Markuis,
Marqise, Marquee, Marqui,
Marquice, Marquie, Marquies,
Marquiss, Marquist, Marquiz,
Marquize

Marquon (American) a com-
bination of Mark + Quon.
Marquin, Marquinn, Marqwan,
Marqwon, Marqwyn

Marr (Spanish) divine. (Arabic)
forbidden.

Mars (Latin) bold warrior.
Mythology: the Roman god
of war.

Marsalis (Italian) a form of
Marcellus.
Marsalius, Marsallis, Marsellis,
Marsellius, Marsellus

Marsden (English) marsh valley.
Marsdon

Marsh (English) swamp land.
(French) a short form of
Marshall.

Marshal (French) a form of
Marshall.
Marschal, Marshel

Marshall (French) caretaker of
the horses; military title.
Marsh, Marshal, Marshell

Marshawn (American) a com-
bination of Mark + Shawn.
Marshaine, Marshaun,
Marshauwn, Marshean,
Marshon, Marshun

Marston (English) town by
the marsh.

Martell (English) hammerer.
Martel, Martele, Martellis

Marten (Dutch) a form of
Martin.
Maarten, Martein

Martez (Spanish) a form of
Martin.
Martaz, Martaze, Martes,
Martese, Marteze, Martice,
Martiece, Marties, Martiese,
Martiez, Martis, Martise,
Martize

Marti (Spanish) a form of
Martin.
Martee, Martie

Martial (French) a form of
Mark.

Martin (Latin, French) a form
of Martinus. History: Martin
Luther King, Jr. led the Civil
Rights movement and won
the Nobel Peace Prize. See
also Tynek.
Maartin, Mairtin, Marciano,
Marcin, Marinos, Marius, Mart,
Martan, Marten, Martez,
Marti, Martijn, Martinas,
Martine, Martinez, Martinho,
Martiniano, Martinien,
Martinka, Martino, Martins,
Marto, Marton, Márton, Marts,
Marty, Martyn, Mattin, Mertin,
Morten, Moss

Martinez (Spanish) a form of
Martin.
Martines

Martinho (Portuguese) a form
of Martin.

Martino (Italian) a form of
Martin.
Martinos

Martins (Latvian) a form of
Martin.

Martinus (Latin) martial, warlike.
Martin

Marty (Latin) a familiar form
of Martin.
Martey, Marti, Martie

Marut (Hindi) Religion: the
Hindu god of the wind.

Marv (English) a short form of
Marvin.
Marve, Marvi, Marvis

Marvin (English) lover of the
sea.
*Marv, Marvein, Marven,
Marvion, Marvn, Marvon,
Marvyn, Marwin, Marwynn,
Mervin*

Marwan (Arabic) history per-
sonage.

Marwood (English) forest
pond.

Masaccio (Italian) twin.
Masaki

Masahiro (Japanese) broad-
minded.

Masamba (Yao) leaves.

Masao (Japanese) righteous.

Masato (Japanese) just.

Mashama (Shona) surprising.

Maska (Native American)
powerful. (Russian) mask.

Maslin (French) little Thomas.
Maslen, Masling

Mason (French) stone worker.
*Mace, Maison, Masson, Masun,
Masyn, Sonny*

Masou (Native American) fire
god.

Massey (English) twin.
Massi

Massimo (Italian) greatest.
Massimiliano

Masud (Arabic, Swahili) fortunate.
Masood, Masoud, Mhasood

Matai (Basque, Bulgarian) a
form of Matthew.
Máté, Matei

Matalino (Filipino) bright.

Mateo (Spanish) a form of
Matthew.
Matías, Matteo

Mateusz (Polish) a form of
Matthew.
Matejs, Mateus

Mathe (German) a short form of Matthew.

Mather (English) powerful army.

Matheu (German) a form of Matthew.
Matheau, Matheus, Mathu

Mathew (Hebrew) a form of Matthew.

Mathias, Matthias (German, Swedish) forms of Matthew.
Maitias, Mathi, Mathia, Mathis, Matías, Matthia, Matthieus, Mattia, Mattias, Matus

Mathieu, Matthieu (French) forms of Matthew.
Mathie, Mathieux, Mathiew, Matthiew, Mattieu, Mattieux

Matías (Spanish) a form of Mathias.
Mattias

Mato (Native American) brave.

Matope (Rhodesian) our last child.

Matoskah (Lakota) white bear.

Mats (Swedish) a familiar form of Matthew.
Matts, Matz

Matson (Hebrew) son of Matt.
Matison, Matsen, Mattison, Mattson

Matt (Hebrew) a short form of Matthew.
Mat

Matteen (Afghan) disciplined; polite.

Matteus (Scandinavian) a form of Matthew.

Matthew (Hebrew) gift of God. Bible: author of the first Gospel of the New Testament.
Mads, Makaio, Maitiú, Mata, Matai, Matek, Mateo, Mateusz, Matfei, Mathe, Matheson, Matheu, Mathew, Mathian, Mathias, Mathieson, Mathieu, Matro, Mats, Matt, Matteus, Matthaeus, Matthaios, Matthaus, Matthäus, Mattheus, Matthews, Mattmias, Matty, Matvey, Matyas, Mayhew

Matty (Hebrew) a familiar form of Matthew.
Mattie

Matus (Czech) a form of Mathias.

Matvey (Russian) a form of Matthew.
Matviy, Matviyko, Matyash, Motka, Motya

Matyas (Polish) a form of Matthew.
Mátyás

Mauli (Hawaiian) a form of Maurice.

Maurice (Latin) dark skinned; moor; marshland. See also Seymour.
Mauli, Maur, Maurance, Maureo, Mauricio, Maurids, Mauriece, Maurikas, Maurin, Maurino, Maurise, Mauritz, Maurius, Maurizio, Mauro, Maurrel, Maurtel, Maury, Maurycy, Meurig, Moore, Morice, Moritz, Morrel, Morrice, Morrie, Morrill, Morris

Mauricio (Spanish) a form of Maurice.
Mauriccio, Mauriceo, Maurico, Maurisio

Mauritz (German) a form of Maurice.

Maurizio (Italian) a form of Maurice.

Mauro (Latin) a short form of Maurice.
Maur, Maurio

Maury (Latin) a familiar form of Maurice.
Maurey, Maurie, Morrie

Maverick (American) independent.
Maverik, Maveryke, Mavric, Mavrick

Mawuli (Ewe) there is a God.

Max (Latin) a short form of Maximilian, Maxwell.
Mac, Mack, Maks, Maxe, Maxx, Maxy, Miksa

Maxfield (English) Mack's field.

Maxi (Czech, Hungarian, Spanish) a familiar form of Maximilian, Máximo.
Makszi, Maxey, Maxie, Maxis, Maxy

Maxim (Russian) a form of Maxime.

Maxime (French) most excellent.
Maxim, Maxyme

Maximilian (Latin) greatest.
Mac, Mack, Maixim, Maksim, Maksym, Max, Maxamillion, Maxemilian, Maxemilion, Maxi, Maximalian, Maximili, Maximilia, Maximiliano, Maximilianus, Maximilien, Maximillian, Máximo, Maximos, Maxmilian, Maxmillion, Maxon, Maxymilian, Maxymillian, Mayhew, Miksa

Maximiliano (Italian) a form of Maximilian.
Massimiliano, Maximiano, Maximino

Maximillian (Latin) a form of Maximilian.
Maximillan, Maximillano, Maximillien, Maximillion, Maxmillian, Maxximillian, Maxximillion

Máximo (Spanish) a form of Maximilian.
Massimo, Maxi, Maximiano,

Maximiliano, Maximino, Máximo

Maximos (Greek) a form of Maximilian.

Maxwell (English) great spring.
Max, Maxwel, Maxwill, Maxxwell, Maxy

Maxy (English) a familiar form of Max, Maxwell.
Maxi

Mayer (Hebrew) a form of Meir. (Latin) a form of Magnus, Major.
Mahyar, Mayeer, Mayor, Mayur

Mayes (English) field.
Mayo, Mays

Mayhew (English) a form of Matthew.

Maynard (English) powerful; brave. See also Meinhard.
May, Mayne, Maynhard, Maynor, Ménard

Mayo (Irish) yew-tree plain. (English) a form of Mayes. Geography: a county in Ireland.

Mayon (Indian) person of black complexion. Religion: another name for the Indian god Mal.

Mayonga (Luganda) lake sailor.

Mazi (Ibo) sir.
Mazzi

Mazin (Arabic) proper.
Mazen, Mazinn, Mazzin

Mbita (Swahili) born on a cold night.

Mbwana (Swahili) master.

McGeorge (Scottish) son of George.
MacGeorge

Mckade (Scottish) son of Kade.
Mccade

Mckay (Scottish) son of Kay.
Mackay, MacKay, Mckae, Mckai, McKay

McKenzie (Irish) a form of Mackenzie.
Mccenzie, Mckennzie, Mckensey, Mckensie, Mckenson, Mckensson, Mckenzi, Mckenzy, Mckinzie

Mckinley (Irish) a form of Mackinnley.
Mckinely, Mckinnely, Mckinnlee, Mckinnley, McKinnley

Mead (English) meadow.
Meade, Meed

Medgar (German) a form of Edgar.

Medwin (German) faithful friend.

Mehetabel (Hebrew) who God benefits.

Mehrdad (Persian) gift of the sun.

Mehtar (Sanskrit) prince.
Mehta

Meinhard (German) strong, firm. See also Maynard.
Meinhardt, Meinke, Meino, Mendar

Meinrad (German) strong counsel.

Meir (Hebrew) one who brightens, shines; enlightener. History: Golda Meir was the prime minister of Israel.
Mayer, Meyer, Muki, Myer

Meka (Hawaiian) eyes.

Mel (English, Irish) a familiar form of Melvin.

Melbourne (English) mill stream.
Melborn, Melburn, Melby, Milborn, Milbourn, Milbourne, Milburn, Millburn, Millburne

Melchior (Hebrew) king.
Meilseoir, Melchor, Melker, Melkior

Meldon (English) mill hill.
Melden

Melrone (Irish) servant of Saint Ruadhan.

Melvern (Native American) great chief.

Melville (French) mill town. Literature: Herman Melville was a well-known nineteenth-century American writer.
Milville

Melvin (Irish) armored chief. (English) mill friend; council friend. See also Vinny.
Malvin, Mel, Melvino, Melvon, Melvyn, Melwin, Melwyn, Melwynn

Menachem (Hebrew) comforter.
Menahem, Nachman

Menassah (Hebrew) cause to forget.
Menashe, Menashi, Menashia, Menashiah, Menashya, Manasseh

Mendel (English) repairman.
Mendeley, Mendell, Mendie, Mendy

Mengesha (Ethiopian) kingdom.

Menico (Spanish) a short form of Domenico.

Mensah (Ewe) third son.

Menz (German) a short form of Clement.

Mercer (English) storekeeper.
Merce

Mered (Hebrew) revolter.

Meredith (Welsh) guardian from the sea.
Meredyth, Merideth, Meridith, Merry

Merion (Welsh) from Merion,
Wales.
Merrion

Merle (French) a short form
of Merlin, Merrill.
Meryl

Merlin (English) falcon.
Literature: the magician who
served as counselor in King
Arthur's court.
*Marlon, Merle, Merlen,
Merlinn, Merlyn, Merlynn*

Merrick (English) ruler of the
sea.
*Merek, Meric, Merick, Merik,
Merric, Merrik, Meryk,
Meyrick, Myrucj*

Merrill (Irish) bright sea.
(French) famous.
*Meril, Merill, Merle, Merrel,
Merrell, Merril, Meryl*

Merritt (Latin, Irish) valuable;
deserving.
Merit, Meritt, Merrett

Merton (English) sea town.
Murton

Merv (Irish) a short form of
Mervin.

Merville (French) sea village.

Mervin (Irish) a form of
Marvin.
*Merv, Mervyn, Mervynn,
Merwin, Merwinn, Merwyn,
Murvin, Murvyn, Myrvyn,
Myrvynn, Myrwyn*

Meshach (Hebrew) artist.
Bible: one of Daniel's three
friends who emerged
unharmed from the fiery
furnace of Babylon.

Mesut (Turkish) happy.

Metikla (Moquelumnan)
reaching a hand underwater
to catch a fish.

Mette (Greek, Danish) pearl.
Almeta, Mete

Meurig (Welsh) a form of
Maurice.

Meyer (German) farmer.
Mayer, Meier, Myer

Mhina (Swahili) delightful.

Micah (Hebrew) a form of
Michael. Bible: a Hebrew
prophet.
*Mic, Micaiah, Michiah, Mika,
Mikah, Myca, Mycah*

Micha (Hebrew) a short form
of Michael.
Mica, Micha, Michah

Michael (Hebrew) who is like
God? See also Micah,
Miguel, Mika, Miles.
*Machael, Machas, Mahail,
Maichail, Maikal, Makael,
Makal, Makel, Makell, Makis,
Meikel, Mekal, Mekhail,
Mhichael, Micael, Micah,
Micahel, Mical, Micha,
Michaele, Michaell, Michail,
Michak, Michal, Michale,*

Michael *(cont.)*
*Michalek, Michalel, Michau,
Micheal, Micheil, Michel,
Michele, Michelet, Michiel,
Micho, Michoel, Mick, Mickael,
Mickey, Mihail, Mihalje,
Mihkel, Mika, Mikael, Mikáele,
Mikal, Mike, Mikeal, Mikel,
Mikelis, Mikell, Mikhail,
Mikkel, Mikko, Miksa, Milko,
Miquel, Misael, Misi, Miska,
Mitchell, Mychael, Mychajlo,
Mychal, Mykal, Mykhas*

Michail (Russian) a form of
Michael.
Mihas, Mikail, Mikale, Misha

Michal (Polish) a form of
Michael.
Michak, Michalek, Michall

Micheal (Irish) a form of
Michael.

Michel (French) a form of
Michael.
*Michaud, Miche, Michee,
Michell, Michelle, Michon*

Michelangelo (Italian) a com-
bination of Michael +
Angelo. Art: Michelangelo
Buonarroti was one of the
greatest Renaissance painters.
Michelange, Miguelangelo

Michele (Italian) a form of
Michael.

Michio (Japanese) man with
the strength of three thousand.

Mick (English) a short form of
Michael, Mickey.
Mickerson

Mickael (English) a form of
Michael.
*Mickaele, Mickal, Mickale,
Mickeal, Mickel, Mickell,
Mickelle, Mickle*

Mickenzie (Irish) a form of
Mackenzie.
Mickenze, Mickenzy, Mikenzie

Mickey (Irish) a familiar form
of Michael.
*Mick, Micki, Mickie, Micky,
Miki, Mique*

Micu (Hungarian) a form of
Nick.

Miguel (Portuguese, Spanish) a
form of Michael.
Migeel, Migel, Miguelly, Migui

Miguelangel (Spanish) a combination of Miguel + Angel.

Mihail (Greek, Bulgarian,
Romanian) a form of
Michael.
Mihailo, Mihal, Mihalis, Mikail

Mika (Ponca) raccoon.
(Hebrew) a form of Micah.
(Russian) a familiar form of
Michael.
Miika, Mikah

Mikael (Swedish) a form of
Michael.
Mikaeel, Mikaele

Mikáele (Hawaiian) a form of Michael.
Mikele

Mikal (Hebrew) a form of Michael.
Mekal, Mikahl, Mikale

Mikasi (Omaha) coyote.

Mike (Hebrew) a short form of Michael.
Mikey, Myk

Mikeal (Irish) a form of Michael.

Mikel (Basque) a form of Michael.
Mekel, Mikele, Mekell, Mikell, Mikelle

Mikelis (Latvian) a form of Michael.
Mikus, Milkins

Mikhail (Greek, Russian) a form of Michael.
Mekhail, Mihály, Mikhael, Mikhale, Mikhalis, Mikhalka, Mikhall, Mikhel, Mikhial, Mikhos

Miki (Japanese) tree.
Mikio

Mikkel (Norwegian) a form of Michael.
Mikkael, Mikle

Mikko (Finnish) a form of Michael.
Mikk, Mikka, Mikkohl, Mikkol, Miko, Mikol

Mikolaj (Polish) a form of Nicholas.
Mikolai

Mikolas (Greek) a form of Nicholas.
Miklós, Milek

Miksa (Hungarian) a form of Max.
Miks

Milan (Italian) northerner. Geography: a city in northern Italy.
Milaan, Milano, Milen, Millan, Millen, Mylan, Mylen, Mylon, Mylynn

Milap (Native American) giving.

Milborough (English) middle borough.
Milbrough

Milek (Polish) a familiar form of Nicholas.

Miles (Greek) millstone. (Latin) soldier. (German) merciful. (English) a short form of Michael.
Milas, Milles, Milo, Milson, Myles

Milford (English) mill by the ford.

Mililani (Hawaiian) heavenly caress.

Milko (Czech) a form of Michael. (German) a familiar form of Emil.
Milkins

Millard (Latin) caretaker of the mill.
Mill, Millar, Miller, Millward, Milward, Myller

Miller (English) miller; grain grinder.
Mellar, Millard, Millen

Mills (English) mills.

Milo (German) a form of Miles. A familiar form of Emil.
Millo, Mylo

Milos (Greek, Slavic) pleasant.

Miloslav (Czech) lover of glory.
Milda

Milt (English) a short form of Milton.

Milton (English) mill town.
Milt, Miltie, Milty, Mylton

Mimis (Greek) a familiar form of Demetrius.

Min (Burmese) king.
Mina

Mincho (Spanish) a form of Benjamin.

Minel (Spanish) a form of Manuel.

Miner (English) miner.

Mingan (Native American) gray wolf.

Mingo (Spanish) a short form of Domingo.

Minh (Vietnamese) bright.
Minhao, Minhduc, Minhkhan, Minhtong, Minhy

Minkah (Akan) just, fair.

Minor (Latin) junior; younger.
Mynor

Minoru (Japanese) fruitful.

Mique (Spanish) a form of Mickey.
Mequel, Mequelin, Miquel

Miron (Polish) peace.

Miroslav (Czech) peace; glory.
Mirek, Miroslaw, Miroslawy

Mirwais (Afghan) noble ruler.

Misael (Hebrew) a form of Michael.
Mischael, Mishael, Missael

Misha (Russian) a short form of Michail.
Misa, Mischa, Mishael, Mishal, Mishe, Mishenka, Mishka

Miska (Hungarian) a form of Michael.
Misi, Misik, Misko, Miso

Mister (English) mister.
Mistur

Misu (Moquelumnan) rippling water.

Mitch (English) a short form of Mitchell.

Mitchel (English) a form of Mitchell.
Mitchael, Mitchal, Mitcheal, Mitchele, Mitchil, Mytchel

Mitchell (English) a form of Michael.
Mitch, Mitchall, Mitchel, Mitchelle, Mitchem, Mytch, Mytchell

Mitsos (Greek) a familiar form of Demetrius.

Modesto (Latin) modest.

Moe (English) a short form of Moses.
Mo

Mogens (Dutch) powerful.
*Mohamad (Arabic) a form of Muhammad.
Mohamid*

Mohamed (Arabic) a form of Muhammad.
Mohamd, Mohameed

Mohamet (Arabic) a form of Muhammad.
Mahomet, Mehemet, Mehmet

Mohammad (Arabic) a form of Muhammad.
Mahammad, Mohammadi, Mohammd, Mohammid, Mohanad, Mohmad

Mohammed (Arabic) a form of Muhammad.
Mahammed, Mahomet,
Mohammad, Mohaned, Mouhamed, Muhammad

Mohamud (Arabic) a form of Muhammad.
Mohammud, Mohamoud

Mohan (Hindi) delightful.

Moises (Portuguese, Spanish) a form of Moses.
Moices, Moise, Moisés, Moisey, Moisis

Moishe (Yiddish) a form of Moses.
Moshe

Mojag (Native American) crying baby.

Molimo (Moquelumnan) bear going under shady trees.

Momuso (Moquelumnan) yellow jackets crowded in their nests for the winter.

Mona (Moquelumnan) gathering jimsonweed seed.

Monahan (Irish) monk.
Monaghan, Monoghan

Mongo (Yoruba) famous.

Monroe (Irish) Geography: the mouth of the Roe River.
Monro, Munro, Munroe

Montague (French) pointed mountain.
Montagne, Montagu, Monte

Montana (Spanish) mountain.
Geography: a U.S. state.
Montaine, Montanna

Montaro (Japanese) big boy.
Montario, Monterio, Montero

Monte (Spanish) a short form
of Montgomery.
*Montae, Montaé, Montay,
Montea, Montee, Monti,
Montoya, Monty*

Montel (American) a form of
Montreal.
Montele, Montell, Montelle

Montez (Spanish) dweller in
the mountains.
*Monteiz, Monteze, Montezz,
Montisze*

Montgomery (English) rich
man's mountain.
Monte, Montgomerie, Monty

Montre (French) show.
*Montra, Montrae, Montray,
Montraz, Montres, Montrey,
Montrez, Montreze*

Montreal (French) royal
mountain. Geography: a city
in Quebec.
*Montel, Monterial, Monterrell,
Montrail, Montrale, Montrall,
Montreall, Montrell, Montrial*

Montrell (French) a form of
Montreal.
*Montral, Montrel, Montrele,
Montrelle*

Montsho (Tswana) black.

Monty (English) a familiar
form of Montgomery.

Moore (French) dark; moor;
marshland.
Moor, Mooro, More

Mordecai (Hebrew) martial,
warlike. Mythology: Marduk
was the Babylonian god of
war. Bible: wise counselor to
Queen Esther.
*Mord, Mordachai, Mordechai,
Mordie, Mordy, Mort*

Mordred (Latin) painful.
Literature: the bastard son of
King Arthur.
Modred

Morel (French) an edible
mushroom.
Morrel

Moreland (English) moor;
marshland.
Moorland, Morland

Morell (French) dark; from
Morocco.
*Moor, Moore, Morelle, Morelli,
Morill, Morrell, Morrill, Murrel,
Murrell*

Morey (Greek) a familiar form
of Moris. (Latin) a form of
Morrie.
Morrey, Morry

Morgan (Scottish) sea warrior.
*Morgen, Morghan, Morgin,
Morgon, Morgun, Morgunn,
Morgwn, Morgyn, Morrgan*

Morio (Japanese) forest.

Moris (Greek) son of the dark one. (English) a form of Morris.
Morey, Morisz, Moriz

Moritz (German) a form of Maurice, Morris.
Morisz

Morley (English) meadow by the moor.
Moorley, Moorly, Morlee, Morleigh, Morlon, Morly, Morlyn, Morrley

Morrie (Latin) a familiar form of Maurice, Morse.
Maury, Morey, Mori, Morie, Morry, Mory, Morye

Morris (Latin) dark skinned; moor; marshland. (English) a form of Maurice.
Moris, Moriss, Moritz, Morrese, Morrise, Morriss, Morry, Moss

Morse (English) son of Maurice.
Morresse, Morrie, Morrison, Morrisson

Mort (French, English) a short form of Morten, Mortimer, Morton.
Morte, Mortey, Mortie, Mortty, Morty

Morten (Norwegian) a form of Martin.
Mort

Mortimer (French) still water.
Mort, Mortymer

Morton (English) town near the moor.
Mort

Morven (Scottish) mariner.
Morvien, Morvin

Mose (Hebrew) a short form of Moses.

Moses (Hebrew) drawn out of the water. (Egyptian) son, child. Bible: the Hebrew law-giver who brought the Ten Commandments down from Mount Sinai.
Moe, Moise, Moïse, Moisei, Moises, Moishe, Mose, Mosese, Moshe, Mosiah, Mosie, Moss, Mosses, Mosya, Mosze, Moszek, Mousa, Moyses, Moze

Moshe (Hebrew, Polish) a form of Moses.
Mosheh

Mosi (Swahili) first-born.

Moss (Irish) a short form of Maurice, Morris. (English) a short form of Moses.

Moswen (African) light in color.

Motega (Native American) new arrow.

Mouhamed (Arabic) a form of Muhammad.
Mouhamad, Mouhamadou, Mouhammed, Mouhamoin

Mousa (Arabic) a form of
Moses.
Moussa

Moze (Lithuanian) a form of
Moses.
Mozes, Mózes

Mpasa (Nguni) mat.

Mposi (Nyakyusa) blacksmith.

Mpoza (Luganda) tax collector.

Msrah (Akan) sixth-born.

Mtima (Nguni) heart.

Muata (Moquelumnan) yellow jackets in their nest.

Mugamba (Runyoro) talks
too much.

Mugisa (Rutooro) lucky.
Mugisha, Mukisa

Muhammad (Arabic) praised.
History: the founder of the
Islamic religion. See also
Ahmad, Hamid,Yasin.
*Mahmoud, Mahmúd,
Mohamad, Mohamed,
Mohamet, Mohamud,
Mohammed, Mouhamed,
Muhamad, Muhamed,
Muhamet, Muhammadali,
Muhammed*

Muhannad (Arabic) sword.
Muhanad

Muhsin (Arabic) beneficent;
charitable.

Muhtadi (Arabic) rightly
guided.

Muir (Scottish) moor; marshland.

Mujahid (Arabic) fighter in
the way of Allah.

Mukasa (Luganda) God's chief
administrator.

Mukhtar (Arabic) chosen.
Mukhtaar

Mukul (Sanskrit) bud, blossom;
soul.

Mulogo (Musoga) wizard.

Mundan (Rhodesian) garden.

Mundo (Spanish) a short form
of Edmundo.

Mundy (Irish) from
Reamonn.

Mungo (Scottish) amiable.

Mun-Hee (Korean) literate;
shiny.

Munir (Arabic) brilliant; shining.

Munny (Cambodian) wise.

Muraco (Native American)
white moon.

Murali (Hindi) flute. Religion:
the instrument the Hindu
god Krishna is usually
depicted as playing.

Murat (Turkish) wish come
true.

Murdock (Scottish) wealthy sailor.
Murdo, Murdoch, Murtagh

Murphy (Irish) sea warrior.
Murfey, Murfy

Murray (Scottish) sailor.
Macmurray, Moray, Murrey, Murry

Murtagh (Irish) a form of Murdock.
Murtaugh

Musa (Swahili) child.

Musád (Arabic) untied camel.

Musoke (Rukonjo) born while a rainbow was in the sky.

Mustafa (Arabic) chosen; royal.
Mostafa, Mostaffa, Moustafa, Mustafaa, Mustafah, Mustafe, Mustaffa, Mustafo, Mustapha, Mustoffa, Mustofo

Mustapha (Arabic) a form of Mustafa.
Mostapha, Moustapha

Muti (Arabic) obedient.

Mwaka (Luganda) born on New Year's Eve.

Mwamba (Nyakyusa) strong.

Mwanje (Luganda) leopard.

Mwinyi (Swahili) king.

Mwita (Swahili) summoner.

Mychajlo (Latvian) a form of Michael.
Mykhaltso, Mykhas

Mychal (American) a form of Michael.
Mychall, Mychalo, Mycheal

Myer (English) a form of Meir.
Myers, Myur

Mykal, Mykel (American) forms of Michael.
Mykael, Mikele, Mykell

Myles (Latin) soldier. (German) a form of Miles.
Myels, Mylez, Mylles, Mylz

Mynor (Latin) a form of Minor.

Myo (Burmese) city.

Myron (Greek) fragrant ointment.
Mehran, Mehrayan, My, Myran, Myrone, Ron

Myung-Dae (Korean) right; great.

Mzuzi (Swahili) inventive.

N

Naaman (Hebrew) pleasant.

Nabiha (Arabic) intelligent.

Nabil (Arabic) noble.
Nabeel, Nabiel

Nachman (Hebrew) a short form of Menachem.
Nachum, Nahum

Nada (Arabic) generous.

Nadav (Hebrew) generous; noble.
Nadiv

Nadidah (Arabic) equal to anyone else.

Nadim (Arabic) friend.
Nadeem

Nadir (Afghan, Arabic) dear, rare.
Nader

Nadisu (Hindi) beautiful river.

Naeem (Arabic) benevolent.
Naem, Naim, Naiym, Nieem

Naftali (Hebrew) wreath.
Naftalie

Nagid (Hebrew) ruler; prince.

Nahele (Hawaiian) forest.

Nahma (Native American) sturgeon.

Nailah (Arabic) successful.

Nairn (Scottish) river with alder trees.
Nairne

Najee (Arabic) a form of Naji.
Najae, Najée, Najei, Najiee

Naji (Arabic) safe.
Najee, Najih

Najíb (Arabic) born to nobility.
Najib, Nejeeb

Najji (Muganda) second child.

Nakia (Arabic) pure.
Nakai, Nakee, Nakeia, Naki, Nakiah, Nakii

Nakos (Arapaho) sage, wise.

Naldo (Spanish) a familiar form of Reginald.

Nalren (Dene) thawed out.

Nam (Vietnamese) scrape off.

Namaka (Hawaiian) eyes.

Namid (Ojibwa) star dancer.

Namir (Hebrew) leopard.
Namer

Nandin (Hindi) Religion: a servant of the Hindu god Shiva.
Nandan

Nando (German) a familiar form of Ferdinand.
Nandor

Nangila (Abaluhya) born while parents traveled.

Nangwaya (Mwera) don't mess with me.

Nansen (Swedish) son of Nancy.

Nantai (Navajo) chief.

Nantan (Apache) spokesman.

Naoko (Japanese) straight, honest.

Napayshni (Lakota) he does not flee; courageous.

Napier (Spanish) new city.
Neper

Napoleon (Greek) lion of the woodland. (Italian) from Naples, Italy. History: Napoleon Bonaparte was a famous nineteenth-century French emperor.
Leon, Nap, Napolean, Napoléon, Napoleone, Nappie, Nappy

Naquan (American) a combination of the prefix Na + Quan.
Naqawn, Naquain, Naquen, Naquon

Narain (Hindi) protector. Religion: another name for the Hindu god Vishnu.
Narayan

Narcisse (French) a form of Narcissus.
Narcis, Narciso, Narkis, Narkissos

Narcissus (Greek) daffodil. Mythology: the youth who fell in love with his own reflection.
Narcisse

Nard (Persian) chess player.

Nardo (German) strong, hardy. (Spanish) a short form of Bernardo.

Narve (Dutch) healthy, strong.

Nashashuk (Fox, Sauk) loud thunder.

Nashoba (Choctaw) wolf.

Nasim (Persian) breeze; fresh air.
Naseem, Nassim

Nasser (Arabic) victorious.
Naseer, Naser, Nasier, Nasir, Nasr, Nassir, Nassor

Nat (English) a short form of Nathan, Nathaniel.
Natt, Natty

Natal (Spanish) a form of Noël.
Natale, Natalie, Natalino, Natalio, Nataly

Natan (Hebrew, Hungarian, Polish, Russian, Spanish) God has given.
Naten

Natanael (Hebrew) a form of Nathaniel.
Natanel, Nataniel

Nate (Hebrew) a short form of Nathan, Nathaniel.

Natesh (Hindi) destroyer. Religion: another name for the Hindu god Shiva.

Nathan (Hebrew) a short form of Nathaniel. Bible: a prophet during the reigns of David and Solomon.
Naethan, Nat, Nate, Nathann, Nathean, Nathen, Nathian, Nathin, Nathon, Nathyn, Natthan, Naythan, Nethan

Nathanael (Hebrew) gift of God. Bible: one of the Twelve Apostles. Also known as Bartholomew.
Nathanae, Nathanal, Nathaneal, Nathaneil, Nathanel, Nathaneol

Nathanial (Hebrew) a form of Nathaniel.
Nathanyal, Nathanual

Nathanie (Hebrew) a familiar form of Nathaniel.
Nathania, Nathanni

Nathaniel (Hebrew) gift of God. Bible: one of the Twelve Apostles.
Nat, Natanael, Nate, Nathan, Nathanael, Nathanial, Nathanie, Nathanielle, Nathanil, Nathanile, Nathanuel, Nathanyel, Nathanyl, Natheal, Nathel, Nathinel, Nethaniel, Thaniel

Nathen (Hebrew) a form of Nathan.

Nav (Gypsy) name.

Navarro (Spanish) plains.
Navarre

Navdeep (Sikh) new light.
Navdip

Navin (Hindi) new, novel.
Naveen, Naven

Nawat (Native American) left-handed.

Nawkaw (Winnebago) wood.

Nayati (Native American) wrestler.

Nayland (English) island dweller.

Nazareth (Hebrew) born in Nazareth, Israel.
Nazaire, Nazaret, Nazarie, Nazario, Nazerene, Nazerine

Nazih (Arabic) pure, chaste.
Nazeeh, Nazeem, Nazeer, Nazieh, Nazim, Nazir, Nazz

Ndale (Nguni) trick.

Neal (Irish) a form of Neil.
Neale, Neall, Nealle, Nealon, Nealy

Neci (Latin) a familiar form of Ignatius.

Nectarios (Greek) saint. Religion: a saint in the Greek Orthodox Church.

Ned (English) a familiar form of Edward, Edwin.
Neddie, Neddym, Nedrick

Nehemiah (Hebrew) compassion of Jehovah. Bible: a Jewish leader.
Nahemiah, Nechemya, Nehemias, Nehemie, Nehemyah, Nehimiah, Nehmia, Nehmiah, Nemo, Neyamia

Nehru (Hindi) canal.

Neil (Irish) champion.
Neal, Neel, Neihl, Neile, Neill, Neille, Nels, Niall, Niele, Niels, Nigel, Nil, Niles, Nilo, Nils, Nyle

Neka (Native American) wild goose.

Nelek (Polish) a form of Cornelius.

Nellie (English) a familiar form of Cornelius, Cornell, Nelson.
Nell, Nelly

Nelius (Latin) a short form of Cornelius.

Nelo (Spanish) a form of Daniel.
Nello, Nilo

Nels (Scandinavian) a form of Neil, Nelson.
Nelse, Nelson, Nils

Nelson (English) son of Neil.
Nealson, Neilsen, Neilson, Nellie, Nels, Nelsen, Nilson, Nilsson

Nemesio (Spanish) just.
Nemi

Nemo (Greek) glen, glade. (Hebrew) a short form of Nehemiah.

Nen (Egyptian) ancient waters.

Neptune (Latin) sea ruler. Mythology: the Roman god of the sea.

Nero (Latin, Spanish) stern. History: a cruel Roman emperor.
Neron, Nerone, Nerron

Nesbit (English) nose-shaped bend in a river.
Naisbit, Naisbitt, Nesbitt, Nisbet, Nisbett

Nestor (Greek) traveler; wise.
Nester

Nethaniel (Hebrew) a form of Nathaniel.
Netanel, Netania, Netaniah, Netaniel, Netanya, Nethanel, Nethanial, Nethaniel, Nethanyal, Nethanyel

Neto (Spanish) a short form of Ernesto.

Nevada (Spanish) covered in snow. Geography: a U.S. state.
Navada, Nevade

Nevan (Irish) holy.
Nevean

Neville (French) new town.
Nev, Nevil, Nevile, Nevill, Nevyle

Nevin (Irish) worshiper of the saint. (English) middle; herb.
Nefen, Nev, Nevan, Neven, Nevins, Nevyn, Niven

Newbold (English) new tree.

Newell (English) new hall.
Newall, Newel, Newyle

Newland (English) new land.
Newlan

Newlin (Welsh) new lake.
Newlyn

Newman (English) newcomer.
Neiman, Neimann, Neimon, Neuman, Numan, Numen

Newton (English) new town.
Newt

Ngai (Vietnamese) herb.

Nghia (Vietnamese) forever.

Ngozi (Ibo) blessing.

Ngu (Vietnamese) sleep.

Nguyen (Vietnamese) a form of Ngu.

Nhean (Cambodian) self-knowledge.

Niall (Irish) a form of Neil. History: Niall of the Nine Hostages was a famous Irish king.
Nial, Nialle

Nibal (Arabic) arrows.
Nibel

Nibaw (Native American) standing tall.

Nicabar (Gypsy) stealthy.

Nicho (Spanish) a form of Dennis.

Nicholas (Greek) victorious people. Religion: Nicholas of Myra is a patron saint of children. See also Caelan, Claus, Cola, Colar, Cole, Colin, Colson, Klaus, Lasse, Mikolaj, Mikolas, Milek.
Niccolas, Nichalas, Nichelas, Nichele, Nichlas, Nichlos, Nichola, Nicholaas, Nicholaes, Nicholase, Nicholaus, Nichole, Nicholias, Nicholl, Nichollas, Nicholos, Nichols, Nicholus, Nick, Nickalus, Nicklaus, Nickolas, Nicky, Niclas, Niclasse, Nico, Nicola, Nicolai, Nicolas, Nicoles, Nicolis, Nicoll, Nicolo, Nikhil, Niki, Nikili, Nikita, Nikko, Niklas, Niko, Nikolai, Nikolas, Nikolaus, Nikolos, Nils, Nioclás, Niocol, Nycholas

Nicholaus (Greek) a form of Nicholas.
Nichalaus, Nichalous, Nichaolas, Nichlaus, Nichloas, Nichlous, Nicholaos, Nicholous

Nichols, Nicholson (English) son of Nicholas.
Nicholes, Nicholis, Nicolls, Nickelson, Nickoles

Nick (English) a short form of Dominic, Nicholas. See also Micu.
Nic, Nik

Nickalus (Greek) a form of Nicholas.
Nickalas, Nickalis, Nickalos, Nickelas, Nickelus

Nicklaus, Nicklas (Greek) forms of Nicholas.
Nickalaus, Nickalous, Nickelous, Nicklauss, Nicklos, Nicklous, Nicklus, Nickolau, Nickolaus, Nicolaus, Niklaus, Nikolaus

Nickolas (Greek) a form of Nicholas.
Nickolaos, Nickolis, Nickolos, Nickolus, Nickolys, Nickoulas

Nicky (Greek) a familiar form of Nicholas.
Nickey, Nicki, Nickie, Niki, Nikki

Nico (Greek) a short form of Nicholas.
Nicco

Nicodemus (Greek) conqueror of the people.
Nicodem, Nicodemius, Nikodem, Nikodema, Nikodemious, Nikodim

Nicola (Italian) a form of Nicholas. See also Cola.
Nicolá, Nikolah

Nicolai (Norwegian, Russian) a form of Nicholas.
Nicholai, Nickolai, Nicolaj,
Nicolau, Nicolay, Nicoly, Nikalai

Nicolas (Italian) a form of Nicholas.
Nico, Nicolaas, Nicolás, Nicolaus, Nicoles, Nicolis, Nicolus

Nicolo (Italian) a form of Nicholas.
Niccolo, Niccolò, Nicol, Nicolao, Nicollo

Niels (Danish) a form of Neil.
Niel, Nielsen, Nielson, Niles, Nils

Nien (Vietnamese) year.

Nigan (Native American) ahead.
Nigen

Nigel (Latin) dark night.
Niegel, Nigal, Nigale, Nigele, Nigell, Nigiel, Nigil, Nigle, Nijel, Nye, Nygel, Nyigel, Nyjil

Nika (Yoruba) ferocious.

Nike (Greek) victorious.
Nikka

Niki (Hungarian) a familiar form of Nicholas.
Nikia, Nikiah, Nikki, Nikkie, Nykei, Nykey

Nikita (Russian) a form of Nicholas.
Nakita, Nakitas, Nikula

Nikiti (Native American) round and smooth like an abalone shell.

Nikko, Niko (Hungarian) forms of Nicholas.
Nikoe, Nyko

Niklas (Latvian, Swedish) a form of Nicholas.
Niklaas, Niklaus

Nikola (Greek) a short form of Nicholas.
Nikolao, Nikolay, Nykola

Nikolai (Estonian, Russian) a form of Nicholas.
Kolya, Nikolais, Nikolaj, Nikolajs, Nikolay, Nikoli, Nikolia, Nikula, Nikulas

Nikolas (Greek) a form of Nicholas.
Nicanor, Nikalas, Nikalis, Nikalus, Nikholas, Nikolaas, Nikolaos, Nikolis, Nikolos, Nikos, Nilos, Nykolas, Nykolus

Nikolaus (Greek) a form of Nicholas.
Nikalous, Nikolaos

Nikolos (Greek) a form of Nicholas. See also Kolya.
Niklos, Nikolaos, Nikolò, Nikolous, Nikolus, Nikos, Nilos

Nil (Russian) a form of Neil.
Nilya

Nila (Hindi) blue.

Niles (English) son of Neil.
Nilesh, Nyles

Nilo (Finnish) a form of Neil.

Nils (Swedish) a short form of Nicholas.

Nimrod (Hebrew) rebel. Bible: a great-grandson of Noah.

Niño (Spanish) young child.

Niran (Tai) eternal.

Nishan (Armenian) cross, sign, mark.
Nishon

Nissan (Hebrew) sign, omen; miracle.
Nisan, Nissim, Nissin, Nisson

Nitis (Native American) friend.
Netis

Nixon (English) son of Nick.
Nixan, Nixson

Nizam (Arabic) leader.

Nkunda (Runyankore) loves those who hate him.

N'namdi (Ibo) his father's name lives on.

Noach (Hebrew) a form of Noah.

Noah (Hebrew) peaceful, restful. Bible: the patriarch who built the ark to survive the Flood.
Noach, Noak, Noe, Noé, Noi

Noam (Hebrew) sweet; friend.

Noble (Latin) born to nobility.
Nobe, Nobie, Noby

Nodin (Native American) wind.
Knoton, Noton

Noe (Czech, French) a form of Noah.

Noé (Hebrew, Spanish) quiet, peaceful. See also Noah.

Noël (French) day of Christ's birth. See also Natal.
Noel, Noél, Noell, Nole, Noli, Nowel, Nowell

Nohea (Hawaiian) handsome.
Noha, Nohe

Nokonyu (Native American) katydid's nose.
Noko, Nokoni

Nolan (Irish) famous; noble.
Noland, Nolande, Nolane, Nolen, Nolin, Nollan, Nolyn

Nollie (Latin, Scandinavian) a familiar form of Oliver.
Noll, Nolly

Norbert (Scandinavian) brilliant hero.
Bert, Norberto, Norbie, Norby

Norberto (Spanish) a form of Norbert.

Norman (French) Norseman. History: a name for the Scandinavians who settled in northern France in the tenth century, and who later conquered England in 1066.
Norm, Normand, Normen, Normie, Normy

Norris (French) northerner. (English) Norman's horse.
Norice, Norie, Noris, Norreys, Norrie, Norry, Norrys

Northcliff (English) northern cliff.
Northcliffe, Northclyff, Northclyffe

Northrop (English) north farm.
North, Northup

Norton (English) northern town.

Norville (French, English) northern town.
Norval, Norvel, Norvell, Norvil, Norvill, Norvylle

Norvin (English) northern friend.
Norvyn, Norwin, Norwinn, Norwyn, Norwynn

Norward (English) protector of the north.
Norwerd

Norwood (English) northern woods.

Notaku (Moquelumnan) growing bear.

Nowles (English) a short form of Knowles.

Nsoah (Akan) seventh-born.

Numa (Arabic) pleasant.

Numair (Arabic) panther.

Nuncio (Italian) messenger.
Nunzi, Nunzio

Nuri (Hebrew, Arabic) my fire.
*Nery, Noori, Nur, Nuris,
Nurism, Nury*

Nuriel (Hebrew, Arabic) fire of
the Lord.
Nuria, Nuriah, Nuriya

Nuru (Swahili) born in daylight.

Nusair (Arabic) bird of prey.

Nwa (Nigerian) son.

Nwake (Nigerian) born on
market day.

Nye (English) a familiar form
of Aneurin, Nigel.

Nyle (English) island. (Irish) a
form of Neil.
Nyal, Nyll

O

Oakes (English) oak trees.
Oak, Oakie, Oaks, Ochs

Oakley (English) oak-tree
field.
*Oak, Oakes, Oakie, Oaklee,
Oakleigh, Oakly, Oaks*

Oalo (Spanish) a form of Paul.

Oba (Yoruba) king.

Obadele (Yoruba) king arrives
at the house.

Obadiah (Hebrew) servant of
God.
*Obadias, Obed, Obediah, Obie,
Ovadiach, Ovadiah, Ovadya*

Obed (English) a short form
of Obadiah.

Oberon (German) noble;
bearlike. Literature: the king
of the fairies in the
Shakespearean play *A
Midsummer Night's Dream*.
See also Auberon, Aubrey.
Oberen, Oberron, Oeberon

Obert (German) wealthy;
bright.

Obie (English) a familiar form
of Obadiah.
Obbie, Obe, Obey, Obi, Oby

Ocan (Luo) hard times.

Octavio (Latin) eighth. See
also Tavey, Tavian.
*Octave, Octavia, Octavian,
Octaviano, Octavien, Octavious,
Octavius, Octavo, Octavous,
Octavus, Ottavio*

Octavious, Octavius (Latin)
forms of Octavio.
*Octavaius, Octaveous, Octaveus,
Octavias, Octaviaus, Octavis,
Octavous, Octavus*

Odakota (Lakota) friendly.
Oda

Odd (Norwegian) point.
Oddvar

Ode (Benin) born along the
road. (Irish, English) a short
form of Odell.
Odey, Odie, Ody

Oded (Hebrew) encouraging.

Odell (Greek) ode, melody.
(Irish) otter. (English)
forested hill.
Dell, Odall, Ode

Odin (Scandinavian) ruler.
Mythology: the Norse god
of wisdom and war.
Oden

Odion (Benin) first of twins.

Odo (Norwegian) a form of
Otto.

Odolf (German) prosperous
wolf.
Odolff

Odom (Ghanaian) oak tree.

Odon (Hungarian) wealthy
protector.
Odi

Odran (Irish) pale green.
*Odhrán, Oran, Oren, Orin,
Orran, Orren, Orrin*

Odysseus (Greek) wrathful.
Literature: the hero of
Homer's epic poem *Odyssey*.

Ofer (Hebrew) young deer.

Og (Aramaic) king. Bible: the
king of Basham.

Ogaleesha (Lakota) red shirt.

Ogbay (Ethiopian) don't take
him from me.

Ogbonna (Ibo) image of his
father.
Ogbonnia

Ogden (English) oak valley.
Literature: Ogden Nash
was a twentieth-century
American writer of light
verse.
Ogdan, Ogdon

Ogima (Chippewa) chief.

Ogun (Nigerian) Mythology:
the god of war.
*Ogunkeye, Ogunsanwo,
Ogunsheye*

Ohanko (Native American)
restless.

Ohannes (Turkish) a form of
John.

Ohanzee (Lakota) comforting
shadow.

Ohin (African) chief.
Ohan

Ohitekah (Lakota) brave.

Oistin (Irish) a form of
Austin.
Osten, Ostyn, Ostynn

OJ (American) a combination of the initials O. + J.
O.J., Ojay

Ojo (Yoruba) difficult delivery.

Okapi (Swahili) an African animal related to the giraffe but having a short neck.

Oke (Hawaiian) a form of Oscar.

Okechuku (Ibo) God's gift.

Okeke (Ibo) born on market day.
Okorie

Okie (American) from Oklahoma.
Okee, Okey

Oko (Ghanaian) older twin. (Yoruba) god of war.

Okorie (Ibo) a form of Okeke.

Okpara (Ibo) first son.

Okuth (Luo) born in a rain shower.

Ola (Yoruba) wealthy, rich.

Olaf (Scandinavian) ancestor. History: a patron saint and king of Norway.
Olaff, Olafur, Olav, Ole, Olef, Olof, Oluf

Olajuwon (Yoruba) wealth and honor are God's gifts.
Olajawon, Olajawun, Olajowuan, Olajuan, Olajuanne, Olajuawon, Olajuwa, Olajuwan, Olaujawon, Oljuwoun

Olamina (Yoruba) this is my wealth.

Olatunji (Yoruba) honor reawakens.

Olav (Scandinavian) a form of Olaf.
Ola, Olave, Olavus, Ole, Olen, Olin, Olle, Olov, Olyn

Ole (Scandinavian) a familiar form of Olaf, Olav.
Olay, Oleh, Olle

Oleg (Latvian, Russian) holy.
Olezka

Oleksandr (Russian) a form of Alexander.
Olek, Olesandr, Olesko

Olés (Polish) a familiar form of Alexander.

Olin (English) holly.
Olen, Olney, Olyn

Olindo (Italian) from Olinthos, Greece.

Oliver (Latin) olive tree. (Scandinavian) kind; affectionate.
Nollie, Oilibhéar, Oliverio, Oliverios, Olivero, Olivier, Oliviero, Oliwa, Ollie, Olliver, Ollivor, Olvan

Olivier (French) a form of Oliver.

Oliwa (Hawaiian) a form of Oliver.

Ollie (English) a familiar form of Oliver.
Olie, Olle, Olley, Olly

Olo (Spanish) a short form of Orlando, Rolando.

Olubayo (Yoruba) highest joy.

Olufemi (Yoruba) wealth and honor favors me.

Olujimi (Yoruba) God gave me this.

Olushola (Yoruba) God has blessed me.

Omar (Arabic) highest; follower of the Prophet. (Hebrew) reverent.
Omair, Omari, Omarr, Omer, Umar

Omari (Swahili) a form of Omar.
Omare, Omaree, Omarey

Omer (Arabic) a form of Omar.
Omeer, Omero

Omolara (Benin) child born at the right time.

On (Burmese) coconut. (Chinese) peace.

Onan (Turkish) prosperous.

Onaona (Hawaiian) pleasant fragrance.

Ondro (Czech) a form of Andrew.
Ondra, Ondre, Ondrea, Ondrey

O'neil (Irish) son of Neil.
Oneal, O'neal, Oneil, O'neill, Onel, Oniel, Onil

Onkar (Hindi) God in his entirety.

Onofrio (German) a form of Humphrey.
Oinfre, Onfre, Onfrio, Onofre, Onofredo

Onslow (English) enthusiast's hill.
Ounslow

Onufry (Polish) a form of Humphrey.

Onur (Turkish) honor.

Ophir (Hebrew) faithful. Bible: an Old Testament people and country.

Opio (Ateso) first of twin boys.

Oral (Latin) verbal; speaker.

Oran (Irish) green.
Odhran, Odran, Ora, Orane, Orran

Oratio (Latin) a form of Horatio.
Orazio

Orbán (Hungarian) born in the city.

Ordell (Latin) beginning.
Orde

Oren (Hebrew) pine tree.
(Irish) light skinned, white.
Oran, Orin, Oris, Orono,
Orren, Orrin

Orestes (Greek) mountain
man. Mythology: the son of
the Greek leader
Agamemnon.
Aresty, Oreste

Ori (Hebrew) my light.
Oree, Orie, Orri, Ory

Orien (Latin) visitor from the
east.
Orian, Orie, Orin, Oris, Oron,
Orono, Orrin, Oryan

Orion (Greek) son of fire.
Mythology: a giant hunter
who was killed by Artemis.
See also Zorion.

Orji (Ibo) mighty tree.

Orlando (German) famous
throughout the land.
(Spanish) a form of Roland.
Lando, Olando, Olo, Orlan,
Orland, Orlanda, Orlandas,
Orlandes, Orlandis, Orlandos,
Orlandus, Orlo, Orlondo,
Orlondon

Orleans (Latin) golden.
Orlean, Orlin

Orman (German) mariner,
seaman. (Scandinavian) ser-
pent, worm.
Ormand

Ormond (English) bear
mountain; spear protector.
Ormande, Ormon, Ormonde

Oro (Spanish) golden.

Orono (Latin) a form of
Oren.
Oron

Orrick (English) old oak tree.
Orric

Orrin (English) river.
Orin, Oryn, Orynn

Orris (Latin) a form of
Horatio.
Oris, Orriss

Orry (Latin) from the Orient.
Oarrie, Orrey, Orrie

Orsino (Italian) a form of
Orson.

Orson (Latin) bearlike.
Orscino, Orsen, Orsin, Orsini,
Orsino, Son, Sonny, Urson

Orton (English) shore town.

Ortzi (Basque) sky.

Orunjan (Yoruba) born under
the midday sun.

Orval (English) a form of
Orville.
Orvel

Orville (French) golden village. History: Orville Wright
and his brother Wilbur were

the first men to fly an airplane.
Orv, Orval, Orvell, Orvie, Orvil

Orvin (English) spear friend.
Orwin, Owynn

Osahar (Benin) God hears.

Osayaba (Benin) God forgives.

Osaze (Benin) whom God likes.

Osbert (English) divine; bright.

Osborn (Scandinavian) divine bear. (English) warrior of God.
Osbern, Osbon, Osborne, Osbourn, Osbourne, Osburn, Osburne, Oz, Ozzie

Oscar (Scandinavian) divine spearman.
Oke, Oskar, Osker, Oszkar

Osei (Fante) noble.
Osee

Osgood (English) divinely good.

O'Shea (Irish) son of Shea.
Oshae, Oshai, Oshane, O'Shane, Oshaun, Oshay, Oshaye, Oshe, Oshea, Osheon

Osip (Russian, Ukrainian) a form of Joseph, Yosef. See also Osya.

Oskar (Scandinavian) a form of Oscar.
Osker, Ozker

Osman (Turkish) ruler. (English) servant of God.
Osmanek, Osmen, Osmin, Otthmor, Ottmar

Osmar (English) divine; wonderful.

Osmond (English) divine protector.
Osmand, Osmonde, Osmont, Osmund, Osmunde, Osmundo

Osric (English) divine ruler.
Osrick

Ostin (Latin) a form of Austin.
Ostan, Osten, Ostyn

Osvaldo (Spanish) a form of Oswald.
Osbaldo, Osbalto, Osvald, Osvalda

Oswald (English) God's power; God's crest. See also Waldo.
Osvaldo, Oswaldo, Oswall, Oswell, Oswold, Oz, Ozzie

Oswaldo (Spanish) a form of Oswald.

Oswin (English) divine friend.
Osvin, Oswinn, Oswyn, Oswynn

Osya (Russian) a familiar form of Osip.

Ota (Czech) prosperous.
Otik

Otadan (Native American) plentiful.

Otaktay (Lakota) kills many; strikes many.

Otek (Polish) a form of Otto.

Otello (Italian) a form of Othello.

Otem (Luo) born away from home.

Othello (Spanish) a form of Otto. Literature: the title character in the Shakespearean tragedy *Othello*.
Otello

Othman (German) wealthy.
Ottoman

Otis (Greek) keen of hearing. (German) son of Otto.
Oates, Odis, Otes, Otess, Otez, Otise, Ottis, Otys

Ottah (Nigerian) thin baby.

Ottar (Norwegian) point warrior; fright warrior.

Ottmar (Turkish) a form of Osman.
Otomars, Ottomar

Otto (German) rich.
Odo, Otek, Otello, Otfried, Othello, Otho, Othon, Otik, Otilio, Otman, Oto, Otón, Otton, Ottone

Ottokar (German) happy warrior.
Otokars, Ottocar

Otu (Native American) collecting seashells in a basket.

Ouray (Ute) arrow. Astrology: born under the sign of Sagittarius.

Oved (Hebrew) worshiper, follower.

Owen (Irish) born to nobility; young warrior. (Welsh) a form of Evan.
Owain, Owens, Owin, Uaine

Owney (Irish) elderly.
Oney

Oxford (English) place where oxen cross the river.
Ford

Oya (Moquelumnan) speaking of the jacksnipe.

Oystein (Norwegian) rock of happiness.
Ostein, Osten, Ostin, Øystein

Oz (Hebrew) a short form of Osborn, Oswald.

Ozturk (Turkish) pure; genuine Turk.

Ozzie (English) a familiar form of Osborn, Oswald.
Ossie, Ossy, Ozee, Ozi, Ozzi, Ozzy

P

Paavo (Finnish) a form of Paul.
Paaveli

Pablo (Spanish) a form of Paul.
Pable, Paublo

Pace (English) a form of Pascal.
Payce

Pacifico (Filipino) peaceful.

Paco (Italian) pack. (Spanish) a familiar form of Francisco. (Native American) bald eagle. See also Quico.
Pacorro, Panchito, Pancho, Paquito

Paddy (Irish) a familiar form of Padraic, Patrick.
Paddey, Paddi, Paddie

Paden (English) a form of Patton.

Padget (English) a form of Page.
Padgett, Paget, Pagett

Padraic (Irish) a form of Patrick.
Paddrick, Paddy, Padhraig, Padrai, Pádraig, Padraigh, Padreic, Padriac, Padric, Padron, Padruig

Page (French) youthful assistant.
Padget, Paggio, Paige, Payge

Paige (English) a form of Page.

Pakelika (Hawaiian) a form of Patrick.

Paki (African) witness.

Pal (Swedish) a form of Paul.

Pál (Hungarian) a form of Paul.
Pali, Palika

Palaina (Hawaiian) a form of Brian.

Palani (Hawaiian) a form of Frank.

Palash (Hindi) flowery tree.

Palben (Basque) blond.

Palladin (Native American) fighter.
Pallaton, Palleten

Palmer (English) palm-bearing pilgrim.
Pallmer, Palmar

Palti (Hebrew) God liberates.
Palti-el

Panas (Russian) immortal.

Panayiotis (Greek) a form of Peter.
Panagiotis, Panajotis, Panayioti, Panayoti, Panayotis

Pancho (Spanish) a familiar form of Francisco, Frank.
Panchito

Panos (Greek) a form of Peter.
Petros

Paolo (Italian) a form of Paul.

Paquito (Spanish) a familiar form of Paco.

Paramesh (Hindi) greatest. Religion: another name for the Hindu god Shiva.

Pardeep (Sikh) mystic light.
Pardip

Paris (Greek) lover. Geography: the capital of France. Mythology: the prince of Troy who started the Trojan War by abducting Helen.
Paras, Paree, Pares, Parese, Parie, Parris, Parys

Park (Chinese) cypress tree. (English) a short form of Parker.
Parke, Parkes, Parkey, Parks

Parker (English) park keeper.
Park

Parkin (English) little Peter.
Perkin

Parlan (Scottish) a form of Bartholomew. See also Parthalán.

Parnell (French) little Peter. History: Charles Stewart Parnell was a famous Irish politician.
Nell, Parle, Parnel, Parrnell, Pernell

Parr (English) cattle enclosure, barn.

Parrish (English) church district.
Parish, Parrie, Parrisch, Parrysh

Parry (Welsh) son of Harry.
Parrey, Parrie, Pary

Parth (Irish) a short form of Parthalán.
Partha, Parthey

Parthalán (Irish) plowman. See also Bartholomew.
Parlan, Parth

Parthenios (Greek) virgin. Religion: a Greek Orthodox saint.

Pascal (French) born on Easter or Passover.
Pace, Pascale, Pascalle, Paschal, Paschalis, Pascoe, Pascow, Pascual, Pasquale

Pascual (Spanish) a form of Pascal.
Pascul

Pasha (Russian) a form of Paul.
Pashenka, Pashka

Pasquale (Italian) a form of Pascal.
Pascuale, Pasqual, Pasquali, Pasquel

Pastor (Latin) spiritual leader.

Pat (Native American) fish. (English) a short form of Patrick.
Pattie, Patty

Patakusu (Moquelumnan) ant biting a person.

Patamon (Native American) raging.

Patek (Polish) a form of Patrick.
Patick

Patric (Latin) a form of Patrick.

Patrice (French) a form of Patrick.

Patricio (Spanish) a form of Patrick.
Patricius, Patrizio

Patrick (Latin) nobleman. Religion: the patron saint of Ireland. See also Fitzpatrick, Ticho.
Paddy, Padraic, Pakelika, Pat, Patek, Patric, Patrice, Patricio, Patrickk, Patrik, Patrique, Patrizius, Patryk, Pats, Patsy, Pattrick

Patrin (Gypsy) leaf trail.

Patryk (Latin) a form of Patrick.
Patryck

Patterson (Irish) son of Pat.
Patteson

Pattin (Gypsy) leaf.

Patton (English) warrior's town.
Paden, Paten, Patin, Paton, Patten, Pattin, Patty, Payton, Peyton

Patwin (Native American) man.

Patxi (Basque, Teutonic) free.

Paul (Latin) small. Bible: Saul, later renamed Paul, was the first to bring the teachings of Christ to the Gentiles.
Oalo, Paavo, Pablo, Pal, Pál, Pall, Paolo, Pasha, Pasko, Pauli, Paulia, Paulin, Paulino, Paulis, Paulo, Pauls, Paulus, Pavel, Pavlos, Pawel, Pol, Poul

Pauli (Latin) a familiar form of Paul.
Pauley, Paulie, Pauly

Paulin (German, Polish) a form of Paul.

Paulino (Spanish) a form of Paul.

Paulo (Portuguese, Swedish, Hawaiian) a form of Paul.

Pavel (Russian) a form of
Paul.
*Paavel, Pasha, Pavils, Pavlik,
Pavlo, Pavlusha, Pavlushenka,
Pawl*

Pavit (Hindi) pious, pure.

Pawel (Polish) a form of Paul.
Pawelek, Pawl

Pax (Latin) peaceful.
Paz

Paxton (Latin) peaceful town.
*Packston, Pax, Paxon, Paxten,
Paxtun*

Payat (Native American) he is
on his way.
Pay, Payatt

Payden (English) a form of
Payton.
Paydon

Payne (Latin) from the country.
Paine, Paynn

Paytah (Lakota) fire.
Pay, Payta

Payton (English) a form of
Patton.
*Paiton, Pate, Payden, Peaton,
Peighton, Peyton*

Paz (Spanish) a form of Pax.

Pearce (English) a form of
Pierce.
Pears, Pearse

Pearson (English) son of
Peter. See also Pierson.
*Pearsson, Pehrson, Peirson,
Peterson*

Peder (Scandinavian) a form
of Peter.
Peadar, Pedey

Pedro (Spanish) a form of
Peter.
Pedrin, Pedrín, Petronio

Peers (English) a form of
Peter.
Peerus, Piers

Peeter (Estonian) a form of
Peter.
Peet

Peirce (English) a form of
Peter.
Peirs

Pekelo (Hawaiian) a form of
Peter.
Pekka

Peleke (Hawaiian) a form of
Frederick.

Pelham (English) tannery
town.

Pelí (Latin, Basque) happy.

Pell (English) parchment.
Pall

Pello (Greek, Basque) stone.
Peru, Piarres

Pelton (English) town by a
pool.

Pembroke (Welsh) headland. (French) wine dealer. (English) broken fence.
Pembrook

Peniamina (Hawaiian) a form of Benjamin.
Peni

Penley (English) enclosed meadow.

Penn (Latin) pen, quill. (English) enclosure. (German) a short form of Penrod.
Pen, Penna, Penney, Pennie, Penny

Penrod (German) famous commander.
Penn, Pennrod, Rod

Pepa (Czech) a familiar form of Joseph.
Pepek, Pepik

Pepe (Spanish) a familiar form of José.
Pepillo, Pepito, Pequin, Pipo

Pepin (German) determined; petitioner. History: Pepin the Short was an eighth-century king of the Franks.
Pepi, Peppie, Peppy

Peppe (Italian) a familiar form of Joseph.
Peppi, Peppo, Pino

Per (Swedish) a form of Peter.

Perben (Greek, Danish) stone.

Percival (French) pierce the valley. Literature: a knight of the Round Table who first appears in Chrétien de Troyes's poem about the quest for the Holy Grail.
Parsafal, Parsefal, Parsifal, Parzival, Perc, Perce, Perceval, Percevall, Percivall, Percy, Peredur, Purcell

Percy (French) a familiar form of Percival.
Pearcey, Pearcy, Percey, Percie, Piercey, Piercy

Peregrine (Latin) traveler; pilgrim; falcon.
Peregrin, Peregryne, Perine, Perry

Pericles (Greek) just leader. History: an Athenian statesman.

Perico (Spanish) a form of Peter.
Pequin, Perequin

Perine (Latin) a short form of Peregrine.
Perino, Perion, Perrin, Perryn

Perkin (English) little Peter.
Perka, Perkins, Perkyn, Perrin

Pernell (French) a form of Parnell.
Perren, Perrnall

Perry (English) a familiar form of Peregrine, Peter.
Parry, Perrie, Perrye

Perth (Scottish) thorn-bush thicket. Geography: a burgh in Scotland; a city in Australia.

Pervis (Latin) passage.
Pervez

Pesach (Hebrew) spared. Religion: another name for Passover.
Pessach

Petar (Greek) a form of Peter.

Pete (English) a short form of Peter.
Peat, Peet, Petey, Peti, Petie, Piet, Pit

Peter (Greek, Latin) small rock. Bible: Simon, renamed Peter, was the leader of the Twelve Apostles. See also Boutros, Ferris, Takis.
Panayiotos, Panos, Peadair, Peder, Pedro, Peers, Peeter, Peirce, Pekelo, Per, Perico, Perion, Perkin, Perry, Petar, Pete, Péter, Peterke, Peterus, Petr, Petras, Petros, Petru, Petruno, Petter, Peyo, Piaras, Pierce, Piero, Pierre, Pieter, Pietrek, Pietro, Piotr, Piter, Piti, Pjeter, Pyotr

Peterson (English) son of Peter.
Peteris, Petersen

Petiri (Shona) where we are.
Petri

Petr (Bulgarian) a form of Peter.

Petras (Lithuanian) a form of Peter.
Petra, Petrelis

Petros (Greek) a form of Peter.
Petro

Petru (Romanian) a form of Peter.
Petrukas, Petrus, Petruso

Petter (Norwegian) a form of Peter.

Peverell (French) piper.
Peverall, Peverel, Peveril

Peyo (Spanish) a form of Peter.

Peyton (English) a form of Patton, Payton.
Peyt, Peyten, Peython, Peytonn

Pharaoh (Latin) ruler. History: a title for the ancient kings of Egypt.
Faroh, Pharo, Pharoah, Pharoh

Phelan (Irish) wolf.

Phelipe (Spanish) a form of Philip.

Phelix (Latin) a form of Felix.

Phelps (English) son of Phillip.

Phil (Greek) a short form of Philip, Phillip.
Fil, Phill

Philander (Greek) lover of mankind.

Philbert (English) a form of
Filbert.
Philibert, Phillbert

Philemon (Greek) kiss.
Phila, Philamina, Phileman,
Philémon, Philmon

Philip (Greek) lover of horses.
Bible: one of the Twelve
Apostles. See also Felipe,
Felippo, Filip, Fillipp, Filya,
Fischel, Flip.
Phelps, Phelipe, Phil, Philipp,
Philippe, Philippo, Phillip,
Phillipos, Phillp, Philly, Philp,
Phylip, Piers, Pilib, Pilipo, Pippo

Philipp (German) a form of
Philip.
Phillipp

Philippe (French) a form of
Philip.
Philipe, Phillepe, Phillipe,
Phillippe, Phillippee, Phyllipe

Phillip (Greek) a form of
Philip.
Phil, Phillipos, Phillipp, Phillips,
Philly, Phyllip

Phillipos (Greek) a form of
Phillip.

Philly (American) a familiar
form of Philip, Phillip.
Phillie

Philo (Greek) love.

Phinean (Irish) a form of
Finian.
Phinian

Phineas (English) a form of
Pinchas.
Fineas, Phinehas, Phinny

Phirun (Cambodian) rain.

Phoenix (Latin) phoenix, a
legendary bird.
Phenix, Pheonix, Phynix

Phuok (Vietnamese) good.
Phuoc

Pias (Gypsy) fun.

Pickford (English) ford at the
peak.

Pickworth (English) wood
cutter's estate.

Pierce (English) a form of
Peter.
Pearce, Peerce, Peers, Peirce,
Piercy, Piers

Piero (Italian) a form of Peter.
Pero, Pierro

Pierre (French) a form of
Peter.
Peirre, Piere, Pierrot

Pierre-Luc (French) a combination of Pierre + Luc.
Piere Luc

Piers (English) a form of
Philip.

Pierson (English) son of Peter.
See also Pearson.
Pierrson, Piersen, Piersson,
Piersun

Pieter (Dutch) a form of Peter.
Pietr

Pietro (Italian) a form of Peter.

Pilar (Spanish) pillar.

Pili (Swahili) second born.

Pilipo (Hawaiian) a form of Philip.

Pillan (Native American) supreme essence.
Pilan

Pin (Vietnamese) faithful boy.

Pinchas (Hebrew) oracle. (Egyptian) dark skinned.
Phineas, Pincas, Pinchos, Pincus, Pinkas, Pinkus, Pinky

Pinky (American) a familiar form of Pinchas.
Pink

Pino (Italian) a form of Joseph.

Piñon (Tupi-Guarani) Mythology: the hunter who became the constellation Orion.

Pio (Latin) pious.

Piotr (Bulgarian) a form of Peter.
Piotrek

Pippin (German) father.

Piran (Irish) prayer. Religion: the patron saint of miners.
Peran, Pieran

Pirro (Greek, Spanish) flaming hair.

Pista (Hungarian) a familiar form of István.
Pisti

Piti (Spanish) a form of Peter.

Pitin (Spanish) a form of Felix.
Pito

Pitney (English) island of the strong-willed man.
Pittney

Pitt (English) pit, ditch.

Placido (Spanish) serene.
Placide, Placidus, Placyd, Placydo

Plato (Greek) broad shouldered. History: a famous Greek philosopher.
Platon

Platt (French) flatland.
Platte

Pol (Swedish) a form of Paul.
Pól, Pola, Poul

Poldi (German) a familiar form of Leopold.
Poldo

Pollard (German) close-cropped head.
Poll, Pollerd, Pollyrd

Pollock (English) a form of Pollux. Art: American artist Jackson Pollock was a leader of abstract expressionism.
Pollack, Polloch

Pollux (Greek) crown. Astronomy: one of the stars in the constellation Gemini.
Pollock

Polo (Tibetan) brave wanderer. (Greek) a short form of Apollo. Culture: a game played on horseback. History: Marco Polo was a thirteenth-century Venetian explorer who traveled throughout Asia.

Pomeroy (French) apple orchard.
Pommeray, Pommeroy

Ponce (Spanish) fifth. History: Juan Ponce de León of Spain searched for the Fountain of Youth in Florida.

Pony (Scottish) small horse.
Poni

Porfirio (Greek, Spanish) purple stone.
Porphirios, Prophyrios

Porter (Latin) gatekeeper.
Port, Portie, Porty

Poshita (Sanskrit) cherished.

Po Sin (Chinese) grand-father elephant.

Poul (Danish) a form of Paul.
Poulos, Poulus

Pov (Gypsy) earth.

Powa (Native American) wealthy.

Powell (English) alert.
Powel

Pramad (Hindi) rejoicing.

Pravat (Tai) history.

Prem (Hindi) love.

Prentice (English) apprentice.
Prent, Prentis, Prentiss, Printes, Printiss

Prescott (English) priest's cottage. See also Scott.
Prescot, Prestcot, Prestcott

Presley (English) priest's meadow. Music: Elvis Presley was an influential American rock 'n' roll singer.
Presleigh, Presly, Presslee, Pressley, Prestley, Priestley, Priestly

Preston (English) priest's estate.
Prestan, Presten, Prestin, Prestyn

Prewitt (French) brave little one.
Preuet, Prewet, Prewett, Prewit, Pruit, Pruitt

Price (Welsh) son of the ardent one.
Brice, Bryce, Pryce

Pricha (Tai) clever.

Primo (Italian) first; premier
quality.
Preemo, Premo

Prince (Latin) chief; prince.
Prence, Prinz, Prinze

Princeton (English) princely
town.
Prenston, Princeston, Princton

Proctor (Latin) official,
administrator.
Prockter, Procter

Prokopios (Greek) declared
leader.

Prosper (Latin) fortunate.
Prospero, Próspero

Pryor (Latin) head of the
monastery; prior.
Prior, Pry

Pumeet (Sanskrit) pure.

Purdy (Hindi) recluse.

Purvis (French, English) pro-
viding food.
Pervis, Purves, Purviss

Putnam (English) dweller by
the pond.
Putnem

Pyotr (Russian) a form of
Peter.
*Petenka, Petinka, Petrusha,
Petya, Pyatr*

Q

Qabil (Arabic) able.

Qadim (Arabic) ancient.

Qadir (Arabic) powerful.
*Qaadir, Qadeer, Quaadir,
Quadeer, Quadir*

Qamar (Arabic) moon.
Quamar, Quamir

Qasim (Arabic) divider.
Quasim

Qimat (Hindi) valuable.

Quaashie (Ewe) born on
Sunday.

Quadarius (American) a
combination of Quan +
Darius.
*Quadara, Quadarious,
Quadaris, Quandarious,
Quandarius, Quandarrius,
Qudarius, Qudaruis*

Quade (Latin) fourth.
*Quadell, Quaden, Quadon,
Quadre, Quadrie, Quadrine,
Quadrion, Quaid, Quayd,
Quayde, Qwade*

Quamaine (American) a com-
bination of Quan +
Jermaine.
*Quamain, Quaman, Quamane,
Quamayne, Quarmaine*

Quan (Comanche) a short form of Quanah.

Quanah (Comanche) fragrant.
Quan

Quandre (American) a combination of Quan + Andre.
Quandrae, Quandré

Quant (Greek) how much?
Quanta, Quantae, Quantai, Quantas, Quantay, Quante, Quantea, Quantey, Quantez, Quantu

Quantavius (American) a combination of Quan + Octavius.
Quantavian, Quantavin, Quantavion, Quantavious, Quantavis, Quantavous, Quatavious, Quatavius

Quashawn (American) a combination of Quan + Shawn.
Quasean, Quashaan, Quashan, Quashaun, Quashaunn, Quashon, Quashone, Quashun, Queshan, Queshon, Qweshawn, Qyshawn

Qudamah (Arabic) courage.

Quenby (Scandinavian) a form of Quimby.

Quennell (French) small oak.
Quenell, Quennel

Quenten (Latin) a form of Quentin.
Quienten

Quentin (Latin) fifth. (English) queen's town.
Qeuntin, Quantin, Quent, Quentan, Quenten, Quentine, Quenton, Quentyn, Quentynn, Quientin, Quinten, Quintin, Quinton, Qwentin

Quenton (Latin) a form of Quentin.
Quienton

Quico (Spanish) a familiar form of many names.
Paco

Quigley (Irish) maternal side.
Quigly

Quillan (Irish) cub.
Quill, Quillen, Quillin, Quillon

Quimby (Scandinavian) woman's estate.
Quenby, Quinby

Quincy (French) fifth son's estate.
Quenci, Quency, Quince, Quincee, Quincey, Quinci, Quinn, Quinncy, Quinnsy, Quinsey, Quinzy

Quindarius (American) a combination of Quinn + Darius.
Quindarious, Quindarrius, Quinderious, Quinderus, Quindrius

Quinlan (Irish) strong; well shaped.
Quindlen, Quinlen, Quinlin, Quinn, Quinnlan, Quinnlin

Quinn (Irish) a short form of
Quincy, Quinlan, Quinton.
Quin

Quintavius (American) a
combination of Quinn +
Octavius.
*Quintavious, Quintavis,
Quintavus, Quintayvious*

Quinten (Latin) a form of
Quentin.
Quinnten

Quintin (Latin) a form of
Quentin.
Quinntin, Quintine, Quintyn

Quinton (Latin) a form of
Quentin.
*Quinn, Quinneton, Quinnton,
Quint, Quintan, Quintann,
Quintin, Quintion, Quintus,
Quitin, Quito, Quiton,
Qunton, Qwinton*

Quiqui (Spanish) a familiar
form of Enrique.
Quinto, Quiquin

Quitin (Latin) a short form of
Quinton.
Quiten, Quito, Quiton

Quito (Spanish) a short form
of Quinton.

Quon (Chinese) bright.

R

Raanan (Hebrew) fresh; luxu-
riant.

Rabi (Arabic) breeze.
*Rabbi, Rabee, Rabeeh, Rabiah,
Rabie, Rabih*

Race (English) race.
Racel, Rayce

Racham (Hebrew) compas-
sionate.
*Rachaman, Rachamim, Rachim,
Rachman, Rachmiel, Rachum,
Raham, Rahamim*

Rad (English) advisor. (Slavic)
happy.
*Raad, Radd, Raddie, Raddy,
Rade, Radee, Radell, Radey,
Radi*

Radbert (English) brilliant
advisor.

Radburn (English) red brook;
brook with reeds.
*Radborn, Radborne, Radbourn,
Radbourne, Radburne*

Radcliff (English) red cliff; cliff
with reeds.
Radcliffe, Radclyffe

Radford (English) red ford;
ford with reeds.

Radley (English) red meadow;
meadow of reeds.
Radlea, Radlee, Radleigh,
Radly

Radman (Slavic) joyful.
Radmen, Radusha

Radnor (English) red shore;
shore with reeds.

Radomil (Slavic) happy peace.

Radoslaw (Polish) happy
glory.
Radik, Rado, Radzmir, Slawek

Raekwon (American) a form
of Raquan.
Raekwan, Raikwan, Rakwane,
Rakwon

Raequan (American) a form
of Raquan.
Raequon, Raeqwon, Raiquan,
Raiquen, Raiqoun

Raeshawn (American) a form
of Rashawn.
Raesean, Raeshaun, Raeshon,
Raeshun

Rafael (Spanish) a form of
Raphael. See also Falito.
Rafaelle, Rafaello, Rafaelo,
Rafal, Rafeal, Rafeé, Rafel,
Rafello, Raffael, Raffaelo,
Raffeal, Raffel, Raffiel, Rafiel

Rafaele (Italian) a form of
Raphael.
Raffaele

Rafal (Polish) a form of
Raphael.

Rafe (English) a short form of
Rafferty, Ralph.
Raff

Rafer (Irish) a short form of
Rafferty.
Raffer

Rafferty (Irish) rich, prosper-
ous.
Rafe, Rafer, Raferty, Raffarty,
Raffer

Rafi (Arabic) exalted.
(Hebrew) a familiar form of
Raphael.
Raffe, Raffee, Raffi, Raffy, Rafi

Rafiq (Arabic) friend.
Raafiq, Rafeeq, Rafic, Rafique

Raghib (Arabic) desirous.
Raquib

Raghnall (Irish) wise power.

Ragnar (Norwegian) powerful
army.
Ragnor, Rainer, Rainier,
Ranieri, Rayner, Raynor,
Reinhold

Rago (Hausa) ram.

Raheem (Punjabi) compassionate God.
Rakeem

Rahim (Arabic) merciful.
Raaheim, Rahaeim, Raheam,
Raheim, Rahiem, Rahiim,
Rahime, Rahium, Rakim

Rahman (Arabic) compassionate.
Rahmatt, Rahmet

Rahul (Arabic) traveler.

Raíd (Arabic) leader.

Raiden (Japanese) Mythology:
the thunder god.
Raidan, Rayden

Raimondo (Italian) a form of
Raymond.
Raymondo, Reimundo

Raimund (German) a form of
Raymond.
Rajmund

Raimundo (Portuguese,
Spanish) a form of
Raymond.
*Mundo, Raimon, Raimond,
Raimonds, Raymundo*

Raine (English) lord; wise.
Rain, Raines, Rayne

Rainer (German) counselor.
*Rainar, Rainey, Rainier, Rainor,
Raynier, Reinier*

Rainey (German) a familiar
form of Rainer.
*Raine, Rainee, Rainie, Rainney,
Rainy, Reiny*

Raini (Tupi-Guarani)
Religion: the god who created the world.

Raishawn (American) a form
of Rashawn.
Raishon, Raishun

Rajabu (Swahili) born in the
seventh month of the Islamic
calendar.

Rajah (Hindi) prince; chief.
*Raj, Raja, Rajaah, Rajae,
Rajahe, Rajan, Raje, Rajeh,
Raji*

Rajak (Hindi) cleansing.

Rajan (Hindi) a form of
Rajah.
Rajaahn, Rajain, Rajen, Rajin

Rakeem (Punjabi) a form of
Raheem.
Rakeeme, Rakeim, Rakem

Rakim (Arabic) a form of
Rahim.
Rakiim

Rakin (Arabic) respectable.
Rakeen

Raktim (Hindi) bright red.

Raleigh (English) a form of
Rawleigh.
Ralegh

Ralph (English) wolf coun-
selor.
*Radolphus, Rafe, Ralf,
Ralpheal, Ralphel, Ralphie,
Ralston, Raoul, Raul, Rolf*

Ralphie (English) a familiar
form of Ralph.
Ralphy

Ralston (English) Ralph's settlement.

Ram (Hindi) god; godlike.
Religion: another name for
the Hindu god Rama.
(English) male sheep. A short
form of Ramsey.
Rami, Ramie, Ramy

Ramadan (Arabic) ninth
month of the Arabic year in
the Islamic calendar.
Rama

Ramanan (Hindi) god; god-
like.
*Raman, Ramandeep, Ramanjit,
Ramanjot*

Rami (Hindi, English) a form
of Ram. (Spanish) a short
form of Ramiro.
Rame, Ramee, Ramey, Ramih

Ramiro (Portuguese, Spanish)
supreme judge.
*Ramario, Rameer, Rameir,
Ramere, Rameriz, Ramero,
Rami, Ramires, Ramirez,
Ramos*

Ramón (Spanish) a form of
Raymond.
*Ramon, Remon, Remone,
Romone*

Ramone (Dutch) a form of
Raymond.
*Raemon, Raemonn, Ramond,
Ramonte, Remone*

Ramsden (English) valley of
rams.

Ramsey (English) ram's island.
Ram, Ramsay, Ramsee, Ramsie,

*Ramsy, Ramzee, Ramzey,
Ramzi, Ramzy*

Rance (English) a short form
of Laurence. (American) a
familiar form of Laurence.
*Rancel, Rancell, Rances, Rancey,
Rancie, Rancy, Ransel, Ransell*

Rand (English) shield; warrior.
Randy

Randal (English) a form of
Randall.
*Randahl, Randale, Randel,
Randl, Randle*

Randall (English) a form of
Randolph.
*Randal, Randell, Randy,
Randyll*

Randolph (English) shield
wolf.
*Randall, Randol, Randolf,
Randolfo, Randolpho, Randy,
Ranolph*

Randy (English) a familiar
form of Rand, Randall,
Randolph.
*Randdy, Randee, Randey,
Randi, Randie, Ranndy*

Ranger (French) forest keeper.
Rainger, Range

Rangle (American) cowboy.
Rangler, Wrangle

Rangsey (Cambodian) seven
kinds of colors.

Rani (Hebrew) my song; my
joy.
Ranen, Ranie, Ranon, Roni

Ranieri (Italian) a form of
Ragnar.
Raneir, Ranier, Rannier

Ranjan (Hindi) delighted;
gladdened.

Rankin (English) small shield.
Randkin

Ransford (English) raven's
ford.

Ransley (English) raven's field.

Ransom (Latin) redeemer.
(English) son of the shield.
Rance, Ransome, Ranson

Raoul (French) a form of
Ralph, Rudolph.
Raol, Raul, Raúl, Reuel

Raphael (Hebrew) God has
healed. Bible: one of the
archangels. Art: a prominent
painter of the Renaissance.
See also Falito, Rafi.
*Rafael, Rafaele, Rafal, Rafel,
Raphaél, Raphale, Raphaello,
Rapheal, Raphel, Raphello,
Raphiel, Ray, Rephael*

Rapheal (Hebrew) a form of
Raphael.
Rafel, Raphiel

Rapier (French) blade-sharp.

Raquan (American) a combi-
nation of the prefix Ra +
Quan.
*Raaquan, Rackwon, Racquan,
Raekwon, Raequan, Rahquan,
Raquané, Raquon, Raquwan,
Raquwn, Raquwon, Raqwan,
Raqwann*

Rashaad (Arabic) a form of
Rashad.

Rashaan (American) a form
of Rashawn.
Rasaan, Rashan, Rashann

Rashad (Arabic) wise coun-
selor.
*Raashad, Rachad, Rachard,
Raeshad, Raishard, Rashaad,
Rashadd, Rashade, Rashaud,
Rasheed, Rashid, Rashod,
Reshad, Rhashad, Rishad,
Roshad*

Rashard (American) a form of
Richard.
Rasharrd

Rashaud (Arabic) a form of
Rashad.
Rachaud, Rashaude

Rashaun (American) a form
of Rashawn.

Rashawn (American) a com-
bination of the prefix Ra +
Shawn.
*Raashawn, Raashen,
Raeshawn, Rahshawn,
Raishawn, Rasaun, Rasawn,
Rashaan, Rashaun, Rashaw,*

Rashon, Rashun, Raushan,
Raushawn, Rhashan,
Rhashaun, Rhashawn

Rashean (American) a combination of the prefix Ra + Sean.
Rahsaan, Rahsean, Rahseen,
Rasean, Rashane, Rasheen,
Rashien, Rashiena

Rasheed (Arabic) a form of Rashad.
Rashead, Rashed, Rasheid,
Rhasheed

Rashid (Arabic) a form of Rashad.
Rasheyd, Rashida, Rashidah,
Rashied, Rashieda, Raushaid

Rashida (Swahili) righteous.

Rashidi (Swahili) wise counselor.

Rashod (Arabic) a form of Rashad.
Rashoda, Rashodd, Rashoud,
Rayshod, Rhashod

Rashon (American) a form of Rashawn.
Rashion, Rashone, Rashonn,
Rashuan, Rashun, Rashunn

Rasmus (Greek, Danish) a short form of Erasmus.

Raul (French) a form of Ralph.

Raulas (Lithuanian) a form of Laurence.

Raulo (Lithuanian) a form of Laurence.
Raulas

Raven (English) a short form of Ravenel.
Ravan, Ravean, Raveen, Ravin,
Ravine, Ravon, Ravyn, Reven,
Rhaven

Ravenel (English) raven.
Raven, Ravenell, Revenel

Ravi (Hindi) sun.
Ravee, Ravijot

Ravid (Hebrew) a form of Arvid.

Raviv (Hebrew) rain, dew.

Ravon (English) a form of Raven.
Raveon, Ravion, Ravone,
Ravonn, Ravonne, Rayvon,
Revon

Rawdon (English) rough hill.

Rawleigh (English) deer meadow.
Raleigh, Rawle, Rawley,
Rawling, Rawly, Rawylyn

Rawlins (French) a form of Roland.
Rawlings, Rawlinson, Rawson

Ray (French) kingly, royal. (English) a short form of Rayburn, Raymond. See also Lei.
Rae, Raye

Rayan (Irish) a form of Ryan.
Rayaun

Rayburn (English) deer brook.
Burney, Raeborn, Raeborne, Raebourn, Ray, Raybourn, Raybourne, Rayburne

Rayce (English) a form of Race.

Rayden (Japanese) a form of Raiden.
Raidin, Raydun, Rayedon

Rayhan (Arabic) favored by God.
Rayhaan

Rayi (Hebrew) my friend, my companion.

Raymon (English) a form of Raymond.
Rayman, Raymann, Raymen, Raymone, Raymun, Reamonn

Raymond (English) mighty; wise protector. See also Aymon.
Radmond, Raemond, Raimondo, Raimund, Raimundo, Ramón, Ramond, Ramonde, Ramone, Ray, Raymand, Rayment, Raymon, Raymont, Raymund, Raymunde, Raymundo, Redmond, Reymond, Reymundo

Raymundo (Spanish) a form of Raymond.
Raemondo, Raimondo, Raimundo, Raymondo

Raynaldo (Spanish) a form of Reynold.
Raynal, Raynald, Raynold

Raynard (French) a form of Renard, Reynard.
Raynarde

Rayne (English) a form of Raine.
Raynee, Rayno

Raynor (Scandinavian) a form of Ragnar.
Rainer, Rainor, Ranier, Ranieri, Raynar, Rayner

Rayshawn (American) a combination of Ray + Shawn.
Raysean, Rayshaan, Rayshan, Rayshaun, Raysheen, Rayshon, Rayshone, Rayshonn, Rayshun, Rayshunn

Rayshod (American) a form of Rashad.
Raychard, Rayshad, Rayshard, Rayshaud

Rayvon (American) a form of Ravon.
Rayvan, Rayvaun, Rayven, Rayvone, Reyven, Reyvon

Razi (Aramaic) my secret.
Raz, Raziel, Raziq

Read (English) a form of Reed, Reid.
Raed, Raede, Raeed, Reaad, Reade

Reading (English) son of the red wanderer.
Redding, Reeding, Reiding

Reagan (Irish) little king. History: Ronald Wilson Reagan was the fortieth U.S. president.
Raegan, Reagen, Reaghan, Reegan, Reegen, Regan, Reigan, Reighan, Reign, Rheagan

Rebel (American) rebel.
Reb

Red (American) red, redhead.
Redd

Reda (Arabic) satisfied.
Ridha

Redford (English) red river crossing.
Ford, Radford, Reaford, Red, Redd

Redley (English) red meadow; meadow with reeds.
Radley, Redlea, Redleigh, Redly

Redmond (German) protecting counselor. (English) a form of Raymond.
Radmond, Radmund, Reddin, Redmund

Redpath (English) red path.

Reece (Welsh) enthusiastic; stream.
Reace, Rece, Reese, Reice, Reyes, Rhys, Rice, Ryese

Reed (English) a form of Reid.
Raeed, Read, Reyde, Rheed

Reese (Welsh) a form of Reece.
Rease, Rees, Reis, Reise, Reiss, Rhys, Riese, Riess

Reeve (English) steward.
Reave, Reaves, Reeves

Reg (English) a short form of Reginald.

Regan (Irish) a form of Reagan.
Regen

Reggie (English) a familiar form of Reginald.
Regi, Regie

Reginal (English) a form of Reginald.
Reginale, Reginel

Reginald (English) king's advisor. A form of Reynold. See also Naldo.
Reg, Reggie, Regginald, Reggis, Reginal, Reginaldo, Reginalt, Reginauld, Reginault, Reginold, Reginuld, Regnauld, Ronald

Regis (Latin) regal.

Rehema (Swahili) second-born.

Rei (Japanese) rule, law.

Reid (English) redhead.
Read, Reed, Reide, Reyd, Ried

Reidar (Norwegian) nest warrior.

Reilly (Irish) a form of Riley.
Reiley, Reilley, Reily, Rielly

Reinaldo (Spanish) a form of Reynold.

Reinhart (German) a form of Reynard.
Rainart, Rainhard, Rainhardt, Rainhart, Reinart, Reinhard, Reinhardt, Renke

Reinhold (Swedish) a form of Ragnar.
Reinold

Reku (Finnish) a form of Richard.

Remi, Rémi (French) forms of Remy.
Remie, Remmie

Remington (English) raven estate.
Rem, Reminton, Tony

Remus (Latin) speedy, quick. Mythology: Remus and his twin brother, Romulus, founded Rome.

Remy (French) from Rheims, France.
Ramey, Remee, Remi, Rémi, Remmy

Renaldo (Spanish) a form of Reynold.
Raynaldo, Reynaldo, Rinaldo

Renard (French) a form of Reynard.
Ranard, Raynard, Reinard, Rennard

Renardo (Italian) a form of Reynard.

Renato (Italian) reborn.

Renaud (French) a form of Reynard, Reynold.
Renauld, Renauldo, Renault, Renould

Rendor (Hungarian) policeman.

René (French) reborn.
Renat, Renato, Renatus, Renault, Renay, Renee, Renny

Renfred (English) lasting peace.

Renfrew (Welsh) raven woods.

Renjiro (Japanese) virtuous.

Renny (Irish) small but strong. (French) a familiar form of René.
Ren, Renn, Renne, Rennie

Reno (American) gambler. Geography: a city in Nevada known for gambling.
Renos, Rino

Renshaw (English) raven woods.
Renishaw

Renton (English) settlement of the roe deer.

Renzo (Latin) a familiar form of Laurence. (Italian) a short form of Lorenzo.
Renz, Renzy, Renzzo

Reshad (American) a form of Rashad.
Reshade, Reshard, Resharrd, Reshaud, Reshawd, Reshead, Reshod

Reshawn (American) a combination of the prefix Re + Shawn.
Reshaun, Reshaw, Reshon, Reshun

Reshean (American) a combination of the prefix Re + Sean.
Resean, Reshae, Reshane, Reshay, Reshayne, Reshea, Resheen, Reshey

Reuben (Hebrew) behold a son.
Reuban, Reubin, Reuven, Rheuben, Rhuben, Rube, Ruben, Rubey, Rubin, Ruby, Rueben

Reuven (Hebrew) a form of Reuben.
Reuvin, Rouvin, Ruvim

Rex (Latin) king.
Rexx

Rexford (English) king's ford.

Rexton (English) king's town.

Rey (Spanish) a short form of Reynaldo, Reynard, Reynold.

Reyes (English) a form of Reece.
Reyce

Reyhan (Arabic) favored by God.
Reyham

Reymond (English) a form of Raymond.
Reymon. Reymound, Reymund

Reymundo (Spanish) a form of Raymond.
Reimond, Reimonde, Reimundo, Reymon

Reynaldo (Spanish) a form of Reynold.
Renaldo, Rey, Reynauldo

Reynard (French) wise; bold, courageous.
Raynard, Reinhard, Reinhardt, Reinhart, Renard, Renardo, Renaud, Rennard, Rey, Reynardo, Reynaud

Reynold (English) king's advisor. See also Reginald.
Rainault, Rainhold, Ranald, Raynald, Raynaldo, Reinald, Reinaldo, Reinaldos, Reinhart, Reinhold, Reinold, Reinwald, Renald, Renaldi, Renaldo, Renaud, Renauld, Rennold, Renold, Rey, Reynald, Reynaldo, Reynaldos, Reynol, Reynolds, Rinaldo, Ronald

Réz (Hungarian) copper; red-head.
Rezsö

Rhett (Welsh) a form of Rhys. Literature: Rhett Butler was the hero of Margaret Mitchell's novel *Gone with the Wind*.
Rhet

Rhodes (Greek) where roses grow. Geography: an island of southeast Greece.
Rhoads, Rhodas, Rodas

Rhyan (Irish) a form of Rian.
Rhian

Rhys (Welsh) a form of Reece, Reese.
Rhett, Rhyce, Rhyse, Rice

Rian (Irish) little king.
Rhyan

Ric (Italian, Spanish) a short form of Rico.
Ricca, Ricci, Ricco

Ricardo (Portuguese, Spanish) a form of Richard.
Racardo, Recard, Ricaldo, Ricard, Ricardoe, Ricardos, Riccardo, Riccarrdo, Ricciardo, Richardo

Rice (English) rich, noble. (Welsh) a form of Reece.
Ryce

Rich (English) a short form of Richard.
Ritch

Richard (English) a form of Richart. See also Aric, Dick, Juku, Likeke.
Rashard, Reku, Ricardo, Rich, Richar, Richards, Richardson, Richart, Richaud, Richer, Richerd, Richie, Richird, Richshard, Rick, Rickard, Rickert, Rickey, Ricky, Rico, Rihardos, Rihards, Rikard, Riocard, Riócard, Risa, Risardas, Rishard, Ristéard, Ritchard, Rostik, Rye, Rysio, Ryszard

Richart (German) rich and powerful ruler.

Richie (English) a familiar form of Richard.
Richey, Richi, Richy, Rishi, Ritchie

Richman (English) powerful.

Richmond (German) powerful protector.
Richmon, Richmound

Rick (German, English) a short form of Cedric, Frederick, Richard.
Ric, Ricke, Rickey, Ricks, Ricky, Rik, Riki, Rykk

Rickard (Swedish) a form of Richard.

Ricker (English) powerful army.

Rickey (English) a familiar form of Richard, Rick, Riqui.

Rickie (English) a form of
Ricky.
Rickee, Ricki

Rickward (English) mighty
guardian.
Rickwerd, Rickwood

Ricky (English) a familiar form
of Richard, Rick.
*Ricci, Rickie, Riczi, Riki,
Rikki, Rikky, Riqui*

Rico (Spanish) a familiar form
of Richard. (Italian) a short
form of Enrico.
Ric, Ricco

Rida (Arabic) favor.

Riddock (Irish) smooth field.
Riddick

Rider (English) horseman.
Ridder, Ryder

Ridge (English) ridge of a
cliff.
Ridgy, Rig, Rigg

Ridgeley (English) meadow
near the ridge.
*Ridgeleigh, Ridglea, Ridglee,
Ridgleigh, Ridgley*

Ridgeway (English) path along
the ridge.

Ridley (English) meadow of
reeds.
*Rhidley, Riddley, Ridlea,
Ridleigh, Ridly*

Riel (Spanish) a short form of
Gabriel.

Rigby (English) ruler's valley.

Rigel (Arabic) foot.
Astronomy: one of the stars
in the constellation Orion.

Rigg (English) ridge.
Rigo

Rigoberto (German) splendid;
wealthy.
Rigobert

Rikard (Scandinavian) a form
of Richard.
Rikárd

Riki (Estonian) a form of
Rick.
Rikkey, Rikki, Riks, Riky

Riley (Irish) valiant.
*Reilly, Rhiley, Rhylee, Rhyley,
Rieley, Rielly, Riely, Rilee,
Rilley, Rily, Rilye, Rylee, Ryley*

Rinaldo (Italian) a form of
Reynold.
Rinald, Rinaldi

Ring (English) ring.
Ringo

Ringo (Japanese) apple.
(English) a familiar form of
Ring.

Rio (Spanish) river.
Geography: Rio de Janeiro is
a city in Brazil.

Riordan (Irish) bard, royal
poet.
Rearden, Reardin, Reardon

Rip (Dutch) ripe; full grown.
(English) a short form of
Ripley.
Ripp

Ripley (English) meadow near
the river.
Rip, Ripleigh, Ripply

Riqui (Spanish) a form of
Rickey.

Rishad (American) a form of
Rashad.
Rishaad

Rishawn (American) a combi-
nation of the prefix Ri +
Shawn.
*Rishan, Rishaun, Rishon,
Rishone*

Rishi (Hindi) sage.

Risley (English) meadow with
shrubs.
*Rislea, Rislee, Risleigh, Risly,
Wrisley*

Risto (Finnish) a short form of
Christopher.

Riston (English) settlement
near the shrubs.
Wriston

Ritchard (English) a form of
Richard.
*Ritcherd, Ritchyrd, Ritshard,
Ritsherd*

Ritchie (English) a form of
Richie.
Ritchy

Rithisak (Cambodian) powerful.

Ritter (German) knight;
chivalrous.
Rittner

River (English) river;
riverbank.
Rivers, Riviera, Rivor

Riyad (Arabic) gardens.
*Riad, Riyaad, Riyadh, Riyaz,
Riyod*

Roald (Norwegian) famous
ruler.

Roan (English) a short form of
Rowan.
Rhoan

Roar (Norwegian) praised
warrior.
Roary

Roarke (Irish) famous ruler.
Roark, Rorke, Rourke, Ruark

Rob (English) a short form of
Robert.
Robb, Robe

Robbie (English) a familiar
form of Robert.
Robie, Robbi

Robby (English) a familiar
form of Robert.
Rhobbie, Robbey, Robhy, Roby

Robert (English) famous bril-
liance. See also Bobek, Dob,
Lopaka.
Bob, Bobby, Rab, Rabbie, Raby,

Riobard, Riobart, Rob, Robars, Robart, Robbie, Robby, Rober, Roberd, Robers, Roberte, Roberto, Roberts, Robin, Robinson, Roibeárd, Rosertas, Rubert, Ruberto, Rudbert, Rupert

Roberto (Italian, Portuguese, Spanish) a form of Robert.

Roberts, Robertson (English) son of Robert.
Roberson, Robertson, Robeson, Robinson, Robson

Robin (English) a short form of Robert.
Robben, Robbin, Robbins, Robbyn, Roben, Robinet, Robinn, Robins, Robyn, Roibín

Robinson (English) a form of Roberts.
Robbinson, Robens, Robenson, Robson, Robynson

Robyn (English) a form of Robin.

Rocco (Italian) rock.
Rocca, Rocio, Rocko, Rocky, Roko, Roque

Rochester (English) rocky fortress.
Chester, Chet

Rock (English) a short form of Rockwell.
Roch, Rocky

Rockford (English) rocky ford.

Rockland (English) rocky land.

Rockledge (English) rocky ledge.

Rockley (English) rocky field.
Rockle

Rockwell (English) rocky spring. Art: Norman Rockwell was a well-known twentieth-century American illustrator.
Rock

Rocky (American) a familiar form of Rocco, Rock.
Rockey, Rockie

Rod (English) a short form of Penrod, Roderick, Rodney.
Rodd

Rodas (Greek, Spanish) a form of Rhodes.

Roddy (English) a familiar form of Roderick.
Roddie, Rody

Roden (English) red valley. Art: Auguste Rodin was an innovative French sculptor.
Rodin

Roderich (German) a form of Roderick.

Roderick (German) famous ruler. See also Broderick.
Rhoderick, Rod, Rodderick, Roddy, Roderic, Roderich, Roderigo, Roderik, Roderrick, Roderyck, Rodgrick, Rodrick, Rodricki, Rodrigo, Rodrigue,

Roderick *(cont.)*
Rodrugue, Roodney, Rory,
Rurik, Ruy

Rodger (German) a form of
Roger.
Rodge, Rodgy

Rodman (German) famous
man, hero.
Rodmond

Rodney (English) island clear-
ing.
Rhodney, Rod, Rodnee, Rodnei,
Rodni, Rodnie, Rodnne, Rodny

Rodolfo (Spanish) a form of
Rudolph.
Rodolpho, Rodulfo

Rodrick (German) a form of
Roderick.
Roddrick, Rodric, Rodrich,
Rodrik, Rodrique, Rodryck,
Rodryk

Rodrigo (Italian, Spanish) a
form of Roderick.

Rodriguez (Spanish) son of
Rodrigo.
Roddrigues, Rodrigues,
Rodriquez

Rodrik (German) famous
ruler.

Rodriquez (Spanish) a form of
Rodriguez.
Rodrigquez, Rodriques,
Rodriquiez

Roe (English) roe deer.
Row, Rowe

Rogan (Irish) redhead.
Rogein, Rogen

Rogelio (Spanish) famous
warrior.
Rojelio

Roger (German) famous spear-
man. See also Lokela.
Rodger, Rog, Rogelio, Rogerick,
Rogerio, Rogers, Rogiero, Rojelio,
Rüdiger, Ruggerio, Rutger

Rogerio (Portuguese, Spanish)
a form of Roger.
Rogerios

Rohan (Hindi) sandalwood.

Rohin (Hindi) upward path.

Rohit (Hindi) big and beautiful fish.

Roi (French) a form of Roy.

Roja (Spanish) red.
Rojay

Roland (German) famous
throughout the land.
Loránd, Orlando, Rawlins, Rolan,
Rolanda, Rolando, Rolek,
Rolland, Rolle, Rollie, Rollin,
Rollo, Rowe, Rowland, Ruland

Rolando (Portuguese, Spanish)
a form of Roland.
Lando, Olo, Roldan, Roldán,
Rolondo

Rolf (German) a form of
Ralph. A short form of
Rudolph.
Rolfe, Rolle, Rolph, Rolphe

Rolle (Swedish) a familiar form of Roland, Rolf.

Rollie (English) a familiar form of Roland.
Roley, Rolle, Rolli, Rolly

Rollin (English) a form of Roland.
Rolin, Rollins

Rollo (English) a familiar form of Roland.
Rolla, Rolo

Rolon (Spanish) famous wolf.

Romain (French) a form of Roman.
Romaine, Romane, Romanne

Roman (Latin) from Rome, Italy.
Roma, Romain, Romann, Romanos, Romman, Romochka, Romy

Romanos (Greek) a form of Roman.
Romano

Romario (Italian) a form of Romeo.
Romar, Romarius, Romaro, Romarrio

Romel (Latin) a short form of Romulus.
Romele, Romell, Romello, Rommel

Romello (Italian) of Romel.
Romelo, Rommello

Romeo (Italian) pilgrim to Rome; Roman. Literature: the title character of the Shakespearean play *Romeo and Juliet*.
Romario, Roméo, Romero

Romero (Latin) a form of Romeo.
Romario, Romeiro, Romer, Romere, Romerio, Romeris, Romeryo

Romney (Welsh) winding river.
Romoney

Romulus (Latin) citizen of Rome. Mythology: Romulus and his twin brother, Remus, founded Rome.
Romel, Romolo, Romono, Romulo

Romy (Italian) a familiar form of Roman.
Rommie, Rommy

Ron (Hebrew) a short form of Aaron, Ronald.
Ronn

Ronald (Scottish) a form of Reginald.
Ranald, Ron, Ronal, Ronaldo, Ronnald, Ronney, Ronnie, Ronnold, Ronoldo

Ronaldo (Portuguese) a form of Ronald.

Rónán (Irish) seal.
Renan, Ronan, Ronat

Rondel (French) short poem.
*Rondal, Rondale, Rondall,
Rondeal, Rondell, Rondey,
Rondie, Rondrell, Rondy, Ronel*

Ronel (American) a form of
Rondel.
*Ronell, Ronelle, Ronnel,
Ronnell, Ronyell*

Roni (Hebrew) my song; my
joy.
*Rani, Roneet, Roney, Ronit,
Ronli, Rony*

Ronnie (Scottish) a familiar
form of Ronald.
Roni, Ronie, Ronnie, Ronny

Ronny (Scottish) a form of
Ronnie.
Ronney

Ronson (Scottish) son of
Ronald.
Ronaldson

Ronté (American) a combination of Ron + the suffix Te.
Rontae, Rontay, Ronte, Rontez

Rooney (Irish) redhead.

Roosevelt (Dutch) rose field.
History: Theodore and
Franklin D. Roosevelt were
the twenty-sixth and thirty-
second U.S. presidents,
respectively.
Roosvelt, Rosevelt

Roper (English) rope maker.

Rory (German) a familiar
form of Roderick. (Irish) red
king.
Rorey, Rori, Rorrie, Rorry

Rosalio (Spanish) rose.
Rosalino

Rosario (Portuguese) rosary.

Roscoe (Scandinavian) deer
forest.
Rosco

Roshad (American) a form of
Rashad.
Roshard

Roshean (American) a combi-
nation of the prefix Ro +
Sean.
*Roshain, Roshan, Roshane,
Roshaun, Roshawn, Roshay,
Rosheen, Roshene*

Rosito (Filipino) rose.

Ross (Latin) rose. (Scottish)
peninsula. (French) red.
*Rosse, Rossell, Rossi, Rossie,
Rossy*

Rosswell (English) springtime
of roses.
Rosvel

Rostislav (Czech) growing
glory.
Rosta, Rostya

Roswald (English) field of
roses.
Ross, Roswell

Roth (German) redhead.

Rothwell (Scandinavian) red spring.

Rover (English) traveler.

Rowan (English) tree with red berries.
Roan, Rowe, Rowen, Rowney, Rowyn

Rowell (English) roe-deer well.

Rowland (English) rough land. (German) a form of Roland.
Rowlando, Rowlands, Rowlandson

Rowley (English) rough meadow.
Rowlea, Rowlee, Rowleigh, Rowly

Rowson (English) son of the redhead.

Roxbury (English) rook's town or fortress.
Roxburghe

Roy (French) king. A short form of Royal, Royce. See also Conroy, Delroy, Fitzroy, Leroy, Loe.
Rey, Roi, Roye, Ruy

Royal (French) kingly, royal.
Roy, Royale, Royall, Royell

Royce (English) son of Roy.
Roice, Roy, Royz

Royden (English) rye hill.
Royd, Roydan

Ruben (Hebrew) a form of Reuben.
Ruban, Rube, Rubean, Rubens, Rubin, Ruby

Rubert (Czech) a form of Robert.

Ruby (Hebrew) a familiar form of Reuben, Ruben.

Rudd (English) a short form of Rudyard.

Ruda (Czech) a form of Rudolph.
Rude, Rudek

Rudi (Spanish) a familiar form of Rudolph.
Ruedi

Rudo (Shona) love.

Rudolf (German) a form of Rudolph.
Rodolf, Rodolfo, Rudolfo

Rudolph (German) famous wolf. See also Dolf.
Raoul, Rezsó, Rodolfo, Rodolph, Rodolphe, Rolf, Ruda, Rudek, Rudi, Rudolf, Rudolpho, Rudolphus, Rudy

Rudolpho (Italian) a form of Rudolph.

Rudy (English) a familiar form of Rudolph.
Roody, Ruddy, Ruddie, Rudey, Rudi, Rudie

Rudyard (English) red enclosure.
Rudd

Rueben (Hebrew) a form of
Reuben.
Rueban, Ruebin

Ruff (French) redhead.

Rufin (Polish) redhead.
Rufino

Ruford (English) red ford; ford
with reeds.
Rufford

Rufus (Latin) redhead.
*Rayfus, Rufe, Ruffis, Ruffus,
Rufino, Rufo, Rufous*

Rugby (English) rook fortress.
History: a famous British
school after which the sport
of Rugby was named.

Ruggerio (Italian) a form of
Roger.
Rogero, Ruggero, Ruggiero

Ruhakana (Rukiga) argumen-
tative.

Ruland (German) a form of
Roland.
Rulan, Rulon, Rulondo

Rumford (English) wide river
crossing.

Runako (Shona) handsome.

Rune (German, Swedish)
secret.

Runrot (Tai) prosperous.

Rupert (German) a form of
Robert.
Ruperth, Ruperto, Ruprecht

Ruperto (Italian) a form of
Rupert.

Ruprecht (German) a form of
Rupert.

Rush (French) redhead.
(English) a short form of
Russell.
Rushi

Rushford (English) ford with
rushes.

Rusk (Spanish) twisted bread.

Ruskin (French) redhead.
Rush, Russ

Russ (French) a short form of
Russell.

Russel (French) a form of
Russell.

Russell (French) redhead; fox
colored. See also Lukela.
*Roussell, Rush, Russ, Russel,
Russelle, Rusty*

Rusty (French) a familiar form
of Russell.
*Ruste, Rusten, Rustie, Rustin,
Ruston, Rustyn*

Rutger (Scandinavian) a form
of Roger.
Ruttger

Rutherford (English) cattle
ford.
Rutherfurd

Rutland (Scandinavian) red land.

Rutledge (English) red ledge.

Rutley (English) red meadow.

Ruy (Spanish) a short form of Roderick.
Rui

Ryan (Irish) little king.
Rayan, Rhyan, Rhyne, Ryane, Ryann, Ryen, Ryian, Ryiann, Ryin, Ryne, Ryon, Ryuan, Ryun, Ryyan

Rycroft (English) rye field.
Ryecroft

Ryder (English) a form of Rider.
Rydder, Rye

Rye (English) a short form of Ryder. A grain used in cereal and whiskey. (Gypsy) gentleman.
Ry.

Ryen (Irish) a form of Ryan.
Ryein, Ryien

Ryerson (English) son of Rider, Ryder.

Ryese (English) a form of Reece.
Reyse, Ryez, Ryse

Ryker (American) a surname used as a first name.
Riker, Ryk

Rylan (English) land where rye is grown.
Ryland, Rylean, Rylen, Rylin, Rylon, Rylyn, Rylynn

Ryland (English) a form of Rylan.
Ryeland, Rylund

Ryle (English) rye hill.
Ryal, Ryel

Rylee (Irish) a form of Riley.
Ryeleigh, Ryleigh, Rylie, Rillie

Ryley (Irish) a form of Riley.
Ryely

Ryman (English) rye seller.

Ryne (Irish) a form of Ryan.
Rynn

Ryon (Irish) a form of Ryan.

S

Sabastian (Greek) a form of Sebastian.
Sabastain, Sabastiano, Sabastien, Sabastin, Sabastion, Sabaston, Sabbastiun, Sabestian

Saber (French) sword.
Sabir, Sabre

Sabin (Basque) ancient tribe of central Italy.
Saban, Saben, Sabian, Sabien, Sabino

Sabiti (Rutooro) born on Sunday.

Sabola (Nguni) pepper.

Saburo (Japanese) third-born son.

Sacha (Russian) a form of Sasha.
Sascha

Sachar (Russian) a form of Zachary.

Saddam (Arabic) powerful ruler.

Sadiki (Swahili) faithful.
Saadiq, Sadeek, Sadek, Sadik, Sadiq, Sadique

Sadler (English) saddle maker.
Saddler

Safari (Swahili) born while traveling.
Safa, Safarian

Safford (English) willow river crossing.

Sage (English) wise. Botany: an herb.
Sagen, Sager, Saige, Saje

Sahale (Native American) falcon.
Sael, Sahal, Sahel, Sahil

Sahen (Hindi) above.
Sahan

Sahil (Native American) a form of Sahale.
Saheel, Sahel

Sahir (Hindi) friend.

Sa'id (Arabic) happy.
Sa'ad, Saaid, Saed, Sa'eed, Saeed, Sahid, Saide, Sa'ied, Saied, Saiyed, Saiyeed, Sajid, Sajjid, Sayed, Sayeed, Sayid, Seyed, Shahid

Sajag (Hindi) watchful.

Saka (Swahili) hunter.

Sakeri (Danish) a form of Zachary.
Sakarai, Sakari

Sakima (Native American) king.

Sakuruta (Pawnee) coming sun.

Sal (Italian) a short form of Salvatore.

Salam (Arabic) lamb.
Salaam

Salamon (Spanish) a form of Solomon.
Saloman, Salomón

Salaun (French) a form of Solomon.

Sálih (Arabic) right, good.
Saleeh, Saleh, Salehe

Salim (Swahili) peaceful.

Salím (Arabic) peaceful, safe.
Saleem, Salem, Saliym, Salman

Salmalin (Hindi) taloned.

Salman (Czech) a form of
Salím, Solomon.
Salmaan, Salmaine, Salmon

Salomon (French) a form of
Solomon.
Salomone

Salton (English) manor town;
willow town.

Salvador (Spanish) savior.
Salvadore

Salvatore (Italian) savior. See
also Xavier.
*Sal, Salbatore, Sallie, Sally,
Salvator, Salvattore, Salvidor,
Sauveur*

Sam (Hebrew) a short form of
Samuel.
*Samm, Sammy, Sem, Shem,
Shmuel*

Sambo (American) a familiar
form of Samuel.
Sambou

Sameer (Arabic) a form of
Samír.

Sami, Samy (Hebrew) forms
of Sammy.
*Sameeh, Sameh, Samie, Samih,
Sammi*

Samír (Arabic) entertaining
companion.
Sameer

Samman (Arabic) grocer.
Saman, Sammon

Sammy (Hebrew) a familiar
form of Samuel.
*Saamy, Samey, Sami, Sammee,
Sammey, Sammie, Samy*

Samo (Czech) a form of
Samuel.
Samho, Samko

Samson (Hebrew) like the
sun. Bible: a judge and pow-
erful warrior betrayed by
Delilah.
*Sampson, Sansao, Sansom,
Sansón, Shem, Shimshon*

Samual (Hebrew) a form of
Samuel.
Samuael, Samuail

Samuel (Hebrew) heard God;
asked of God. Bible: a
famous Old Testament
prophet and judge. See also
Kamuela, Zamiel, Zanvil.
*Sam, Samael, Samaru,
Samauel, Samaul, Sambo,
Sameul, Samiel, Sammail,
Sammel, Sammuel, Sammy,
Samo, Samouel, Samu, Samual,
Samuele, Samuelis, Samuell,
Samuello, Samuil, Samuka,
Samule, Samuru, Samvel,
Sanko, Saumel, Schmuel, Shem,
Shmuel, Simão, Simuel,
Somhairle, Zamuel*

Samuele (Italian) a form of
Samuel.
Samulle

Samuru (Japanese) a form of
Samuel.

Sanat (Hindi) ancient.

Sanborn (English) sandy brook.
Sanborne, Sanbourn, Sanbourne, Sanburn, Sanburne, Sandborn, Sandbourne

Sanchez (Latin) a form of Sancho.
Sanchaz, Sancheze

Sancho (Latin) sanctified; sincere. Literature: Sancho Panza was Don Quixote's squire.
Sanchez, Sauncho

Sandeep (Punjabi) enlightened.
Sandip

Sander (English) a short form of Alexander, Lysander.
Sandor, Sándor, Saunder

Sanders (English) son of Sander.
Sanderson, Saunders, Saunderson

Sándor (Hungarian) a short form of Alexander.
Sanyi

Sandro (Greek, Italian) a short form of Alexander.
Sandero, Sandor, Sandre, Saundro, Shandro

Sandy (English) a familiar form of Alexander.
Sande, Sandey, Sandi, Sandie

Sanford (English) sandy river crossing.
Sandford

Sani (Hindi) the planet Saturn. (Navajo) old.

Sanjay (American) a combination of Sanford + Jay.
Sanjaya, Sanje, Sanjey, Sanjo

Sanjiv (Hindi) long lived.
Sanjeev

Sankar (Hindi) a form of Shankara, another name for the Hindu god Shiva.

Sansón (Spanish) a form of Samson.
Sanson, Sansone, Sansun

Santana (Spanish) History: Antonio López de Santa Anna was a Mexican general and political leader.
Santanna

Santiago (Spanish) a form of James.

Santino (Spanish) a form of Santonio.
Santion

Santo (Italian, Spanish) holy.
Santos

Santon (English) sandy town.

Santonio (Spanish) Geography: a short form of San Antonio, a city in Texas.
Santino, Santon, Santoni

Santos (Spanish) saint.
Santo

Santosh (Hindi) satisfied.

Sanyu (Luganda) happy.

Saqr (Arabic) falcon.

Saquan (American) a combination of the prefix Sa + Quan.
Saquané, Saquin, Saquon, Saqwan, Saqwone

Sarad (Hindi) born in the autumn.

Sargent (French) army officer.
Sargant, Sarge, Sarjant, Sergeant, Sergent, Serjeant

Sarito (Spanish) a form of Caesar.
Sarit

Sariyah (Arabic) clouds at night.

Sarngin (Hindi) archer; protector.

Sarojin (Hindi) like a lotus.
Sarojun

Sasha (Russian) a short form of Alexander.
Sacha, Sash, Sashenka, Sashka, Sashok, Sausha

Sasson (Hebrew) joyful.
Sason

Satchel (French) small bag.
Satch

Satordi (French) Saturn.
Satori

Saul (Hebrew) asked for, borrowed. Bible: in the Old Testament, a king of Israel and the father of Jonathan; in the New Testament, Saint Paul's original name was Saul.
Saül, Shaul, Sol, Solly

Saverio (Italian) a form of Xavier.

Saville (French) willow town.
Savelle, Savil, Savile, Savill, Savylle, Seville, Siville

Savon (Spanish) a treeless plain.
Savan, Savaughn, Saveion, Saveon, Savhon, Saviahn, Savian, Savino, Savion, Savo, Savone, Sayvon, Sayvone

Saw (Burmese) early.

Sawyer (English) wood worker.
Sawyere

Sax (English) a short form of Saxon.
Saxe

Saxon (English) swordsman. History: the Roman name for the Teutonic raiders who ravaged the Roman British coasts.
Sax, Saxen, Saxsin, Saxxon

Sayer (Welsh) carpenter.
Say, Saye, Sayers, Sayr, Sayre,
Sayres

Sayyid (Arabic) master.
Sayed, Sayid, Sayyad, Sayyed

Scanlon (Irish) little trapper.
Scanlan, Scanlen

Schafer (German) shepherd.
Schaefer, Schaffer, Schiffer,
Shaffar, Shäffer

Schmidt (German)
blacksmith.
Schmid, Schmit, Schmitt,
Schmydt

Schneider (German) tailor.
Schnieder, Snider, Snyder

Schön (German) handsome.
Schoen, Schönn, Shon

Schuyler (Dutch) sheltering.
Schuylar, Schyler, Scoy, Scy,
Skuyler, Sky, Skylar, Skyler,
Skylor

Schyler (Dutch) a form of
Schuyler.
Schylar, Schylre, Schylur

Scorpio (Latin) dangerous,
deadly. Astronomy: a southern constellation near Libra
and Sagittarius. Astrology: the
eighth sign of the zodiac.
Scorpeo

Scott (English) from Scotland.
A familiar form of Prescott.
Scot, Scottie, Scotto, Scotty

Scottie (English) a familiar
form of Scott.
Scotie, Scotti

Scotty (English) a familiar
form of Scott.
Scottey

Scoville (French) Scott's town.

Scully (Irish) town crier.

Seabert (English) shining sea.
Seabright, Sebert, Seibert

Seabrook (English) brook
near the sea.

Seamus (Irish) a form of
James.
Seamas, Seumas, Shamus

Sean (Hebrew) God is gra-
cious. (Irish) a form of John.
Seaghan, Séan, Seán, Seanán,
Seane, Seann, Shaan, Shaine,
Shane, Shaun, Shawn, Shayne,
Shon, Siôn

Searlas (Irish, French) a form
of Charles.
Séarlas, Searles, Searlus

Searle (English) armor.

Seasar (Latin) a form of Caesar.
Seasare, Seazar, Sesar, Sesear,
Sezar

Seaton (English) town near
the sea.
Seeton, Seton

Sebastian (Greek) venerable.
(Latin) revered.
Bastian, Sabastian, Sabastien,

Sebashtian, Sebastain,
Sebastiane, Sebastiano,
Sebastien, Sébastien, Sebastin,
Sebastine, Sebastion, Sebbie,
Sebestyén, Sebo, Sepasetiano

Sebastien, Sébastien
(French) forms of Sebastian.
Sebasten, Sebastyen

Sebastion (Greek) a form of
Sebastian.

Sedgely (English) sword
meadow.
Sedgeley, Sedgly

Sedric (Irish) a form of Cedric.
Seddrick, Sederick, Sedrick,
Sedrik, Sedriq

Seeley (English) blessed.
Sealey, Seely, Selig

Sef (Egyptian) yesterday.
Mythology: one of the two
lions that make up the
Akeru, guardian of the gates
of morning and night.

Sefton (English) village of
rushes.

Sefu (Swahili) sword.

Seger (English) sea spear; sea
warrior.
Seager, Seeger, Segar

Segun (Yoruba) conqueror.

Segundo (Spanish) second.

Seibert (English) bright sea.
Seabert, Sebert

Seif (Arabic) religion's sword.

Seifert (German) a form of
Siegfried.

Sein (Basque) innocent.

Sekaye (Shona) laughter.

Selby (English) village by the
mansion.
Selbey, Shelby

Seldon (English) willow tree
valley.
Selden, Sellden

Selig (German) a form of
Seeley.
Seligman, Seligmann, Zelig

Selwyn (English) friend from
the palace.
Selvin, Selwin, Selwinn,
Selwynn, Selwynne, Wyn

Semanda (Luganda) cow clan.

Semer (Ethiopian) a form of
George.
Semere, Semier

Semon (Greek) a form of
Simon.
Semion

Sempala (Luganda) born in
prosperous times.

Sen (Japanese) wood fairy.
Senh

Sener (Turkish) bringer of joy.

Senior (French) lord.

Sennett (French) elderly.
Sennet

Senon (Spanish) living.

Senwe (African) dry as a grain stalk.

Sepp (German) a form of Joseph.
Seppi

Septimus (Latin) seventh.

Serafino (Portuguese) a form of Seraphim.

Seraphim (Hebrew) fiery, burning. Bible: the highest order of angels, known for their zeal and love.
Saraf, Saraph, Serafim, Serafin, Serafino, Seraphimus, Seraphin

Sereno (Latin) calm, tranquil.

Serge (Latin) attendant.
Seargeoh, Serg, Sergei, Sergio, Sergios, Sergius, Sergiusz, Serguel, Sirgio, Sirgios

Sergei (Russian) a form of Serge.
Sergey, Sergeyuk, Serghey, Sergi, Sergie, Sergo, Sergunya, Serhiy, Serhiyko, Serjiro, Serzh

Sergio (Italian) a form of Serge.
Serginio, Serigo, Serjio

Servando (Spanish) to serve.
Servan, Servio

Seth (Hebrew) appointed. Bible: the third son of Adam.
Set, Sethan, Sethe, Shet

Setimba (Luganda) river dweller. Geography: a river in Uganda.

Seumas (Scottish) a form of James.
Seaumus

Severiano (Italian) a form of Séverin.

Séverin (French) severe.
Seve, Sevé, Severan, Severian, Severiano, Severo, Sevien, Sevrin, Sevryn

Severn (English) boundary.
Sevearn, Sevren, Sevrnn

Sevilen (Turkish) beloved.

Seward (English) sea guardian.
Sewerd, Siward

Sewati (Moquelumnan) curved bear claws.

Sexton (English) church official; sexton.

Sextus (Latin) sixth.
Sixtus

Seymour (French) prayer. Religion: name honoring Saint Maur. See also Maurice.
Seamor, Seamore, Seamour, See

Shabouh (Armenian) king, noble. History: a fourth-century Persian king.

Shad (Punjabi) happy-go-lucky.
Shadd

Shadi (Arabic) singer.
Shadde, Shaddi, Shaddy, Shade, Shadee, Shadeed, Shadey, Shadie, Shady, Shydee, Shydi

Shadrach (Babylonian) god; godlike. Bible: one of three companions who emerged unharmed from the fiery furnace of Babylon.
Shad, Shadrack, Shadrick, Sheddrach, Shedrach, Shedrick

Shadwell (English) shed by a well.

Shah (Persian) king. History: a title for rulers of Iran.

Shaheem (American) a combination of Shah + Raheem.
Shaheim, Shahiem, Shahm

Shahid (Arabic) a form of Sa'id.
Shahed, Shaheed

Shai (Hebrew) a short form of Yeshaya.
Shaie

Shaiming (Chinese) life; sunshine.

Shaine (Irish) a form of Sean.
Shain

Shaka (Zulu) founder, first. History: Shaka Zulu was the founder of the Zulu empire.

Shakeel (Arabic) a form of Shaquille.
Shakeil, Shakel, Shakell, Shakiel, Shakil, Shakille, Shakyle

Shakir (Arabic) thankful.
Shaakir, Shakeer, Shakeir, Shakur

Shakur (Arabic) a form of Shakir.
Shakuur

Shalom (Hebrew) peace.
Shalum, Shlomo, Sholem, Sholom

Shalya (Hindi) throne.

Shaman (Sanskrit) holy man, mystic, medicine man.
Shamaine, Shamaun, Shamin, Shamine, Shammon, Shamon, Shamone

Shamar (Hebrew) a form of Shamir.
Shamaar, Shamare, Shamari

Shamir (Hebrew) precious stone.
Shahmeer, Shahmir, Shamar, Shameer, Shamyr

Shamus (American) slang for detective.
Shamas, Shames, Shamos, Shemus

Shan (Irish) a form of Shane.
Shann, Shanne

Shanahan (Irish) wise, clever.

Shandy (English) rambunctious.
Shandey, Shandie

Shane (Irish) a form of Sean.
Shan, Shayn, Shayne

Shangobunni (Yoruba) gift from Shango.

Shanley (Irish) small; ancient.
Shaneley, Shannley

Shannon (Irish) small and wise.
Shanan, Shannan, Shannen, Shannin, Shannone, Shanon

Shantae (French) a form of Chante.
Shant, Shanta, Shantai, Shante, Shantell, Shantelle, Shanti, Shantia, Shantie, Shanton, Shanty

Shap (English) a form of Shep.

Shaquan (American) a combination of the prefix Sha + Quan.
Shaqaun, Shaquand, Shaquane, Shaquann, Shaquaunn, Shaquawn, Shaquen, Shaquian, Shaquin, Shaqwan

Shaquell (American) a form of Shaquille.
Shaqueal, Shaqueil, Shaquel, Shaquelle, Shaquiel, Shaquiell, Shaquielle

Shaquille (Arabic) handsome.
Shakeel, Shaquell, Shaquil, Shaquile, Shaquill, Shaqul

Shaquon (American) a combination of the prefix Sha + Quon.
Shaikwon, Shaqon, Shaquoin, Shaquoné

Sharad (Pakistani) autumn.
Sharod

Sharíf (Arabic) honest; noble.
Shareef, Sharef, Shareff, Shareif, Sharief, Sharife, Shariff, Shariyf, Sharrif, Sharyif

Sharod (Pakistani) a form of Sharad.
Sharrod

Sharron (Hebrew) flat area, plain.
Sharon, Sharone, Sharonn, Sharonne

Shattuck (English) little shad fish.

Shaun (Irish) a form of Sean.
Shaughan, Shaughn, Shaugn, Shauna, Shaunahan, Shaune, Shaunn, Shaunne

Shavar (Hebrew) comet.
Shavit

Shavon (American) a combination of the prefix Sha + Yvon.
Shauvan, Shauvon, Shavan, Shavaughn, Shaven, Shavin,

Shavone, Shawan, Shawon, Shawun

Shaw (English) grove.

Shawn (Irish) a form of Sean.
Shawen, Shawne, Shawnee, Shawnn, Shawon

Shawnta (American) a combination of Shawn + the suffix Ta.
Shawntae, Shawntel, Shawnti

Shay (Irish) a form of Shea.
Shae, Shai, Shaya, Shaye, Shey

Shayan (Cheyenne) a form of Cheyenne.
Shayaan, Shayann, Shayon

Shayne (Hebrew) a form of Sean.
Shayn, Shaynne, Shean

Shea (Irish) courteous.
Shay

Shedrick (Babylonian) a form of Shadrach.
Shadriq, Shederick, Shedric, Shedrique

Sheehan (Irish) little; peaceful.
Shean

Sheffield (English) crooked field.
Field, Shef, Sheff, Sheffie, Sheffy

Shel (English) a short form of Shelby, Sheldon, Shelton.

Shelby (English) ledge estate.
Shel, Shelbe, Shelbey, Shelbie, Shell, Shellby, Shelley, Shelly

Sheldon (English) farm on the ledge.
Shel, Sheldan, Shelden, Sheldin, Sheldyn, Shell, Shelley, Shelly, Shelton

Shelley (English) a familiar form of Shelby, Sheldon, Shelton. Literature: Percy Bysshe Shelley was a nineteenth-century British poet.
Shell, Shelly

Shelton (English) town on a ledge.
Shel, Shelley, Shelten

Shem (Hebrew) name; reputation. (English) a short form of Samuel. Bible: Noah's oldest son.

Shen (Egyptian) sacred amulet. (Chinese) meditation.

Shep (English) a short form of Shepherd.
Shap, Ship, Shipp

Shepherd (English) shepherd.
Shep, Shepard, Shephard, Shepp, Sheppard, Shepperd

Shepley (English) sheep meadow.
Sheplea, Sheplee, Shepply, Shipley

Sherborn (English) clear brook.
Sherborne, Sherbourn, Sherburn, Sherburne

Sheridan (Irish) wild.
*Dan, Sheredan, Sheriden,
Sheridon, Sherridan*

Sherill (English) shire on a
hill.
Sheril, Sherril, Sherrill

Sherlock (English) light
haired. Literature: Sherlock
Holmes is a famous British
detective character, created
by Sir Arthur Conan Doyle.
Sherlocke, Shurlock, Shurlocke

Sherman (English) sheep
shearer; resident of a shire.
*Scherman, Schermann, Sherm,
Shermain, Shermaine,
Shermann, Shermie, Shermon,
Shermy*

Sherrod (English) clearer of
the land.
*Sherod, Sherrad, Sherrard,
Sherrodd*

Sherwin (English) swift run-
ner, one who cuts the wind.
*Sherveen, Shervin, Sherwan,
Sherwind, Sherwinn, Sherwyn,
Sherwynd, Sherwynne, Win*

Sherwood (English) bright
forest.
Sherwoode, Shurwood, Woody

Shihab (Arabic) blaze.

Shilín (Chinese) intellectual.
Shilan

Shiloh (Hebrew) God's gift.
*Shi, Shile, Shiley, Shilo, Shiloe,
Shy, Shyle, Shylo, Shyloh*

Shimon (Hebrew) a form of
Simon.
Shymon

Shimshon (Hebrew) a form
of Samson.
Shimson

Shing (Chinese) victory.
Shingae, Shingo

Shipton (English) sheep village; ship village.

Shiquan (American) a combi-
nation of the prefix Shi +
Quan.
*Shiquane, Shiquann, Shiquawn,
Shiquoin, Shiqwan*

Shiro (Japanese) fourth-born
son.

Shiva (Hindi) life and death.
Religion: the most common
name for the Hindu god of
destruction and reproduc-
tion.
Shiv, Shivan, Siva

Shlomo (Hebrew) a form of
Solomon.
*Shelmu, Shelomo, Shelomoh,
Shlomi, Shlomot*

Shmuel (Hebrew) a form of
Samuel.
*Shem, Shemuel, Shmelke,
Shmiel, Shmulka*

Shneur (Yiddish) senior.
Shneiur

Shon (German) a form of Schön. (American) a form of Sean.
Shoan, Shoen, Shondae, Shondale, Shondel, Shone, Shonn, Shonntay, Shontae, Shontarious, Shouan, Shoun

Shunnar (Arabic) pheasant.

Si (Hebrew) a short form of Silas, Simon.
Sy

Sid (French) a short form of Sidney.
Cyd, Siddie, Siddy, Sidey, Syd

Siddel (English) wide valley.
Siddell

Siddhartha (Hindi) History: Siddhartha Gautama was the original name of Buddha, the founder of Buddhism.
Sida, Siddartha, Siddhaarth, Siddhart, Siddharth, Sidh, Sidharth, Sidhartha, Sidhdharth

Sidney (French) from Saint-Denis, France.
Cydney, Sid, Sidnee, Sidny, Sidon, Sidonio, Sydney, Sydny

Sidonio (Spanish) a form of Sidney.

Sidwell (English) wide stream.

Siegfried (German) victorious peace. See also Zigfrid, Ziggy.
Seifert, Seifried, Siegfred, Siffre, Sig, Sigfrid, Sigfried, Sigfroi, Sigfryd, Siggy, Sigifredo, Sigvard, Singefrid, Sygfried, Szygfrid

Sierra (Irish) black. (Spanish) saw-toothed.
Siera

Sig (German) a short form of Siegfried, Sigmund.

Sigifredo (German) a form of Siegfried.
Sigefriedo, Sigfrido, Siguefredo

Siggy (German) a familiar form of Siegfried, Sigmund.

Sigmund (German) victorious protector. See also Ziggy, Zsigmond, Zygmunt.
Siegmund, Sig, Siggy, Sigismond, Sigismondo, Sigismund, Sigismundo, Sigismundus, Sigmond, Sigsmond, Szygmond

Sigurd (German, Scandinavian) victorious guardian.
Sigord, Sjure, Syver

Sigwald (German) victorious leader.

Silas (Latin) a short form of Silvan.
Si, Sias, Sylas

Silvan (Latin) forest dweller.
Silas, Silvain, Silvano, Silvaon,
Silvie, Silvio, Sylvain, Sylvan,
Sylvanus, Sylvio

Silvano (Italian) a form of
Silvan.
Silvanos, Silvanus, Silvino

Silvester (Latin) a form of
Sylvester.
Silvestr, Silvestre, Silvestro, Silvy

Silvestro (Italian) a form of
Sylvester.

Silvio (Italian) a form of
Silvan.

Simão (Portuguese) a form of
Samuel.

Simba (Swahili) lion. (Yao) a
short form of Lisimba.
Sim

Simcha (Hebrew) joyful.
Simmy

Simeon (French) a form of
Simon.
Simione, Simone

Simms (Hebrew) son of
Simon.
Simm, Sims

Simmy (Hebrew) a familiar
form of Simcha, Simon.
Simmey, Simmi, Simmie,
Symmy

Simon (Hebrew) he heard.
Bible: one of the Twelve
Disciples. See also

Symington, Ximenes.
Saimon, Samien, Semon,
Shimon, Si, Sim, Simao, Simen,
Simeon, Simion, Simm,
Simmon, Simmonds, Simmons,
Simms, Simmy, Simonas,
Simone, Simson, Simyon,
Slomón, Symon, Szymon

Simpson (Hebrew) son of
Simon.
Simonson, Simson

Sinclair (French) prayer.
Religion: name honoring
Saint Clair.
Sinclare, Synclair

Singh (Hindi) lion.
Sing

Sinjon (English) saint, holy
man. Religion: name honoring Saint John.
Sinjin, Sinjun, Sjohn, Syngen,
Synjen, Synjon

Sipatu (Moquelumnan) pulled
out.

Sipho (Zulu) present.

Siraj (Arabic) lamp, light.

Siseal (Irish) a form of Cecil.

Sisi (Fante) born on Sunday.

Siva (Hindi) a form of Shiva.
Siv

Sivan (Hebrew) ninth month
of the Jewish year.

Siwatu (Swahili) born during a time of conflict.
Siwazuri

Siwili (Native American) long fox's tail.

Skah (Lakota) white.
Skai

Skee (Scandinavian) projectile.
Ski, Skie

Skeeter (English) swift.
Skeat, Skeet, Skeets

Skelly (Irish) storyteller.
Shell, Skelley, Skellie

Skelton (Dutch) shell town.

Skerry (Scandinavian) stony island.

Skip (Scandinavian) a short form of Skipper.

Skipper (Scandinavian) ship-master.
Skip, Skipp, Skippie, Skipton

Skiriki (Pawnee) coyote.

Skule (Norwegian) hidden.

Skye (Dutch) a short form of Skylar, Skyler, Skylor.
Sky

Skylar (Dutch) a form of Schuyler.
Skilar, Skkylar, Skye, Skyelar, Skylaar, Skylare, Skylarr, Skylayr

Skyler (Dutch) a form of Schuyler.
Skieler, Skiler, Skye, Skyeler, Skylee, Skyller

Skylor (Dutch) a form of Schuyler.
Skye, Skyelor, Skyloer, Skylore, Skylour, Skylur, Skylyr

Slade (English) child of the valley.
Slaide, Slayde

Slane (Czech) salty.
Slan

Slater (English) roof slater.
Slader, Slate, Slayter

Slava (Russian) a short form of Stanislav, Vladislav, Vyacheslav.
Slavik, Slavoshka

Slawek (Polish) a short form of Radoslaw.

Slevin (Irish) mountaineer.
Slaven, Slavin, Slawin

Sloan (Irish) warrior.
Sloane, Slone

Smedley (English) flat meadow.
Smedleigh, Smedly

Smith (English) blacksmith.
Schmidt, Smid, Smidt, Smitt, Smitty, Smyth, Smythe

Snowden (English) snowy hill.
Snowdon

Socrates (Greek) wise,
learned. History: a famous
ancient Greek philosopher.
Socratis, Sokrates, Sokratis

Sofian (Arabic) devoted.

Sohrab (Persian) ancient hero.

Soja (Yoruba) soldier.

Sol (Hebrew) a short form of
Saul, Solomon.
Soll, Sollie, Solly

Solly (Hebrew) a familiar
form of Saul, Solomon.
Sollie, Zollie, Zolly

Solomon (Hebrew) peaceful.
Bible: a king of Israel famous
for his wisdom. See also
Zalman.
*Salamen, Salamon, Salamun,
Salaun, Salman, Salomo,
Salomon, Selim, Shelomah,
Shlomo, Sol, Solamh, Solaman,
Solly, Solmon, Soloman,
Solomonas, Sulaiman*

Solon (Greek) wise. History: a
noted ancient Athenian lawmaker.

Somerset (English) place of
the summer settlers.
Literature: William Somerset
Maugham was a well-known
British writer.
*Sommerset, Sumerset,
Summerset*

Somerville (English) summer
village.
*Somerton, Summerton,
Summerville*

Son (Vietnamese) mountain.
(Native American) star.
(English) son, boy. A short
form of Madison, Orson.
Sonny

Songan (Native American)
strong.
Song

Sonny (English) a familiar
form of Grayson, Madison,
Orson, Son.
Soni, Sonnie, Sony

Sono (Akan) elephant.

Sören (Danish) thunder; war.
Sorren

Sorrel (French) reddish
brown.
Sorel, Sorell, Sorrell

Soroush (Persian) happy.

Soterios (Greek) savior.
Soteris, Sotero

Southwell (English) south
well.

Sovann (Cambodian) gold.

Sowande (Yoruba) wise healer
sought me out.

Spalding (English) divided
field.
Spaulding

Spangler (German) tinsmith.
Spengler

Spark (English) happy.
Sparke, Sparkie, Sparky

Spear (English) spear carrier.
Speare, Spears, Speer, Speers, Spiers

Speedy (English) quick; successful.
Speed

Spence (English) a short form of Spencer.
Spense

Spencer (English) dispenser of provisions.
Spence, Spencre, Spenser

Spenser (English) a form of Spencer. Literature: Edmund Spenser was the British poet who wrote *The Faerie Queene*.
Spanser, Spense

Spike (English) ear of grain; long nail.
Spyke

Spiro (Greek) round basket; breath.
Spiridion, Spiridon, Spiros, Spyridon, Spyros

Spoor (English) spur maker.
Spoors

Sproule (English) energetic.
Sprowle

Spurgeon (English) shrub.

Spyros (Greek) a form of Spiro.

Squire (English) knight's assistant; large landholder.

Stacey, Stacy (English) familiar forms of Eustace.
Stace, Stacee

Stafford (English) riverbank landing.
Staffard, Stafforde, Staford

Stamford (English) a form of Stanford.

Stamos (Greek) a form of Stephen.
Stamatis, Stamatos

Stan (Latin, English) a short form of Stanley.

Stanbury (English) stone fortification.
Stanberry, Stanbery, Stanburghe, Stansbury

Stancio (Spanish) a form of Constantine.
Stancy

Stancliff (English) stony cliff.
Stanclife, Stancliffe

Standish (English) stony parkland. History: Miles Standish was a leader in colonial America.

Stane (Slavic) a short form of Stanislaus.

Stanfield (English) stony field.
Stansfield

Stanford (English) rocky ford.
Sandy, Stamford, Stan,
Standford, Stanfield

Stanislaus (Latin) stand of
glory. See also Lao, Tano.
Slavik, Stana, Standa, Stane,
Stanislao, Stanislas, Stanislau,
Stanislav, Stanislus, Stannes,
Stano, Stasik, Stasio

Stanislav (Slavic) a form of
Stanislaus. See also Slava.
Stanislaw

Stanley (English) stony
meadow.
Stan, Stanely, Stanlea, Stanlee,
Stanleigh, Stanly

Stanmore (English) stony
lake.

Stannard (English) hard as
stone.

Stanton (English) stony farm.
Stan, Stanten, Staunton

Stanway (English) stony road.

Stanwick (English) stony village.
Stanwicke, Stanwyck

Stanwood (English) stony
woods.

Starbuck (English) challenger
of fate. Literature: a character
in Herman Melville's novel
Moby-Dick.

Stark (German) strong, vigorous.
Starke, Stärke, Starkie

Starling (English) bird.
Sterling

Starr (English) star.
Star, Staret, Starlight, Starlon,
Starwin

Stasik (Russian) a familiar
form of Stanislaus.
Stas, Stash, Stashka, Stashko,
Stasiek

Stasio (Polish) a form of
Stanislaus.
Stas, Stasiek, Stasiu, Staska,
Stasko

Stavros (Greek) a form of
Stephen.

Steadman (English) owner of
a farmstead.
Steadmann, Stedman, Stedmen,
Steed

Steel (English) like steel.
Steele

Steen (German, Danish)
stone.
Steenn, Stein

Steeve (Greek) a short form
of Steeven.

Steeven (Greek) a form of
Steven.
Steaven, Steavin, Steavon,
Steevan, Steeve, Steevn

Stefan (German, Polish, Swedish) a form of Stephen.
Steafan, Steafeán, Stefaan, Stefane, Stefanson, Stefaun, Stefawn, Steffan

Stefano (Italian) a form of Stephen.
Stefanos, Steffano

Stefanos (Greek) a form of Stephen.
Stefans, Stefos, Stephano, Stephanos

Stefen (Norwegian) a form of Stephen.
Steffen, Steffin, Stefin

Steffan (Swedish) a form of Stefan.
Staffan

Stefon (Polish) a form of Stephon.
Staffon, Steffon, Steffone, Stefone, Stefonne

Stein (German) a form of Steen.
Steine, Steiner

Steinar (Norwegian) rock warrior.

Stepan (Russian) a form of Stephen.
Stepa, Stepane, Stepanya, Stepka, Stipan

Steph (English) a short form of Stephen.

Stephan (Greek) a form of Stephen.
Stepfan, Stephanas, Stephano, Stephanos, Stephanus, Stephaun

Stéphane (French) a form of Stephen.
Stefane, Stepháne, Stephanne

Stephen (Greek) crowned.
See also Estéban, Estebe, Estevan, Estevao, Étienne, István, Szczepan, Tapani, Teb, Teppo, Tiennot.
Stamos, Stavros, Stefan, Stefano, Stefanos, Stefen, Stenya, Stepan, Stepanos, Steph, Stephan, Stephanas, Stéphane, Stephens, Stephenson, Stephfan, Stephin, Stephon, Stepven, Steve, Steven, Stevie

Stephon (Greek) a form of Stephen.
Stefon, Stepfon, Stepfone, Stephfon, Stephion, Stephone, Stephonne

Sterling (English) valuable; silver penny. A form of Starling.
Sterlen, Sterlin, Stirling

Stern (German) star.

Sterne (English) austere.
Stearn, Stearne, Stearns

Stetson (Danish) stepson.
Steston, Steton, Stetsen, Stetzon

Stevan (Greek) a form of
Steven.
*Stevano, Stevanoe, Stevaughn,
Stevean*

Steve (Greek) a short form of
Stephen, Steven.
Steave, Stevie, Stevy

Steven (Greek) a form of
Stephen.
*Steeven, Steiven, Stevan, Steve,
Stevens, Stevie, Stevin, Stevon,
Stiven*

Stevens (English) son of
Steven.
Stevenson, Stevinson

Stevie (English) a familiar
form of Stephen, Steven.
Stevey, Stevy

Stevin, Stevon (Greek) forms
of Steven.
Stevieon, Stevion, Stevyn

Stewart (English) a form of
Stuart.
Steward, Stu

Stian (Norwegian) quick on
his feet.

Stig (Swedish) mount.

Stiggur (Gypsy) gate.

Stillman (English) quiet.
Stillmann, Stillmon

Sting (English) spike of grain.

Stockman (English) tree-
stump remover.

Stockton (English) tree-stump
town.

Stockwell (English) tree-
stump well.

Stoddard (English) horse
keeper.

Stoffel (German) a short form
of Christopher.

Stoker (English) furnace tender.
Stoke, Stokes, Stroker

Stone (English) stone.
*Stoen, Stoner, Stoney, Stonie,
Stonie, Stoniy, Stony*

Storm (English) tempest,
storm.
*Storme, Stormey, Stormi,
Stormmie, Stormy*

Storr (Norwegian) great.
Story

Stover (English) stove tender.

Stowe (English) hidden;
packed away.

Strahan (Irish) minstrel.
Strachan

Stratford (English) bridge
over the river. Literature:
Stratford-upon-Avon was
Shakespeare's birthplace.
Stradford

Stratton (Scottish) river valley
town.
Straten, Straton

Strephon (Greek) one who turns.

Strom (Greek) bed, mattress. (German) stream.

Strong (English) powerful.

Stroud (English) thicket.

Struthers (Irish) brook.

Stu (English) a short form of Stewart, Stuart.
Stew

Stuart (English) caretaker, steward. History: a Scottish and English royal family.
Stewart, Stu, Stuarrt

Studs (English) rounded nail heads; shirt ornaments; male horses used for breeding. History: Louis "Studs" Terkel is a famous American journalist.
Stud, Studd

Styles (English) stairs put over a wall to help cross it.
Stiles, Style, Stylz

Subhi (Arabic) early morning.

Suck Chin (Korean) unshakable rock.

Sudi (Swahili) lucky.
Su'ud

Sued (Arabic) master, chief.
Suede

Suffield (English) southern field.

Sugden (English) valley of sows.

Suhail (Arabic) gentle.
Sohail, Sohayl, Souhail, Suhael, Sujal

Suhuba (Swahili) friend.

Sukru (Turkish) grateful.

Sulaiman (Arabic) a form of Solomon.
Sulaman, Sulay, Sulaymaan, Sulayman, Suleiman, Suleman, Suleyman, Sulieman, Sulman, Solomon, Sulyman

Sullivan (Irish) black eyed.
Sullavan, Sullevan, Sully

Sully (Irish) a familiar form of Sullivan. (French) stain, tarnish. (English) south.
Sulleigh, Sulley

Sultan (Swahili) ruler.
Sultaan

Sum (Tai) appropriate.

Summit (English) peak, top.
Sumeet, Sumit, Summet, Summitt

Sumner (English) church officer; summoner.
Summer

Sundeep (Punjabi) light; enlightened.
Sundip

Sunny (English) sunny, sunshine.
Sun, Sunni

Sunreep (Hindi) pure.
Sunrip

Sutcliff (English) southern cliff.
Sutcliffe

Sutherland (Scandinavian) southern land.
Southerland, Sutherlan

Sutton (English) southern town.

Sven (Scandinavian) youth.
Svein, Svend, Svenn, Swen, Swenson

Swaggart (English) one who sways and staggers.
Swaggert

Swain (English) herdsman; knight's attendant.
Swaine, Swane, Swanson, Swayne

Swaley (English) winding stream.
Swail, Swailey, Swale, Swales

Sweeney (Irish) small hero.
Sweeny

Swinbourne (English) stream used by swine.
Swinborn, Swinborne, Swinburn, Swinburne, Swinbyrn, Swynborn

Swindel (English) valley of the swine.
Swindell

Swinfen (English) swine's mud.

Swinford (English) swine's crossing.
Swynford

Swinton (English) swine town.

Sy (Latin) a short form of Sylas, Symon.
Si

Sydney (French) a form of Sidney.
Syd, Sydne, Sydnee, Syndey

Syed (Arabic) happy.
Syeed, Syid

Sying (Chinese) star.

Sylas (Latin) a form of Silas.
Sy, Syles, Sylus

Sylvain (French) a form of Silvan, Sylvester.
Sylvan, Sylvian

Sylvester (Latin) forest dweller.
Silvester, Silvestro, Sly, Syl, Sylvain, Sylverster, Sylvestre

Symington (English) Simon's town, Simon's estate.

Symon (Greek) a form of Simon.
Sy, Syman, Symeon, Symion, Symms, Symon, Symone

Szczepan (Polish) a form of Stephen.

Szygfrid (Hungarian) a form
of Siegfried.
Szigfrid

Szymon (Polish) a form of
Simon.

T

Taaveti (Finnish) a form of
David.
Taavi, Taavo

Tab (German) shining, brilliant. (English) drummer.
Tabb, Tabbie, Tabby

Tabari (Arabic) he remembers.
*Tabahri, Tabares, Tabarious,
Tabarius, Tabarus, Tabur*

Tabib (Turkish) physician.
Tabeeb

Tabo (Spanish) a short form of
Gustave.

Tabor (Persian) drummer.
(Hungarian) encampment.
*Tabber, Taber, Taboras, Taibor,
Tayber, Taybor, Taver*

Tad (Welsh) father. (Greek,
Latin) a short form of
Thaddeus.
Tadd, Taddy, Tade, Tadek, Tadey

Tadan (Native American)
plentiful.
Taden

Tadarius (American) a combi-
nation of the prefix Ta +
Darius.
*Tadar, Tadarious, Tadaris,
Tadarrius*

Taddeo (Italian) a form of
Thaddeus.
Tadeo

Taddeus (Greek, Latin) a form
of Thaddeus.
*Taddeous, Taddeusz, Taddius,
Tadeas, Tades, Tadeusz, Tadio,
Tadious*

Tadi (Omaha) wind.

Tadzi (Carrier) loon.

Tadzio (Polish, Spanish) a
form of Thaddeus.
Taddeusz

Taffy (Welsh) a form of David.
(English) a familiar form of
Taft.

Taft (English) river.
Taffy, Tafton

Tage (Danish) day.
Tag

Taggart (Irish) son of the
priest.
Tagart, Taggert

Tahír (Arabic) innocent, pure.
Taheer

Tai (Vietnamese) weather;
prosperous; talented.

Taima (Native American)
born during a storm.

Taishawn (American) a combination of Tai + Shawn.
Taisen, Taishaun, Taishon

Tait (Scandinavian) a form of Tate.
Taite, Taitt

Taiwan (Chinese) island; island dweller. Geography: a country off the coast of China.
Taewon, Tahwan, Taivon, Taiwain, Tawain, Tawan, Tawann, Tawaun, Tawon, Taywan, Tywan

Taiwo (Yoruba) first-born of twins.

Taj (Urdu) crown.
Taje, Tajee, Tajeh, Tajh, Taji

Tajo (Spanish) day.
Taio

Tajuan (American) a combination of the prefix Ta + Juan.
Taijuan, Taijun, Taijuon, Tájuan, Tajwan, Taquan, Tyjuan

Takeo (Japanese) strong as bamboo.
Takeyo

Takis (Greek) a familiar form of Peter.
Takias, Takius

Takoda (Lakota) friend to everyone.

Tal (Hebrew) dew; rain.
Tali, Talia, Talley, Talor, Talya

Talbert (German) bright valley.

Talbot (French) boot maker.
Talbott, Tallbot, Tallbott, Tallie, Tally

Talcott (English) cottage near the lake.

Tale (Tswana) green.

Talen (English) a form of Talon.
Talin, Tallen

Talib (Arabic) seeker.

Taliesin (Welsh) radiant brow.
Tallas, Tallis

Taliki (Hausa) fellow.

Talli (Delaware) legendary hero.

Talmadge (English) lake between two towns.
Talmage

Talmai (Aramaic) mound; furrow.
Telem

Talman (Aramaic) injured; oppressed.
Talmon

Talon (French, English) claw, nail.
Taelon, Taelyn, Talen, Tallin, Tallon, Talyn

Talor (English) a form of Tal, Taylor.
Taelor, Taelur

Tam (Vietnamese) number
eight. (Hebrew) honest.
(English) a short form of
Thomas.
Tama, Tamas, Tamás, Tameas,
Tamlane, Tammany, Tammas,
Tammen, Tammy

Taman (Slavic) dark, black.
Tama, Tamann, Tamin, Tamon,
Tamone

Tamar (Hebrew) date; palm
tree.
Tamarie, Tamario, Tamarr, Timur

Tambo (Swahili) vigorous.

Tamir (Arabic) tall as a palm
tree.
Tameer

Tammy (English) a familiar
form of Thomas.
Tammie

Tamson (Scandinavian) son of
Thomas.
Tamsen

Tan (Burmese) million.
(Vietnamese) new.
Than

Tanek (Greek) immortal. See
also Atek.

Taneli (Finnish) God is my
judge.
Taneil, Tanell, Tanella

Taner (English) a form of
Tanner.
Tanar

Tanguy (French) warrior.

Tani (Japanese) valley.

Tanmay (Sanskrit) engrossed.

Tanner (English) leather
worker; tanner.
Tan, Taner, Tanery, Tann, Tannar,
Tannir, Tannor, Tanny

Tannin (English) tan colored;
dark.
Tanin, Tannen, Tannon, Tanyen,
Tanyon

Tanny (English) a familiar
form of Tanner.
Tana, Tannee, Tanney, Tannie,
Tany

Tano (Spanish) camp glory.
(Ghanaian) Geography: a
river in Ghana. (Russian) a
short form of Stanislaus.
Tanno

Tanton (English) town by the
still river.

Tapan (Sanskrit) sun; summer.

Tapani (Finnish) a form of
Stephen.
Tapamn, Teppo

Täpko (Kiowa) antelope.

Taquan (American) a combi-
nation of the prefix Ta +
Quan.
Taquann, Taquawn, Taquon,
Taqwan

Tarak (Sanskrit) star; protector.

Taran (Sanskrit) heaven.
Tarran

Tarek (Arabic) a form of
Táriq.
Tareek, Tareke

Tarell (German) a form of
Terrell.
Tarelle, Tarrel, Tarrell, Taryl

Taren (American) a form of
Taron.
Tarren, Tarrin

Tarif (Arabic) uncommon.
Tareef

Tarik (Arabic) a form of Táriq.
*Taric, Tarick, Tariek, Tarikh,
Tarrick, Tarrik, Taryk*

Táriq (Arabic) conqueror.
History: Tariq bin Ziyad was
the Muslim general who
conquered Spain.
*Tareck, Tarek, Tarik, Tarique,
Tarreq, Tereik*

Tarleton (English) Thor's settlement.
Tarlton

Taro (Japanese) first-born
male.

Taron (American) a combina-
tion of Tad + Ron.
*Taeron, Tahron, Taren, Tarone,
Tarrion, Tarron, Taryn*

Tarrant (Welsh) thunder.
Terrant

Tarun (Sanskrit) young, youth.
Taran

Tarver (English) tower; hill;
leader.
Terver

Taryn (American) a form of
Taron.
Tarryn, Taryon

Tas (Gypsy) bird's nest.

Tashawn (American) a combi-
nation of the prefix Ta +
Shawn.
*Tashaan, Tashan, Tashaun,
Tashon, Tashun*

Tass (Hungarian) ancient
mythology name.

Tasunke (Dakota) horse.

Tate (Scandinavian, English)
cheerful. (Native American)
long-winded talker.
Tait, Tayte

Tatius (Latin) king, ruler.
History: a Sabine king.
Tatianus, Tazio, Titus

Tatum (English) cheerful.

Tau (Tswana) lion.

Tauno (Finnish) a form of
Donald.

Taurean (Latin) strong; force-
ful. Astrology: born under the
sign of Taurus.
*Tauraun, Taurein, Taurin,
Taurion, Taurone, Taurus*

Taurus (Latin) Astrology: the second sign of the zodiac.
Taurice, Tauris

Tavares (Aramaic) a form of Tavor.
Tarvarres, Tavarres, Taveress

Tavaris (Aramaic) a form of Tavor.
Tarvaris, Tavar, Tavaras, Tavari, Tavarian, Tavarious, Tavarius, Tavarous, Tavarri, Tavarris, Tavars, Tavarse, Tavarus, Tevaris, Tevarius, Tevarus

Tavey (Latin) a familiar form of Octavio.

Tavi (Aramaic) good.

Tavian (Latin) a form of Octavio.
Taveon, Taviann, Tavien, Tavieon, Tavin, Tavio, Tavion, Tavionne, Tavon, Tayvon

Tavish (Scottish) a form of Thomas.
Tav, Tavi, Tavis

Tavo (Slavic) a short form of Gustave.

Tavon (American) a form of Tavian.
Tavonn, Tavonne, Tavonni

Tavor (Aramaic) misfortune.
Tarvoris, Tavares, Tavaris, Tavores, Tavorious, Tavoris, Tavorise, Tavorres, Tavorris, Tavuris

Tawno (Gypsy) little one.
Tawn

Tayib (Hindi) good; delicate.

Tayler (English) a form of Taylor.
Tailer, Taylar, Tayller, Teyler

Taylor (English) tailor.
Tailor, Talor, Tayler, Tayllor, Taylour, Taylr, Teylor

Tayshawn (American) a combination of Taylor + Shawn.
Taysean, Tayshan, Tayshun, Tayson

Tayvon (American) a form of Tavian.
Tayvan, Tayvaughn, Tayven, Tayveon, Tayvin, Tayvohn, Taywon

Taz (Arabic) shallow ornamental cup.
Tazz

Tazio (Italian) a form of Tatius.

Teagan (Irish) a form of Teague.
Teagen, Teagun, Teegan

Teague (Irish) bard, poet.
Teag, Teagan, Teage, Teak, Tegan, Teige

Tearence (Latin) a form of Terrence.
Tearance, Tearnce, Tearrance

Tearlach (Scottish) a form of Charles.

Tearle (English) stern, severe.

Teasdale (English) river dweller. Geography: a river in England.

Teb (Spanish) a short form of Stephen.

Ted (English) a short form of Edward, Edwin, Theodore.
Tedd, Tedek, Tedik, Tedson

Teddy (English) a familiar form of Edward, Theodore.
Teddey, Teddie, Tedy

Tedmund (English) protector of the land.
Tedman, Tedmond

Tedorik (Polish) a form of Theodore.
Teodoor, Teodor, Teodorek

Tedrick (American) a combination of Ted + Rick.
Teddrick, Tederick, Tedric

Teetonka (Lakota) big lodge.

Tefere (Ethiopian) seed.

Tegan (Irish) a form of Teague.
Teghan, Teigan, Tiegan

Tej (Sanskrit) light; lustrous.

Tejas (Sanskrit) sharp.

Tekle (Ethiopian) plant.

Telek (Polish) a form of Telford.

Telem (Hebrew) mound; furrow.
Talmai, Tel

Telford (French) iron cutter.
Telek, Telfer, Telfor, Telfour

Teller (English) storyteller.
Tell, Telly

Telly (Greek) a familiar form of Teller, Theodore.

Telmo (English) tiller, cultivator.

Telutci (Moquelumnan) bear making dust as it runs.

Telvin (American) a combination of the prefix Te + Melvin.
Tellvin, Telvan

Tem (Gypsy) country.

Teman (Hebrew) on the right side; southward.

Tembo (Swahili) elephant.

Tempest (French) storm.

Temple (Latin) sanctuary.

Templeton (English) town near the temple.
Temp, Templeten

Tennant (English) tenant, renter.
Tenant, Tennent

Tennessee (Cherokee) mighty warrior. Geography: a southern U.S. state.
Tennessee, Tennesy, Tennysee

Tennyson (English) a form of Dennison. Literature: Alfred, Lord Tennyson was a nine-

teenth-century British poet.
Tenney, Tenneyson, Tennie,
Tennis, Tennison, Tenny, Tenson

Teo (Vietnamese) a form of
Tom.

Teobaldo (Italian, Spanish) a
form of Theobald.

Teodoro (Italian, Spanish) a
form of Theodore.
Teodore, Teodorico

Teppo (French) a familiar
form of Stephen.

Tequan (American) a combination of the prefix Te + Quan.
Tequinn, Tequon

Terance (Latin) a form of
Terrence.
Terriance

Terell (German) a form of
Terrell.
Tarell, Tereall, Terel, Terelle, Tyrel

Teremun (Tiv) father's accept-
ance.
Terence (Latin) a form of
Terrence.
Teren, Teryn

Terencio (Spanish) a form of
Terrence.

Terran (Latin) a short form of
Terrance.
Teran, Teren, Terran, Terren

Terrance (Latin) a form of
Terrence.
Tarrance, Terran

Terrell (German) thunder
ruler.
Terell, Terrail, Terral, Terrale,
Terrall, Terreal, Terrel, Terrelle,
Terrill, Terryal, Terryel, Tirel,
Tirrel, Tirrell, Turrell, Tyrel,
Tyrell

Terrence (Latin) smooth.
Tarrance, Tearence, Terance,
Terence, Terencio, Terrance, Terren,
Terrin, Terry, Torrence, Tyreese

Terrick (American) a combi-
nation of the prefix Te +
Derrick.
Teric, Terick, Terik, Teriq, Terric,
Terrik, Tirek, Tirik

Terrill (German) a form of
Terrell.
Teriel, Teriell, Terril, Terryl,
Terryll, Teryll, Teryl, Tyrill

Terrin (Latin) a short form of
Terrence.
Terin, Terrien, Terryn, Teryn,
Tiren

Terris (Latin) son of Terry.

Terron (American) a form of
Tyrone.
Tereon, Terion, Terione, Teron,
Terone, Terrion, Terrione,
Terriyon, Terrone, Terronn,
Terryon, Tiron

Terry (English) a familiar form
of Terrence. See also Keli.
Tarry, Terrey, Terri, Terrie, Tery

Tertius (Latin) third.

Teshawn (American) a combination of the prefix Te + Shawn.
Tesean, Teshaun, Teshon

Teva (Hebrew) nature.

Tevan (American) a form of Tevin.
Tevaughan, Tevaughn, Teven, Tevvan

Tevel (Yiddish) a form of David.

Tevin (American) a combination of the prefix Te + Kevin.
Teavin, Teivon, Tevan, Tevien, Tevinn, Tevon, Tevvin, Tevyn

Tevis (Scottish) a form of Thomas.
Tevish

Tevon (American) a form of Tevin.
Tevion, Tevohn, Tevone, Tevonne, Tevoun, Teyvon

Tewdor (German) a form of Theodore.

Tex (American) from Texas.
Tejas

Thabit (Arabic) firm, strong.

Thad (Greek, Latin) a short form of Thaddeus.
Thadd, Thade, Thadee, Thady

Thaddeus (Greek) courageous. (Latin) praiser. Bible: one of the Twelve Apostles. See also Fadey.
Tad, Taddeo, Taddeus, Thaddis, Thadeaus, Tadzio, Thad, Thaddaeus, Thaddaus, Thaddeau, Thaddeaus, Thaddeo, Thaddeous, Thaddiaus, Thaddius, Thadeaou, Thadeous, Thadeus, Thadieus, Thadious, Thadius, Thadus

Thady (Irish) praise.
Thaddy

Thai (Vietnamese) many, multiple.

Thaman (Hindi) god; godlike.

Than (Burma) million.
Tan, Thanh

Thane (English) attendant warrior.
Thain, Thaine, Thayne

Thang (Vietnamese) victorious.

Thanh (Vietnamese) finished.

Thaniel (Hebrew) a short form of Nathaniel.

Thanos (Greek) nobleman; bear-man.
Athanasios, Thanasis

Thatcher (English) roof thatcher, repairer of roofs.
Thacher, Thatch, Thaxter

Thaw (English) melting ice.

Thayer (French) nation's army.
Thay

Thel (English) upper story.

Thenga (Yao) bring him.

Theo (English) a short form of Theodore.

Theobald (German) people's prince. See also Dietbald.
Teobaldo, Thebault, Theòbault, Thibault, Tibalt, Tibold, Tiebold, Tiebout, Toiboid, Tybald, Tybalt, Tybault

Theodore (Greek) gift of God. See also Feodor, Fyodor.
Téadóir, Téador, Ted, Teddy, Tedor, Tedorek, Tedorik, Telly, Teodomiro, Teodoro, Teodus, Teos, Tewdor, Theo, Theodor, Theódor, Theodors, Theodorus, Theodosios, Theodrekr, Tivadar, Todor, Tolek, Tudor

Theodoric (German) ruler of the people. See also Dedrick, Derek, Dirk.
Teodorico, Thedric, Thedrick, Thierry, Till

Theophilus (Greek) loved by God.
Teofil, Théophile, Theophlous, Theopolis

Theron (Greek) hunter.
Theran, Theren, Thereon, Therin, Therion, Therrin, Therron, Theryn, Theryon

Thian (Vietnamese) smooth.
Thien

Thibault (French) a form of Theobald.
Thibaud, Thibaut

Thierry (French) a form of Theodoric.
Theirry, Theory

Thom (English) a short form of Thomas.
Thomy

Thoma (German) a form of Thomas.

Thomas (Greek, Aramaic) twin. Bible: one of the Twelve Apostles. See also Chuma, Foma, Maslin.
Tam, Tammy, Tavish, Tevis, Thom, Thoma, Thomason, Thomaz, Thomeson, Thomison, Thommas, Thompson, Thomson, Tom, Toma, Tomas, Tomás, Tomasso, Tomcy, Tomey, Tomey, Tomi, Tommy, Toomas

Thompson (English) son of Thomas.
Thomason, Thomison, Thomsen, Thomson

Thor (Scandinavian) thunder. Mythology: the Norse god of thunder.
Thorin, Tor, Tyrus

Thorald (Scandinavian) Thor's follower.
Terrell, Terrill, Thorold, Torald

Thorbert (Scandinavian) Thor's brightness.
Torbert

Thorbjorn (Scandinavian)
Thor's bear.
Thorburn, Thurborn, Thurburn

Thorgood (English) Thor is
good.

Thorleif (Scandinavian) Thor's
beloved.
Thorlief

Thorley (English) Thor's
meadow.
*Thorlea, Thorlee, Thorleigh,
Thorly, Torley*

Thorndike (English) thorny
embankment.
*Thorn, Thorndyck, Thorndyke,
Thorne*

Thorne (English) a short form
of names beginning with
"Thorn."
Thorn, Thornie, Thorny

Thornley (English) thorny
meadow.
*Thorley, Thorne, Thornlea,
Thornleigh, Thornly*

Thornton (English) thorny
town.
Thorne

Thorpe (English) village.
Thorp

Thorwald (Scandinavian)
Thor's forest.
Thorvald

Thuc (Vietnamese) aware.

Thurlow (English) Thor's hill.
Thurlo

Thurmond (English) defended
by Thor.
Thormond, Thurmund

Thurston (Scandinavian)
Thor's stone.
*Thorstan, Thorstein, Thorsten,
Thurstain, Thurstan, Thursten,
Torsten, Torston*

Tiago (Spanish) a form of
Jacob.

Tiberio (Italian) from the
Tiber River region.
*Tiberias, Tiberious, Tiberiu,
Tiberius, Tibius, Tyberious,
Tyberius, Tyberrius*

Tibor (Hungarian) holy place.
Tiburcio

Tichawanna (Shona) we shall
see.

Ticho (Spanish) a short form
of Patrick.

Tieler (English) a form of
Tyler.
Tielar, Tielor, Tielyr

Tiennot (French) a form of
Stephen.
Tien

Tiernan (Irish) lord.

Tierney (Irish) lordly.
Tiarnach, Tiernan

Tige (English) a short form of Tiger.
Ti, Tig, Tighe, Ty, Tyg, Tyge, Tygh, Tyghe

Tiger (American) tiger; powerful and energetic.
Tige, Tigger, Tyger

Tiimu (Moquelumnan) caterpillar coming out of the ground.

Tilden (English) tilled valley.
Tildon

Tiktu (Moquelumnan) bird digging up potatoes.

Tilford (English) prosperous ford.

Till (German) a short form of Theodoric.
Thilo, Til, Tillman, Tilman, Tillmann, Tilson

Tilton (English) prosperous town.

Tim (Greek) a short form of Timothy.
Timmie, Timmy

Timin (Arabic) born near the sea.

Timmothy (Greek) a form of Timothy.
Timmathy, Timmithy, Timmoty, Timmthy

Timmy (Greek) a familiar form of Timothy.
Timmie

Timo (Finnish) a form of Timothy.
Timio

Timofey (Russian) a form of Timothy.
Timofei, Timofej, Timofeo

Timon (Greek) honorable.

Timoteo (Portuguese, Spanish) a form of Timothy.

Timothy (Greek) honoring God. See also Kimokeo.
Tadhg, Taidgh, Tiege, Tim, Tima, Timithy, Timka, Timkin, Timmothy, Timmy, Timo, Timofey, Timok, Timon, Timontheo, Timonthy, Timót, Timote, Timotei, Timoteo, Timoteus, Timothé, Timothée, Timotheo, Timotheos, Timotheus, Timothey, Timothie, Timthie, Tiomóid, Tisha, Tomothy, Tymon, Tymothy

Timur (Hebrew) a form of Tamar. (Russian) conqueror.
Timour

Tin (Vietnamese) thinker.

Tino (Spanish) venerable, majestic. (Italian) small. A familiar form of Antonio. (Greek) a short form of Augustine.
Tion

Tinsley (English) fortified field.

Tiquan (American) a combination of the prefix Ti + Quan.
Tiquawn, Tiquine, Tiquon, Tiquwan, Tiqwan

Tisha (Russian) a form of Timothy.
Tishka

Tishawn (American) a combination of the prefix Ti + Shawn.
Tishaan, Tishaun, Tishean, Tishon, Tishun

Tito (Italian) a form of Titus.
Titas, Titis, Titos

Titus (Greek) giant. (Latin) hero. A form of Tatius. History: a Roman emperor.
Tite, Titek, Tito, Tytus

Tivon (Hebrew) nature lover.

TJ (American) a combination of the initials T. + J.
Teejay, Tj, T.J., T Jae, Tjayda

Tobal (Spanish) a short form of Christopher.
Tabalito

Tobar (Gypsy) road.

Tobi (Yoruba) great.

Tobias (Hebrew) God is good.
Tobia, Tobiah, Tobiás, Tobiath, Tobin, Tobit, Toby, Tobyas, Tuvya

Tobin (Hebrew) a form of Tobias.
Toben, Tobian, Tobyn, Tovin

Toby (Hebrew) a familiar form of Tobias.
Tobbie, Tobby, Tobe, Tobee, Tobey, Tobie

Todd (English) fox.
Tod, Toddie, Toddy

Todor (Basque, Russian) a form of Theodore.
Teodor, Todar, Todas, Todos

Toft (English) small farm.

Tohon (Native American) cougar.

Tokala (Dakota) fox.

Toland (English) owner of taxed land.
Tolan

Tolbert (English) bright tax collector.

Toller (English) tax collector.

Tom (English) a short form of Tomas, Thomas.
Teo, Thom, Tommey, Tommie, Tommy

Toma (Romanian) a form of Thomas.
Tomah

Tomas (German) a form of Thomas.
Tom, Tomaisin, Tomaz, Tomcio, Tome, Tomek, Tomelis, Tomico,

Tomik, Tomislaw, Tommas, Tomo, Tomson

Tomás (Irish, Spanish) a form of Thomas.
Tomas, Tómas, Tomasz

Tomasso (Italian) a form of Thomas.
Tomaso, Tommaso

Tombe (Kakwa) northerners.

Tomey (Irish) a familiar form of Thomas.
Tome, Tomi, Tomie, Tomy

Tomi (Japanese) rich. (Hungarian) a form of Thomas.

Tomlin (English) little Tom.
Tomkin, Tomlinson

Tommie (Hebrew) a form of Tommy.
Tommi

Tommy (Hebrew) a familiar form of Thomas.
Tommie, Tomy

Tonda (Czech) a form of Tony.
Tonek

Tong (Vietnamese) fragrant.

Toni (Greek, German, Slavic) a form of Tony.
Tonee, Tonie, Tonio, Tonis, Tonnie

Tonio (Portuguese) a form of Tony. (Italian) a short form of Antonio.
Tono, Tonyo

Tony (Greek) flourishing. (Latin) praiseworthy. (English) a short form of Anthony. A familiar form of Remington.
Tonda, Tonek, Toney, Toni, Tonik, Tonio, Tonny

Tooantuh (Cherokee) spring frog.

Toomas (Estonian) a form of Thomas.
Toomis, Tuomas, Tuomo

Topher (Greek) a short form of Christopher, Kristopher.
Tofer, Tophor

Topo (Spanish) gopher.

Topper (English) hill.

Tor (Norwegian) thunder. (Tiv) royalty, king.
Thor

Torian (Irish) a form of Torin.
Toran, Torean, Toriano, Toriaun, Torien, Torrian, Torrien, Torryan

Torin (Irish) chief.
Thorfin, Thorstein, Torian, Torion, Torrin, Toryn

Torkel (Swedish) Thor's cauldron.

Tormey (Irish) thunder spirit.
Tormé, Tormee

Tormod (Scottish) north.

Torn (Irish) a short form of Torrence.
Toran

Torquil (Danish) Thor's kettle.
Torkel

Torr (English) tower.
Tory

Torrance (Irish) a form of
Torrence.
Torance

Torren (Irish) a short form of
Torrence.
Torehn, Toren

Torrence (Irish) knolls. (Latin)
a form of Terrence.
*Tawrence, Toreence, Torence,
Torenze, Torey, Torin, Torn, Torr,
Torrance, Torren, Torreon, Torrin,
Torry, Tory, Torynce, Tuarence,
Turance*

Torrey (English) a form of Tory.
*Toreey, Torie, Torre, Torri, Torrie,
Torry*

Toru (Japanese) sea.

Tory (English) familiar form
of Torr, Torrence.
Torey, Tori, Torrey

Toshi-Shita (Japanese) junior.

Tovi (Hebrew) good.
Tov

Townley (English) town
meadow.
*Townlea, Townlee, Townleigh,
Townlie, Townly*

Townsend (English) town's
end.
*Town, Townes, Towney, Townie,
Townsen, Townshend, Towny*

Trace (Irish) a form of Tracy.
Trayce

Tracey (Irish) a form of Tracy.
Traci

Tracy (Greek) harvester.
(Latin) courageous. (Irish)
battler.
Trace, Tracey, Tracie, Treacy

Trader (English) well-trodden
path; skilled worker.

Trae (English) a form of Trey.
Trai, Traie, Tre, Trea

Trahern (Welsh) strong as
iron.
Traherne, Tray

Tramaine (Scottish) a form of
Tremaine, Tremayne.
*Tramain, Traman, Tramane,
Tramayne, Traymain, Traymon*

Traquan (American) a combi-
nation of Travis + Quan.
*Traequan, Traqon, Traquon,
Traqwan, Traqwaun, Trayquan,
Trayquane, Trayqwon*

Trashawn (American) a com-
bination of Travis + Shawn.
*Trasen, Trashaun, Trasean,
Trashon, Trashone, Trashun,
Trayshaun, Trayshawn*

Traugott (German) God's
truth.

Travaris (French) a form of Travers.
Travares, Travaress, Travarious, Travarius, Travarous, Travarus, Travauris, Traveress, Traverez, Traverus, Travoris, Travorus

Travell (English) traveler.
Travail, Travale, Travel, Travelis, Travelle, Trevel, Trevell, Trevelle

Traven (American) a form of Trevon.
Travin, Travine, Trayven

Travers (French) crossroads.
Travaris, Traver, Travis

Travion (American) a form of Trevon.
Traveon, Travian, Travien, Travione, Travioun

Travis (English) a form of Travers.
Travais, Travees, Traves, Traveus, Travious, Traviss, Travius, Travous, Travus, Travys, Trayvis, Trevais, Trevis

Travon (American) a form of Trevon.
Traevon, Traivon, Travone, Travonn, Travonne

Tray (English) a form of Trey.
Traye

Trayton (English) town full of trees.
Trayten

Trayvon (American) a combination of Tray + Von.
Trayveon, Trayvin, Trayvion, Trayvond, Trayvone, Trayvonne, Trayvyon

Treavon (American) a form of Trevon.
Treavan, Treavin, Treavion

Tredway (English) well-worn road.
Treadway

Tremaine, Tremayne (Scottish) house of stone.
Tramaine, Tremain, Tremane, Treymaine, Trimaine

Trent (Latin) torrent, rapid stream. (French) thirty. Geography: a city in northern Italy.
Trente, Trentino, Trento, Trentonio

Trenton (Latin) town by the rapid stream. Geography: the capital of New Jersey.
Trendon, Trendun, Trenten, Trentin, Trentton, Trentyn, Trinten, Trintin, Trinton

Trequan (American) a combination of Trey + Quan.
Trequanne, Trequaun, Trequian, Trequon, Trequon, Treyquane

Treshawn (American) a combination of Trey + Shawn.
Treshaun, Treshon, Treshun, Treysean, Treyshawn, Treyshon

Treston (Welsh) a form of
Tristan.
Trestan, Trestin, Trestton, Trestyn

Trev (Irish, Welsh) a short
form of Trevor.

Trevaughn (American) a com-
bination of Trey + Vaughn.
*Trevaughan, Trevaugn, Trevaun,
Trevaune, Trevaunn, Treyvaughn*

Trevelyan (English) Elian's
homestead.

Trevin (American) a form of
Trevon.
*Trevian, Trevien, Trevine,
Trevinne, Trevyn, Treyvin*

Trevion (American) a form of
Trevon.
*Trevione, Trevionne, Trevyon,
Treyveon, Treyvion*

Trevis (English) a form of
Travis.
Treves, Trevez, Treveze, Trevius

Trevon (American) a combi-
nation of Trey + Von.
*Traven, Travion, Travon, Tre,
Treavon, Trévan, Treveyon,
Trevin, Trevion, Trevohn,
Trevoine, Trévon, Trevone,
Trevonn, Trevonne, Treyvon*

Trevor (Irish) prudent. (Welsh)
homestead.
*Travor, Treavor, Trebor, Trefor, Trev,
Trevar, Trevares, Trevarious,
Trevaris, Trevarius, Trevaros,
Trevarus, Trever, Trevore, Trevores,*

*Trevoris, Trevorus, Trevour, Trevyr,
Treyvor*

Trey (English) three; third.
Trae, Trai, Tray, Treye, Tri, Trie

Treyvon (American) a form of
Trevon.
*Treyvan, Treyven, Treyvenn,
Treyvone, Treyvonn, Treyvun*

Trigg (Scandinavian) trusty.

Trini (Latin) a short form of
Trinity.

Trinity (Latin) holy trinity.
Trenedy, Trini, Trinidy

Trip, Tripp (English) traveler.

Tristan (Welsh) bold.
Literature: a knight in the
Arthurian legends who fell
in love with his uncle's wife.
*Treston, Tris, Trisan, Tristain,
Tristano, Tristen, Tristian, Tristin,
Triston, Tristyn, Trystan*

Tristano (Italian) a form of
Tristan.

Tristen (Welsh) a form of
Tristan.
Trisden, Trissten

Tristin (Welsh) a form of
Tristan.
Tristian, Tristinn

Triston (Welsh) a form of
Tristan.

Tristram (Welsh) sorrowful.
Literature: the title character
in Laurence Sterne's eigh-

teenth-century novel *Tristram Shandy*.
Tristam

Tristyn (Welsh) a form of Tristan.
Tristynne

Trot (English) trickling stream.

Trowbridge (English) bridge by the tree.

Troy (Irish) foot soldier. (French) curly haired. (English) water. See also Koi.
Troi, Troye, Troyton

True (English) faithful, loyal.
Tru

Truesdale (English) faithful one's homestead.

Truitt (English) little and honest.
Truett

Truman (English) honest. History: Harry S. Truman was the thirty-third U.S. president.
Trueman, Trumain, Trumaine, Trumann

Trumble (English) strong; bold.
Trumball, Trumbell, Trumbull

Trustin (English) trustworthy.
Trustan, Trusten, Truston

Trygve (Norwegian) brave victor.

Trystan (Welsh) a form of Tristan.
Tryistan, Trysten, Trystian, Trystin, Trystn, Tryston, Trystyn

Tsalani (Nguni) good-bye.

Tse (Ewe) younger of twins.

Tu (Vietnamese) tree.

Tuaco (Ghanaian) eleventh-born.

Tuan (Vietnamese) goes smoothly.

Tucker (English) fuller, tucker of cloth.
Tuck, Tuckie, Tucky, Tuckyr

Tudor (Welsh) a form of Theodore. History: an English ruling dynasty.
Todor

Tug (Scandinavian) draw, pull.
Tugg

Tuketu (Moquelumnan) bear making dust as it runs.

Tukuli (Moquelumnan) caterpillar crawling down a tree.

Tulio (Italian, Spanish) lively.
Tullio

Tullis (Latin) title, rank.
Tullius, Tullos, Tully

Tully (Irish) at peace with God. (Latin) a familiar form of Tullis.
Tull, Tulley, Tullie, Tullio

Tumaini (Mwera) hope.

Tumu (Moquelumnan) deer thinking about eating wild onions.

Tung (Vietnamese) stately, dignified. (Chinese) everyone.

Tungar (Sanskrit) high; lofty.

Tupi (Moquelumnan) pulled up.

Tupper (English) ram raiser.

Turi (Spanish) a short form of Arthur.
Ture

Turk (English) from Turkey.

Turner (Latin) lathe worker; wood worker.

Turpin (Scandinavian) Finn named after Thor.

Tut (Arabic) strong and courageous. History: a short form of Tutankhamen, an Egyptian king.
Tutt

Tutu (Spanish) a familiar form of Justin.

Tuvya (Hebrew) a form of Tobias.
Tevya, Tuvia, Tuviah

Tuwile (Mwera) death is inevitable.

Tuyen (Vietnamese) angel.

Twain (English) divided in two. Literature: Mark Twain (whose real name was Samuel Langhorne Clemens) was one of the most prominent nineteenth-century American writers.
Tawine, Twaine, Twan, Twane, Tway, Twayn, Twayne

Twia (Fante) born after twins.

Twitchell (English) narrow passage.
Twytchell

Twyford (English) double river crossing.

Txomin (Basque) like the Lord.

Ty (English) a short form of Tyler, Tyrone, Tyrus.
Tye

Tyee (Native American) chief.

Tyger (English) a form of Tiger.
Tige, Tyg, Tygar

Tylar (English) a form of Tyler.
Tyelar, Tylarr

Tyler (English) tile maker.
Tieler, Tiler, Ty, Tyel, Tyeler, Tyelor, Tyhler, Tylar, Tyle, Tylee, Tylere, Tyller, Tylor, Tylyr

Tylor (English) a form of Tyler.
Tylour

Tymon (Polish) a form of Timothy. (Greek) a form of Timon.
Tymain, Tymaine, Tymane, Tymeik, Tymek, Tymen

Tymothy (English) a form of
Timothy.
*Tymithy, Tymmothy, Tymoteusz,
Tymothee, Timothi*

Tynan (Irish) dark.
Ty

Tynek (Czech) a form of
Martin.
Tynko

Tyquan (American) a combi-
nation of Ty + Quan.
*Tykwan, Tykwane, Tykwon,
Tyquaan, Tyquane, Tyquann,
Tyquine, Tyquinn, Tyquon,
Tyquone, Tyquwon, Tyqwan*

Tyran (American) a form of
Tyrone.
Tyraine, Tyrane

Tyree (Scottish) island dweller.
Geography: Tiree is an island
off the west coast of
Scotland.
*Tyra, Tyrae, Tyrai, Tyray, Tyre,
Tyrea, Tyrée*

Tyreese (American) a form of
Terrence.
*Tyreas, Tyrease, Tyrece, Tyreece,
Tyreice, Tyres, Tyrese, Tyresse,
Tyrez, Tyreze, Tyrice, Tyriece,
Tyriese*

Tyrel, Tyrell (American) forms
of Terrell.
Tyrelle, Tyrrel, Tyrrell

Tyrick (American) a combination of Ty + Rick.
Tyreck, Tyreek, Tyreik, Tyrek,

*Tyreke, Tyric, Tyriek, Tyrik,
Tyriq, Tyrique*

Tyrin (American) a form of
Tyrone.
Tyrinn, Tyrion, Tyrrin, Tyryn

Tyron (American) a form of
Tyrone.
*Tyrohn, Tyronn, Tyronna,
Tyronne*

Tyrone (Greek) sovereign.
(Irish) land of Owen.
*Tayron, Tayrone, Teirone, Terron,
Ty, Tyerone, Tyhrone, Tyran,
Tyrin, Tyron, Tyroney, Tyronne,
Tyroon, Tyroun*

Tyrus (English) a form of
Thor.
Ty, Tyruss, Tyryss

Tyshawn (American) a combi-
nation of Ty + Shawn.
*Tyshan, Tyshaun, Tyshauwn,
Tyshian, Tyshinn, Tyshion,
Tyshon, Tyshone, Tyshonne,
Tyshun, Tyshunn, Tyshyn*

Tyson (French) son of Ty.
*Tison, Tiszon, Tyce, Tycen,
Tyesn, Tyeson, Tysen, Tysie,
Tysin, Tysne, Tysone*

Tytus (Polish) a form of Titus.
Tyus

Tyvon (American) a combina-
tion of Ty + Von.
*Tyvan, Tyvin, Tyvinn, Tyvone,
Tyvonne*

Tywan (Chinese) a form of Taiwan.
Tywain, Tywaine, Tywane, Tywann, Tywaun, Tywen, Tywon, Tywone, Tywonne

Tzadok (Hebrew) righteous.
Tzadik, Zadok

Tzion (Hebrew) sign from God.
Zion

Tzuriel (Hebrew) God is my rock.
Tzuriya

Tzvi (Hebrew) deer.
Tzevi, Zevi

U

Uaine (Irish) a form of Owen.

Ubadah (Arabic) serves God.

Ubaid (Arabic) faithful.

Uberto (Italian) a form of Hubert.

Uche (Ibo) thought.

Uday (Sanskrit) to rise.

Udell (English) yew-tree valley.
Dell, Eudel, Udale, Udall, Yudell

Udit (Sanskrit) grown; shining.

Udo (Japanese) ginseng plant. (German) a short form of Udolf.

Udolf (English) prosperous wolf.
Udo, Udolfo, Udolph

Ugo (Italian) a form of Hugh, Hugo.

Ugutz (Basque) a form of John.

Uilliam (Irish) a form of William.
Uileog, Uilleam, Ulick

Uinseann (Irish) a form of Vincent.

Uistean (Irish) intelligent.
Uisdean

Uja (Sanskrit) growing.

Uku (Hawaiian) flea, insect; skilled ukulele player.

Ulan (African) first-born twin.

Ulbrecht (German) a form of Albert.

Ulf (German) wolf.

Ulfred (German) peaceful wolf.

Ulger (German) warring wolf.

Ulises (Latin) a form of Ulysses.
Ulishes, Ulisse, Ulisses

Ullock (German) sporting wolf.

Ulmer (English) famous wolf.
Ullmar, Ulmar

Ulmo (German) from Ulm, Germany.

Ulric (German) a form of Ulrich.
Ullric

Ulrich (German) wolf ruler; ruler of all. See also Alaric.
Uli, Ull, Ulric, Ulrick, Ulrik, Ulrike, Ulu, Ulz, Uwe

Ultman (Hindi) god; godlike.

Ulyses (Latin) a form of Ulysses.
Ulysee, Ulysees

Ulysses (Latin) wrathful. A form of Odysseus.
Eulises, Ulick, Ulises, Ulyses, Ulysse, Ulyssees, Ulysses, Ulyssius

Umang (Sanskrit) enthusiastic.
Umanga

Umar (Arabic) a form of Omar.
Umair, Umarr, Umayr, Umer

Umberto (Italian) a form of Humbert.
Uberto

Umi (Yao) life.

Umit (Turkish) hope.

Unai (Basque) shepherd.
Una

Uner (Turkish) famous.

Unika (Lomwe) brighten.

Unique (Latin) only, unique.
Uneek, Unek, Unikque, Uniqué, Unyque

Unwin (English) nonfriend.
Unwinn, Unwyn

Upshaw (English) upper wooded area.

Upton (English) upper town.

Upwood (English) upper forest.

Urban (Latin) city dweller; courteous.
Urbain, Urbaine, Urbane, Urbano, Urbanus, Urvan, Urvane

Urbane (English) a form of Urban.

Urbano (Italian) a form of Urban.

Uri (Hebrew) a short form of Uriah.
Urie

Uriah (Hebrew) my light. Bible: a soldier and the husband of Bathsheba. See also Yuri.
Uri, Uria, Urias, Urijah

Urian (Greek) heaven.
Urihaan

Uriel (Hebrew) God is my light.
Urie

Urson (French) a form of
Orson.
Ursan, Ursus

Urtzi (Basque) sky.

Usamah (Arabic) like a lion.
Usama

Useni (Yao) tell me.
Usene, Usenet

Usi (Yao) smoke.

Ustin (Russian) a form of
Justin.

Utatci (Moquelumnan) bear
scratching itself.

Uthman (Arabic) companion
of the Prophet.
Usman, Uthmaan

Uttam (Sanskrit) best.

Uwe (German) a familiar form
of Ulrich.

Uzi (Hebrew) my strength.
Uzzia

Uziel (Hebrew) God is my
strength; mighty force.
Uzie, Uzziah, Uzziel

Uzoma (Nigerian) born during a journey.

Uzumati (Moquelumnan)
grizzly bear.

V

Vachel (French) small cow.
Vache, Vachell

Vaclav (Czech) wreath of
glory.
Vasek

Vadin (Hindi) speaker.
Vaden

Vail (English) valley.
Vaile, Vaill, Vale, Valle

Val (Latin) a short form of
Valentin.

Valborg (Swedish) mighty
mountain.

Valdemar (Swedish) famous
ruler.

Valentin (Latin) strong;
healthy.
*Val, Valencio, Valenté, Valentijn,
Valentine, Valentino, Valenton,
Valentyn, Velentino*

Valentino (Italian) a form of
Valentin.

Valerian (Latin) strong;
healthy.
Valeriano, Valerii, Valerio, Valeryn

Valerii (Russian) a form of
Valerian.
*Valera, Valerie, Valerij, Valerik,
Valeriy, Valery*

Valfrid (Swedish) strong peace.

Valin (Hindi) a form of Balin.
Mythology: a tyrannical
monkey king.

Vallis (French) from Wales.
Valis

Valter (Lithuanian, Swedish) a
form of Walter.
Valters, Valther, Valtr, Vanda

Van (Dutch) a short form of
Vandyke.
Vander, Vane, Vann, Vanno

Vance (English) thresher.

Vanda (Lithuanian) a form of
Walter.
Vander

Vandyke (Dutch) dyke.
Van

Vanya (Russian) a familiar
form of Ivan.
*Vanechka, Vanek, Vanja, Vanka,
Vanusha, Wanya*

Vardon (French) green knoll.
*Vardaan, Varden, Verdan, Verdon,
Verdun*

Varian (Latin) variable.

Varick (German) protecting
ruler.
Varak, Varek, Warrick

Vartan (Armenian) rose pro-
ducer; rose giver.

Varun (Hindi) rain god.
Varron

Vasant (Sanskrit) spring.
Vasanth

Vashawn (American) a combi-
nation of the prefix Va +
Shawn.
*Vashae, Vashan, Vashann,
Vashaun, Vashawnn, Vashon,
Vashun, Vishon*

Vasilis (Greek) a form of Basil.
*Vas, Vasaya, Vaselios, Vashon,
Vasil, Vasile, Vasileior, Vasileios,
Vasilios, Vasilius, Vasilos, Vasilus,
Vasily, Vassilios, Vasylko, Vasyltso,
Vazul*

Vasily (Russian) a form of
Vasilis.
*Vasilek, Vasili, Vasilii, Vasilije,
Vasilik, Vasiliy, Vassili, Vassilij,
Vasya, Vasyenka*

Vasin (Hindi) ruler, lord.

Vasu (Sanskrit) wealth.

Vasyl (German, Slavic) a form
of William.
*Vasos, Vassily, Vassos, Vasya,
Vasyuta, VaVaska, Wassily*

Vaughn (Welsh) small.
*Vaughan, Vaughen, Vaun, Vaune,
Von, Voughn*

Veasna (Cambodian) lucky.

Ved (Sanskrit) sacred knowledge.

Vedie (Latin) sight.

Veer (Sanskrit) brave.

Vegard (Norwegian) sanctuary; protection.

Velvel (Yiddish) wolf.

Vencel (Hungarian) a short form of Wenceslaus.
Venci, Vencie

Venedictos (Greek) a form of Benedict.
Venedict, Venediktos, Venka, Venya

Veniamin (Bulgarian) a form of Benjamin.
Venyamin, Verniamin

Venkat (Hindi) god; godlike. Religion: another name for the Hindu god Vishnu.

Venya (Russian) a familiar form of Benedict.
Venedict, Venka

Vere (Latin, French) true.

Vered (Hebrew) rose.

Vergil (Latin) a form of Virgil. Literature: a Roman poet best known for his epic poem *Aenid*.
Verge

Vern (Latin) a short form of Vernon.
Verna, Vernal, Verne, Verneal, Vernel, Vernell, Vernelle, Vernial, Vernine, Vernis, Vernol

Vernados (German) courage of the bear.

Verner (German) defending army.
Varner

Verney (French) alder grove.
Vernie

Vernon (Latin) springlike; youthful.
Vern, Varnan, Vernen, Verney, Vernin

Verrill (German) masculine. (French) loyal.
Verill, Verrall, Verrell, Verroll, Veryl

Vian (English) full of life.

Vic (Latin) a short form of Victor.
Vick, Vicken, Vickenson

Vicente (Spanish) a form of Vincent.
Vicent, Visente

Vicenzo (Italian) a form of Vincent.

Victoir (French) a form of Victor.

Victor (Latin) victor, conqueror.
Vic, Victa, Victer, Victoir, Victoriano, Victorien, Victorin, Victorio, Viktor, Vitin, Vittorio, Vitya, Wikoli, Wiktor, Witek

Victorio (Spanish) a form of Victor.
Victorino

Vidal (Spanish) a form of Vitas.
Vida, Vidale, Vidall, Videll

Vidar (Norwegian) tree warrior.

Vidor (Hungarian) cheerful.

Vidur (Hindi) wise.

Viho (Cheyenne) chief.

Vijay (Hindi) victorious.

Vikas (Hindi) growing.
Vikash, Vikesh

Vikram (Hindi) valorous.
Vikrum

Vikrant (Hindi) powerful.
Vikran

Viktor (German, Hungarian, Russian) a form of Victor.
Viktoras, Viktors

Vilhelm (German) a form of William.
Vilhelms, Vilho, Vilis, Viljo, Villem

Vili (Hungarian) a short form of William.
Villy, Vilmos

Viliam (Czech) a form of William.
Vila, Vilek, Vilém, Viliami, Viliamu, Vilko, Vilous

Viljo (Finnish) a form of William.

Ville (Swedish) a short form of William.

Vimal (Hindi) pure.

Vin (Latin) a short form of Vincent.
Vinn

Vinay (Hindi) polite.

Vince (English) a short form of Vincent.
Vence, Vint

Vincent (Latin) victor, conqueror. See also Binkentios, Binky.
Uinseann, Vencent, Vicente, Vicenzo, Vikent, Vikenti, Vikesha, Vin, Vince, Vincence, Vincens, Vincente, Vincentius, Vincents, Vincenty, Vincenzo, Vinci, Vincien, Vincient, Vinciente, Vincint, Vinny, Vinsent, Vinsint, Wincent

Vincente (Spanish) a form of Vincent.
Vencente

Vincenzo (Italian) a form of Vincent.
Vincenz, Vincenza, Vincenzio, Vinchenzo, Vinzenz

Vinci (Hungarian, Italian) a familiar form of Vincent.
Vinci, Vinco, Vincze

Vinny (English) a familiar form of Calvin, Melvin, Vincent.
Vinnee, Vinney, Vinni, Vinnie

Vinod (Hindi) happy, joyful.
Vinodh, Vinood

Vinson (English) son of Vincent.
Vinnis

Vipul (Hindi) plentiful.

Viraj (Hindi) resplendent.

Virat (Hindi) very big.

Virgil (Latin) rod bearer, staff bearer.
Vergil, Virge, Virgial, Virgie, Virgilio

Virgilio (Spanish) a form of Virgil.
Virjilio

Virote (Tai) strong, powerful.

Vishal (Hindi) huge; great.
Vishaal

Vishnu (Hindi) protector.

Vitas (Latin) alive, vital.
Vidal, Vitus

Vito (Latin) a short form of Vittorio.
Veit, Vidal, Vital, Vitale, Vitalis, Vitas, Vitin, Vitis, Vitus, Vitya, Vytas

Vittorio (Italian) a form of Victor.
Vito, Vitor, Vitorio, Vittore, Vittorios

Vitya (Russian) a form of Victor.
Vitenka, Vitka

Vivek (Hindi) wisdom.
Vivekinan

Vladimir (Russian) famous prince. See also Dima, Waldemar, Walter.
Bladimir, Vimka, Vlad, Vladamir, Vladik, Vladimar, Vladimeer, Vladimer, Vladimere, Vladimire, Vladimyr, Vladjimir, Vladka, Vladko, Vladlen, Vladmir, Volodimir, Volodya, Volya, Vova, Wladimir

Vladislav (Slavic) glorious ruler. See also Slava.
Vladik, Vladya, Vlas, Vlasislava, Vyacheslav, Wladislav

Vlas (Russian) a short form of Vladislav.

Volker (German) people's guard.
Folke

Volney (German) national spirit.

Von (German) a short form of many German names.

Vova (Russian) a form of Walter.
Vovka

Vuai (Swahili) savior.

Vyacheslav (Russian) a form of Vladislav. See also Slava.

Waban (Ojibwa) white.
Wabon

Wade (English) ford; river crossing.
Wad, Wadesworth, Wadi, Wadie, Waed, Waid, Waide, Wayde, Waydell, Whaid

Wadley (English) ford meadow.
Wadleigh, Wadly

Wadsworth (English) village near the ford.
Waddsworth

Wagner (German) wagoner, wagon maker. Music: Richard Wagner was a famous nineteenth-century German composer.
Waggoner

Wahid (Arabic) single; exclusively unequaled.
Waheed

Wahkan (Lakota) sacred.

Wahkoowah (Lakota) charging.

Wain (English) a short form of Wainwright. A form of Wayne.

Wainwright (English) wagon maker.
Wain, Wainright, Wayne, Wayneright, Waynewright, Waynright, Wright

Waite (English) watchman.
Waitman, Waiton, Waits, Wayte

Wakefield (English) wet field.
Field, Wake

Wakely (English) wet meadow.

Wakeman (English) watchman.
Wake

Wakiza (Native American) determined warrior.

Walcott (English) cottage by the wall.
Wallcot, Wallcott, Wolcott

Waldemar (German) powerful; famous. See also Vladimir.
Valdemar, Waldermar, Waldo

Walden (English) wooded valley. Literature: Henry David Thoreau made Walden Pond famous with his book *Walden*.
Waldi, Waldo, Waldon, Welti

Waldo (German) a familiar form of Oswald, Waldemar, Walden.
Wald, Waldy

Waldron (English) ruler.

Waleed (Arabic) newborn.
Waled, Walid

Walerian (Polish) strong; brave.

Wales (English) from Wales.
Wael, Wail, Wali, Walie, Waly

Walford (English) Welshman's ford.

Walfred (German) peaceful ruler.
Walfredo, Walfried

Wali (Arabic) all-governing.

Walker (English) cloth walker;
cloth cleaner.
Wallie, Wally

Wallace (English) from Wales.
*Wallach, Wallas, Wallie, Wallis,
Wally, Walsh, Welsh*

Wallach (German) a form of
Wallace.
Wallache

Waller (German) powerful.
(English) wall maker.

Wally (English) a familiar form
of Walter.
Walli, Wallie

Walmond (German) mighty
ruler.

Walsh (English) a form of
Wallace.
Welch, Welsh

Walt (English) a short form of
Walter, Walton.
Waltey, Waltli, Walty

Walter (German) army ruler,
general. (English) woodsman.
See also Gautier, Gualberto,
Gualtiero, Gutierre, Ladislav,
Vladimir.
*Valter, Vanda, Vova, Walder,
Wally, Walt, Waltli, Walther,
Waltr, Wat, Waterio, Watkins
Watson, Wualter*

Walther (German) a form of
Walter.

Walton (English) walled town.
Walt

Waltr (Czech) a form of
Walter.

Walworth (English) fenced-in
farm.

Walwyn (English) Welsh
friend.
*Walwin, Walwinn, Walwynn,
Walwynne, Welwyn*

Wamblee (Lakota) eagle.

Wang (Chinese) hope; wish.

Wanikiya (Lakota) savior.

Wanya (Russian) a form of
Vanya.
Wanyai

Wapi (Native American) lucky.

Warburton (English) fortified
town.

Ward (English) watchman,
guardian.
Warde, Warden, Worden

Wardell (English) watchman's
hill.

Wardley (English) watchman's
meadow.
Wardlea Wardleigh

Ware (English) wary, cautious.

Warfield (English) field near
the weir or fish trap.

Warford (English) ford near
the weir or fish trap.

Warley (English) meadow near the weir or fish trap.

Warner (German) armed defender. (French) park keeper.
Werner

Warren (German) general; warden; rabbit hutch.
Ware, Waring, Warrenson, Warrin, Warriner, Worrin

Warton (English) town near the weir or fish trap.

Warwick (English) buildings near the weir or fish trap.
Warick, Warrick

Washburn (English) overflowing river.

Washington (English) town near water. History: George Washington was the first U.S. president.
Wash

Wasili (Russian) a form of Basil.
Wasyl

Wasim (Arabic) graceful; good-looking.
Waseem, Wasseem, Wassim

Watende (Nyakyusa) there will be revenge.

Waterio (Spanish) a form of Walter.
Gualtiero

Watford (English) wattle ford; dam made of twigs and sticks.

Watkins (English) son of Walter.
Watkin

Watson (English) son of Walter.
Wathson, Whatson

Waverly (English) quaking aspen-tree meadow.
Waverlee, Waverley

Wayland (English) a form of Waylon.
Weiland, Weyland

Waylon (English) land by the road.
Wallen, Walon, Way, Waylan, Wayland, Waylen, Waylin, Weylin

Wayman (English) road man; traveler.
Waymon

Wayne (English) wagon maker. A short form of Wainwright.
Wain, Wanye, Wayn, Waynell, Waynne, Wene, Whayne

Wazir (Arabic) minister.

Webb (English) weaver.
Web, Weeb

Weber (German) weaver.
Webber, Webner

Webley (English) weaver's meadow.
Webbley, Webbly, Webly

Webster (English) weaver.

Weddel (English) valley near the ford.

Wei-Quo (Chinese) ruler of the country.
Wei

Welborne (English) spring-fed stream.
Welborn, Welbourne, Welburn, Wellborn, Wellborne, Wellbourn, Wellburn

Welby (German) farm near the well.
Welbey, Welbie, Wellbey, Wellby

Weldon (English) hill near the well.
Weldan

Welfel (Yiddish) a form of William.
Welvel

Welford (English) ford near the well.

Wells (English) springs.
Welles

Welsh (English) a form of Wallace, Walsh.
Welch

Welton (English) town near the well.

Wemilat (Native American) all give to him.

Wemilo (Native American) all speak to him.

Wen (Gypsy) born in winter.

Wenceslaus (Slavic) wreath of honor.
Vencel, Wenceslao, Wenceslas, Wenzel, Wenzell, Wiencyslaw

Wendell (German) wanderer. (English) good dale, good valley.
Wandale, Wendall, Wendel, Wendle, Wendy

Wene (Hawaiian) a form of Wayne.

Wenford (English) white ford.
Wynford

Wentworth (English) pale man's settlement.

Wenutu (Native American) clear sky.

Werner (English) a form of Warner.
Wernhar, Wernher

Wes (English) a short form of Wesley.
Wess

Wesh (Gypsy) woods.

Wesley (English) western meadow.
Wes, Weseley, Wesle, Weslee, Wesleyan, Weslie, Wesly, Wessley, Westleigh, Westley, Wezley

West (English) west.

Westbrook (English) western brook.
Brook, West, Westbrooke

Westby (English) western farmstead.

Westcott (English) western cottage.
Wescot, Wescott, Westcot

Westley (English) a form of Wesley.
Westlee, Westly

Weston (English) western town.
West, Westen, Westin

Wetherby (English) wether-sheep farm.
Weatherbey, Weatherbie, Weatherby, Wetherbey, Wetherbie

Wetherell (English) wether-sheep corner.

Wetherly (English) wether-sheep meadow.

Weylin (English) a form of Waylon.
Weylan, Weylyn

Whalley (English) woods near a hill.
Whaley

Wharton (English) town on the bank of a lake.
Warton

Wheatley (English) wheat field.
Whatley, Wheatlea, Wheatleigh, Wheatly

Wheaton (English) wheat town.

Wheeler (English) wheel maker; wagon driver.

Whistler (English) whistler, piper.

Whit (English) a short form of Whitman, Whitney.
Whitt, Whyt, Whyte, Wit, Witt

Whitby (English) white house.

Whitcomb (English) white valley.
Whitcombe, Whitcumb

Whitelaw (English) small hill.
Whitlaw

Whitey (English) white skinned; white haired.

Whitfield (English) white field.

Whitford (English) white ford.

Whitley (English) white meadow.
Whitlea, Whitlee, Whitleigh

Whitman (English) white-haired man.
Whit

Whitmore (English) white moor.
Whitmoor, Whittemore, Witmore, Wittemore

Whitney (English) white
island; white water.
Whit, Whittney, Widney, Widny

Whittaker (English) white field.
Whitacker, Whitaker, Whitmaker

Wicasa (Dakota) man.

Wicent (Polish) a form of
Vincent.
Wicek, Wicus

Wichado (Native American)
willing.

Wickham (English) village
enclosure.
Wick

Wickley (English) village
meadow.
Wilcley

Wid (English) wide.

Wies (German) renowned
warrior.

Wikoli (Hawaiian) a form of
Victor.

Wiktor (Polish) a form of
Victor.

Wilanu (Moquelumnan) pour-
ing water on flour.

Wilbert (German) brilliant;
resolute.
Wilberto, Wilburt

Wilbur (English) wall fortifica-
tion; bright willows.
*Wilber, Wilburn, Wilburt,
Willbur, Wilver*

Wilder (English) wilderness,
wild.
Wylder

Wildon (English) wooded hill.
Wilden, Willdon

Wile (Hawaiian) a form of
Willie.

Wiley (English) willow
meadow; Will's meadow.
Whiley, Wildy, Willey, Wylie

Wilford (English) willow-tree
ford.
Wilferd

Wilfred (German) determined
peacemaker.
*Wilferd, Wilfredo, Wilfrid,
Wilfride, Wilfried, Wilfryd, Will,
Willfred, Willfried, Willie, Willy*

Wilfredo (Spanish) a form of
Wilfred.
*Fredo, Wifredo, Wilfrido,
Willfredo*

Wilhelm (German)
determined guardian.
Wilhelmus, Willem

Wiliama (Hawaiian) a form of
William.
Pila, Wile

Wilkie (English) a familiar
form of Wilkins.
Wikie, Wilke

Wilkins (English) William's kin.
*Wilkens, Wilkes, Wilkie, Wilkin,
Wilks, Willkes, Willkins*

Wilkinson (English) son of little William.
Wilkenson, Willkinson

Will (English) a short form of William.
Wil, Wilm, Wim

Willard (German) determined and brave.
Williard

Willem (German) a form of William.
Willim

William (English) a form of Wilhelm. See also Gilamu, Guglielmo, Guilherme, Guillaume, Guillermo, Gwilym, Liam, Uilliam, Wilhelm.
Bill, Billy, Vasyl, Vilhelm, Vili, Viliam, Viljo, Ville, Villiam, Welfel, Wilek, Wiliam, Wiliama, Wiliame, Wiliame, Will, Willaim, Willam, Willeam, Willem, Williams, Willie, Willil, Willis, Willium, Williw, Willyam, Wim

Williams (German) son of William.
Wilams, Willaims, Williamson, Wuliams

Willie (German) a familiar form of William.
Wile, Wille, Willi, Willia, Willy

Willis (German) son of Willie.
Willice, Wills, Willus, Wyllis

Willoughby (English) willow farm.
Willoughbey, Willoughbie

Wills (English) son of Will.

Willy (German) a form of Willie.
Willey, Wily

Wilmer (German) determined and famous.
Willimar, Willmer, Wilm, Wilmar, Wylmar, Wylmer

Wilmot (Teutonic) resolute spirit.
Willmont, Willmot, Wilm, Wilmont

Wilny (Native American) eagle singing while flying.

Wilson (English) son of Will.
Wilkinson, Willson, Wilsen, Wolson

Wilt (English) a short form of Wilton.

Wilton (English) farm by the spring.
Will, Wilt

Wilu (Moquelumnan) chicken hawk squawking.

Win (Cambodian) bright. (English) a short form of Winston and names ending in "win."
Winn, Winnie, Winny

Wincent (Polish) a form of Vincent.
Wicek, Wicenty, Wicus, Wince, Wincenty

Winchell (English) bend in the road; bend in the land.

Windsor (English) riverbank with a winch. History: the surname of the British royal family.
Wincer, Winsor, Wyndsor

Winfield (English) friendly field.
Field, Winfred, Winfrey, Winifield, Winnfield, Wynfield, Wynnfield

Winfried (German) friend of peace.

Wing (Chinese) glory.
Wing-Chiu, Wing-Kit

Wingate (English) winding gate.

Wingi (Native American) willing.

Winslow (English) friend's hill.

Winston (English) friendly town; victory town.
Win, Winsten, Winstin, Winstonn, Winton, Wynstan, Wynston

Winter (English) born in winter.
Winterford, Wynter

Winthrop (English) victory at the crossroads.

Winton (English) a form of Winston.
Wynten, Wynton

Winward (English) friend's guardian; friend's forest.

Wit (Polish) life. (English) a form of Whit. (Flemish) a short form of DeWitt.
Witt, Wittie, Witty

Witek (Polish) a form of Victor.

Witha (Arabic) handsome.

Witter (English) wise warrior.

Witton (English) wise man's estate.

Wladislav (Polish) a form of Vladislav.
Wladislaw

Wolcott (English) cottage in the woods.

Wolf (German, English) a short form of Wolfe, Wolfgang.
Wolff, Wolfie, Wolfy

Wolfe (English) wolf.
Wolf, Woolf

Wolfgang (German) wolf quarrel. Music: Wolfgang Amadeus Mozart was a famous eighteenth-century Austrian composer.
Wolf, Wolfegang, Wolfgans

Wood (English) a short form of Elwood, Garwood, Woodrow.
Woody

Woodfield (English) forest meadow.

Woodford (English) ford through the forest.

Woodrow (English) passage in the woods. History: Thomas Woodrow Wilson was the twenty-eighth U.S. president.
Wood, Woodman, Woodroe, Woody

Woodruff (English) forest ranger.

Woodson (English) son of Wood.
Woods, Woodsen

Woodward (English) forest warden.
Woodard

Woodville (English) town at the edge of the woods.

Woody (American) a familiar form of Elwood, Garwood, Woodrow.
Wooddy, Woodie

Woolsey (English) victorious wolf.

Worcester (English) forest army camp.

Wordsworth (English) wolf-guardian's farm. Literature: William Wordsworth was a famous British poet.
Worth

Worie (Ibo) born on market day.

Worth (English) a short form of Wordsworth.
Worthey, Worthington, Worthy

Worton (English) farm town.

Wouter (German) powerful warrior.

Wrangle (American) a form of Rangle.
Wrangler

Wray (Scandinavian) corner property. (English) crooked.
Wreh

Wren (Welsh) chief, ruler. (English) wren.

Wright (English) a short form of Wainwright.

Wrisley (English) a form of Risley.
Wrisee, Wrislie, Wrisly

Wriston (English) a form of Riston.
Wryston

Wuliton (Native American) will do well.

Wunand (Native American) God is good.

Wuyi (Moquelumnan) turkey vulture flying.

Wyatt (French) little warrior.
Wiatt, Wyat, Wyatte, Wye,
Wyeth, Wyett, Wyitt, Wytt

Wybert (English) battle
bright.

Wyborn (Scandinavian) war
bear.

Wyck (Scandinavian) village.

Wycliff (English) white cliff;
village near the cliff.
Wyckliffe, Wycliffe

Wylie (English) charming.
Wiley, Wye, Wyley, Wyllie, Wyly

Wyman (English) fighter, warrior.

Wymer (English) famous in
battle.

Wyn (Welsh) light skinned;
white. (English) friend. A
short form of Selwyn.
Win, Wyne, Wynn, Wynne

Wyndham (Scottish) village
near the winding road.
Windham, Wynndham

Wynono (Native American)
first-born son.

Wythe (English) willow tree.

Xabat (Basque) savior.

Xaiver (Basque) a form of
Xavier.
Xajavier, Xzaiver

Xan (Greek) a short form of
Alexander.
Xane

Xander (Greek) a short form
of Alexander.
Xande, Xzander

Xanthus (Latin) golden
haired.
Xanthos

Xarles (Basque) a form of
Charles.

Xavier (Arabic) bright.
(Basque) owner of the new
house. See also Exavier,
Javier, Salvatore, Saverio.
Xabier, Xaiver, Xavaeir, Xaver,
Xavian, Xaviar, Xavior, Xavon,
Xavyer, Xever, Xizavier,
Xxavier, Xzavier, Zavier

Xenophon (Greek) strange
voice.
Xeno, Zennie

Xenos (Greek) stranger; guest.
Zenos

Xerxes (Persian) ruler. History:
a king of Persia.
Zerk

Ximenes (Spanish) a form of
Simon.
Ximenez, Ximon, Ximun,
Xymenes

Xylon (Greek) forest.

Xzavier (Basque) a form of Xavier.
Xzavaier, Xzaver, Xzavion, Xzavior, Xzvaier

Y

Yadid (Hebrew) friend; beloved.
Yedid

Yadon (Hebrew) he will judge.
Yadean, Yadin, Yadun

Yael (Hebrew) a form of Jael.

Yafeu (Ibo) bold.

Yagil (Hebrew) he will rejoice.

Yago (Spanish) a form of James.

Yahto (Lakota) blue.

Yahya (Arabic) living.
Yahye

Yair (Hebrew) he will enlighten.
Yahir

Yakecen (Dene) sky song.

Yakez (Carrier) heaven.

Yakov (Russian) a form of Jacob.
Yaacob, Yaacov, Yaakov, Yachov, Yacoub, Yacov, Yakob, Yashko

Yale (German) productive. (English) old.

Yan, Yann (Russian) forms of John.
Yanichek, Yanick, Yanka, Yannick

Yana (Native American) bear.

Yancy (Native American) Englishman, Yankee.
Yan, Yance, Yancey, Yanci, Yansey, Yansy, Yantsey, Yauncey, Yauncy, Yency

Yanick, Yannick (Russian) familiar forms of Yan.
Yanic, Yanik, Yannic, Yannik, Yonic, Yonnik

Yanka (Russian) a familiar form of John.
Yanikm

Yanni (Greek) a form of John.
Ioannis, Yani, Yannakis, Yannis, Yanny, Yiannis, Yoni

Yanton (Hebrew) a form of Johnathon, Jonathon.

Yao (Ewe) born on Thursday.

Yaphet (Hebrew) a form of Japheth.
Yapheth, Yefat, Yephat

Yarb (Gypsy) herb.

Yardan (Arabic) king.

Yarden (Hebrew) a form of Jordan.

Yardley (English) enclosed
meadow.
Lee, Yard, Yardlea, Yardlee,
Yardleigh, Yardly

Yarom (Hebrew) he will raise
up.
Yarum

Yaron (Hebrew) he will sing;
he will cry out.
Jaron, Yairon

Yasashiku (Japanese) gentle;
polite.

Yash (Hindi) victorious; glory.

Yasha (Russian) a form of
Jacob, James.
Yascha, Yashka, Yashko

Yashwant (Hindi) glorious.

Yasin (Arabic) prophet.
Yasine, Yasseen, Yassin, Yassine,
Yazen

Yasir (Afghan) humble; takes it
easy. (Arabic) wealthy.
Yasar, Yaser, Yashar, Yasser

Yasuo (Japanese) restful.

Yates (English) gates.
Yeats

Yatin (Hindi) ascetic.

Yavin (Hebrew) he will under-
stand.
Jabin

Yawo (Akan) born on
Thursday.

Yazid (Arabic) his power will
increase.
Yazeed, Yazide

Yechiel (Hebrew) God lives.

Yedidya (Hebrew) a form of
Jedidiah. See also Didi.
Yadai, Yedidia, Yedidiah, Yido

Yegor (Russian) a form of
George. See also Egor, Igor.
Ygor

Yehoshua (Hebrew) a form of
Joshua.
Yeshua, Yeshuah, Yoshua, Y'shua,
Yushua

Yehoyakem (Hebrew) a form
of Joachim, Joaquín.
Yakim, Yehayakim, Yokim,
Yoyakim

Yehudi (Hebrew) a form of
Judah.
Yechudi, Yechudit, Yehuda,
Yehudah, Yehudit

Yelutci (Moquelumnan) bear
walking silently.

Yeoman (English) attendant;
retainer.
Yoeman, Youman

Yeremey (Russian) a form of
Jeremiah.
Yarema, Yaremka, Yeremy, Yerik

Yervant (Armenian) king,
ruler. History: an Armenian
king.

Yeshaya (Hebrew) gift. See also Shai.

Yeshurun (Hebrew) right way.

Yeska (Russian) a form of Joseph.
Yesya

Yestin (Welsh) just.

Yevgenyi (Russian) a form of Eugene.
Gena, Yevgeni, Yevgenij, Yevgeniy

Yigal (Hebrew) he will redeem.
Yagel, Yigael

Yirmaya (Hebrew) a form of Jeremiah.
Yirmayahu

Yishai (Hebrew) a form of Jesse.

Yisrael (Hebrew) a form of Israel.
Yesarel, Yisroel

Yitro (Hebrew) a form of Jethro.

Yitzchak (Hebrew) a form of Isaac. See also Itzak.
Yitzak, Yitzchok, Yitzhak

Yngve (Swedish) ancestor; lord, master.

Yo (Cambodian) honest.

Yoakim (Slavic) a form of Jacob.
Yoackim

Yoan (German) a form of Johan, Johann.
Yoann

Yoav (Hebrew) a form of Joab.

Yochanan (Hebrew) a form of John.
Yohanan

Yoel (Hebrew) a form of Joel.

Yogesh (Hindi) ascetic. Religion: another name for the Hindu god Shiva.

Yohance (Hausa) a form of John.

Yohan, Yohann (German) forms of Johan, Johann.
Yohane, Yohanes, Yohanne, Yohannes, Yohans, Yohn

Yonah (Hebrew) a form of Jonah.
Yona, Yonas

Yonatan (Hebrew) a form of Jonathan.
Yonathan, Yonathon, Yonaton, Yonattan

Yong (Chinese) courageous.
Yonge

Yong-Sun (Korean) dragon in the first position; courageous.

Yoni (Greek) a form of Yanni.
Yonis, Yonnas, Yonny, Yony

Yoofi (Akan) born on Friday.

Yooku (Fante) born on Wednesday.

Yoram (Hebrew) God is high.
Joram

Yorgos (Greek) a form of
George.
Yiorgos, Yorgo

York (English) boar estate;
yew-tree estate.
Yorick, Yorke, Yorker, Yorkie,
Yorrick

Yorkoo (Fante) born on
Thursday.

Yosef (Hebrew) a form of
Joseph. See also Osip.
Yoceph, Yoosuf, Yoseff, Yoseph,
Yosief, Yosif, Yosuf, Yosyf, Yousef,
Yusif

Yóshi (Japanese) adopted son.
Yoshiki, Yoshiuki

Yoshiyahu (Hebrew) a form
of Josiah.
Yoshia, Yoshiah, Yoshiya,
Yoshiyah, Yosiah

Yoskolo (Moquelumnan)
breaking off pine cones.

Yosu (Hebrew) a form of
Jesus.

Yotimo (Moquelumnan) yellow jacket carrying food to
its hive.

Yottoko (Native American)
mud at the water's edge.

Young (English) young.
Yung

Young-Jae (Korean) pile of
prosperity.

Young-Soo (Korean) keeping
the prosperity.

Youri (Russian) a form of
Yuri.

Yousef (Yiddish) a form of
Joseph.
Yousaf, Youseef, Yousef, Youseph,
Yousif, Youssef, Yousseff, Yousuf

Youssel (Yiddish) a familiar
form of Joseph.
Yussel

Yov (Russian) a short form of
Yoakim.

Yovani (Slavic) a form of
Jovan.
Yovan, Yovanni, Yovanny, Yovany,
Yovni

Yoyi (Hebrew) a form of
George.

Yrjo (Finnish) a form of
George.

Ysidro (Greek) a short form
of Isidore.

Yu (Chinese) universe.
Yue

Yudell (English) a form of
Udell.
Yudale, Yudel

Yuki (Japanese) snow.
Yukiko, Yukio, Yuuki

Yul (Mongolian) beyond the horizon.

Yule (English) born at Christmas.

Yuli (Basque) youthful.

Yuma (Native American) son of a chief.

Yunus (Turkish) a form of Jonah.

Yurcel (Turkish) sublime.

Yuri (Russian, Ukrainian) a form of George. (Hebrew) a familiar form of Uriah.
Yehor, Youri, Yura, Yure, Yuric, Yurii, Yurij, Yurik, Yurko, Yurri, Yury, Yusha

Yusif (Russian) a form of Joseph.
Yuseph, Yusof, Yussof, Yusup, Yuzef, Yuzep

Yustyn (Russian) a form of Justin.
Yusts

Yusuf (Arabic, Swahili) a form of Joseph.
Yusef, Yusuff

Yutu (Moquelumnan) coyote out hunting.

Yuval (Hebrew) rejoicing.

Yves (French) a form of Ivar, Ives.
Yvens, Yvon, Yyves

Yvon (French) a form of Ivar, Yves.
Ivon, Yuvon, Yvan, Yvonne

Z

Zac (Hebrew) a short form of Zachariah, Zachary.
Zacc

Zacarias (Portuguese, Spanish) a form of Zachariah.
Zacaria, Zacariah

Zacary (Hebrew) a form of Zachary.
Zac, Zacaras, Zacari, Zacariah, Zacarias, Zacarie, Zacarious, Zacery, Zacory, Zacrye

Zaccary (Hebrew) a form of Zachary.
Zac, Zaccaeus, Zaccari, Zaccaria, Zaccariah, Zaccary, Zaccea, Zaccharie, Zacchary, Zacchery, Zaccury

Zaccheus (Hebrew) innocent, pure.
Zacceus, Zacchaeus, Zacchious

Zach (Hebrew) a short form of Zachariah, Zachary.

Zachari (Hebrew) a form of Zachary.
Zacheri

Zacharia (Hebrew) a form of Zachary.
Zacharya

Zachariah (Hebrew) God remembered.
Zac, Zacarias, Zacarius, Zacary, Zaccary, Zach, Zacharias, Zachary, Zacharyah, Zachory, Zachury, Zack, Zakaria, Zako, Zaquero, Zecharia, Zechariah, Zecharya, Zeggery, Zeke, Zhachory

Zacharias (German) a form of Zachariah.
Zacarías, Zacharais, Zachariaus, Zacharius, Zackarias, Zakarias, Zecharias, Zekarias

Zacharie (Hebrew) a form of Zachary.
Zachare, Zacharee, Zachurie, Zecharie

Zachary (Hebrew) a familiar form of Zachariah. History: Zachary Taylor was the twelfth U.S. president. See also Sachar, Sakeri.
Xachary, Zac, Zacary, Zaccary, Zach, Zacha, Zachaery, Zachaios, Zacharay, Zacharey, Zachari, Zacharia, Zacharias, Zacharie, Zacharry, Zachaury, Zachery, Zachory, Zachrey, Zachry, Zachuery, Zachury, Zack, Zackary, Zackery, Zackory, Zakaria, Zakary, Zakery, Zakkary, Zechary, Zechery, Zeke

Zachery (Hebrew) a form of Zachary.
Zacheray, Zacherey, Zacheria,

Zacherias, Zacheriah, Zacherie, Zacherius, Zackery

Zachory (Hebrew) a form of Zachary.

Zachry (Hebrew) a form of Zachary.
Zachre, Zachrey, Zachri

Zack (Hebrew) a short form of Zachariah, Zachary.
Zach, Zak, Zaks

Zackary (Hebrew) a form of Zachary.
Zack, Zackari, Zacharia, Zackare, Zackaree, Zackariah, Zackarie, Zackery, Zackhary, Zackie, Zackree, Zackrey, Zackry

Zackery (Hebrew) a form of Zachery.
Zackere, Zackeree, Zackerey, Zackeri, Zackeria, Zackeriah, Zackerie, Zackerry

Zackory (Hebrew) a form of Zachary.
Zackoriah, Zackorie, Zacorey, Zacori, Zacory, Zacry, Zakory

Zadok (Hebrew) a short form of Tzadok.
Zaddik, Zadik, Zadoc, Zaydok

Zadornin (Basque) Saturn.

Zafir (Arabic) victorious.
Zafar, Zafeer, Zafer, Zaffar

Zahid (Arabic) self-denying, ascetic.
Zaheed

Zahir (Arabic) shining, bright.
*Zahair, Zahar, Zaheer, Zahi,
Zair, Zaire, Zayyir*

Zahur (Swahili) flower.

Zaid (Arabic) increase, growth.
Zaied, Zaiid, Zayd

Zaide (Hebrew) older.

Zaim (Arabic) brigadier general.

Zain (English) a form of Zane.
Zaine

Zakaria (Hebrew) a form of
Zachariah.
*Zakaraiya, Zakareeya,
Zakareeyah, Zakariah,
Zakariya, Zakeria, Zakeriah*

Zakariyya (Arabic) prophet.
Religion: an Islamic prophet.

Zakary (Hebrew) a form of
Zachery.
*Zak, Zakarai, Zakare, Zakaree,
Zakari, Zakarias, Zakarie,
Zakarius, Zakariye, Zake,
Zakhar, Zaki, Zakir, Zakkai,
Zako, Zakqary, Zakree, Zakri,
Zakris, Zakry*

Zakery (Hebrew) a form of
Zachary.
Zakeri, Zakerie, Zakiry

Zaki (Arabic) bright; pure.
(Hausa) lion.
*Zakee, Zakia, Zakie, Zakiy,
Zakki*

Zakia (Swahili) intelligent.

Zakkary (Hebrew) a form of
Zachary.
*Zakk, Zakkari, Zakkery,
Zakkyre*

Zako (Hungarian) a form of
Zachariah.

Zale (Greek) sea strength.
Zayle

Zalmai (Afghan) young.

Zalman (Yiddish) a form of
Solomon.
Zaloman

Zamiel (German) a form of
Samuel.
Zamal, Zamuel

Zamir (Hebrew) song; bird.
Zameer

Zan (Italian) clown.
*Zann, Zanni, Zannie, Zanny,
Zhan*

Zander (Greek) a short form
of Alexander.
*Zandore, Zandra, Zandrae,
Zandy*

Zane (English) a form of
John.
Zain, Zayne, Zhane

Zanis (Latvian) a form of
Janis.
Zannis

Zanvil (Hebrew) a form of
Samuel.
Zanwill

Zaquan (American) a combination of the prefix Za + Quan.
Zaquain, Zaquon, Zaqwan

Zareb (African) protector.

Zared (Hebrew) ambush.
Zaryd

Zarek (Polish) may God protect the king.
Zarik, Zarrick, Zerek, Zerick, Zerric, Zerrick

Zavier (Arabic) a form of Xavier.
Zavair, Zaverie, Zavery, Zavierre, Zavior, Zavyr, Zayvius, Zxavian

Zayit (Hebrew) olive.

Zayne (English) a form of Zane.
Zayan, Zayin, Zayn

Zdenek (Czech) follower of Saint Denis.

Zeb (Hebrew) a short form of Zebediah, Zebulon.
Zev

Zebediah (Hebrew) God's gift.
Zeb, Zebadia, Zebadiah, Zebedee, Zebedia, Zebidiah, Zedidiah

Zebedee (Hebrew) a familiar form of Zebediah.
Zebadee

Zebulon (Hebrew) exalted, honored; lofty house.
Zabulan, Zeb, Zebulan, Zebulen, Zebulin, Zebulun, Zebulyn, Zev, Zevulon, Zevulun, Zhebulen, Zubin

Zechariah (Hebrew) a form of Zachariah.
Zecharia, Zecharian, Zecheriah, Zechuriah, Zekariah, Zekarias, Zeke, Zekeria, Zekeriah, Zekerya

Zed (Hebrew) a short form of Zedekiah.

Zedekiah (Hebrew) God is mighty and just.
Zed, Zedechiah, Zedekias, Zedikiah

Zedidiah (Hebrew) a form of Zebediah.

Zeeman (Dutch) seaman.

Zeév (Hebrew) wolf.
Zeévi, Zeff, Zif

Zeheb (Turkish) gold.

Zeke (Hebrew) a short form of Ezekiel, Zachariah, Zachary, Zechariah.

Zeki (Turkish) clever, intelligent.
Zeky

Zelgai (Afghan) heart.

Zelig (Yiddish) a form of Selig.
Zeligman, Zelik

Zelimir (Slavic) wishes for peace.

Zemar (Afghan) lion.

Zen (Japanese) religious. Religion: a form of Buddhism.

Zenda (Czech) a form of Eugene.
Zhek

Zeno (Greek) cart; harness. History: a Greek philosopher.
Zenan, Zenas, Zenon, Zino, Zinon

Zephaniah (Hebrew) treasured by God.
Zaph, Zaphania, Zeph, Zephan

Zephyr (Greek) west wind.
Zeferino, Zeffrey, Zephery, Zephire, Zephram, Zephran, Zephrin

Zero (Arabic) empty, void.

Zeroun (Armenian) wise and respected.

Zeshawn (American) a combination of the prefix Ze + Shawn.
Zeshan, Zeshaun, Zeshon, Zishaan, Zishan, Zshawn

Zesiro (Luganda) older of twins.

Zeus (Greek) living. Mythology: chief god of the Greek pantheon.

Zeusef (Portuguese) a form of Joseph.

Zev (Hebrew) a short form of Zebulon.

Zevi (Hebrew) a form of Tzvi.
Zhvie, Zhvy, Zvi

Zhek (Russian) a short form of Evgeny.
Zhenechka, Zhenka, Zhenya

Zhìxin (Chinese) ambitious.
Zhi, Zhìhuán, Zhipeng, Zhi-yang, Zhìyuan

Zhuàng (Chinese) strong.

Zhora (Russian) a form of George.
Zhorik, Zhorka, Zhorz, Zhurka

Zia (Hebrew) trembling; moving. (Arabic) light.
Ziah

Zigfrid (Latvian, Russian) a form of Siegfried.
Zegfrido, Zigfrids, Ziggy, Zygfryd, Zygi

Ziggy (American) a familiar form of Siegfried, Sigmund.
Ziggie

Zigor (Basque) punishment.

Zikomo (Nguni) thank-you.

Zilaba (Luganda) born while sick.
Zilabamuzale

Zimra (Hebrew) song of praise.
Zemora, Zimrat, Zimri, Zimria, Zimriah, Zimriya

Zimraan (Arabic) praise.

Zinan (Japanese) second son.

Zindel (Yiddish) a form of Alexander.
Zindil, Zunde

Zion (Hebrew) sign, omen; excellent. Bible: the name used to refer to Israel and to the Jewish people.
Tzion, Zyon

Ziskind (Yiddish) sweet child.

Ziv (Hebrew) shining brightly. (Slavic) a short form of Ziven.

Ziven (Slavic) vigorous, lively.
Zev, Ziv, Zivka, Zivon

Ziyad (Arabic) increase.
Zayd, Ziyaad

Zlatan (Czech) gold.
Zlatek, Zlatko

Zohar (Hebrew) bright light.
Zohair

Zollie, Zolly (Hebrew) forms of Solly.
Zoilo

Zoltán (Hungarian) life.

Zorba (Greek) live each day.

Zorion (Basque) a form of Orion.
Zoran, Zoren, Zorian, Zoron, Zorrine, Zorrion

Zorya (Slavic) star; dawn.

Zotikos (Greek) saintly, holy. Religion: a saint in the Eastern Orthodox Church.

Zotom (Kiowa) a biter.

Zsigmond (Hungarian) a form of Sigmund.
Ziggy, Zigmund, Zsiga

Zuberi (Swahili) strong.

Zubin (Hebrew) a short form of Zebulon.
Zubeen

Zuhayr (Arabic) brilliant, shining.
Zyhair, Zuheer

Zuka (Shona) sixpence.

Zuriel (Hebrew) God is my rock.

Zygmunt (Polish) a form of Sigmund.